Movement, stability and low back pain
The essential role of the pelvis

For Churchill Livingstone:

Editorial director (Nursing and Allied Health): Mary Law
Project manager: Valerie Burgess
Project development editor: Dinah Thom
Design direction: Judith Wright
Project controller: Derek Robertson
Copy editor: Carrie Walker
Indexer: Jill Halliday
Promotions manager: Hilary Brown

Movement, stability and low back pain

The essential role of the pelvis

Edited by

Andry Vleeming PhD
Director, Spine and Joint Centre, Rotterdam and Head of Musculoskeletal Research Group,
Department of Anatomy, Faculty of Medicine and Health Sciences, Erasmus University
Rotterdam, The Netherlands

Vert Mooney MD
Professor of Orthopedic Surgery, University of California at San Diego, California, USA

Chris J Snijders PhD
Professor of Medical Technology and Head of Department, Biomedical Physics and
Technology, Faculty of Medicine, Erasmus University Rotterdam, The Netherlands

Thomas A Dorman MD
Internal and Orthopedic Medicine, San Louis Obispo, California, USA

Rob Stoeckart PhD
Department of Anatomy, Faculty of Medicine and Health Sciences,
Erasmus University Rotterdam, The Netherlands

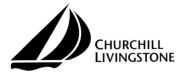
CHURCHILL
LIVINGSTONE

NEW YORK   EDINBURGH   LONDON   MADRID   MELBOURNE   SAN FRANCISCO   AND   TOKYO   1997

CHURCHILL LIVINGSTONE
Medical Division of Pearson Professional Limited

Distributed in the United States of America by Churchill
Livingstone, 650 Avenue of the Americas, New York, N.Y.
10011, and by associated companies, branches and
representatives throughout the world.

First published 1997

ISBN 0 443 05574 2

British Library Cataloguing in Publication Data
A catalogue record for this book is available from the British
Library.

Library of Congress Cataloging in Publication Data
A catalog record for this book is avaailable from the Library
of Congress.

Medical knowledge is constantly changing. As new
information becomes available, changes in treatment,
procedures, equipment and the use of drugs become
necessary. The editors, contributors and publishers have, as
far as it is possible, taken care to ensure that the information
given in this text is accurate and up to date. However, readers
are strongly advised to confirm that information, especially
with regard to drug usage, complies with the latest legislation
and standards of practice.

The
publisher's
policy is to use
paper manufactured
from sustainable forests

Printed and bound in Great Britain by
The Bath Press, Bath

Contents

Contributors

Sidsel Platou Aarseth MA is currently Director of the Centre for Women's Research, University of Oslo, Norway. She has been mothering full time, raising three children. She obtained a Master of Sociology from the University of Oslo in 1992, related to the topic of pelvic pain in pregnancy.

M. Maurice Abitbol MA FACS is Clinical Associate Professor of Obstetrics and Gynecology at the State University of New York, Stony Brook, Long Island, New York, USA. He is the Chairman of the Department of Obstetrics and Gynecology and Director of the Residency Program at the Jamaica Hospital Medical Center, Queens, New York.

He has studied extensively and published numerous articles on the pelvis and on obstetric mechanics in prehuman species. This work is summarized in *Birth and Human Evolution: Anatomical and Obstetrical Mechanics in Primates*, published by Greenwood Publishing Group, Connecticut, USA.

Michael A. Adams BSc PhD is a physicist, currently working as a Senior Research Fellow in the Department of Anatomy at the University of Bristol, UK. During the past 18 years, he has published over 50 papers on spinal mechanics, many of them concerned with mechanical function and failure in cadaver spines. More recently he has joined forces with his wife, Patricia Dolan, to investigate spinal movements and muscle (dys)function in living people. He is a member of the editorial board of *Spine*, *Clinical Biomechanics*, and the *European Spine Journal*.

Mark D. Avillar MSESS received his graduate degree from the University of Florida, USA, in Exercise Science, with an emphasis on exercise physiology. His research interest centered on low back strength and cross-sectional area adaptations in healthy and chronic low back pain populations. In Mr Avillar's clinical experience, his interests have shifted to low back pain and strength training within those populations. His main areas of interest are evaluation of the sacroiliac joint and rehabilitation of patients with non-operative and operative chronic low back pain.

Richard M. Bachrach DO is engaged in the private practice of orthopedic, sports, and dance medicine in New York City. He is the founder and President of the not-for-profit Center for Dance Medicine, and is the President and Medical Director of the Center for Sports and Osteopathic Medicine. His practice encompasses osteopathic manipulation, prolotherapy, acupuncture, trigger point injection, and a program for back pain management, education, rehabilitation, and prevention.

Dr Bachrach has authored many scientific papers and textbook chapters on back pain and dance-related injuries, and lectured nationally and internationally on these subjects. He is consultant to many dance companies, and aerobic and fitness studios in the New York area. He has been continuing education provider to the American Council on Exercise and to the International Dance and Exercise Association. Dr Bachrach is an American Running and Fitness Association clinic advisor and holds the Certificate of Special Competence in Sports Medicine conferred by the American Osteopathic Academy of Sports Medicine. He is a Clinical Assistant Professor at the College of Osteopathic

Medicine of the Pacific and at the New York College of Osteopathic Medicine.

Thomas N. Bernard Jr MD is a native of New Orleans, Louisiana, USA. After graduating from Tulane University, he served three years with the United States Navy and returned to Tulane University School of Medicine, where he completed both medical school and orthopedic residency. He studied with the late Dr S. Henry LaRocca as a spine fellow and then completed his spine fellowship with Dr W. H. Kirkaldy-Willis at the Royal University of Saskatchewan, Canada. His interest in the sacroiliac joint began while working with Drs Kirkaldy-Willis and J. D. Cassidy, culminating in 1991 in the publication of a chapter entitled *Sacroiliac joint syndrome, pathophysiology, diagnosis and management*, in the *Adult Spine: Principles and Practice*, edited by J. W. Frymoyer. Dr Bernard has been appointed Clinical Assistant Professor of Orthopedic Surgery, Tulane University School of Medicine, and is currently in private practice in Anderson, South Carolina, USA.

Norman A. Broadhurst MD PhD practices full time as a musculoskeletal physician with a special interest in dysfunction of the musculosketal structures of the pelvis. He is part-time Senior Visiting Medical Specialist to The Queen Elizabeth Hospital, University of Adelaide, South Australia and half-time senior lecturer and honorary Visiting Medical Specialist in musculoskeletal medicine at the Flinders Medical Centre and Flinders University, South Australia.

Dr Broadhurst has a special role in medical education and conducts postgraduate diplomas and certificates as well as weekend workshops in all Australian states. Over the past 2 years, he has written regular articles and provided case studies on musculoskeletal problems in *Australian Doctor*, a weekly publication with special relevance for general practitioners, and he is currently the President of the Australian Association of Musculoskeletal Medicine.

Muzaffer Buyruk MD PhD was born in Istanbul, Turkey, in 1963. He received the Doctor of Medicine degree in 1987 and the Specialist in

Anatomy degree in 1991, both from Istanbul University Faculty of Medicine. After working as a member of the teaching staff in the same faculty, he completed his PhD study at the Department of Rehabilitation, Erasmus University Rotterdam, The Netherlands in 1996 and is now working in the same department. His research interests include Doppler imaging of the musculoskeletal system, the physical properties of the pelvic girdle, the biomechanics of the lumbar spine and pelvis, the relation of low back pain to the sacroiliac joints and the biomechanics of the hand and wrist.

Steven A Caruso MEng graduated from The Cooper Union School for the Advancement of Science and Art-Albert Neiken School of Engineering with both a Bachelor's and Master's degree in Engineering. He has directed the research efforts of the Biomechanical Engineering Laboratory at St Vincents Hospital and Medical Center of New York, USA (a major teaching affiliate of New York Medical College) since 1994. Although the majority of his interests lie in the field of orthopedic spinal biomechanics, he is actively involved in the investigation of many orthopedic and biomechanical concerns.

Michel Dalstra MSc PhD became interested in biomechanics during his mechanical engineering study at the Twente University of Technology, The Netherlands. He obtained his MSc degree in 1986 with a project on adaptive bone remodeling, which was performed in the Biomechanics Section of the Institute of Orthopedics at the University of Nijmegen. After a year of military service, he returned to Nijmegen to start a PhD project on pelvic biomechanics under the tutorship of Professor Rik Huiskes. In November 1993 this was completed by publicly defending his thesis entitled *Biomechanical aspects of the pelvic bone and design criteria for acetabular prostheses*. He then started work as an assistant professor at the Biomechanics Laboratory of the Aarhus University Hospital, Denmark. His current work involves teaching, supervising, and research, the latter predominantly in the field of bone mechanics, finite element modeling, and biomechanics of the shoulder and elbow.

Howard J. Dananberg DPM FACFOAM is a podiatrist and Director of the Walking Clinic in New Hamsphire, USA, performing gait analysis on chronic postural pain patients. He graduated from the Ohio College of Podiatric Medicine in 1975. He serves as contributing editor for *The Journal of the American Podiatric Medical Association* and is a Fellow in the American College of Foot & Ankle Orthopedics and Medicine. Dr Dananberg has lectured extensively to various medical groups worldwide on the subject of gait-related lower back pain as well as non-surgical treatment of chronic foot and limb pain. He has published over 25 papers and text chapters on this subject, and in 1994 was awarded the Outstanding Clinical Paper of the Year Award in *Podiatric Medicine* by the American Podiatric Medical Association and the Scholl's Corporation. He resides in Bedford, New Hampshire with his wife, Margie, and his two sons, Ross and Geoffrey.

Vincent J. Devlin MD is Attending Orthopedic Surgeon at the Southern California Permanente Medical Group, USA. His specialty is pediatric and adult reconstructive spinal surgery. Clinical duties include management of both a regional scoliosis clinic and the Complex Multidisciplinary Spine Clinic. Dr Devlin is also a Clinical Instructor of Orthopedic Surgery at Loma Linda University Medical Center. He has published numerous papers on clinical aspects of spinal disorders as well as on biomechanics of the spine.

P. F. Dijkstra MD DIC PhD has, since 1975, been a radiologist at the Academic Medical Centre, Amsterdam, The Netherlands, and member and Chairman of the medical staff and Head of Department of Radiology at the Jan van Breemen Institute for Skeletal Disease, Amsterdam. In 1973/74 he attended the Medical Engineering course at Imperial College of Science and Technology, London, UK, and later received a PhD from the University of Amsterdam.

Dr Dijkstra's publications cover a range of skeletal and other radiologic subjects, sialography in rheumatic disease being an area of special interest. His current work focuses on the radiology of rheumatic disease and the sacroiliac joints, the dynamics of wrist pathology, and skeletal dysplasia.

Patricia Dolan BSc PhD is a muscle physiologist working as an A. R. C. Research Fellow in the Department of Anatomy, University of Bristol, UK. Her research mostly concerns posture, spinal movements, and the electromyographic analysis of trunk muscle function and fatigue. A particular interest is the putative role of muscle dysfunction in chronic back pain. She has published over 30 papers, and is a member of the Editorial Board of the *European Spine Journal*.

Richard L. DonTigny BS PT is a physical therapist in Havre, Montana, USA, now retired after 38 years of practice. He has conducted a personal investigation into the sacroiliac joint and its relationship to idiopathic low back pain for nearly all of that time, and has published several articles on the functional biomechanics, pathomechanics, and treatment of the sacroiliac joint.

Thomas Dorman MD is an internist in private practice in California, USA. From outside academe, he has conducted research into orthopedic medicine and prolotherapy. From this, there has developed a new understanding of the role of ligaments as stores of elastic energy. He has analyzed the human pelvis as a transductor of the forces of locomotion. Dr Dorman has written a modern textbook on injection techniques in orthopedic medicine and has published in other fields of alternative medicine.

Frank J. E. Falco MD is a physiatrist (physical medicine & rehabilitation physician) who specializes in the evaluation and non-surgical treatment of spinal disorders. He is board certified in physical medicine & rehabilitation, electrodiagnostic medicine and pain medicine. Dr Falco is the founder of Comprehensive Spine & Sports Medicine, P. A., which is an outpatient musculoskeletal medical practice serving patient needs in the states of Delaware, Maryland and

Pennyslvania. Dr Falco is actively involved in teaching and research. He maintains a faculty appointment as clinical assistant professor at Temple University Medical School in Philadelphia, Pennsylvania. Dr Falco is an accomplished author who lectures nationally and internationally on a variety of musculoskeletal topics. Dr Falco also hosts a weekly 'call-in' radio talk show where he discusses current medical issues with guests and listeners.

Joseph D. Fortin DO is a physiatrist (physical medicine and rehabilitation) who specializes in the evaluation and non-surgical treatment of spinal disorders. He is board certified in physical medicine and rehabilitation and electrodiagnostic medicine. Dr Fortin is currently the Medical Director of the Rehabilitation Hospital of Fort Wayne, Indiana, an Associate at the Imaging Center, and the President of Spine Technology and Rehabilitation, P.C. Through the application of the entire spectrum of spinal injection procedures, Dr Fortin has concentrated work in spinal imaging analysis and research. He has given numerous national and international lectures, as well as scientific presentations. Dr Fortin has authored numerous scientific reports, five chapters on spinal imaging and image-guided injection procedures as well as several on spinal injury mechanisms in athletes. Dr Fortin is a member of several professional organizations including the North American Spine Society, American Academy of Physical Medicine and Rehabilitation, and The International Society for Study of the Lumbar Spine, and the American Association of Electrodiagnostic Medicine. He is co-editing a medical text entitled, *Functional Biomechanics and Rehabilitation of Sports Injuries.*

Lawrence Friedman MB BCh FFRad(D)SA FRCP(C) FACR is Chief of Diagnostic Imaging, Guelph General Hospital, Guelph, Ontario, Canada; Clinical Associate, McMaster University Medical Centre, Hamilton, Ontario; and Clinical Associate, Guelph University, Guelph, Ontario; and was previously Chief CT, Musculoskeletal Radiology and MRI, McMaster University Medical Centre, Hamilton, Ontario.

John M. Gorup MD is an Assistant Clinical Instructor at the State University of New York at Brooklyn, USA. He is also a Spine Fellow at the Lakewood Orthopaedic Clinic in Lakewood, Colorado.

Serge Alain Gracovetsky PEng PhD is Associate Professor of Engineering at Concordia University, Montreal, Canada, and President of Spinex Technologies, Inc., a company dedicated to understanding the function of the human spine. This knowledge is applied to the design of non-invasive tools and methodologies for the objective and comparable assessment of back function in a free and dynamic environment. The ideas Dr Gracovetsky has contributed to the understanding of spinal function are the subject of numerous books and publications.

Philip E. Greenman DO FAAO is currently Professor of Biomechanics, and Professor of Physical Medicine and Rehabilitation at the College of Osteopathic Medicine at Michigan State University, East Lansing, Michigan, USA. His research has been in the failed low back pain syndrome, post-traumatic cervicocranial syndrome, and suboccipital muscle atrophy. He is past president of the North American Association of Musculoskeletal Medicine and Vice President of the American Back Society. The author of the acclaimed text *Principles of Manual Medicine*, he directs a comprehensive course series in the field of manual medicine, which attracts clinicians throughout the world.

Jennifer K Gullick BS is currently working in clinical research and student programs at the Department of Orthopaedics, OrthoMed, University of California, San Diego, USA. She has worked on physiological testing in healthy people, elite athletes and diseased populations at the Center for Exercise Research at the University of Florida. She received her Bachelor's degree in exercise science from the University of Florida. She is continuing her education in a Master's of education program.

Eli Heiberg MA is currently a researcher and senior supervisor at the Norwegian Centre for Physiotherapy Research and Development, Oslo,

Norway. She is both a physiotherapist and a Master of Social Anthropology (obtained from the University of Oslo, Norway, 1986), and has over the past 15 years written several books on pregnancy, childbirth, and breastfeeding issues. She is the mother of four children.

Jerry Hesch BS PT graduated from the University of New Mexico, USA, in 1981. He is a member of the Orthopedic and Obstetrics/Gynecology Sections of the American Physical Therapy Association. He has 15 years' experience in treating the spine and pelvic girdle and has developed a unique and practical evaluation and treatment approach over that time. He has discovered 12 new types of pelvic joint dysfunction that have not been described in the literature. His method challenges traditional approaches to the pelvic girdle and spine.

Mr Hesch has presented over 60 workshops on his approach to the spine and pelvic girdle. He has presented his approach at several state, national, and international conferences, including The First Interdisciplinary World Congress on Low Back Pain and its Relationship to the Sacroiliac Joint in 1992 and The Second Congress in 1995. He has published a workbook entitled *The Hesch Method of Treating the Sacroiliac Joint: Integrating the Pelvis and Lumbar Spine*, an article in *Physical Therapy Today*, and a paper entitled 'The pitfalls associated with traditional evaluation of sacroiliac dysfunction and their proposed solutions', which was presented at the APTA National Conference in 1990. Mr Hesch was the keynote speaker at the Canadian National Athletic Therapist Convention in 1994 and presented the 10th Annual Rex McMorris Memorial Lecture on Rehabilitation. He is self-employed.

Peter Heuts MD is rehabilitation physician and head of the Department of Chronic Pain at the Rehabilitation Centre at Hoensbroek, The Netherlands. He practices full-time and works mainly with patients suffering from chronic pain disability, including spinal disorders, fibromyalgia, and rheumatoid arthritis. Dr Heuts also has a part-time appointment at the Pain Knowledge Centre of the Maastricht University Hospital. Over the

past 3 years, he has been involved in the treatment of patients who participated in a number of clinical trials concerning the effects of behavioral rehabilitation programs.

Wim Holland MSc has been a Physicist at the Central Instrumentation Department of the Medical Faculty at Erasmus University Rotterdam since 1970. He received his Degree in Electrical Engineering at Eindhoven University of Technology in Control Engineering in 1968. He is engaged in the utilization of physical measurement techniques and methods for medical application and in the development of medical instrumentation.

Anthony Huson MD PhD is Professor Emeritus of Anatomy and Embryology at the University of Leiden and Professor of Movements Sciences at Limburg University, The Netherlands. His research centered around kinematical analysis of the lower limbs, with special emphasis on the knee joint and the foot. He is currently Professor of Functional Anatomy in the Faculty of Mechanical Engineering at Eindhoven University of Technology. He is associated with the Center for Biomedical and Health Care Technology of the Eindhoven University as advisor for the bioengineering curriculum under development.

Robert Irvin DO practices as a musculoskeletal physician with a special interest in factors predisposing to chronic pain and dysfunction without specific cause. He is Adjunct Associate Professor of the Department of Ballet and Modern Dance, Texas Christian University. He has been Associate Professor of General Medicine in the Department of Osteopathic Principles and Practice, Oklahoma State University, College of Osteopathic Medicine, and Assistant Professor of Manipulative Medicine, North Texas State University Health Science Center, USA.

Hilaire A. C. Jacob PhD is Head of the Biomechanical Unit of the Department of Orthopaedic Surgery, Balgrist, University of Zurich, Switzerland. He began his professional career in the field of stress analysis in heavy industrial engineering at Sulzer Bros Ltd in Winterthur, which in the 1970s first brought him in contact with structural problems pertaining to hip endoprostheses.

After completely moving over to biomechanics in 1982, Dr Jacob has carried out research on the lumbar spine, the knee joint, the foot (which enabled him to obtain a PhD from the University of Strathclyde, Glasgow, UK), the wrist, and the glenohumeral joint, without, however, ever losing his deep interest in the hip. He has read papers on his research work at symposia in many countries of the world, and is author or co-author of over 100 scientific publications.

Dr Jacob's present occupation is mainly guidance of postgraduate medical students and research workers in the field of orthopedic biomechanics.

Erik Jurriaans BSc MB ChB DTM&H FRCR FRCP(C) is Assistant Professor and Chief of Musculoskeletal Radiology, McMaster University Medical Centre, Hamilton, Ontario, Canada.

John Geoffrey Keating MD was raised in Greenville, Mississippi, USA, and then attended Bowdoin College, Brunswick, Maine from 1964 to 1968. After Bowdoin College, he pursued his interests in running and the martial arts, afterwards attending Tulane Medical School from 1977 to 1981. Dr Keating then went into a general surgery internship at the Ochsner Foundation, after which he fulfilled his orthopedic residency at Georgia Baptist Hospital. Dr Keating is a Board-certified orthopedic surgeon and Diplomate of the American Board of Orthopedic Surgery.

Dr Keating has continuing interests in karate, Muay Thai, Brazilian Jiu Jitsu, running, and weight-training, and he has worked more rounds as a ring physician for full-contact karate than has any other physician in the USA. Dr Keating's specialty areas are sports medicine, occupational orthopedics, non-operative neck/lower back treatment, and orthopedic rehabilitation using MedX. He is extremely interested in researching the sacroiliac joint and its related problems, with a special interest in operative treatment of the sacroiliac joint.

Rudolf Kissling MD is a rheumatologist and currently Head of the Section of Rheumatology, Physical Medicine and Rehabilitation at the Orthopaedic University Hospital, Balgrist, Zurich, Switzerland. He is present President of the League Against Rheumatism in Zurich and Secretary of the Swiss Association for the Study of Pain.

His research centres around the biomechanics of the pelvic girdle, epidemiologic studies in ankylosing spondylitis, and cartilage research in osteoarthritis.

Dr Kissling is a tutor in medical education and a supervisor and consultant for several theses, postgraduate diplomas, and certificates. He is also author or co-author of over 60 scientific publications.

Gerrit Jan Kleinrensink PhD is an Assistant Professor of Anatomy at the Erasmus University Rotterdam, Faculty of Medicine, The Netherlands. He is involved in developing and administering postgraduate education courses in The Netherlands and Germany. His research centers on the influence of posture and motion on peripheral nerve tension and the influence of peripheral nerve lesions on joint stability. Furthermore he studies functional anatomical relationships in the human lumbar and cervical spine.

Ank M. J. Kole-Snijders MSc works as a psychologist and behaviour therapist at the Department of Chronic Pain of the Rehabilitation Centre at Hoensbroek, The Netherlands, and in private practice. She has a special interest in the behavioral assessment and rehabilitation of pain patients and has been involved in clinical trials evaluating the effects of behavioral rehabilitation programs for chronic low back pain patients.

Per Kristiansson MD PhD graduated in medicine from Uppsala University, Sweden, in 1981 and became a Licensed Specialist in Family Medicine in 1980. He is now a general practitioner and chairman of a group practice. Dr Kristiansson has a special interest in gynecology and dysfunction of the musculoskeletal system. He completed his PhD studies on back pain during pregnancy and its relation to hormonal changes at the Department of Family Medicine at the Uppsala University Hospital, Uppsala in 1996. He is also affiliated with the Department of Obstetrics and Gynecology at the Karolinska Hospital, Stockholm, Sweden.

Michael L. Kuchera DO FAAO is Professor and Chairman of Osteopathic Manipulative Medicine at the Kirksville College of Osteopathic Medicine, USA. His research centers around postural decompensation. He is currently President of the American Academy of Osteopathy and a board member of the American Association of Orthopaedic Medicine. He also serves on the Board of the American Osteopathic Association's Bureau of Research, where he chairs the Council on Research Grants and the Special Outcomes Research Committee. He is a Governors' Appointee to the Missouri Arthritis Advisory Board, which he also chairs.

Dr Kuchera has coauthored two standard osteopathic textbooks and numerous book chapters. He lectures nationally and internationally on manual medicine and gravitational strain. He is a leader in educational activities, chairing the Osteopathic Principles in Practice section of the National Board of Osteopathic Medical Examiners, coordinating OMM residencies nationwide, and advising on educational standards for MDs and DOs both nationally and internationally.

J. S. Laméris MD PhD has been a Radiologist at the Department of Radiology at the University Hospital Rotterdam Dijkzigt since 1979. His PhD studied ultrasound guided interventions. At present he is Professor in Radiology. Special fields of interest are non-vascular interventional radiology and ultrasound.

Mark Laslett NZRP DipMT DipMDT first registered as a physiotherapist in New Zealand in 1971. He gained the postgraduate Diploma in Manipulative Therapy in 1976 and the Diploma in Mechanical Diagnosis and Therapy in 1991. He is a senior international lecturer for the McKenzie Institute International and past President and senior lecturer in manipulative therapy for the New Zealand Manipulative

Therapists Association. Mr Laslett is a part-time tutor in clinical science at the Auckland Institute of Technology at undergraduate level and for the Advanced Diploma in Manual Therapy. He has been presenting manipulative therapy workshops and McKenzie Institute Courses internationally since 1985, and his own courses in Mechanical Diagnosis and Therapy for the Upper and Lower Limbs internationally since 1993. Mr Laslett has presented papers at many conferences on a wide variety of subjects relating to musculoskeletal pain, and has been the principal investigator in several research projects into epidemiology and clinical science.

Bruce Latimer PhD is Director of the Collections and Research Division and Curator and Head of the Department of Physical Anthropology at the Cleveland Museum of Natural History, Ohio, USA. He is also Director of the Biological Anthropology Program in the Department of Anatomy at the Case Western Reserve University School of Medicine. He holds additional appointments at Cleveland State University and in the School of Biomedical Sciences of Kent State University. He has published widely on the evolution of the lower limb in primates and human ancestors.

Diane Lee BSR COMP is an instructor and chief examiner for the Orthopaedic Division of the Canadian Physiotherapy Association as well as the North American Institute of Orthopaedic Manual Therapy. She is the director of the Delta Orthopaedic Physiotherapy Clinic, which specializes in the rehabilitation of musculoskeletal dysfunction, in particular spinal and pelvic girdle disorders. She teaches postgraduate courses in orthopedic manual therapy throughout North America and is currently an editorial advisor for the journal *Manual Therapy* and on the Board of Associate Editors of the *Journal of Manual and Manipulative Therapy*.

Stephen M. Levin MD FACS FACOS is a board-certified orthopedic surgeon and is Director of the Potomac Back Center, Vienna, Virginia, USA. He began his orthopedic practice as a general orthopedic surgeon in Alexandria, VA and was Chief Orthopedic Surgeon at Alexandria Hospital. In the past 10 years, he has limited his practice to the diagnosis and treatment of back pain, initially including both surgical and non-surgical methods; the practice is now solely non-surgical.

Dr Levin is Past President of the North American Academy of Musculoskeletal Medicine and a member of the North American Spine Society, The American Back Society, the American Society of Biomechanics, and several other professional and research organizations. Academic appointments include being a former Associate Clinical Professor of Orthopedic Surgery, Michigan State University; Assistant Clinical Professor of Orthopedic Surgery, Howard University; Distinguished Visiting Professor Orthopedic Surgery, Louisiana State University, USA.

His research interest has been biomechanics and he has presented papers and lectured in the USA, Canada and Europe on biomechanics of the spine.

Alan B. Lippitt MD is an attending Orthopedic Surgeon at the Georgia Baptist Medical Center in Atlanta, Georgia, USA, and a clinical instructor in their orthopedic residency program. Dr Lippitt received a BS from Trinity College, Connecticut, and an MD from New York Medical College. His orthopedic residency was at the Hospital for Joint Diseases in New York City. He has published articles in the literature concerning vertebral apophyseal end-plate injuries in adolescents, the treatment of back pain with facet joint injections, recurrent subluxation of the sacroiliac joint, and saphenous nerve injuries as a cause of knee pain. He is certified by the American Board of Orthopedic Surgery and a member of the American Association of Orthopedic Medicine.

C. Owen Lovejoy MA PhD is University Professor of Biological Anthropology at Kent State University, Ohio, USA. He also holds appointments in the Department of Anatomy at the Northeast Ohio University College of Medicine, the Department of Orthopedic Surgery at Case Western Reserve University, and at the Cleveland Museum of Natural History.

His research has centered around the origin of early hominids, with special reference to the anatomic and behavioral role of upright walking, including the anatomy and kinematics of the lower limb in humans and their ancestors. He has served on the scientific boards of the Institute for Human Origins, the Foundation for Research into the Origins of Man and the Human Biology Council, and on the board of editors of *American Anthropologist*.

R. McNeill Alexander DSc FRS is Professor of Zoology in the University of Leeds and Secretary of the Zoological Society of London. His research is principally on the mechanics of walking, running, and jumping, not only in humans but also in animals ranging from mice to elephants and dinosaurs. His many books include *The Human Machine* (1992) and *Exploring Biomechanics: Animals in Motion* (1992).

Dr Jean-Yves Maigne MD is currently head of the Department of Rehabilitation and Orthopedic Medicine in the Hotel-Dieu Hospital, Paris, France. He conducts a postgraduate Diploma of Orthopedic Medicine and is Editor-in-Chief of the *Revue de Médecine Orthopédique*. His research has centered around the anatomy of dorsal primary rami, the natural history of disc herniations, spinal manipulations, the sacroiliac syndrome, and coccodynia.

Joseph Y. Margulies MD, PhD is an Assistant Professor of Orthopedic Surgery at the Albert Einstein College of Medicine and a member of the Spine Service in the Department of Orthopedic Surgery at Montefiore Medical Center in the Bronx, New York, USA. His main fields of research are the biomechanical issues of spinal implants, as well as the mechanical properties of the bony structures in the spine. In collaboration with other colleagues, he has edited a book, *Lumbosacral and Spinopelvic Fixation*, published by Lippincott.

Jan M. A. Mens MD is a pupil of James Cyriax, the founder of orthopedic medicine in Europe. He is currently a member of the Musculoskeletal Research Group of the Erasmus University

Rotterdam, The Netherlands. As a medical doctor, he has been working in general practice and in outpatient clinics for rheumatology, rehabilitation medicine, and orthopedic medicine. His research has centered around the biomechanical impact of impairments of the locomotor system. Dr Mens is President of the Dutch Association of Physicians for Orthopedic Medicine and chief consultant for the Dutch Association for Patients with Pelvic Pain in Relation to Symphysiolysis.

Vert Mooney MD is currently Professor of Orthopedic Surgery at the University of California, San Diego, USA. He also serves as Medical Director of the clinical facility for the orthopedic faculty, which includes the Spine and Joint Conditioning Centers. He is Past President of the North American Spine Society and the International Society for the Study of Lumbar Spine. Dr Mooney has been Secretary and Vice President of the American Orthopaedic Association and is currently President of the International Intradiscal Therapy Society. He was a Governor's Appointee to the California Industrial Medical Council.

Michael R. Moore MD BSc is one of the founding physicians of the Colorado Spine Center, PC, USA. He is a graduate of the Johns Hopkins University School of Medicine and completed his residency training at the University of California, San Diego. He is Assistant Clinical Instructor of Orthopedics at the University of Colorado Health Sciences Center.

Hans C. Östgaard MD PhD is chief of the Department of Orthopedics and Surgery at Skene Hospital, Sweden. He practices orthopedic surgery full-time and has an interest in posterior pelvic pain. Over the past 5 years, he has published 10 articles on the subject. He is part-time Senior Visiting Orthopedic surgeon at the Social Insurance Office with a special interest in workers' compensation claims. He is a scientific board member of the Medical Research and Development Unit in Borås, Sweden.

Stanley V. Paris PhD PT, founder and Chairman of the Institute of Physical Therapy in St

Augustine, Florida, USA, graduated from the New Zealand School of Physiotherapy in 1958 and obtained his PhD from the Union Institute in 1984. A noted author of more than 30 articles and books, he is currently active in researching spinal anatomy and joint mechanics.

Dr Paris has been elected to membership of the International Society for the Study of the Lumbar Spine and Orthopaedic Research Society, and is a Fellow of the North American Spine Society, and an honorary life member of the New Zealand Society of Manipulative Therapy. He has been recognized by the Council on Specialization of the American Physical Therapy Association for his work in developing the specializations, and the Orthopedic Section have named the Annual Founders' Award and Address after him.

John Pier MD is a physical medicine rehabilitation physician specializing in treatment of spine, occupational and sports medicine injuries. He is board certified in physical medicine and rehabilitation. Dr Pier is presently Outpatient Medical Director for Healthsouth Rehabilitation in Portland, Maine. He is also in private practice serving the Southern Maine area. Dr Pier also assists in providing medical coverage for the US Ski Team, in regional competition. He continues to lecture regionally and nationally, with a special interest in cost-effective and time-efficient paradigms for spine, occupational and sports-related injuries.

Robert Pozos BS MA PhD is Professor of Biology and Assistant Dean at San Diego State University, San Diego, USA. He received his BS from St Mary's College, his MA and PhD from Southern Illinois University and his post-doc from the University of Tennessee. For 17 years, Dr Pozos was Chairman of the Physiology Department at the University of Minnesota in Duluth. He was also Vice President for Minority Affairs at the University of Washington in Seattle. In addition, he has been Director of Physiological Performance and Operational Medicine at the Naval Health Research Center in San Diego. He is presently working on developing telecommunication links between institutes in Mexico and SDSU. He is also developing a research program on the head and neck and on the neck and back in female helicopter pilots. Dr Pozos has been the author of 19 publications, including studies on the electrophysiological effects of acute ethanol exposure, inflight SEMG, video analysis of Navy helicopter pilots, and accidental hypothermia.

Michael M. Price MD attended undergraduate school in Atlanta, USA, at the Georgia Institute of Technology. He received his medical education at the Medical College of Georgia, in nearby Augusta. He is currently an orthopedic resident at Georgia Baptist Medical Center in Atlanta. After graduation, Dr Price is going into private practice in Douglas, Georgia, where he is interested in spinal implant developments and the general conditions that afflict the sacroiliac joint.

Tom Ravin MD practices full time as a musculoskeletal physician in Denver, Colorado, USA. At one time, he was a diagnostic radiologist and a nuclear medicine physician, but his interest in hands-on patient care led him into a medical practice that includes manipulation and injection therapies as well as some radiography. His background in radiology has been translated into an interest in imaging of the musculoskeletal system, particularly of the spine, ankles, and wrists.

Dr Ravin's special interests are in teaching ligamentous injection techniques and how to use imaging to aid in diagnosis of ligamentous laxity. He has written numerous articles and taught seminars on these subjects for the American Association of Orthopedic Medicine and the American Academy of Osteopathy. He is the immediate Past President of the AAOM.

Vicki Sims PT is director of a physical therapy practice and works in orthopedic offices in Atlanta, Athens, and Gainesville, Georgia, USA. A graduate of Georgia State University, Ms Sims brings with her 19 years of clinical experience in hospital and outpatient orthopedic physical therapy. She was invited to speak at the 1995 Second Interdisciplinary World Congress on Low Back Pain in San Diego, California, USA.

Gary L. Smidt PhD PT FAPTA is former long-time Director of the Physical Therapy Graduate Program and Professor in the College of Medicine at The University of Iowa. His research has centered around biomechanics, with widespread basic and clinical investigations involving gait, muscle function, joint mechanics, and development-objective clinical measurement of physical function. Dr Smidt is currently a Professor Emeritus in the College of Medicine at the University of Iowa, USA, and Editor-in-Chief of the *Journal of Orthopaedic and Sports Physical Therapy*.

Chris J. Snijders PhD is currently Professor of Medical Technology at the Erasmus University Rotterdam, and at the University of Technology, Delft, The Netherlands. His research focuses on biomechanics related to arm and hand problems, neck and low back pain, and foot dysfunction. As a mechanical engineer, he is involved in the design of professional and consumer products.

Henk J. Stam MD PhD graduated as specialist in physical medicine and rehabilitation from Erasmus University, Faculty of Medicine, Rotterdam in 1983. His PhD thesis (1990) concentrated on isokinetic measurements of the knee extensors. At present he is Head of the Department of Rehabilitation Medicine of the University Hospital and Institute of Rehabilitation Medicine, Erasmus University. The research fields of this institute focus on the development of measurement instruments and methods in physical medicine and rehabilitation.

Rob Stoeckart PhD specialized in morphology, biochemistry, and brain research during his training at the University of Amsterdam, The Netherlands, although he was in fact mainly interested in sports and politics. At the Erasmus University Rotterdam, being a member of the anatomy department, he became interested in university politics and in teaching medical students and others. For many years, he was chairman of Studium Generale, an organization providing 'culture' to students and members of the University. In organizing specific symposia (e.g. on 'Priorities in health care', 'Euthanasia', and 'The nature of reality'), combined with his experiences in the dissecting room, Dr Stoeckart became more and more interested in death, disease, and life. His research focused on ultrastructural aspects of the hypothalamus.

After his PhD thesis, his attention shifted to the pelvis. For over 15 years, Dr Stoeckart has been working with Andry Vleeming and Chris Snijders on anatomic and biomechanical aspects of the low(er) back. Together with Corrie, his wife, he organizes 3-day workshops for couples wanting to deepen their relationships. In his spare time, he writes poems.

Bengt Sturesson MD is currently consultant in spine surgery and general orthopedics at the county hospital of Angelholm, Sweden. His research on mobility in the sacroiliac joints is connected with Malmö General Hospital, Lund University, Sweden.

David D Swenski MA is currently earning a clinical doctorate degree in physical therapy at the University of Southern California, San Diego, USA. He received his Master's degree in exercise physiology from San Diego State University and his Bachelor's degree in exercise science and nutrition from Arizona State University. He has worked in spine patient care and clinical research in the Department of Orthopedics at the University of California San Diego and has served as assistant strength and conditioning coach for the San Diego Chargers.

Hugo van Eek MSc works as a clinical psychologist and behaviour therapist at the departments of rheumatology and orthopedics of the Rehabilitation Centre at Hoensbroek, The Netherlands. He has a special interest in the behavioral rehabilitation of chronic pain patients, and has been involved in the behavioral treatment of patients who participated in a number of clinical trials concerning the effects of behavioral rehabilitation programs.

Jan-Paul van Wingerden PT BSc is currently working at the Spine and Joint Center as a coordinator of functional assessment. Over the

past 7 years, he has cooperated in several articles on functional anatomy of the spine and pelvis, as well as on ergonomics. He has been teaching ergonomics and biomechanics to physical therapy students and contributes to postacademic education in the field of functional anatomy.

Johan W. S. Vlaeyen PhD is clinical psychologist and senior lecturer at the Department of Medical Psychology of the University of Limburg, Maastricht, The Netherlands, as well as clinical researcher at the interacademic Postgraduate School of Experimental Psychopathology and the Institute for Rehabilitation Research at Hoensbroek, The Netherlands. He is a member of the Flemish Associations for Behavior Therapy and Hypnotherapy and the Dutch and Belgian Chapters of the International Association for the Study of Pain. Dr Vlaeyen's research mainly focuses on the assessment and treatment of chronic musculoskeletal pain syndromes, including back pain and fibromyalgia, from a behavioral rehabilitation perspective.

Andre Vleeming PhD is a clinical anatomist working in the medical faculty, Erasmus University Rotterdam, The Netherlands. He did his doctorate study, at the same medical faculty, on a biomechanical, anatomical and radiological study of the function of the pelvis. New studies of the pelvis and anatomy in general are the subject of his several books and articles. He lectures extensively on these subjects nationally and internationally.

Frank H. Willard PhD is an Associate Professor of Anatomy at the University of New England, USA, and a visiting lecturer in anatomy at the European School of Osteopathy in Maidstone, UK. He is Director of Medical Curriculum at the University of New England, USA, and is involved in developing and administering postgraduate education courses in the UK, Belgium, Australia, and New Zealand. His research centers on the nervous system and functional anatomic relationships in the human back.

Introduction

This book has its origins in two world congresses on low back and pelvic pain. The congresses were characterized by their interdisciplinary approach, and included speakers ranging from internationally renowned clinical groups to departments dealing with the basic sciences; the same applies to this book. The contributions are from different disciplines embracing anthropology, orthopedic surgery, biomechanical engineering, chiropractic practice, anatomy, osteopathy, physical therapy, podiatry, gynecology, rehabilitation medicine and several others. The new ideas put forward in this book will hopefully lead to wide acceptance amongst the several disciplines. If we are right, this will considerably reduce the multitude of therapies used to treat lumbopelvic pain.

The human pelvis is unique in the animal kingdom as the human being is the only biped amongst mammals. Even our closest living animal relatives, the African great apes, are inherently quadrupeds and only temporarily rise on their hind legs. Through identical terminology, based on comparative anatomy, similarities in the framework of pelvic anatomy between mammals and humans have been fixed in our consciousness. However, the function of the human pelvis is quite different from that of quadrupeds. Perhaps it is better to think of the human as swivelling on one leg, except, of course, that the legs alternate. When one thinks of the mechanics of the transfer of weight and forces through the human pelvis, the reader will begin to appreciate the uniqueness of the human pelvis in walking. Because of this unique feature of humans, we, as editors of this book, have agreed that an understanding of the role of the pelvis is essential if we are to appreciate fully the

new knowledge dealing with the musculoskeletal system.

Early in the century, ligaments in general, and those governing the sacroiliac joints (SIJ) in particular, were recognized as a source of back pain, sometimes accompanied by radiating pain down one lower limb or the other. However, in clinical orthopedics the role of the pelvis, and especially the role of the SIJ, have been largely denied. This is primarily due to the description of the prolapse of the intervertebral disc by Mixter & Barr in 1934.

With the advent of imaging techniques for intervertebral disc degeneration in its multiple forms, lumbopelvic pain has been mainly ascribed to that which can be seen. From this has developed the mind set of 'believing is seeing'. As a result, a host of naturally occurring changes, for example aging and wear and tear, have been wrongly blamed for back pain.

The potential for the abnormalities of the disc to be visualized with constantly improving imaging technology has distracted many contemporary surgeons from the role of the pelvis and the function of ligaments in the lumbopelvic area. But gradually it has become clear that structural abnormalities involving the intervertebral disc, facet joints or SIJ are not necessarily sources of low back or pelvic pain.

In this book, convincing evidence is presented that the SIJ and its surrounding ligaments are capable of producing pain. This is clinically relevant, since a large number of studies show evidence of movement in the SIJ. Thus, in the case of, for example, hypermobility of the SIJ, certain surrounding ligaments can become overstretched. However, we should not make the same mistake as with the intervertebral disc by exclusively featuring the SIJ as the major source of pain.

Therefore, when trying to understand the causes of lumpopelvic pain, we do not consider it realistic any more to divide the body into separate parts, based on topographical and structural anatomical concepts. We all feel that true understanding of the function and dysfunction of the locomotor system must be based on the integration of knowledge of how the torso, pelvis, legs and arms act together.

From the surgeon's point of view, the most important aspect of this book is the redefinition of anatomy. This fresh look at structural relationships, provided by careful anatomic dissection with its projected mechanical relationships, has been illuminating. We must realize that the pelvis has to be capable of allowing long levers like the trunk and legs to act on it. A central hypothesis of this book is, therefore, that without adequate muscle and ligament function, pelvic stability is not guaranteed. The combination of anatomic findings and biomechanical modelling led to the concept that lumbopelvic pain can only be understood if we also have a proper insight into the role of the SIJ and of the action of muscles and fascia that participate in load transfer from shoulder to feet. In this approach, biomechanical modelling is important since it has shown explanatory as well as predictive power. The clinical significance is that for treatment and prevention of lumbopelvic pain primary attention should be shifted to understanding load transfer and to the combined action of muscle systems. This holds especially true for the role of muscles, such as the oblique and transverse abdominals, the coupled action of the gluteus maximus and latissimus dorsi, and of the erector spinae and multifidus muscle. This approach might lead to a deviating view on some surgical interventions.

A rational treatment program traverses many therapeutic boundaries. We anticipate that these boundaries will turn out to be increasingly small when we become more receptive to each other's point of view. Most of the concepts presented here are based on well-substantiated anatomic and biomechanic principles referred to in the text. The varied chapters are only building blocks of an educational edifice which is incomplete. Scientific validity is the cement which allows this structure to enlarge. Many more pieces of the jigsaw still have to fit together before the structure is complete; however, provided that the fresh, documented concepts which are the 'leitmotif' of this book are correct, we are convinced that new effective approaches for the management of lumbopelvic pain will arise.

The studies reviewed in this book reflect the specialities of the contributors, their backgrounds, styles and approaches. To maintain a varied approach, we invited both authors with a long history of sound clinical work and relatively young researchers. The editors have studiously avoided the trend to mold the contributions into a uniform format. What matters to us is the advance of ideas.

It is clinicians, in dealing with their patients, who first encounter problems in adhering to traditional medical concepts, but very few practitioners persist in asking and in challenging. In this respect we would like to express our appreciation for all the work done by Richard DonTigny, who never ceased to vigorously draw attention to the neglected role of the pelvis.

Lumpopelvic pain is a significant scourge on our civilization, predominantly affecting productive members of our society. Every person has a back and pelvis; clinicians, epidemiologists and even politicians must be aware of the prevalence of lumbopelvic pain; can any of us ignore this problem?

REFERENCES

Mixter WJ, Barr JS 1934 Rupture of the intervertebral disc with involvement of the spinal canal. New England Journal of Medicine 211: 210–215

Abbreviations and terminology

ABBREVIATIONS

SI	sacroiliac
SIJ	sacroiliac joint(s)
SIJD	sacroiliac joint dysfunction
LBP	low back pain
ASIS	anterior superior iliac spine(s)
PSIS	posterior superior iliac spine(s)
AP	anterior posterior/anteroposterior
PA	posterior anterior/posteroanterior
PPP	peripartum pelvic pain or pregnancy related pelvic pain

SYNONYMS

anterior – ventral
posterior – dorsal
superior – cranial
inferior – caudal
coronal – frontal

long dorsal sacroiliac ligament – long posterior sacroiliac ligament – (long ligament)

thoracolumbar fascia – lumbodorsal fascia

TERMINOLOGY

For the terminology the contributors of this book were asked to use the Glossary of osteopathic terminology* which was kindly provided by William A. Kuchera, DO, FAAO.
*Glossary of osteopathic terminology 1996 In: Allen T. W (ed) AOA Yearbook and Directory, American Osteopathic Association, Chicago, IL

Anatomy and pathophysiology

PART I

Basic research

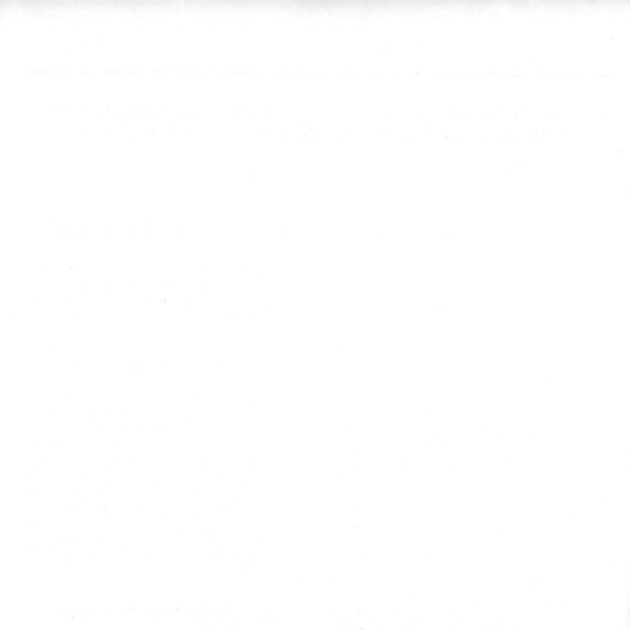

1. The muscular, ligamentous and neural structure of the low back and its relation to back pain

F. H. Willard

INTRODUCTION

The lumbosacral spinal column performs a key role in the transfer of weight from the torso and upper body into the lower extremities, both in static positions and during mobility. The primary bony structures involved in the transduction are five lumbar vertebrae, a sacrum, and two innominate bones. Critical to the stability of these bony components is a complex arrangement of dense connective tissue. Although typically described as separate entities in most textbooks of anatomy, these soft tissue, fibrous structures actually form a continuous ligamentous stocking in which the lumbar vertebrae and sacrum are positioned. The major muscles representing the prime movers in this region, such as the multifidus, gluteus maximus, and biceps femoris, have various attachments to this elongated, ligamentous stocking. The muscular and ligamentous relationships composing the lumbosacral connection are of extreme importance in stabilizing the lumbar vertebrae and sacrum during the transfer of energy from the upper body to the lower extremities. This arrangement has been termed a self-locking mechanism (Vleeming et al 1995c) and, as such, its dysfunction is critical to the failure of the lower back.

A critical relationship also exists between the neural components of the lumbosacral region and the surrounding ligamentous structures. Current research, using immunohistochemical techniques to identify specific types of axons, suggests that all of these connective tissue structures receive a supply of small-caliber, primary afferent fibers, typical of those involved in nociception. Irritation of these primary afferent nociceptive axons initiates the release of neuropeptides that interact with fibroblasts, mast cells and immune cells present in the surrounding connective tissue (Levine et al 1993). The resultant cascade of events, referred to as a neurogenic inflammatory response, is thought to play a major role in degenerative diseases and the development of low back pain (Garrett et al 1992, Kidd et al 1990, Weidenbaum & Farcy 1990, Weinstein 1992). Sensitization of these small-caliber, primary afferent fibers, along with sensitization of their central connections in the dorsal horn of the spinal cord, appears to play a critical role in the evolution of chronic painful conditions (Coderre et al 1993, Woolf & Chong 1993). This chapter will examine recent advances in our knowledge of the lumbosacral region structure and its innervation.

LIGAMENTOUS STRUCTURE OF THE LUMBAR REGION

The various ligaments of the lumbar vertebral column form a continuous dense connective tissue stocking surrounding the vertebrae and extending into the sacral area. For ease of description, the vertebral connective tissue sheath will be divided into three parts: (1) the neural arch structures, (2) the capsular structures, and (3) the ventral or vertebral body structures (Fig. 1.1). However, it should be noted that the partitions between each of these three divisions are for convenience only, since the connective tissue of the dorsal and ventral

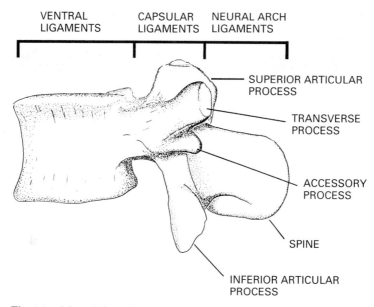

VENTRAL LIGAMENTS   CAPSULAR LIGAMENTS   NEURAL ARCH LIGAMENTS

SUPERIOR ARTICULAR PROCESS

TRANSVERSE PROCESS

ACCESSORY PROCESS

SPINE

INFERIOR ARTICULAR PROCESS

Fig. 1.1   A lateral view of a lumbar vertebra illustrating the position of the neural arch ligaments, capsular ligaments, and ventral ligaments.

components is essentially continuous across the pedicles of the vertebrae.

Neural arch ligaments

The neural arch of each lumbar vertebra is composed of the pedicles, laminae, transverse processes, and spine. There are two major ligaments that participate in surrounding the neural arch: the ligamentum flavum and the interspinous ligament. Two additional small ligaments are also present: the supraspinous ligament posteriorly and the intertransverse ligament laterally. To view the ligaments of the neural arch, the multifidus muscle must be removed from the lumbosacral region (Figs 1.2 and 1.3). Although most of these ligaments have a distinct biochemical

make-up when isolated (Ballard & Weinstein 1992, Fujii et al 1993, Yahia et al 1990), in the

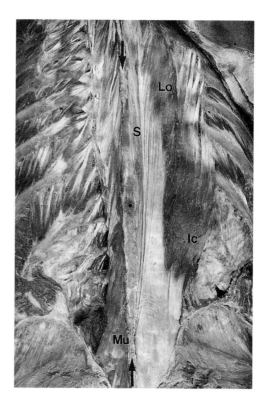

Fig. 1.2   The three lumbar paravertebral muscles in a male. On the individual's right side is the iliocostalis muscle (Ic) laterally and the longissimus muscle (Lo) medially. Note that the spinalis muscle (S) does not extend into the lumbar region beyond L2 or L3. On his left side, the iliocostalis and longissimus have been removed to reveal the medially positioned multifidus muscle (Mu). Arrows top and bottom are aligned along the spinous processes of the thoracic and lumbar vertebrae (midline). The thick lumbar multifidus muscle is seen differentiating into the thin, flattened semispinalis muscle at the superior end of the lumbar vertebral column (asterisk).

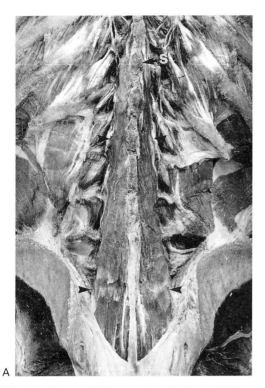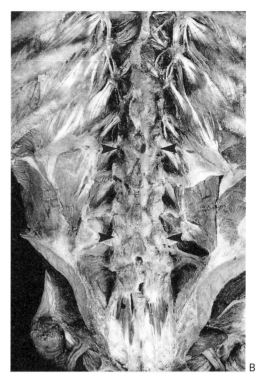

Fig. 1.3 The multifidus muscle and its bed. (A) The pyramidal-shaped multifidus muscle is demonstrated between the four arrowheads (S, lumbar spinous processes). (B) The multifidus muscle has been removed to reveal a continuous ligamentous stocking surrounding the neural arch components of the lumbar vertebrae (between arrowheads). On the sacrum, only the deepest laminae of the multifidus remains (asterisk).

composition (Ballard & Weinstein 1992, Fujii et al 1993, Yahia et al 1990) they grade together at their boundaries to unite and function as a single unit. To demonstrate this concept, the osseous components of the neural arch were removed with minimal disturbance to the associated ligamentous structures (Figs 1.4 and 1.5). The unitary nature of the supraspinous and intraspinous ligaments and the ligamentum flavum is obvious since these soft tissue structures maintain their continuity despite the lack of supporting osseous material.

The ligamentum flavum represents a medialward continuation of the articular capsule of the facet joint (Fig. 1.4). This ligament stretches between the laminae of adjacent vertebra, forming a roof over the spinal canal. This distensible ligament is composed of elastic fibers (80%) and collagenous fibers (20%), the elastic fibers imparting the ligament its yellow color and flexible nature (Bogduk & Twomey 1991). The medial fibers of the ligament bridge the gap between the laminae of adjacent vertebra, while the lateral fibers attach to the facet joint capsule (Figs 1.4B and 1.5; (Behrsin & Briggs 1988, Bogduk & Twomey 1991, Ramsey 1966). The medial border of the ligamentum flavum turns posteriorly and decreases in elastic fiber content to become the interspinous ligament. A significant function for the ligamentum flavum is to provide a roof for the vertebral canal that will not buckle during extension–flexion movements of the vertebral column (Bogduk & Twomey 1991). At rest (in a neutral position), the ligaments have a pre-tension, keeping the ligaments from buckling (Nachemson & Evans 1968). Failure of the elastic properties of this ligament has been related to the development of adolescent idiopathic scoliosis (Hadley-Miller et al 1994). Unfortunately, there is little or no regenerative capacity in the elastic tissue of the ligamentum flavum; thus a damaged ligament is replaced by a cicatrix (Ramsey 1966). In addition, there is an age-related loss of elastic fibers and

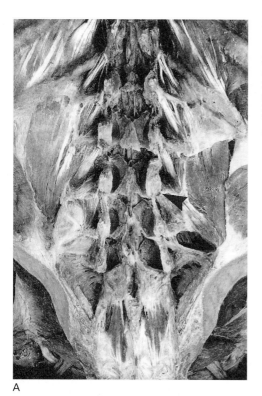

A

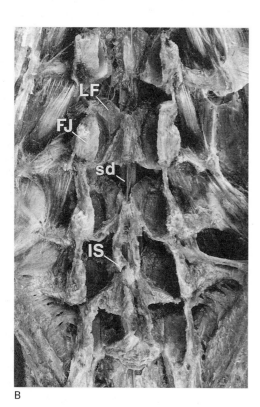

B

Fig. 1.4 The ligamentous stocking of the lumbar vertebrae.
(A) This orientation photograph is a posterior view of the lumbar
spinal column, similar to that in Fig. 1.3. The spinous processes,
laminae, and inferior articular processes of the facet joint have been
removed. (B) This detailed view of the ligamentous stocking
illustrates the ligamentum flavum (LF) extending between the
interspinous ligament (IS) medially and the facet joint capsule (FJ)
laterally. The arrowhead indicates the same facet joint capsule in
both photographs. Between the flaval ligaments, the epidural space
and spinal dural (sd) can be seen.

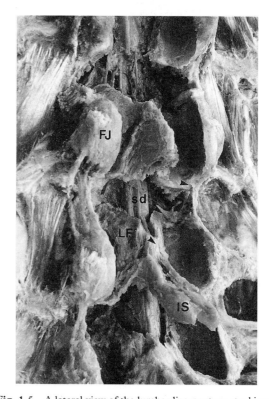

Fig. 1.5 A lateral view of the lumbar ligamentous stocking.
The facet joint marked FJ is the same as that marked FJ in
Fig. 1.4B. The continuity of the flaval ligament (LF) with the
facet joint capsule and interspinous ligament (IS) is indicated
by the arrowheads. The spinal dura (sd) can be seen in the
epidural space.

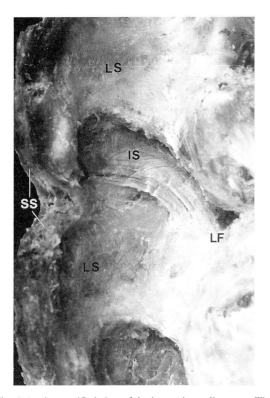

Fig. 1.6 A magnified view of the interspinous ligament. The lumbar spinous processes (LS) are seen superior and inferior to the ligament. Note the fan-like orientation of the collagenous fibers in the ligament. The proximal end of the ligament is continuous with the ligamentum flavum (LF) and the distal end of the ligament is embedded in the supraspinous ligament (SS). This latter structure is attached to the thoracolumbar fascia. This arrangement would serve to transform any increased tension in the thoracolumbar fascia into increased tension on the ligamentum flavum, resulting in an alignment of the lumbar vertebrae (see Fig. 1.7).

related changes in the ligamentum flavum have been related to specific neurologic sequelae such as the cauda equina syndrome and lumbar radiculopathy (Baba et al 1995, Ryan 1993).

The interspinous ligament extends between borders of the spines of adjacent vertebrae (Figs 1.5 and 1.6). Its anterior border is a continuation of the ligamentum flavum. The posterior border of the ligament thickens to form the supraspinous ligament, which is, in turn, anchored to the thoracolumbar fascia. The orientation of fibers in the interspinous ligament has been given multiple, conflicting descriptions. In humans, the ligament can best be described as a fan (Fig. 1.6; see also Fig. 1.11 below). The narrow or proximal end of the fan blends with the ligamentum flavum and contains elastic fibers (Yahia et al 1990), while the broad end of the fan extends in a posterior direction towards the tips of the spines and is composed primarily of collagen fibers. In the center of the ligament, the collagen fibers are oriented parallel to the vertebral spines; distally, the peripheral collagen fibers flare posterocranially and posterocaudally (Aspden et al 1987, Hukins et al 1990). This fan-like arrangement allows the ligament to expand without rupture as the vertebral spines separate during flexion. The fibers of this ligament are described as resisting the separation of the vertebral spines during flexion (Bogduk & Twomey 1991); however, the most likely function of these ligaments, given their anteroposterior fiber orientation, is to act as an anchor, transmitting the anteroposterior pull of the thoracolumbar fascia, into which it is attached via the supraspinous ligament (Hukins et al 1990), into an increased tension in the ligamentum flavum (Fig. 1.7). This increased tension would assist in preventing the latter ligament from buckling onto the spinal cord and would also serve to assist in alignment of the lumbar vertebrae. Along the osseous borders of the interspinous ligaments, chondrocytes are present, and age-related chondrification of the interspinous ligament occurs after the third decade of life (Yahia et al 1990). Degenerative processes in the motion segment of the vertebrae appear to enhance the chondrification of the ligament. All of these pathologic events occurring to the interspinous ligament should diminish the ability of the thoracolumbar fascia to influence the alignment

elasticity of the ligamentum flavum, contributing to their progressive loss of tension in the elderly (Nachemson & Evans 1968; Ramsey 1966). Specifically, there is a decrease in elastic fibers and a concomitant increase in the density of collagen fibers, along with a shift to high molecular weight proteoglycans (Kashiwagi 1993, Okada et al 1993). These events favor the deposition of calcium, so an ossification of the ligament often occurs with the increased presence of calcium pyrophosphate dihydrate and hydroxyapatite crystals (Kashiwagi 1993). Calcification of the ligament leads to its hypertrophy and to subsequent lumbar spinal stenosis (Yoshida et al 1992). These age-

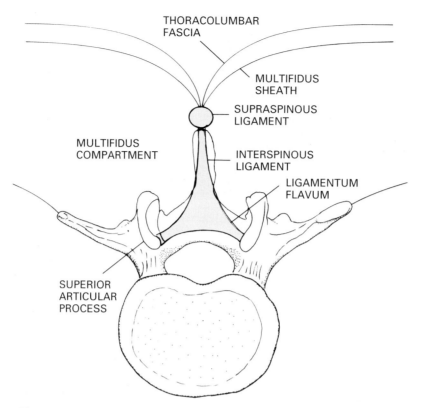

Fig. 1.7 A horizontal view of a lumbar vertebra illustrating the interspinous–supraspinous–thoracolumbar (IST) ligamentous complex. By anchoring the thoracolumbar fascia and multifidus sheath to the facet joint capsules, the IST complex becomes the central support system for the lumbar spine.

of the lumbar vertebrae, and thereby increase their risk of destructive injury.

Of the two small ligaments associated with the neural arch, the supraspinous ligament, the most prominent, forms the posterior border of the interspinous ligament (Fig. 1.8). Throughout its lumbar course, it is tightly adherent to the posterior border of the lumbar spines and to the interspinous ligament. This creates an interspinous–supraspinous–thoracolumbar (IST) ligamentous complex that anchors the major fascial planes of the back to the lumbar spines. Traction placed on the thoracolumbar fascia will destroy the thoracolumbar sheath before it will separate the IST complex (Fig. 1.8). Thus it is possible for the interspinous and supraspinous ligaments to act as force transducers, translating the tension of the thoracolumbar fascia, developed in the extremities and torso, into the lumbar vertebral

column. At lower lumbar levels, the supraspinous ligament becomes progressively less organized as it grades into the distal attachments of the thoracolumbar fascia, and in some individuals it may not be recognizable caudal to L4 (Bogduk & Twomey 1991). This ligament often presents with fatty involution late in life (Heylings 1978) and can also ossify (Mine & Kawai 1995). Finally, the small, intertransverse ligament arises from the periosteal tissue surrounding the transverse processes and pedicle of the lumbar vertebrae. Caudally, this tissue expands to represent the iliolumbar ligament.

Articular capsular ligament

The articular processes of the lumbar vertebrae form the facet or zygapophyseal joints. Each joint consist of two opposed and vertically oriented

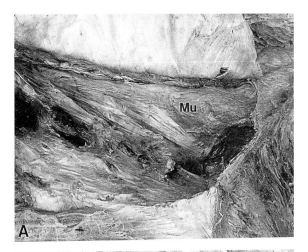

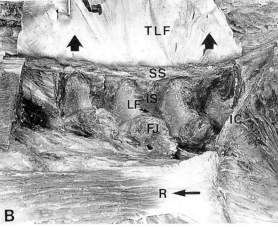

Fig. 1.8 The attachment of the multifidus sheath to the supraspinous ligament. The thoracolumbar fascia (TLF) and multifidus sheath have been sectioned longitudinally to reveal the multifidus muscle (Mu). (A) The iliocostalis and longissimus muscles have been removed. (B) The multifidus muscle has also been removed to illustrate the continuity between the thoracolumbar fascia (and multifidus sheath), supraspinous ligament (SS), ligamentum flavum (LF), and facet joint capsule (FJ). Traction in the posterior direction on the TLF (see hemostat tips) shreds the fascial sheath long before it ever separates this fascial complex. The arrow in the lower right points rostral (R) and the iliac crest (IC) is seen on the right side of the photograph.

plates surrounded by a dense connective tissue fibrous capsule (Lewin et al 1962). The plates are curved such that the inferior articular process (from the above vertebrae) presents a convex process to the concave superior articular process (of the vertebrae below) (Fig. 1.9). These joints contain a true synovial space, a connective tissue

rim and a complicated array of surrounding adipose tissue pads and fibroadipose menisci (Engel & Bogduk 1982). The articular surface of the facet joints is covered with a hyaline cartilage. The joint capsule represents a connective tissue bridge between the neural arch ligaments and those of the vertebral body. As such, the capsule is encased in a thin sheet of dense, irregular investing fascia, which is continuous dorsally with that surrounding the ligamentum flavum and ventrally with the investing fascia of the vertebral body. The main component of the capsule is composed of dense, regularly arranged connective tissue in which the predominant orientation of the collagenous fibers is orthogonal to the joint line (the plane on which the two facet plates oppose each other (Fig. 1.10). The capsule is bound tightly to the articular processes with the exception of its inferior and superior recesses, each of which consists of a loosened fold in the capsule wall (Figs 1.9C and 1.11). This arrangement of the capsule allows for a gliding movement in the sagittal plane, but restricts its range of motion in the horizontal plane. Each recess has a small defect that is capable of transmitting fat from the capsular space outward (Bogduk & Twomey 1991). The capsule is reinforced dorsally by the multifidus muscle and ventrally by the ligamentum flavum. It is weakest around the superior recess, which can burst from effusion during arthrography (Dory 1981). The inferior border of the capsule is continuous with the ligamentum flavum, the medial border with the periosteum of the lamina, and the lateral border with the periosteum of the pedicle and body.

The facet joint is subject to an age-related process of degeneration. Unlike the intervertebral discs, facet joints maintain the proteoglycans of their articular cartilage surface, which actually thickens through a process of increase hydration with age (Tobias et al 1992). These changes are accompanied by an increase in coarse fibrillation of the facet joint surface, more pronounced on the superior than the inferior process (Tobias et al 1992, Ziv et al 1993), osteophyte formation, and sclerosis of the subchondral bone (Vernon-Roberts 1992). The degenerative changes are regional (Swanepoel et al 1995, Taylor & Twomey 1986), being greatest for the articular surface of

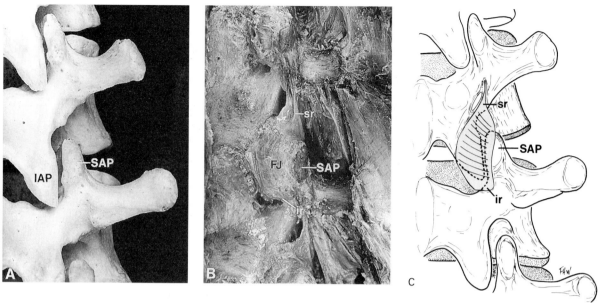

Fig. 1.9   The lumbar facet joint capsule recesses. (A) This is an orientation view of an articulated lumbar column illustrating the superior articular process (SAP) and inferior articular process (IAP) of the lumbar facet joint (rostal is towards the top of the figure). (B) This photograph has the same orientation as Fig. 1.9A. The facet joint (FJ) capsule is seen with the superior (sr) and inferior (ir) recesses. (C) A schematic diagram illustrating the facet joint capsule (shading) with the superior (sr) and inferior (ir) recesses.

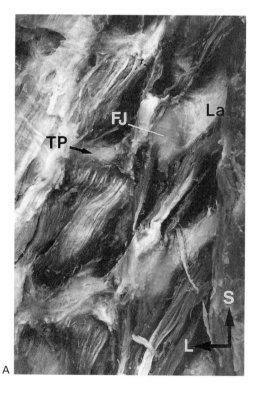
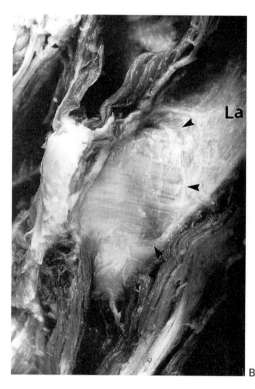

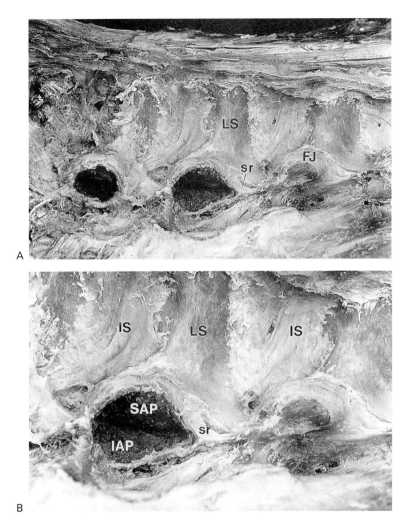

Fig. 1.11 The lumbar facet joint cavity. (A) This is a lateral view of the middle lumbar vertebra after removing the multifidus muscle. The spines (LS) of the lumbar vertebrae are oriented vertically, the cadaver is prone, with rostral positioned toward the right of the photograph. The lower two facet joints (FJ) have had the superior articular process drilled away to expose the joint cavity and its superior recesses (sr). (B) A magnified view of the middle facet joint from Fig. 1.11A. The superior articular process (SAP) can be seen forming the posteromedial wall of the joint and the remains of the inferior articular process (IAP) can be seen in an anterolateral position. The superior recess (sr) extend upward toward the facet joint above. A lumbar spine (LS) and two interspinous ligaments are visible. Note the orientation of the fibers in the interspinous ligament, parallel to the long axis of the lumbar spine.

Fig. 1.10 (*Facing page*) The lumbar facet joint capsule (A) This is a dorsal view of the lumbar spinal column with all but the deepest laminae of the multifidus muscle removed to reveal the facet joint capsule (FJ), vertebral laminae (La), and transverse processes (TP) of a lumbar vertebra. The right side of the photograph is aligned along the midline of the body. The orientation figure in the lower right of the photograph indicates superior (S) and lateral (L) directions. (B) This is an enlarged view of the lumbar facet joint capsule marked FJ in photograph Fig. 1.10A. The arrowheads mark the medial border of the capsule as it attaches to the vertebral laminae (La). Note the horizontal orientation to the collagenous fibers in the capsule. This orientation is orthogonal to the long axis of the joint. The capsule is strongest on its posterior (current view) and anterior sides, and weakest superiorly and inferiorly. The deepest laminae of the multifidus muscle can be seen attaching to the inferior and superior recesses of the capsule.

the superior process peripherally, superiorly and inferiorly; but in the inferior process it is peripheral and posterior (Swanepoel et al 1995). The intervertebral disc and its two associated facet joints make up a triad representing the load-bearing joint surfaces at each lumbar vertebral level (Lewin et al 1962). It has been noted that there is a correlation between the degenerative events occurring in the intervertebral joint and those in the accompanying facet joints (Vernon-Roberts 1992). This correlation has been supported quantitatively with the demonstration that there is increasing coarse fibrillation of the facet joint surface as one progresses from grade I to grade III degeneration of the associated intervertebral disc (Ziv et al 1993). However, recent attempts to demonstrate this same relationship using computer-assisted methods have proven only a very weak correlation (Swanepoel et al 1995). Based on these results, it has been suggested that disc degeneration is not the only means of placing stress on the facet joints and that inadequate conditioning on surrounding muscles may also be a prime cause of fibrillation in the facet joint (Swanepoel et al 1995).

Ligaments ventral to the facet joints

The vertebral bodies are surrounded by a well-developed periosteum. This sheath can be envisioned as a dense connective tissue stocking that houses the vertebrae and the annular ligaments of the intervertebral discs. Dorsally, the periosteum of the body is continuous with that of the pedicles, facet joint capsule and laminae. Embedded in the periosteal sheath of the vertebrae are two longitudinal thickenings: the anterior longitudinal ligament and the posterior longitudinal ligament.

The anterior longitudinal ligament, the stronger of the two vertebral body ligaments (Panjabi & White 1990), consists of a thickened band of vertically oriented collagenous fibers that extends from the basiocciput to the sacrum, where it is continuous with the anteromedial aspect of the sacroiliac joint (SIJ) capsule. The deepest bands of collagenous fibers are the shortest and extend from one vertebral body to the next, forming only loose attachments to the annular ligament of the

intervertebral disc. The more superficial bands of the ligament span longer distances (Bogduk & Twomey 1991). In the lumbar region, the fibrous organization of the anterior longitudinal ligament is disrupted where it serves as an attachment for the two crura of the diaphragm. Although the main attachments of the crura are in the region of the upper three lumbar vertebrae, some of the crural fibers extend to the lower lumbar region as well. The anterior longitudinal ligament undergoes age-related changes. Its energy-absorbing and elastic properties decrease with age, as does the strength of the bone into which it is attached (Neumann et al 1994, Panjabi & White 1990). As the mineral content of the surrounding bone decreases with age, the strength of the ligament also decreases (Neumann et al 1993). Rarely, the anterior longitudinal ligament can calcify, extreme cases resulting in spinal cord compression and peripheral nerve entrapment (McCafferty et al 1995).

The posterior longitudinal ligament is also embedded in the periosteum of the vertebrae and extends from the basiocciput (as the membrana tectoria) to the periosteum of the sacrum. As this ligament descends along the anterior wall of the vertebral canal, it narrows to pass around the bases of the pedicles and expands over the annular ligament of the intervertebral discs. This undulating margin imparts a serrated appearance to the longitudinal profile of the ligament. In contradistinction to its anterior counterpart, the attachments of the posterior longitudinal ligament are strongest to the outer layer of the annulus fibrosis of the intervertebral disc and weakest to the vertebral body. The lumbar posterior longitudinal ligament is much thinner, both in width and thickness, than its anterior counterpart; therefore, the main opposition to flexion of the lumbar spine comes from the ligamentum flavum (Panjabi & White 1990). Throughout its lumbosacral distribution, the posterior longitudinal ligament acts as an attachment site for the spinal dural sac (Dupuis 1992, Parke & Watanabe 1990, Spencer et al 1983). These attachments are accomplished though a series of ventral adhesions referred to as Hofmann's ligaments. Medial and lateral dural attachment ligaments are recognized (Firooznia et al 1993).

The two longitudinal ligaments and the ligamentum flavum function to stabilize the lumbar vertebral column in flexion (posterior longitudinal ligament and ligamentum flavum) and extension (anterior longitudinal ligament). The ligaments, especially the anterior longitudinal ligament, are most vulnerable to injury when in rotation (Roaf 1960). Of particular interest is the observation that data on load–deformation values for the anterior longitudinal ligament are similar to those data obtained from the ligamentum flavum, suggesting that the two major stabilizing ligaments are balanced in their design (Panjabi & White 1990). The anterior longitudinal ligament comes under its greatest strain in extension (Panjabi et al 1982) and its injury is associated with instability of the spinal column in extension (Oxland et al 1991).

LIGAMENTS OF THE SACRAL REGION

Iliolumbar ligament

The iliolumbar ligament is a complex structure that extends from the transverse processes of the lower two lumbar vertebrae to reach the ileal crest superolaterally and blend with the interosseous ligaments of the SIJ inferolaterally (Figs 1.12 and 1.13). It has received numerous and varied descriptions. 'Gray's Anatomy' (Williams 1995) describes superior and inferior bands in the ligament, the inferior band being called the lumbosacral ligament. Kapandji (1974) describes superior and inferior bands with an occasional sacral band below the inferior band. O'Rahilly (1986) describes anterior, superior, and inferior bands, whereas Bogduk and Twomey (1991) describe anterior, posterior, superior, inferior, and vertical iliolumbar divisions. A recent study

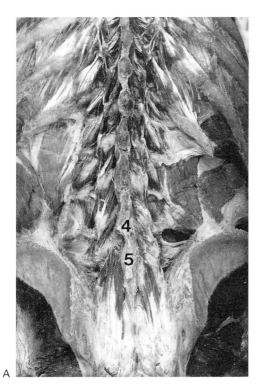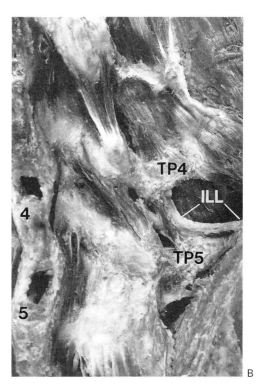

Fig. 1.12 A dorsal view of the sacrum and iliolumbar ligament. (A) In this orientation view, note that the multifidus muscle, except for its deepest laminae, has been removed. The spinous processes of L4 and L5 are indicated. (B) This is an enlarged view of the iliolumbar ligament (ILL) from the photograph in Fig. 1.12A. The ligament (ILL) can be seen attaching to the transverse processes of L4 and L5 (TP4 and TP5). The spinous processes of L4 and L5 are indicated.

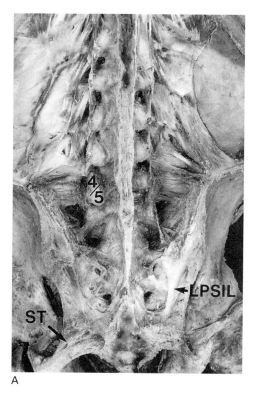

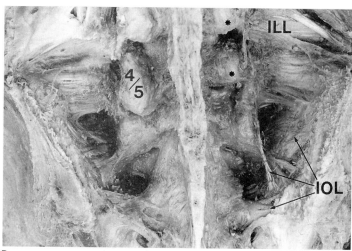

Fig. 1.13   A dorsal view of the female SIJ. (A) In this orientation view, the multifidus muscle has been entirely removed to reveal the interosseous ligaments of the SIJ. The long dorsal (posterior) SI ligament (LPSIL), the facet joint between the 4th and 5th lumbar vertebrae (4/5), and the sacrotuberous ligament (ST) are indicated as landmarks. (B) In this enlarged view of the SIJ, the interosseous ligaments (IOL), the facet joint between the 4th and 5th lumbar vertebrae (4/5), and the iliolumbar ligaments (ILL) are indicated. The iliolumbar ligament is seen attaching to the transverse processes of L4 and L5. Each process is located opposite the facet joint capsule marked with an asterisk.

based on 100 specimens reported only two parts to the ligament: anterior and posterior (Hanson & Sonesson 1994). My experience with this ligament is that the individual bands of fascia are highly variable in their number and their form, but that they consistently blend superiorly with the intertransverse ligaments of the lumbar vertebrae and inferiorly with the sacroiliac (SI) ligaments.

The iliolumbar ligament arises from the transverse processes of L4 and L5 in some individuals (Figs 1.12 and 1.13), contrary to the observations of Hanson and Sonesson (1994) that it only attaches to L5. The iliolumbar ligament has previously been described as developing out of the inferior border of the quadratus lumborum muscle in the second decade of life (Luk et al 1986). However, this has recently been refuted with the observation that the ligament is present in the fetus as early as 11–15 weeks gestational age (Uhthoff 1993), a finding that has been verified by Hanson and Sonesson (1994). The taut bands of the iliolumbar ligament form hoods over the L4 and L5 nerve roots. These hoods are

capable of compressing the associated nerve roots (Briggs & Chandraraj 1995). The iliolumbar ligament is subject to fatty degeneration after the first decade of life and has been reported to ossify on occasion (Lapadula et al 1991).

The major function of this ligament is to restrict motion at the lumbosacral junction, particularly that of side-bending (Chow et al 1989, Leong et al 1987, Yamamoto et al 1990). After bilateral transection of the iliolumbar ligament, rotation about the vertebral axis is increased by 18%, extension by 20%, flexion by 23%, and lateral bending by 29% (Yamamoto et al 1990). Thus the iliolumbar ligament represents a critical structure for stabilizing the lumbar vertebrae on the sacral base.

Articular capsule of the SIJ

At the caudal end of the lumbar ligaments lies the capsular structure surrounding the SIJ (Figs 1.13–1.15). This joint is synovial, having a C-shaped articular surface, with the longer limb of the joint oriented posteriorly and the shorter

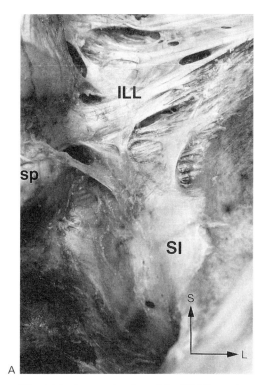
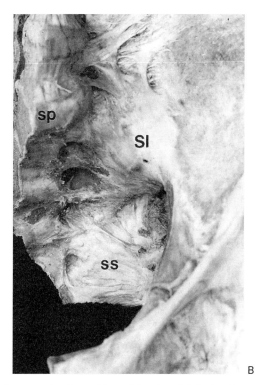

Fig. 1.14 An anterior view of the SIJ. These photographs were taken into a bisected female pelvic basin after removing all of the pelvic contents and endopelvic fascia. The photograph in Fig. 1.14A illustrates the superior portion of the SIJ (SI), demonstrating its smooth surface and its continuity with the iliolumbar ligament (ILL). Fig. 1.14B illustrates the inferior portion of the SIJ (SI), demonstrating its continuity with the sacrospinous ligament (SS). In both photographs, the sacral promontory (sp) is marked for reference. The orientation figure in the lower right of Fig. 1.14A indicates superior (S) and lateral (L) directions.

limb superiorly (Fig. 1.15). As such, the joint has a limited range of motion (Brunner et al 1991, Vleeming et al 1992). There is a renewed interest in understanding the structure (Bernard & Cassidy 1991) and biomechanics (Jacob & Kissling 1995, Kissling 1995) of this joint since it is now realized that dysfunction of this joint represents a major source of low back pain (Daum 1995, Fortin et al 1994a, 1994b; Vleeming et al 1995c, Schwarzer et al 1995). The joint surface is derived, in part, from the first three sacral vertebrae; its sacral surface is lined with hyaline cartilage and its ileal surface with fibrocartilage (Fig. 1.15). The joint is surrounded by a tough capsule presenting several remarkably different surfaces (Figs 1.13–1.15). The superior aspect of the joint capsule is a caudal extension of the iliolumbar ligament. The anterior aspect of this capsule is composed of a smooth sheet of dense connective tissue stretched between the ventral surface of the sacral alar and that of the ilium (Fig. 1.15). The caudal border of the anterior SI capsule blends with the rostral edge of the sacrospinous ligament. The posterior aspect of the joint capsule is much more complex than its anterior counterpart (see Fig. 1.13). It consists of numerous, discontinuous interwoven bands of dense connective tissue. The short interosseous SI ligaments arise on the intermediate and lateral sacral crest and attach to the rough sacropelvic surface of the ilium. The long interosseous SI ligaments extend from the median and lateral sacral crests, diagonally in a superior direction across the sacral gutter, and attach to the posterior superior spine of the ilium. Particularly prominent is the long dorsal SI ligament, which is a thickened band extending from the posterior superior iliac spine to the lower transverse tubercle on the lateral sacral crest (Fig. 1.16). Several

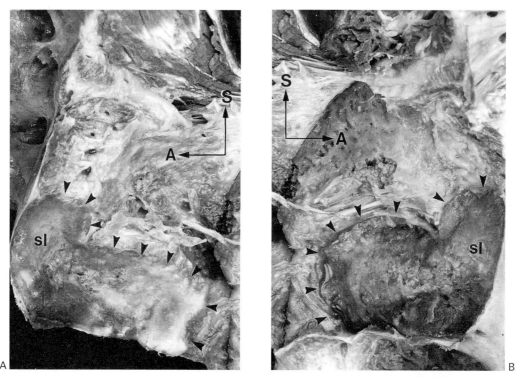

Fig. 1.15 The internal features of the SIJ. The female SIJ seen in Fig. 1.14 was opened to display its medial or sacral (A) and lateral or ilial (B) surfaces. The boundaries of the joint are marked with arrowheads in both photographs. The anterior boundary is formed by a precise capsule, the posterior boundary being formed by the interweaving of the interosseous ligaments. The joint has a superior limb (sl) and inferior limb. The orientation arrows in both photographs indicate the superior (S) and anterior (A) directions. The medial surface is concave and covered with hyaline cartilage with associated fatty deposits; the lateral surface is convex and covered with fibrocartilage.

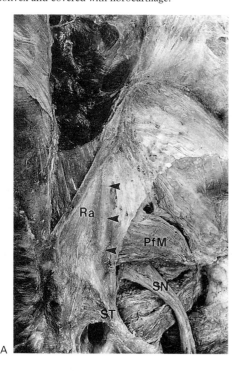

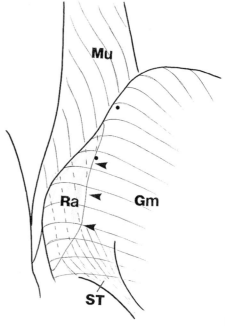

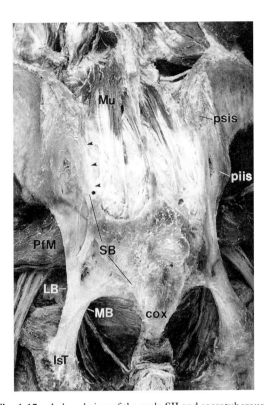

Fig. 1.17 A dorsal view of the male SIJ and sacrotuberous ligament. All but the deepest laminae of the multifidus muscle (Mu) have been removed. The sacrotuberous ligaments seen stretching from the ischial tuberosity (IsT) to the coccyx (cox) medially and the posterior iliac spines superolaterally. The posterior superior iliac spine (psis) and the posterior inferior iliac spine (piis) are marked on the contralateral side. The asterisk marks the transverse tuberosity of the lateral sacral crest and the arrowheads mark the course of the long posterior interosseous ligament under the lateral band of the sacrotuberous ligament. Three major bands of the ligament are seen: lateral (LB), medial (MB), and superior (SB). The lateral band spans the piriformis muscle (PfM) to reach the ilium inferior to the (piis). As the lateral band climbs toward the psis, it blends with the raphe (see Fig. 1.16). The medial band attaches to the coccyx, and the superior band courses superficial to the long dorsal SI ligament to connect the coccyx with the posterior ileal spines. Tendons of the multifidus pass between the superior band and the long dorsal SI ligament to insert into the body of the sacrotuberous ligament.

structures anchor into these tough ligaments of the SIJ. A portion of the sacrotuberous ligament attaches to the transverse crest of the sacrum where its fibers blend with the long dorsal SI ligaments of the joint capsule (Figs 1.17 and 1.18), and the thoracolumbar fascia anchors to these same interosseous ligaments from its medial side. This anchoring portion of the thoracolumbar fascia also forms a prominent raphe separating the multifidus and gluteus maximus muscle (see Fig. 1.20 below).

The articular surfaces of the SIJ are smooth and flattened at birth, and the long axis of the joint is oriented parallel to that of the lumbar spine (Bernard & Cassidy 1991). Remodeling of the joint into the adult, C-shaped orientation with roughened surface occurs through puberty. The ileal surface develops a crescent-shaped ridge along its long axis (see Fig. 1.15A above), while the sacral surface forms a concavity complementary to the convexity of the ileal surface in the second decade of life (see Fig. 1.15B above). These changes in the surface of the joint contribute to its stability and limited range of motion (Simonian et al 1994). The interlocking surfaces of the joint form the centerpiece in the self-bracing model of SIJ function (Snijders et al 1993, Vleeming et al 1995c). A series of age-related degenerative changes occur to the joint, especially after the fifth decade of life. In this age range, the cartilaginous surfaces of the joints begin to degenerate and ossification occurs between the two articular surfaces, especially in males (Bernard & Cassidy 1991). These changes eventually lead to further restricted motion of the joint.

Sacrotuberous ligament

The sacrotuberous ligament is a specialization derived from the posteroinferior aspect of the SIJ capsule. It is a triangular-shaped structure extending between the posterior iliac spines, the SIJ capsule, the coccygeal vertebrae, and the ischial tuberosity

Fig. 1.16 (*Facing page*) The posterior attachments of the SIJ. (A) This is a posterior view of the sacral region with the multifidus sheath open. Most of the multifidus muscle has been removed as has the entire gluteus maximus muscle. The raphe (Ra) overlaying the inferior end of the multifidus muscle is present. The posterior surface of the raphe is the attachment of the gluteus maximus muscle. A ridge in the raphe (arrowheads) indicates its attachment to the long posterior interosseous ligament of the SIJ. The inferior border of the raphe blends into the sacrotuberous ligament (ST). The piriformis muscle (PfM) and sciatic nerve (SN) are seen emerging from greater sciatic foramen under the raphe. (B) An illustration of the raphe (Ra) as it separates the multifidus (Mu) and gluteus maximus (Gm) muscles. The deep border of the raphe lies along the long posterior interosseous ligament (arrowheads). The posterior superior iliac spine and posterior inferior iliac spine are indicated by the black dots.

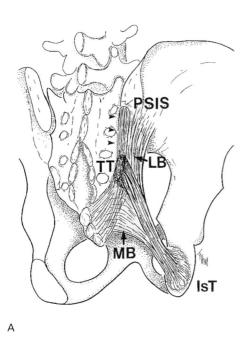

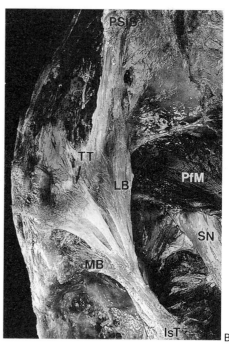

Fig. 1.18   The relationships of the sacrotuberous ligament with the SIJ. (A) This schematic diagram illustrates the three groups of bands forming the sacrotuberous ligament. The lateral band (LB) overlays the long posterior interosseous ligament (arrowheads) and reaches upward toward the posterior superior iliac spine. The firmest attachment of the lateral band is to the transverse tubercle (TT) of the lateral sacral crest. The medial band (MB) bends toward the coccygeal vertebra. Both of these bands arise on the ischial tuberosity (IsT). A superior band courses upward from the coccygeal attachments to blend with the lateral band over the long posterior interosseous ligament. (B) Photograph of the sacrotuberous ligament similar to that seen in (A). The piriformis muscle (PfM) and sciatic nerve (SN) are marked for reference.

(see Fig. 1.17). The tendon of the biceps femoris often reaches over the tuberosity to attach to the sacrotuberous ligament (Vleeming et al 1989a), and an occasional aberrant muscle derived from the biceps femoris establishes the attachment of its entire superior head to this ligament (Akita et al 1992). The tendons of the deepest laminae of the multifidus often extend into the sacrotuberous ligament from its superior surface (see Fig. 1.17 above). The sacrotuberous ligament can be divided into several large fibrous bands (Fig. 1.18). Its prominent lateral band reaches from the posterior inferior iliac spine to the ischial tuberosity, and its medial band connects the coccygeal vertebrae with the ischial tuberosity. The superior band is the thinnest and forms a plate stretching between the posterior iliac spines and the coccygeal vertebrae. Several central bands arise

from the lateral band and attach to the lower transverse tubercle of the lateral sacral crest. They share this attachment with the inferior border of the long dorsal SI ligament. Along its medial and superior borders, the sacrotuberous ligament merges with the interosseous ligaments of the SIJ capsule. The body of the sacrotuberous ligament is made up from the fusion of its multiple bands and is occasionally penetrated by branches from the inferior gluteal neurovascular bundle. This ligament is positioned to resist nutation of the sacrum and is opposed by the long dorsal SI ligament that is portioned to resist counternutation (Vleeming et al 1995a). Occasional ossification of the sacrotuberous ligament has been reported outside the more obvious cases of general ossification, such as occurs in diffuse idiopathic skeletal hyperostosis (Prescher & Bohndorf 1993).

Sacrospinous ligament

The sacrospinous ligament is a specialization of the anteroinferior aspect of the SIJ capsule. It is a triangular-shaped structure (see Fig. 1.14B above) arising from the lateral margin of the lower sacral and coccygeal vertebrae and the inferior aspect of the SIJ capsule. Its distal attachment is to the spine of the ischium. Proximally, its superior fibers blend with those of the SIJ capsule. Its anterior surface is closely related to the coccygeus muscle (Williams 1995). Although initially involved in movements of the tail in quadrupeds, this ligament has evolved into a support mechanism for the pelvic floor in humans (Abitbol 1988). As such, the ligament forms the posterolateral border of the pelvic outlet and has been used as an anchor into which the pelvic floor is secured in situations involving eversion of the vagina (Dofferhof & Vink 1985, Morley & DeLancey 1988, Nichols 1985, Porges & Smilen 1994).

SUMMARY OF THE LIGAMENTOUS STRUCTURES

The ligamentous structures of the lumbosacral connection form a continuous, dense connective tissue stocking that houses the lumbar vertebrae and sacrum and provides attachment sites for the associated muscles. This complicated ligamentous structure plays a key role in the self-bracing mechanism of the pelvis, a mechanism that functions to maintain the integrity of the low back and pelvis during the transfer of energy from the spine to the lower extremities (Vleeming et al 1989a, 1989b). Tension in the sacrotuberous and long dorsal SI ligaments varies with rocking movements of the sacrum in its joint capsule (Vleeming et al 1995a), and unilateral lesions of the SIJ capsule increase the range of motion (decrease the stability) of the joint under compressive loads (Simonian et al 1994). The ligamentous support mechanism of the lumbosacral region is influenced by several major muscle groups in the low back and pelvis; each of these groups will be discussed below.

MAJOR MUSCLE GROUPS ASSOCIATED WITH THE LUMBOSACRAL LIGAMENTOUS STRUCTURES

Multifidus muscle

The paravertebral muscles in the lumbar region are represented by three large muscles (Fig. 1.2), each in its own fascial compartment and arranged from lateral to medial: the iliocostalis, longissimus, and multifidus (Bogduk 1980). The lateral two muscles, iliocostalis and longissimus, arise from the iliac crest and thoracolumbar fascia, but, with the exception of a few medial slips from the longissimus, do not attach to the lumbar vertebrae. The multifidus is divided into five bands (Fig. 1.19), each band arising from the spine of a lumbar vertebrae and associated tissues (Macintosh et al 1986). Its distal attachments are the sacral crest, interosseous SI ligaments, thoracolumbar fascia,

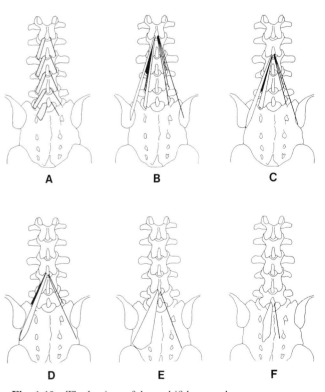

Fig. 1.19 The laminae of the multifidus muscle. (A) represents the shortest laminae of the multifidus muscle. (B–F) represent the five laminae of the multifidus muscle (B, L1; C, L2; D, L3; E, L4; F, L5). Each lamina arises from a lumbar spine and attachment to the sacrum. (Adapted from Macintosh et al 1986.)

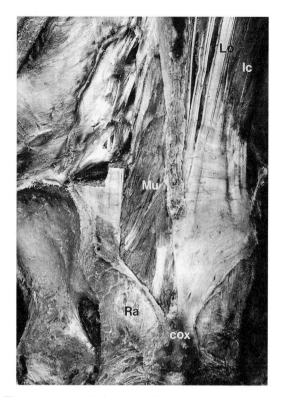

Fig. 1.20   A dorsal view of the SI region with the gluteus maximus muscle removed. The thoracolumbar fascia and the tendinous insertion of the iliocostalis (Ic) and longissimus (Lo) muscles have been opened to expose the multifidus muscle (Mu). The raphe (Ra) separating the multifidus and gluteus muscles is seen stretching from the coccyx (cox) to the posterior superior ileal spine (asterisk). Its anterior border is blended with the SIJ capsule and its posterior border with the thoracolumbar fascia. The rough surface visible on this raphe represents the attachment site for the gluteal muscle.

and extreme medial edge of the iliac crest. The attachment of the muscles to the thoracolumbar fascia represents a raphe separating the multifidus from the gluteus maximus muscle (Fig. 1.16 and Fig. 1.20 above). The anterior border of the raphe is anchored in the SIJ capsule, and the posterior border of the raphe becomes part of the thoracolumbar fascia. Finally, tendinous slips of the multifidus muscle pass under the long dorsal SI ligament to join with the sacrotuberous ligament (see Fig. 1.17 above). These connections integrate the multifidus into the ligamentous support system of the SIJ.

The fibers of the multifidus are aligned in the vertical plane with only very slight horizontal deviations. This arrangement is superior for move-ment in the sagittal plane, making the multifidus a significant extensor muscle, along with the erector spinae muscles, for the lumbar spine (Bogduk et al 1992, Macintosh & Bogduk 1986). However, owing to its geometry, only slight movements in the horizontal plane can be accomplished by this muscle. The long fibers in the body of the muscle span multiple segments, thus giving the multifidus muscle the additional role of a prime stabilizer of the lumbar spine (Crisco & Panjabi 1991, Macintosh & Bogduk 1986). Finally, by increasing tension on the thoracolumbar fascia, SI ligaments and sacrotuberous ligaments, activation of the multifidus also contributes to the self-bracing mechanism of the pelvis and to the transfer of energy from the upper body to the lower extremities.

Alteration in the structure of the multifidus muscle occurs either with aging or in association with pathologic processes. Size changes have been reported for the multifidus muscle in idiopathic scoliosis, the side of the lumbar spinal convexity being reduced in cross-sectional area on imaging (Kennelly & Stokes 1993). In addition, structural changes in the muscle histochemistry, the muscle fiber type, and the myotendenous junction have been reported for the multifidus on the concave side of the lumbar scoliotic curve (Khosla et al 1980). Lumbar disc herniation is also associated with histochemical changes in the multifidus muscle consistent with atrophy and fibrosis (Lehto et al 1989, Mattila et al 1986). Finally, there is with aging a pronounced fatty metaplasia in the muscle, this event being exacerbated in neuromuscular diseases involving the multifidus (Hadar et al 1983). Reduced size of the muscle and increased fatty deposits typified a population of low back pain patients when compared with a population of healthy volunteers (Parkkola et al 1993).

Latissimus dorsi muscle

The upper extremity is anchored to the body through an anterior muscular hood, the pectoralis muscles, and a posterior muscular hood, the latissimus dorsi. This latter muscle has its axial attachment to the thoracolumbar fascia (Fig. 1.21), the iliac crest, and to the caudal three or four ribs. Its appendicular attachment is to the intertubercular groove of the humerus. This arrangement allows the activation of the latissimus dorsi, expressed through the thoracolumbar fascia, to influence the supraspinous and interspinous ligaments, and the spines in the lumbar region (see Fig. 1.7 above). It is through the actions of this muscle, expressed via the thoracolumbar fascia, that the upper extremity can assist the lower extremity during locomotion.

Gluteus maximus muscle

The gluteus maximus is the largest muscle of the body. It is attached to the posterior surface of the iliac blade and crest, the thoracolumbar fascia (Fig. 1.21) and its associated raphe (which also functions as an attachment for the multifidus), the sacrotuberous ligament, and the lateral crest of the sacrum and coccygeal vertebrae. Its appendicular attachment involves the iliotibial band and the gluteal tuberosity of the femur. This muscle, through its attachment to the raphe of the thoracolumbar fascia, is also opposed to the ipsilateral multifidus muscle and coupled to the contralateral latissimus dorsi muscle (Vleeming et al 1995b). Thus, through its attachments to the ligaments and fascia of the SIJ, the gluteus maximus muscle can become a contributing force to the self-bracing mechanism of the pelvis (Snijders et al 1993).

Biceps femoris muscle (long head)

In many individuals, the long head of the biceps femoris muscle reaches over the posterior surface of the ischial tuberosity to attach to the sacrotuberous ligament (Vleeming et al 1989a). Its inferior attachment is to the lateral aspect of the fibular head, to the lateral condyle of the tibia, and to a sheet of fascia covering the lateral aspect of the leg. Thus, this muscle represents a continuum from the SI ligaments to the fibula and investing fascia of the leg. Contraction of the biceps femoris, along with extending the thigh, will pull the sacrum against the ilium, compressing the SIJ. As such, it contributes to the self-bracing mechanism in the pelvis and assists in stabilizing the SIJ during the force transfer from spine to lower extremity (Vleeming et al 1989a).

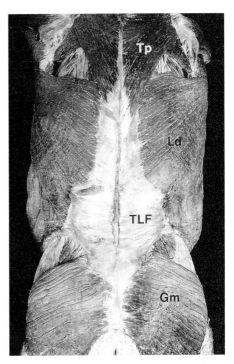

Fig. 1.21   A posterior view of the thoracolumbar fascia in a male cadaver. The superficial fat and fascia have been removed to demonstrate the diamond shape of the thoracolumbar fascia (TLF). A small window is present in the fascial sheath on the left of the photograph, revealing the paravertebral muscles underneath. Large muscles of the upper extremity (trapezius, Tp; Latissimus dorsi, Ld) and lower extremity (gluteus maximus, Gm) attach along the borders of the thoracolumbar fascia. The iliac crest and gluteus medius muscle can be seen emerging from under the superolateral border of the gluteus maximus.

Piriformis muscle

Inside the pelvic basin, another extremity muscle, the piriformis, influences the integrity of the SIJ. Proximally, the piriformis muscle attaches to the sacrum, the sacrotuberous ligament, the margin of the greater sciatic foramen, and the medial edge of the SIJ capsule. Distally, the muscle reaches out through the greater sciatic foramen to attach to the greater trochanter of the femur. Contraction of the piriformis, besides laterally rotating the thigh and stabilizing the head of the femur in the acetabulum, also places tension on the SIJ capsule, pulling the sacrum against the ilium and thereby contributing to the self-bracing mechanism (Vleeming et al 1989a).

Summary of the muscular and ligamentous structures

The ligamentous stocking of the lumbar spine and the SIJ capsule fuse to the anterior surface of the thoracolumbar fascia. This large sheet of fascia and these lumbosacral ligaments serve as attachment sites for the major prime movers and stabilizing muscles of the spine. Activation of these muscles helps to tighten the connective tissue support structures, stabilizing the lumbosacral spine, and thereby contributing to a mechanism that has been referred to as self-bracing (Snijders et al 1993). In addition, large muscles of the extremities such as the latissimus dorsi and the gluteus maximus attach to the borders of the thoracolumbar fascia, and the cross-hatched structural organization of the multilayer, collagenous fiber bundles in this facial sheet are ideally arranged to resist tension from several directions (Bednar et al 1995, Bogduk & Macintosh 1984). This arrangement of muscles and fascia facilitates the transfer of energy, generated by movement of the upper extremities, through the spine and into the lower extremities. The close coupling of these extremity and back muscles through the thoracolumbar fascia and its attachments to the ligamentous stocking of the spine, allow the motion in the upper limbs to assist in rotation of the trunk and movement of the lower extremities in gait, creating an integrated system (Vleeming et al 1995b).

INNERVATION OF THE LUMBOSACRAL REGION

The ligaments of the lumbosacral region are innervated predominantly with small-caliber primary afferent fibers and sympathetic efferent fibers, carried by branches of the dorsal rami of lumbar and sacral spinal nerve roots. The primary afferent fibers are typical of those involved with the detection of nociception and the initiation of inflammatory processes; they have been termed primary afferent nociceptors (Levine et al 1993). Thus the nerve supply to the lumbosacral ligaments plays a key role in the integrity of this region. There are three separate sources of innervation to the tissue of the lumbosacral region:

the dorsal rami of the spinal nerves, the sinu vertebral nerve (or recurrent meningeal nerve), and the somatosympathetic nerves (Bogduk 1983, Groen et al 1990, Imai et al 1995, Jinkins et al 1989, Stilwell 1956). Each nerve supply covers a different area of tissue and, based on its distribution, creates a different pattern of pain perception when irritated.

Spinal nerve roots and spinal nerves

The lumbosacral spinal cord gives rise to numerous small nerve rootlets from its dorsolateral and ventrolateral borders. In the subarachnoid space of the vertebral canal, between five and seven dorsal rootlets from each lumbar segment bundle together to form a dorsal spinal nerve root, which joins with a similarly derived ventral spinal nerve root (de Peretti et al 1989). These nerve roots descend in the vertebral canal, exiting at each intervertebral foramen. At the level of the foramen, a complex relationship occurs. The nerve roots enter a funnel-shaped lateral recess of the spinal canal that narrows to form the lumbar nerve root canal (Firooznia et al 1993). The distal end of the root canal is the intervertebral foramen. The walls of the nerve root canal are composed of the pedicle and pars interarticularis of the vertebra, the ligamentum flavum, and the lateral aspect of the intervertebral disc (Bose & Balasubramanian 1984). From L1 to S1, the obliquity of the canals and their length increase (Bose & Balasubramanian 1984). As the nerve root enters this canal, it is enveloped by a sheath of spinal dura termed the epineurium. In the canal, the nerve root is deflected laterally around the pedicle and over the surface of the intervertebral disc. In the foramen, the dorsal root has its ganglion of primary afferent cell bodies and subsequently fuses with the ventral root to form the spinal nerve. In the lumbar region, as the spinal nerves leave their canals, they are attached to the foramen by several fibrous expansions of the canal wall (de Peretti et al 1989). As the nerve root traverses the canal and foramen, it is at risk from several structures: the pedicles and intervertebral discs (Hasegawa et al 1995, Hasue et al 1983), the ligamentum flavum (Yoshida et al 1992), the capsule of the facet joint (Kirkaldy-Willis 1984), and the foramenal ligaments (Golub & Silverman 1969, Nowicki & Haughton 1992).

In addition, the canal transmits branches of the spinal artery to the vertebral canal, veins draining the epidural plexus and associated lymphatic vessels (Garfin et al 1995, Nohara et al 1991, Olmarker et al 1989, Rydevik 1992, Rydevik et al 1984, Sato et al 1994). Venous congestion, arteriovenous malformation, and epidural hematoma have all been demonstrated to mimic disc herniation or lumbar spinal stenosis (Hanley et al 1994, Parke 1991). Whether by mechanical compression or fluid congestion, the traumatized lumbosacral nerve roots experience edema and ischemia (Garfin et al 1995, Olmarker et al 1989, Rydevik 1992, Rydevik et al 1984, Sato et al 1994), which lead to inflammatory and fibrotic alterations in the neural tissue with concomitant loss of motor function, paresthesia, and hypesthesia (Garfin et al 1995, Olmarker & Rydevik 1991, Rydevik 1992, Rydevik et al 1984).

Finally, an additional non-mechanical method for irritating neural tissue in the foraminal area appears to involve the release of fluids containing such proinflammatory compounds as the proteoglycans from the nucleus pulposus (Olmarker et al 1993, 1995).

Lumbosacral dorsal rami

The dorsal ramus leaves the spinal nerve as the nerves exits the lumbar intervertebral canals. As it wraps around the facet joint directly below, it divides into several main branches: the lateral branch, which innervates the lateral fascial compartment containing the iliocostalis muscle; the intermediate branch, which innervates the intermediate fascial compartment containing the longissimus muscle; and several medial branches, which innervate the medial fascial compartment containing the multifidus muscle, as well as the ligaments and intrinsic muscles of the lumbar and sacral vertebrae (Fig. 1.22) (Bogduk 1983). Specifically, the medial compartment contains the multifidus, interspinalis, and intertransversarii medialis muscles; it also contains skeletal elements such as the interspinous ligament, the facet joints, and the ligament flavum. Inferiorly, the dorsal and ventral rami of L5 and of the sacral roots provide innervation of the SIJ capsule

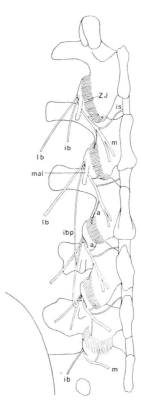

Fig. 1.22   A dorsal view of the lumbar spine illustrating the three major branches of the dorsal ramus. a, articular twigs from medial branch; ib, intermediate branch; ibp, intermediate branch plexus; is, interspinous twig from medial branch; lb, lateral branch; m, medial branch; mal, mamillio-accessory ligament; ZJ, zygoapophyseal joint. (Reproduced from Bogduk 1983.)

(Ikeda 1991). More recent study has confirmed the innervation of the joint from dorsal rami, but not from branches of the ventral rami (Grob et al 1995; see also Chapter 12). Irritation of the small-caliber, primary afferent fibers of the dorsal ramus innervating these tissue results in the perception of pain. This perception is usually a sharp, burning pain, similar to spinal root pain, and can refer to the area supplied by the corresponding ventral ramus, thus mimicking sciatica. Since the dorsal ramus also innervates muscle groups in the back, compression or damage to this nerve can present with signs of denervation weakness, as well as with pain.

Sinu vertebral or recurrent meningeal nerves

Distal to the dorsal root ganglion, but prior to the

division into dorsal and ventral rami, the spinal nerve gives off a small branch that curves back into the intervertebral foramen to reach the vertebral canal (Pedersen et al 1956b) (Fig. 1.23). This

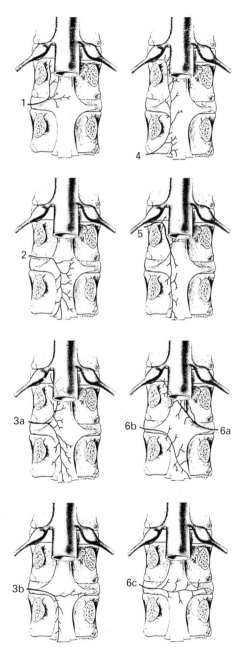

Fig. 1.23 The sinu vertebral nerve. The eight diagrams represent variations in the distribution of the sinu vertebral nerve. See text for discussion. (Reproduced from Groen et al 1990.)

small branch is termed the sinu vertebral or recurrent meningeal nerve. The terminal branches of this nerve service the posterior longitudinal ligament, the periosteum on the posterior aspect of the vertebral body, the outer layers of the intervertebral discs, and the anterior surface of the spinal dura (Bogduk 1983, Groen et al 1990, Pedersen et al 1956a, Stilwell 1956). In an elegant study of the sinu vertebral nerve, Groen et al (1990) have demonstrated that this nerve can travel up and/or down the vertebral canal at least two or three segments from the point of entry (Fig. 1.23, parts 1–5). In addition, it can cross the midline to innervate tissue on the contralateral side (Fig. 1.23, parts 6a–c). Notably, some sinu vertebral fibers cross the vertebral canal and subsequently pass outward through the contralateral intervertebral foramina (Fig. 1.23, part 6c).

Based on this pattern of innervation, irritation of the small-caliber, primary afferent fibers in the sinu vertebral nerve can refer pain several segments up or down the spinal cord, as well as referring pain to the contralateral side of the body. In addition, very slight movements of any obstacle in the vertebral canal or intervertebral foramina could irritate sinu vertebral fibers from either or both of the left or right sides of the body. This arrangement also offers a possible explanation for the shifting of pain presentation patterns from side to side in a given patient. Finally, the sinu vertebral nerve does not supply any skeletal muscle, so compression or other damage to this nerve alone does not present with the signs of denervation weakness.

Somatosympathetic nerves

There are no somatic nerves (direct branches of the dorsal or ventral rami or spinal nerves) that reach the anterior aspect of the vertebral bodies. However, this area is serviced by sensory fibers traveling in branches of the sympathetic trunk (Bogduk 1983, Groen et al 1990, Jinkins 1993, Stilwell 1956). These small-caliber, primary afferent fibers wrap around the anterior longitudinal ligament and the periosteum on the anterior aspect of the vertebral body, and reach into the outer layers of the intervertebral discs (Fig. 1.24). To return to the spinal cord, these sensory fibers follow the sympathetic trunk. They appear primarily

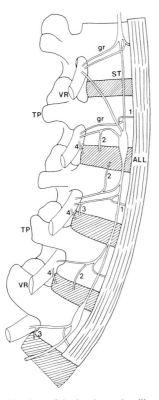

Fig. 1.24 A side view of the lumbar spine illustrating the somatosympathetic nerves. The sympathetic trunk communicates with the ventral ramus (VR) through grey rami (gr). Small branches (1) from the sympathetic trunk provide sympathetic efferent and primary afferent fibers to the anterior longitudinal ligament (ALL). Small branches (2 and 3) from the grey rami and ventral ramus (4) reach the intervertebral disc. TP, transverse process. (Reproduced from Bogduk 1983.)

diffuse, dense, boring pain that refers to the zones of Head in the thoracolumbar region (Jinkins et al 1989). In a population chosen because they were experiencing pain, individuals with vertebral lesions involving the anterior territory (anterior longitudinal ligament) generally described the pain as deep, dense, and hard to localize. The referral zones involved upper lumbar segments along the flank of the body extending downward onto the thigh. This pattern was present even in individuals with anterior disc lesions as low as L5. The somatosympathetic pattern of pain was in contrast to that in patients suffering pain and having posterior lesions that irritated axons in the sinu vertebral nerve or dorsal ramus. The pain pattern in these latter patients was better related to the segment of injury and was of a sharp or burning quality. As with the sinu vertebral nerve, the somatosympathetic axons do not supply any skeletal muscle, so damage to these nerves alone will not present with signs of denervation weakness.

INNERVATION OF SPECIFIC LUMBOSACRAL STRUCTURES

The general innervation patterns described in the previous section demonstrate that most structures in the lumbosacral region receive a generous nerve supply. However, a critical question involves the exact types of axons and terminals found in specific connective tissues. The types of nerve fiber present will influence the function of the tissue as well as its susceptibility to neurogenic inflammatory processes (Basbaum & Levine 1991, Levine et al 1993, Schaible & Grubb 1993). There are three general innervation types for tissue other than skeletal muscle: large, myelinated sensory axons with encapsulated endings involved with discriminative touch and proprioception; small, lightly myelinated or unmyelinated sensory axons with naked nerve endings involved in nociception; and small, lightly myelinated efferent axons involved in the autonomic nervous system. Of the latter two types of axon, the small primary afferent axons often contain neuropeptides such as substance P, calcitonin gene-related polypeptide, or somatostatin. Axons associated with the autonomic nervous system often contain norepinephrine (which can be indicated by the

to use white rami when gaining access to the spinal nerve and dorsal root ganglia. Therefore the sensory fibers pass superiorly in the sympathetic trunk to reach the lowest white rami located at the thoracolumbar junction (Jinkins et al 1989). Thus, noxious stimuli in the lower lumbar and sacral levels will ascend in the sympathetic trunk, presenting to the spinal cord at the thoracolumbar junction (the region of the lowest white rami). This circuitous route results in referral of pain and subsequent facilitation of spinal segments in the lower thoracic and upper lumbar region from dysfunction of lumbosacral and pelvic structures.

Noxious stimuli activating somatosympathetic fibers result in what has been described as a presence of tyrosine hydroxylase) and neuropeptide Y. Both small, primary afferent fibers and sympathetic efferent fibers play critical roles in the induction and maintenance of neurogenic inflammatory processes (Basbaum & Levine 1991, Levine et al 1993).

Neural arch ligaments

The use of immunohistochemical procedures to label and identify axons found in connective tissue has allowed the characterization of the innervation of neural arch ligaments. These ligaments are serviced by the medial branch of the dorsal ramus. Small-caliber axons from this nerve have been detected in the supraspinous ligament and interspinous ligament (Jiang et al 1995, Rhalmi et al 1993), and ligamentum flavum (Rhalmi et al 1993), these fibers being identified with an antibody for neurofilament protein, which is a nonspecific marker for the neural process. In addition, similar fibers have also been found in the thoracolumbar fascia (Rhalmi et al 1993, Yahia et al 1992). Frequently, the small axons were seen to leave the areas of the blood vessels and course through the matrix of the surrounding connective tissue. Small-caliber fibers containing substance P, suggesting a role in nociception, have been demonstrated in the supraspinous ligament (El-Bohy et al 1988). Larger-caliber fibers in the supraspinous and interspinous ligaments, reactive for neurofilament protein, were seen associated with Pacinian and Ruffini endings (Jiang et al 1995), suggesting a role in proprioception. In addition, fibers positive for tyrosine hydroxylase and neuropeptide Y, suggesting that they are sympathetic efferent axons, have been described in the interspinous ligaments (Ahmed et al 1993a). Electrophysiologic recordings from neural processes in the supraspinous and interspinous ligaments and in the ligamentum flavum have been described (Yamashita et al 1990), and, based on their activation thresholds and conduction velocities, both proprioceptive and nociceptive axons were present. These results collectively demonstrate the presence of both primary afferent proprioceptors and nociceptors and efferent sympathetic axons in the neural arch ligaments of the lumbar spine.

Articular capsule ligaments

The facet joint is innervated by branches from the medial divisions of the dorsal rami above and below the joint (Bogduk & Long 1979). This observation suggests that inflammatory or degenerative diseases of any facet joint will activate multiple segments in the spinal cord. Neurophysiologic studies of the lumbar facet joints of rabbits have demonstrated the presence of both high-threshold, slow-conducting fibers and low-threshold, fast-conducting fibers (Avramov et al 1992, Yamashita et al 1990). The former represent potential nociceptive axons, and the latter are potential proprioceptive axons. Electrophysiologic recordings of primary afferent fibers from joints under varying loads also demonstrate the presence of proprioceptive and nociceptive components (Avramov et al 1992). Encapsulated nerve endings, suggestive of proprioceptors, have been observed histologically in facet joint capsules (Jackson et al 1966). The presence of small-caliber, primary afferent fibers containing sensory neuropeptides, such as substance P and calcitonin gene-related polypeptide, in the joint capsule and synovial plica has also been confirmed in several anatomical studies (Ahmed et al 1993b, Beaman et al 1993, El-Bohy et al 1988). Many of these primary afferent fibers are present in the connective tissue of the joint capsule, separate from the vasculature (Ahmed et al 1993b). In addition, fibers containing tyrosine hydroxylase and neuropeptide Y – markers for sympathetic axons – have been reported in the joint capsule; however, these axons remain close to the vasculature (Ahmed et al 1993b). Facet joints contain proinflammatory cells such as monocytes and reactive fibroblasts (cells positive for CD11 antigens) (Konttinen et al 1990b). When an inflammatory substance, such as carrageenan, is injected into these joints, it produces sensitized primary afferent fibers (increased firing rates) and recruits 'silent nociceptors', the smallest of the primary afferent fibers and those typically associated with pain (Ozaktay et al 1994). The presence of small-caliber, primary afferent fibers in the capsule of the facet joints, responding to inflammatory challenge, supports the contention that dysfunction of these joints is a source of low back pain (Bernard & Kirkaldy-Willis 1987, Carette et al 1991, Mooney & Robertson 1976). This is consistent with the relief of pain experienced by some patients following anesthetization of the lumbar facet joints (Schwarzer et al 1994).

The bone and articular cartilage of normal human facet joints contains small-caliber fibers, positive for the neuropeptide substance P, but these have been shown to be present only in very low numbers (Beaman et al 1993). However, neuropeptide-containing axons were present in increased quantity in specimens that were undergoing degenerative diseases involving the facet joints. These fibers were found in erosion channels accompanying the vasculature deep into the bone underlying the articular surface. These observations suggest that normal facet joints may be refractive to pain owing to a limited supply of small-caliber fibers under pressure-bearing surfaces, and that degenerative joints become painful owing to the increase in nociceptive fibers associated with pressure-bearing surfaces.

Vertebral body ligaments and intervertebral discs

An extensive nerve plexus is present in the posterior and anterior longitudinal ligaments of the lumbar region (Bogduk 1983, Cavanaugh et al 1995, Groen et al 1988, 1990, Imai et al 1995, Jackson et al 1966, Kojima et al 1990a, 1990b, Korkala et al 1985, Pedersen et al 1956b, Pionchon et al 1986, Stilwell 1956, von During et al 1995). Despite the density of small-caliber fibers present along these ligaments, very few large fibers with encapsulate endings have been demonstrated to date (Cavanaugh et al 1995, Jackson et al 1966). Small primary afferent axons, containing neuropeptides, have been identified in the posterior longitudinal ligament and the peripheral portion of the annulus fibrosus (Imai et al 1995, Konttinen et al 1990a, Korkala et al 1985). Since many of these axons travel in the sinu vertebral nerve, these observations support the theory that this nerve is capable of nociception (Korkala et al 1985). Axons positive for tyrosine hydroxylase and neuropeptide Y – suggesting that they are sympathetic efferent axons – have also been detected in the posterior longitudinal ligament (Imai et al 1995), the ventral dura, the periosteum

of the vertebral body, the intervertebral disc, and the vertebral body, where they reach into the marrow cavities (Ahmed et al 1993a).

Imai et al (1995) have described a dual plexus of fibers in the rat posterior longitudinal ligament. The superficial plexus ascends and descends along the margins of the ligament while the deep plexus is present only over the intervertebral segments of the ligament and reaches inward to serve the outer layers of the annulus fibrosus. Axons containing calcitonin gene-related polypeptide, suggesting nociceptive sensory functions, are present in both plexuses, whereas axons containing tyrosine hydroxylase, suggesting sympathetic activity, were present only in the superficial plexus.

Based on the density of small-caliber fiber (nociceptive) innervation for the longitudinal ligaments, one would expect that the commonly observed large disc and osteophyte distortions present in these ligaments would be painful. This is, however, not often the case, since these large protrusions are frequently 'clinically silent' when detected in imaging studies. An explanation of this conundrum may lie in the possibility that the degree of pain perceived from injury of the spinal ligaments is related to the speed of the injury and not to its extent; thus a slow-growing distortion could give the neural plexus ample time to accommodate and not trigger afferent barrages on nociceptive afferent fibers. Support for this concept comes from the observation that the degree of nerve injury in experimental compression neuropathies is proportional to the speed of onset of the compressive force (Olmarker et al 1990).

The intervertebral discs are innervated by fibers from an elaborate plexus composed of the sinu vertebral nerve posteriorly and the somatosympathetic nerve anterolaterally (Bogduk 1983, Bogduk et al 1981, Groen et al 1990, Jinkins et al 1989, Stilwell 1956). Branches from this plexus penetrate the disc through the outer one-third of the annulus fibrosus. These branches are primarily composed of small-caliber fibers having unencapsulated endings (Jackson et al 1966). Many of these fibers contain neuropeptides such as substance P and calcitonin gene-related polypeptide, as demonstrated through immunohistochemical staining of discal tissue from rats (Ahmed et al

1993a, von During et al 1995), rabbits (Cavanaugh et al 1995), and humans (Konttinen et al 1990a). There is no evidence of any of these fibers innervating the nucleus pulposus in the central portion of the disc. The recent findings demonstrating neuropeptides in the outer one-third of the annulus support a sensory role for the sinu vertebral–somatosympathetic plexus present in the periosteum and ligaments surrounding the vertebral column. This raises the problem of why discography is generally a non-painful procedure in normal individuals but a painful one in patients with degenerative discs. It is possible that this is due to the distance separating the nuclear material in the normal individual from the nerve endings in the outer portion of the disc. However, an additional consideration could be that most of the disc fibers are 'silent nociceptors', that is, they are normally unexcitable even by some noxious stimuli. If provoked by prolonged exposure to proinflammatory chemical insult, they can become active and have a threshold of activation well within the range of non-noxious stimuli. This concept is supported by the observation that autologous material from the nucleus pulposus is proinflammatory and an irritant to nerve endings (McCarron et al 1987, Olmarker et al 1993, 1995, Saal 1995, Saal et al 1990). Thus discographic materials delivered to the center of a normal disc for a temporary period of time would not be expected to activate the normally quite silent nociceptors. The same material delivered to a degenerative disc may be reaching and activating previously sensitized primary afferent nociceptors.

Sacral region ligaments

The SIJ has only recently become a focus of attention in low back pain studies, and very few studies have examined its innervation. Ikeda reports that the anterior superior aspect of the joint receives twigs from spinal nerve L5, and the inferior anterior aspect of the joint is supplied by sacral spinal nerve S2 and other sacral nerves (Ikeda 1991). The posterior superior aspect of the joint is supplied by lateral branches from the 5th lumbar dorsal ramus and the inferior posterior aspect from a plexus of lateral branches from the sacral dorsal rami. In a similar study, Grob et al (1995) identified fine branches from the dorsal rami S1–S4 servicing the joint, but were unable to confirm any innervation from the ventral rami. Thick myelinated fibers, thin lightly myelinated fibers, and unmyelinated fibers are all present in the SI branches (Grob et al 1995). These nerves reach the joint capsule and invade the surrounding ligaments. Axons in the nerves to the SIJ were approximately 0.2–2.5 µm in diameter, placing them well within the range of the group IV (C-fibers) and possibly within the smaller end of the group III (A-delta) fiber range (Ikeda 1991). Axons of this size are associated with nociception and could be involved in the perception of pain from the SIJ. The role of the SIJ in the generation of chronic low back pain has previously been described (Beal 1982) and has received recent renewed attention (Schwarzer et al 1995; see also Chapter 12). The finding of small-caliber, primary afferent fibers in the joint capsule provides further support for this concept.

NEUROGENIC INFLAMMATION

The recent studies of the lumbosacral ligamentous structure using immunohistochemical techniques have provided evidence that many regions of this structure, if not the entire connective tissue stocking, receive a small-caliber, primary afferent fiber innervation. Not only are these sensory neurons organized to supply the spinal cord with nociceptive stimuli, but they are also typical of the B-afferent neural system (Prechtl & Powley 1990), that is, many of them are capable of secreting proinflammatory neuropeptides from their distal processes. Irritation of these primary afferent nociceptor fibers and the subsequent release of such peptides as substance P and calcitonin gene-related polypeptide can result in the degranulation of mast cells and the release of histamine (Fig. 1.25). This biogenic amine promotes vasodilation, leukocyte recruitment, and proliferation, and can further irritate primary afferent fibers, initiating the release of more substance P (Basbaum & Levine 1991). In addition, substance P stimulates macrophages and monocytes to increase phagocytosis, to release proinflammatory compounds such as thromboxane and hydrogen peroxide, and to increase the production

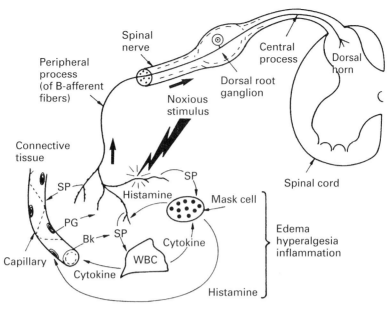

Fig. 1.25   The cascade effect of a neurogenic inflammation. The diagram illustrates a primary afferent nociceptor, its central termination in the dorsal horn of the spinal cord and its peripheral termination near a blood vessel in the local tissue. A noxious stimulus has irritated the terminal end of the primary afferent, causing it to depolarize. Action potentials are being sent to the central nervous system and neuropeptides (such as substance P, SP) are being released into the tissue surrounding the terminal. In response to the neuropeptides, mast cells degranulate, releasing histamine, and in response to this neuropeptide and histamine cocktail, blood vessels dilate, extravasating fluid and initiating edema and swelling. Prostaglandins (PG) and bradykinin (Bk) are released into the tissue. This chemical cocktail is chemoattractant for white blood cells, which then release cytokines (such as interleukins-1 and 6), furthering the inflammatory process. The chemical soup so created is irritating to the primary afferent nociceptor, thereby propagating the neurogenic inflammation. (Adapted from Willard 1995.)

of cytokines such as interleukin-1 (Payan 1989, 1992). Thus a vicious cycle of events is begun, the final product of this sequence being tissue inflammation and edema (Willard 1995). This cascade of events, involving neural-immune interactions, typifies the neurogenic inflammatory process (Levine et al 1993, Payan 1992). Interestingly, inflammatory cells are present in the synovial plica of lumbar facet joints (Konttinen et al 1990b) and in the nucleus pulposus of herniated disc material (Gronblad et al 1994). In addition, the proteoglycan rich fluid in the nucleus pulposus is inflammatory to non-disc tissue (Olmarker et al 1995). Thus the elements are present in the lumbosacral musculoskeletal system to facilitate chronic inflammatory processes (Weinstein 1991), leading to tissue degeneration and chronic pain syndromes.

Several recent observations suggest that the population of sensory neurons innervating connective tissue is dynamic and can respond to changing states of the tissue. The thoracolumbar fascia in non-back pain patients has both fibers with small, naked nerve endings and larger fibers with encapsulated endings (Pedersen et al 1956a, Yahia et al 1992), whereas patients who required surgery for treatment of low back pain were missing the myelinated fibers and encapsulated endings in the thoracolumbar fascia (Bednar et al 1995). Small, unmyelinated fibers with naked endings remained detectable in the fascia of the surgical cohort. From this study, it is impossible to say which happened first, the initiation of low back pain or the shift in sensory fiber population. However, studies of normal tissue that has been deafferented suggest that the loss of sensory innervation destabilizes the tissue, predisposing it to other damage such as degenerative disease processes (O'Connor et al 1985).

In addition to the primary afferent fibers, sympathetic efferent axons have been detected in much of the connective tissue of the lumbosacral spine. A balanced interaction between these two neural systems is thought to be important for the maintenance of normal tissue texture and the normal trafficking of cells through the extracellular matrix of the tissue (Holzer 1988, Kidd et al 1992, Levine et al 1990). Abnormal activity in either or both of these systems, increasing the output of neuropeptides and catecholamines, has been associated with increased susceptibility to degenerative connective tissue diseases (Basbaum & Levine 1991, Garrett et al 1992, Kidd et al 1989, 1990, 1992, Lam & Ferrell 1991, Levine et al 1985a, 1985b, 1993). Thus the activity of the primary afferent nociceptors and sympathetic efferent fiber systems represents an important consideration in maintenance of the integrity of the lumbosacral ligamentous structures. Finally, evidence has accumulated suggesting that sympathetic fibers can activate, either directly or indirectly, sensitized primary afferent fibers (Roberts & Kramis 1990). These findings raise the possibility that the sympathetic efferent fiber is involved in either the genesis and/or the maintenance of chronic pain states in connective tissue of the lumbosacral spine.

CONCLUSIONS

1. This chapter has examined the anatomy and innervation of the ligamentous stocking that forms the lumbosacral connection. Although there are numerous regional ligaments in this stocking, I have emphasized their continuity with each other, thereby giving the structure a unitary function.

2. The ligamentous stocking supports the osseous elements of the lumbosacral spine. In turn, this stocking is anchored to the thoracolumbar fascia of the back. This large sheet of aponeurotic fascia serves as an attachment site for the major muscle groups of the spine, the abdomen, and the upper and lower extremities. Through these connections, the thoracolumbar fascia can assist

in the transfer of energy from the upper to the lower body, minimizing stress on the lumbosacral spine. It can also facilitate the upper body's ability to assist in lower body motion, forming the integrated system described by Vleeming et al (1995b).

3. Not surprisingly, the thoracolumbar fascia has been demonstrated to contain both a small-caliber fiber system, typical of nociceptors and sympathetic axons, and a large-caliber fiber system with encapsulated endings typical of mechanoreception and proprioception. Thus the force transformation occurring through the thoracolumbar fascia may be under proprioceptive control by neural elements in this tissue.

4. It has also been demonstrated that most of the component tissues in the ligamentous stocking of the lumbosacral spine receive a primary afferent nociceptor and sympathetic efferent axon supply.

5. There are at least three separate sources of the small-caliber, primary afferent fibers in the lumbosacral region. Each fiber source has a differential distribution within the tissues of the back. Thus several different pain presentation patterns in the low back are established.

6. A possible interactive role of these neural elements in the normal trophic activity of the tissue has also been proposed. Besides their role in the maintenance of normal tissue, it is clear that these neural systems are also instrumental in orchestrating neurogenic inflammatory processes when they become irritated and sensitized.

7. Thus the tissues of the lumbosacral connection receive a nerve supply that is capable of sustaining a prolonged inflammatory response, contributing to the progressive breakdown of function in the back and the initiation of chronic pain conditions.

Acknowledgement

I would like to thank Jane Carreiro, DO for critical discussion and reading of this paper and Suezan Moore for assistance in preparation of the manuscript. I would also like to thank Ralph Theime, Gretchen Sibley, Dense Frigon and Tom Scott for their assistance in the preparation of anatomical specimens.

REFERENCES

Abitbol M M 1988 Evolution of the ischial spine and of the pelvic floor in the Hominoidea. American Journal of Physical Anthropology 75: 53–67

Ahmed M, Bjurholm A, Kreicbergs A, Schultzberg M 1993a Neuropeptide Y, tyrosine hydroxylase and vasoactive intestinal polypeptide-immunoreactive nerve fibers in the vertebral bodies, disc, dura mater, and spinal ligaments of the rat lumbar spine. Spine 18: 268–273

Ahmed M, Bjurholm A, Kreicbergs A, Schultzberg M 1993b Sensory and autonomic innervation of the facet joint in the rat lumbar spine. Spine 18: 2121–2126

Akita K, Sakamoto H, Sato T 1992 Innervation of an aberrant digastric muscle in the posterior thigh: statified relationships between branches of the inferior gluteal nerve. Journal of Anatomy 181: 503–506

Aspden R M, Bornstein N H, Hukins D W L 1987 Collagen organisation in the interspinous ligament and its relationship to tissue function. Journal of Anatomy 155: 141–151

Avramov A I, Cavanaugh J M, Ozaktay C A, Getchell T V, King A I 1992 The effects of controlled mechanical loading on group-II, III, and IV afferent units from the lumbar facet joint and surrounding tissue. An in vitro study. Journal of Bone and Joint Surgery (US) 74: 1464–1471

Baba H, Maezawa Y, Furusawa N, Imura S, Tomita K 1995 The role of calcium deposition in the ligamentum flavum causing a cauda equina syndrome and lumbar radiculopathy. Paraplegia 33: 219–223

Ballard W T, Weinstein J N 1992 Biochemistry of the intervertebral disc. In: Kirkaldy-Willis W H and Burton C V (eds) Managing low back pain. Churchill Livingstone, New York, pp 39–48

Basbaum A I, Levine J D 1991 The contributions of the nervous system to inflammation and inflammatory disease. Canadian Journal of Physiology and Pharmacology 69: 647–651

Beal M C 1982 The sacroiliac problem: review of anatomy, mechanics, and diagnosis. Journal of the American Osteopathic Association 81: 667–679

Beaman D N, Graziano G P, Glover R A, Wojtys E M, Vhang V 1993 Substance P innervation of lumbar spine facet joints. Spine 18: 1044–1049

Bednar D A, Orr F W, Simon G T 1995 Observations on the pathomorphology of the thoracolumbar fascia in chronic mechanical back pain: a microscopic study. Spine 20: 1161–1164

Behrsin J F, Briggs C A 1988 Ligaments of the lumbar spine: a review. Surgical and Radiologic Anatomy 10: 211–219

Bernard T N, Cassidy J D 1991 The sacroiliac joint syndrome: pathophysiology, diagnosis, and management. In: Frymoyer J W (ed.) The adult spine: principles and practices. Raven Press, New York, pp 2107–2130

Bernard T N, Kirkaldy-Willis W H 1987 Recognizing specific characteristics of nonspecific low back pain. Clinical Orthopaedics and Related Research 217: 266–280

Bogduk N 1980 A reappraisal of the anatomy of the human lumbar erector spinae. Journal of Anatomy 131: 525–540

Bogduk N 1983 The innervation of the lumbar spine. Spine 8: 286–293

Bogduk N, Long D M 1979 The anatomy of the so-called 'articular nerves' and their relationship to facet denervation in the treatment of low-back pain. Journal of Neurosurgery 51: 172–177

Bogduk N, Macintosh J E 1984 The applied anatomy of the thoracolumbar fascia. Spine 9: 164–170

Bogduk N, Twomey L T 1991 Clinical anatomy of the lumbar spine. Churchill Livingstone, Melbourne

Bogduk N, Tynan W, Wilson A S 1981 The nerve supply to the human lumbar intervertebral discs. Journal of Anatomy 132: 39–56

Bogduk N, Macintosh J E, Pearcy M J 1992 A universal model of the lumbar back muscles in the upright position. Spine 17: 897–913

Bose K, Balasubramanian P 1984 Nerve root canals of the lumbar spine. Spine 9: 16–18

Briggs C A, Chandraraj S 1995 Variations in the lumbosacral ligament and associated changes in the lumbosacral region resulting in compression of the fifth dorsal root ganglion and spinal nerve. Clinical Anatomy 8: 339–346

Brunner C, Kissling R O, Jacob H A C 1991 The effects of morphology and histopathologic findings on the mobility of the sacroiliac joint. Spine 16: 1111–1117

Carette S, Marcoux S, Truchon R et al 1991 A controlled trial of corticosteroid injections into facet joints for chronic low back pain. New England Journal of Medicine 325: 1002–1007

Cavanaugh J M, Kallakuri S, Özaktay A C 1995 Innervation of the rabbit lumbar intervertebral disc and posterior longitudinal ligament. Spine 20: 2080–2085

Chow D H, Luk K D K, Leong J C, Woo C W 1989 Torsional stability of the lumbosacral junction. Significance of the iliolumbar ligament. Spine 14: 611–615

Coderre T J, Katz J, Vaccarina A L, Melzack R 1993 Contribution of central neuroplasticity to pathological pain: review of clinical and experimental evidence. Pain 52: 259–285

Crisco J J, Panjabi M M 1991 The intersegmental and multisegmental muscles of the lumbar spine: a biomechanical model comparing lateral stabilizing potential. Spine 16: 793–799

Daum W J 1995 The sacroiliac joint: an underappreciated pain generator. American Journal of Orthopedics 24: 475–478

de Peretti F, Micalef J P, Bourgeon A, Argenson C, Rabischong P 1989 Biomechanics of the lumbar spinal nerve roots and the first sacral root within the intervertebral foramina. Surgical and Radiologic Anatomy 11: 221–225

Dofferhof A S, Vink P 1985 The stabilising function of the mm. iliocostales and mm. multifidi during walking. Journal of Anatomy 140: 329–336

Dory M A 1981 Arthrography of the lumbar facet joints. Radiology 140: 23–27

Dupuis P 1992 The anatomy of the lumbosacral spine. In: Kirkaldy-Willis W H and Burton C V (eds) Managing low back pain. Churchill Livingstone, New York, pp 7–25

El-Bohy A A, Cavanaugh J M, Getchell M L, Bulas J, Getchell T V, King A I 1988 Localization of substance P and neurofilament immunoreactive fibers in the lumbar facet joint capsule and supraspinous ligament of the rabbit. Brain Research 460: 379–382

Engel R, Bogduk N 1982 The menisci of the lumbar zygoapophysial joints. Journal of Anatomy 135: 795–809

Firooznia H, Rauschning W, Rafii M, Golimbu C 1993 Normal correlative anatomy of the lumbosacral spine and its contents. Neuroimaging Clinics of North America 3: 411–423

Fortin J D, April C N, Ponthieux B, Pier J 1994a Sacroiliac joint: pain referral maps upon applying a new injection/arthrography technique. Part II: Clinical evaluation. Spine 19: 1483–1489

Fortin J D, Dwyer A P, West S, Pier J 1994b Sacroiliac joint: pain referral maps upon applying a new injection/arthrography technique. Part I: Asymptomatic volunteers. Spine 19: 1475–1482

Fujii Y, Yoshida H, Sakou T 1993 Immunohistochemical studies on tenascin in human yellow ligament. In Vivo 7: 143–146

Garfin S R, Rydevik B L, Lind B, Massie J 1995 Spinal nerve root compression. Spine 20: 1810–1820

Garrett N E, Mapp P I, Cruwys S C, Kidd B L, Blake D R 1992 Role of substance P in inflammatory arthritis. Annals of the Rheumatic Diseases 51: 1014–1018

Golub B S, Silverman B 1969 Transforaminal ligaments of the lumbar spine. Journal of Bone and Joint Surgery (US) 51: 947–956

Grob K R, Neuhuber W L, Kissling R O 1995 Innervation of the sacroiliac joint of the human. Zeitschrift fur Rheumatologie 54: 117–122

Groen G J, Baljet B, Drukker J 1988 The innervation of the spinal dura mater: anatomy and clinical implications. Acta Neurochirurgica 92: 39–46

Groen G J, Baljet B, Drukker J 1990 Nerves and nerve plexuses of the human vertebral column. American Journal of Anatomy 188: 282–296

Gronblad M, Virri J, Tolonen J et al 1994 A controlled immunohistochemical study of inflammatory cells in disc herniation tissue. Spine 19: 2744–2751

Hadar H, Gadoth N, Heifetz M 1983 Fatty replacement of lower paraspinal muscles: normal and neuromuscular disorders. American Journal of Roentgenology 5: 895–898

Hadley-Miller N, Mims B, Milewicz D M 1994 The potential role of the elastic fiber system in adolescent idiopathic scoliosis. Journal of Bone and Joint Surgery (US) 76: 1193–1206

Hanley E N, Howard B H, Brigham C D, Chapman T M, Guilford W B, Coumas J M 1994 Lumbar epidural varix as a cause of radiculopathy. Spine 19: 2122–2126

Hanson P, Sonesson B 1994 The anatomy of the iliolumbar ligament. Archives of Physical Medicine and Rehabilitation 75: 1245–1246

Hasegawa T, An H S, Haughton V M, Nowicki B H 1995 Lumbar foraminal stenosis: critical heights of the intervertebral discs and foramina. A cryomicrotome study in cadavera. Journal of Bone and Joint Surgery (US) 77: 32–38

Hasue M, Kikuchi S, Sakuyama Y, Ito T 1983 Anatomic study of the interrelation between lumbosacral nerve roots and their surrounding tissues. Spine 8: 50–58

Heylings D J A 1978 Supraspinous and interspinous ligaments of the human lumbar spine. Journal of Anatomy 125: 127–131

Holzer P 1988 Local effector functions of capsaicin-sensitive sensory nerve endings: involvement of tachykinins, calcitonin gene-related polypeptide and other neuropeptides. Neuroscience 24: 739–768

Hukins D W L, Kirby M C, Sikoryn T A, Aspden R M, Cox A J 1990 Comparison of structure, mechanical properties, and function of lumbar spinal ligaments. Spine 15: 787–795

Ikeda R 1991 Innervation of the sacroiliac joint. Macroscopical and histological studies. Nippon Ika Daigaku Zasshi 58: 587–596

Imai S, Hukuda S, Maeda T 1995 Dually innervating nociceptive networks in the rat lumbar posterior longitudinal ligaments. Spine 20: 2086–2092

Jackson H C, Winkelmann R K, Bickel W H 1966 Nerve endings in the human lumbar spinal column and related structures. Journal of Bone and Joint Surgery (US) 48: 1272–1281

Jacob H A C, Kissling R O 1995 The mobility of the sacroiliac joints in healthy volunteers between 20 and 50 years of age. Clinical Biomechanics 10: 352–361

Jiang H X, Russell G, Raso V J, Moreau M J, Hill D L, Bagnall K M 1995 The nature and distribution of the innervation of human supraspinal and interspinal ligaments. Spine 20: 869–876

Jinkins J R 1993 The pathoanatomic basis of somatic and autonomic syndromes originating in the lumbosacral spine. Neuroimaging Clinics of North America 3: 443–463

Jinkins J R, Whittermore A R, Bradley W G 1989 The anatomic basis of vertebrogenic pain and the autonomic syndrome associated with lumbar disk extrusion. American Journal of Radiology 152: 1277–1289

Kapandji I A 1974 The physiology of the joints, vol. 3, The trunk and the vertebral column. Churchill Livingstone, Edinburgh

Kashiwagi K 1993 Histological changes of the lumbar ligamentum flavum with age. Nippon Seikeigeka Gakkai Zasshi 67: 221–229

Kennelly K P, Stokes M J 1993 Pattern of asymmetry of paraspinal muscle size in adolescent idiopathic scoliosis examined by real-time ultrasound imaging. A preliminary study. Spine 18: 913–917

Khosla S, Tredwell S J, Day B, Shinn S L, Ovalle W K Jr 1980 An ultrastructural study of multifidus muscle in progressive idiopathic scoliosis. Changes resulting from a sarcolemmal defect at the myotendinous junction. Journal of the Neurological Sciences 46: 13–31

Kidd B L, Gibson S J, O'Higgins F et al 1989 A neurogenic mechanism for symmetrical arthritis. Lancet 1128: 1131–1989

Kidd B L, Mapp P I, Blake D R, Gibson J S, Polak J M 1990 Neurogenic influences in arthritis. Annals of the Rheumatic Diseases 49: 649–652

Kidd B L, Cruwys S, Mapp P I, Blake D R 1992 Role of the sympathetic nervous system in chronic joint pain and inflammation. Annals of the Rheumatic Diseases 51: 1188–1191

Kirkaldy-Willis W H 1984 The relationship of structural pathology to the nerve root. Spine 9: 49–52

Kissling R O 1995 The mobility of the sacro-iliac joint in healthy subjects. In: Vleeming A, Mooney V, Dorman T, Snijders C J (eds) Second interdisciplinary world congress on low back pain. San Diego, CA, 9–11 November, pp 411–422

Kojima Y, Maeda T, Arai R, Shichikawa K 1990a Nerve supply to the posterior longitudinal ligament and the intervertebral disc of the rat vertebral column as studied by acetylcholinesterase histochemistry. II: Regional differences in the distribution of the nerve fibres and their origins. Journal of Anatomy 169: 247–255

Kojima Y, Maeda T, Arai R, Shichikawa K 1990b Nerve supply to the posterior longitudinal ligament and the intervertebral disc of the rat vertebral column as studied by acetylcholinesterase histochemistry. I: Distribution in the lumbar region. Journal of Anatomy 169: 237–246

Konttinen Y T, Gronblad M, Antti-Poika I et al 1990a Neuroimmunohistochemical analysis of peridiscal nociceptive neural elements. Spine 15: 383–386

Konttinen Y T, Gronblad M, Korkala O, Tolvanen E, Polak J M 1990b Immunohistochemical demonstration of subclasses of inflammatory cells and active, collagen-producing fibroblasts in the synovial plicae of lumbar facet joints. Spine 15: 387–390

Korkala O, Gronblad M, Liesi P, Karaharju E 1985 Immunohistochemical demonstration of nociceptors in the ligamentous structures of the lumbar spine. Spine 10: 156–157

Lam F Y, Ferrell W R 1991 Neurogenic component of different models of acute inflammation in the knee joint. Annals of the Rheumatic Disease 50: 747–751

Lapadula G, Covelli M, Numo R, Pipitone V 1991 Iliolumbar ligament ossification as a radiologic feature of reactive arthritis. Journal of Rheumatology 18: 1760–1762

Lehto M, Hurme M, Alaranta H et al 1989 Connective tissue changes of the multifidus muscle in patients with lumbar disc herniation. An immunohistologic study of collagen types I and III and fibronectin. Spine 14: 302–309

Leong J C, Luk K D, Chow D H, Woo C W 1987 The biomechanical functions of the iliolumbar ligament in maintaining stability of the lumbosacral junction. Spine 12: 669–674

Levine J D, Collier D H, Basbaum A I, Moskowitz M A, Helms C A 1985a Hypothesis: the nervous system may contribute to the pathophysiology of rheumatoid arthritis. Journal of Rheumatology 12: 406–411

Levine J D, Moskowitz M A, Basbaum A I 1985b The contribution of neurogenic inflammation in experimental arthritis. Journal of Immunology 135: 843s–847s

Levine J D, Coderre T J, Covinsky K, Basbaum A I 1990 Neural influences on synovial mast cell density in rat. Journal of Neuroscience Research 26: 301–307

Levine J D, Fields H L, Basbaum A I 1993 Peptides and the primary afferent nociceptor. Journal of Neuroscience 13: 2273–2286

Lewin T, Moffett B, Viidik A 1962 The morphology of the lumbar synovial intervertebral joints. Acta Morphologica Neerl Scandinavia 4: 299–319

Luk K D K, Ho H C, Leong J C Y 1986 The iliolumbar ligament a study of its anatomy development and clinical significance. Journal of Bone and Joint Surgery (UK) 68: 197–200

McCafferty R R, Harrison M J, Tamas L B, Larkins M V 1995 Ossification of the anterior longitudinal ligament and Forestier's disease: an analysis of seven cases. Journal of Neurosurgery 83: 13–17

McCarron R F, Wimpee M W, Hudkins P G, Laros G S 1987 The inflammatory effects of the nucleus pulposus: a possible element in the pathogenesis of low back pain. Spine 12: 760–764

Macintosh J E, Bogduk N 1986 The biomechanics of the lumbar multifidus. Clinical Biomechanics 1: 205–213

Macintosh J E, Valencia F, Bogduk N, Munro R R 1986 The morphology of the human lumbar multifidus. Clinical Biomechanics 1: 196–204

Mattila M, Hurme M, Alaranta H et al 1986 The multifidus muscle in patients with lumbar disc herniation. A histochemical and morphometric analysis of intraoperative biopsies. Spine 11: 732–738

Mine T, Kawai S 1995 Ultrastructural observations on the ossification of the supraspinous ligament. Spine 20: 297–302

Mooney V, Robertson J 1976 The facet syndrome. Clinical Orthopaedics and Related Research 115: 149–156

Morley G W, DeLancey J O L 1988 Sacrospinous ligament fixation for eversion of the vagina. American Journal of Obstetrics and Gynecology 158: 872–881

Nachemson A, Evans J 1968 Some mechanical properties of the third lumbar intervertebral ligament (ligamentum flavum). Journal of Biomechanics 1: 211

Neumann P, Keller T, Ekstrom L, Hult E, Hansson T 1993 Structural properties of the anterior longitudinal ligament. Correlation with lumbar bone mineral content. Spine 18: 637–645

Neumann P, Ekstrom L A, Keller T S, Perry L, Hansson T H 1994 Aging, vertebral density, and disc degeneration alter the tensile stress–strain characteristics of the human anterior longitudinal ligament. Journal of Orthopaedic Research 12: 103–112

Nichols D H 1985 Vaginal prolapse affecting bladder function. Urologic Clinics of North America 12: 329–338

Nohara Y, Brown M D, Eurell J A 1991 Lymphatic drainage of epidural space in rabbits. Orthopedic Clinics of North America 22: 189–194

Nowicki B H, Haughton V M 1992 Neural foraminal ligaments of the lumbar spine: appearance at CT and MR imaging. Radiology 183: 257–264

O'Connor B L, Palmoski M J, Brandt K D 1985 Neurogenic acceleration of degenerative joint lesions. Journal of Bone and Joint Surgery (US) 67: 562–572

Okada A, Harata S, Takeda Y, Nakamura T, Takagaki K, Endo M 1993 Age-related changes in proteoglycans of human ligamentum flavum. Spine 18: 2261–2266

Olmarker K, Rydevik B L 1991 Pathophysiology of sciatica. Orthopedic Clinics of North America 22: 223–234

Olmarker K, Rydevik B L, Holm S 1989 Edema formation in spinal nerve roots induced by experimental, graded compression: an experimental study on the pig cauda equina with special reference to the differences in effects between rapid and slow onset of compression. Spine 14: 569–573

Olmarker K, Holm S, Rydevik B L 1990 Importance of compression onset rate for the degree of impairment of impulse propergation in experimental compression of the porcine cauda equina. Spine 15: 416–419

Olmarker K, Rydevik B L, Nordborg C 1993 Autologous nucleus pulposus induces neurophysiologic and histologic changes in porcine cauda equina nerve roots. Spine 18: 1425–1432

Olmarker K, Blomquist J, Strömberg J, Nannmark U, Thomsen P, Rydevik B L 1995 Inflammatogenic properties of nucleus pulposus. Spine 20: 665–669

O'Rahilly R 1986 Anatomy: a regional study of human structure. WB Saunders, Philadelphia

Oxland T R, Panjabi M M, Southern E P, Duranceau J S 1991 An anatomic basis for spinal instability: a porcine trauma model. Journal of Orthopaedic Research 9: 452–462

Ozaktay A C, Cavanaugh J M, Blagoev D C, Getchell T V, King A I 1994 Effects of a carrageenan-induced inflammation in rabbit lumbar facet joint capsule and adjacent tissues. Neuroscience Research 20: 355–364

Panjabi M M, White A A 1990 Physical properties and functional biomechanics of the spine. In: White A A, Panjabi M M (eds) Clinical Biomechanics of the Spine. JB Lippincott, Philadelphia, pp 1–84

Panjabi M M, Goel V K, Takata K 1982 Physiologic strains in the lumbar spinal ligaments. An in vitro biomechanical study. Spine 7: 192–203

Parke W W 1991 The significance of venous return impairment in ischemic radiculopathy and myelopathy. Orthopedic Clinics of North America 22: 213–221

Parke W W, Watanabe R 1990 Adhesions of the ventral lumbar dura: an adjunct source of discogenic pain? Spine 15: 300–303

Parkkola R, Rytokoski U, Kormano M 1993 Magnetic resonance imaging of the discs and trunk muscles in patients with chronic low back pain and healthy control subjects. Spine 18: 830–836

Payan D G 1989 Substance P: a neuroendocrine-immune modulator. Hospital Practice 24(2): 67–80

Payan D G 1992 The role of neuropeptides in inflammation. In: Gallin J I, Goldstein I M, Snyderman R (eds) Inflammation: basic principles and clinical correlations. Raven Press, New York, pp 177–192

Pedersen H E, Blunck C J F, Gardner E 1956a Innervation of the lumbar spine. Journal of Bone and Joint Surgery (US) 38: 377–391

Pedersen H E, Blunck F J, Gardner E 1956b The anatomy of lumbosacral posterior rami and meningeal branches of spinal nerves (sinu-vertebral nerves). Journal of Bone and Joint Surgery (US) 38: 377–391

Pionchon H, Tommasi M, Pialat J et al 1986 [Study of the innervation of the spinal ligaments at the lumbar level.] Bulletin de l'Association des Anatomistes 70: 63–67 (French)

Porges R, Smilen S W 1994 Long-term analysis of the surgical management of pelvic support defects. American Journal of Obstetrics and Gynecology 171: 1518–1528

Prechtl J C, Powley T L 1990 B-afferents: a fundamental division of the nervous system mediating homeostasis? Behavioral and Brain Science 13: 289–331

Prescher A, Bohndorf K 1993 Anatomical and radiological observations concerning ossification of the sacrotuberous ligament: is there a relation to spinal diffuse idiopathic skeletal hyperostosis (DISH)? Skeletal Radiology 22: 581–585

Ramsey R H 1966 The anatomy of the ligamenta flava. Clinical Orthopaedics and Related Research 44: 129–140

Rhalmi S, Yahia L H, Newman N, Isler M 1993 Immunohistochemical study of nerves in lumbar spinae ligaments. Spine 18: 264–267

Roaf R 1960 A study of the mechanics of spinal injuries. Journal of Bone and Joint Surgery (UK) 42: 810

Roberts W J, Kramis R C 1990 Sympathetic nervous system influence on acute and chronic pain. In: Fields H L (ed.) Pain syndromes in neurology. Butterworth Heineman, Oxford, pp 85–106

Ryan L M 1993 Calcium pyrophosphate dihydrate crystal deposition and other crystal deposition diseases. Current Opinion in Rheumatology 5: 517–521

Rydevik B L 1992 The effects of compression on the physiology of nerve roots. Journal of Manipulative and Physiological Therapeutics 15: 62–66

Rydevik B L, Brown M D, Lundborg G 1984 Pathoanatomy and pathophysiology of nerve root compression. Spine 9: 7–15

Saal J S 1995 The role of inflammation in lumbar pain. Spine 20: 1821–1827

Saal J S, Franson R C, Dobrow R, Saal J A, White A H 1990 High levels of inflammatory phospholipase A2 activity in lumbar disc herniation. Spine 15: 674–678

Sato K, Olmarker K, Cornefjord M, Rydevik B L, Lilucji S 1994 Effects of chronic nerve root compression on intraradicular blood flow: an experimental study in pigs. Neuro-Orthopedics 16: 1–7

Schaible H G, Grubb B D 1993 Afferent and spinal mechanisms of joint pain. Pain 55: 5–54

Schwarzer A C, Aprill C N, Derby R, Fortin J, Kine G, Bogduk N 1994 Clinical features of patients with pain stemming from the lumbar zygapophysial joints. Is the lumbar facet syndrome a clinical entity? Spine 19: 1132–1137

Schwarzer A C, Aprill C N, Bogduk N 1995 The sacroiliac joint in chronic low back pain. Spine 20: 31–37

Simonian P T, Routt M L C, Harrington R M, Mayo K A, Tencer A F 1994 Biomechanical simulation of the anteroposterior compression injury of the pelvis. Clinical Orthopaedics and Related Research 309: 245–256

Snijders C J, Vleeming A, Stoeckart R 1993 Transfer of lumbosacral load to iliac bones and legs. Part I: Biomechanics of self-bracing of the sacroiliac joints and its significance for treatment and exercise. Clinical Biomechanics 8: 285–294

Spencer D L, Irwin G S, Miller J A A 1983 Anatomy and significance of fixation of the lumbosacral nerve roots in sciatica. Spine 8: 672–679

Stilwell D L 1956 The nerve supply of the vertebral column and its associated structures in the monkey. Anatomical Record 125: 139–169

Swanepoel M W, Adams L M, Smeathers J E 1995 Human lumbar apophyseal joint damage and intervertebral disc degeneration. Annals of the Rheumatic Diseases 54: 182–188

Taylor J R, Twomey L T 1986 Age changes in lumbar zygapophyseal joints. Observations on structure and function. Spine 11: 739–745

Tobias D, Ziv I, Maroudas A 1992 Human facet cartilage: swelling and some physico-chemical characteristics as a function of age. Part I: Swelling of human facet joint cartilage. Spine 17: 694–700

Uhthoff H K 1993 Prenatal development of the iliolumbar ligament. Journal of Bone and Joint Surgery (UK) 75: 93–95

Vernon-Roberts B 1992 Age-related and degenerative pathology of intervertebral discs and apophyseal joints. In: Jayson M I V (ed.) The lumbar spine and back pain. Churchill Livingstone, Edinburgh, pp 17–41

Vleeming A, Stoeckart R, Snijders C J 1989a The sacrotuberous ligament: a conceptual approach to its dynamic role in stabilizing the sacroiliac joint. Clinical Biomechanics 4: 201–203

Vleeming A, van Wingerden J P, Snijders C J, Stoeckart R, Stijnen T 1989b Load application to the sacrotuberous ligament: influences on sacroiliac joint mechanics. Clinical Biomechanics 4: 204–209

Vleeming A, Stoeckart R, Snijders C J 1992 General introduction (to the sacroiliac joint). In: Vleeming A, Mooney V, Snijders C J, Dorman T (eds) First interdisciplinary world congress on low back pain and its relation to the sacroiliac joints. San Diego, CA, 5–6 November, pp 3–63

Vleeming A, Pool-Goudzwaard A L, Hammudoghlu D, Stoeckart R, Snijders C J, Mens J M A 1995a The function of the long dorsal sacroiliac ligament: its implication for understanding low back pain. In: Vleeming A, Mooney V, Dorman T, Snijders C J (eds) Second interdisciplinary world congress on low back pain. San Diego, CA, 9–10 November, pp 125–137

Vleeming A, Pool-Goudzwaard A L, Stoeckart R, van Wingerden J P, Snijders C J 1995b The posterior layer of the thoracolumbar fascia: its function in load transfer from spine to legs. Spine 20: 753–758

Vleeming A, Snijders C J, Stoeckart R, Mens J M A 1995c A new light on low back pain: the selflocking mechanism of the sacroiliac joints and its implication for sitting, standing and walking. In: Vleeming A, Mooney V, Dorman T, Snijders C J (eds) Second interdisciplinary world congress on low back pain. San Diego, CA, 9–11 November, pp 149–168

von During M, Fricke B, Dahlmann A 1995 Topography and distribution of nerve fibers in the posterior longitudinal ligament of the rat: an immunocytochemical and electron-microscopical study. Cell and Tissue Research 281: 325–338

Weidenbaum M, Farcy J-P 1990 Pain syndromes of the lumbar spine. In: Floman Y (ed.) Disorders of the lumbar spine. Aspen Publishing, Rockville, MD, pp 85–115

Weinstein J N 1991 Neurogenic and nonneurogenic pain and inflammatory mediators. Orthopedic Clinics of North America 22: 235–246

Weinstein J N 1992 The role of neurogenic and non-neurogenic mediators as they relate to pain and the development of osteoarthritis. Spine 105: S356–S361

Willard F H 1995 Neuroendocrine–immune network, nociceptive stress, and the general adaptive response. In: Everett T, Dennis M, Ricketts E (eds) Physiotherapy in mental health: a practical approach. Butterworth

Heinemann, Oxford, pp 102–126

Williams P L 1995 Gray's anatomy: the anatomical basis of medicine and surgery. Churchill Livingstone, Edinburgh

Woolf C J, Chong M-S 1993 Preemptive analgesia – treating postoperative pain by preventing the establishment of central sensitization. Anesthesia and Analgesia 77: 362–379

Yahia L H, Garzon S, Strykowski H, Rivard C-H 1990 Ultrastructure of the human interspinous ligament and ligamentum flavum: a preliminary study. Spine 15: 262–268

Yahia L H, Rhalmi S, Newman N, Isler M 1992 Sensory innervation of the human thoracolumbar fascia. Acta Orthopedica Scandinavia 63: 195–197

Yamamoto I, Panjabi M M, Oxland T R, Crisco J J 1990 The role of the iliolumbar ligament in the lumbosacral junction. Spine 15: 1138–1141

Yamashita T, Cavanaugh J M, El-Bohy A A, Getchell T V, King A I 1990 Mechanosensitive afferent units in the lumbar facet joint. Journal of Bone and Joint Surgery (US) 72: 865–870

Yoshida M, Shima K, Taniguchi Y, Tamaki T, Tanaka T 1992 Hypertrophied ligamentum flavum in lumbar spinal canal stenosis. Pathogenesis and morphologic and immunohistochemical observation. Spine 17: 1353–1360

Ziv I, Maroudas C, Robin G, Maroudas A 1993 Human facet cartilage: swelling and some physio-chemical characteristics as a function of age. Part 2: Age changes in some biophysical parameters of human facet joint cartilage. Spine 18: 136–146

2. Sacroiliac joint dysfunction

V. Mooney

INTRODUCTION

The sacroiliac joint (SIJ) has had a varied history of interest as a significant source of persistent back pain. At the beginning of the century, perhaps due to its location in the buttock, where frequent back pain complaints are common, it was considered to be the primary source of chronic back pain (Albee 1909, Goldthwait & Osgood 1905). This early enthusiasm for the SIJ as the major source of back problems, however, faded for several reasons. By the 1930s, it became apparent that the lumbar disc could create sciatica and apparently also lumbago. It could be approached surgically and its pathoanatomy visualized. In addition, radiographic procedures gradually emerged which confirmed the clinical syndromes associated with disc herniations. Thus, objective testing became available. For several decades, the disc was thought to be the only clinically significant pain generator.

The absence of a clear-cut clinical syndrome to explain the majority of persistent back pain was confirmed by the Quebec Task Force report (1987) which could not give a specific diagnostic picture for most back and leg syndromes, and had to resort to classification by only pain location and duration. In addition, with improved fluoroscopic equipment, pain reproduction, and ablation at specific anatomic sites, clinical pain source alternatives to the disc could be demonstrated (Mooney & Robertson 1976).

Thus, with the recognition that physical examination itself seldom offers a consensus on the structural diagnosis, and that imaging studies may be specific as to the symptomatic pain generator in the spine, it is once again reasonable to look to other inverted structures that may be sources of painful spinal disorders. The most controversial source is probably the SIJ. As this chapter will explain, the clinical findings are often subtle, the potential for imaging confirmation somewhat controversial, and the definitive treatment program not yet clearly defined. Nonetheless, as will be demonstrated, it is now incontrovertible that some proportion of painful spinal disorders is secondary to SIJ dysfunction.

STRUCTURAL ANATOMY

The SIJ is a unique articulation in the human body. It is a diarthrodial joint because it contains synovial fluid and matching articular surfaces. The articular surfaces, however, are different from those in any other joint in the body. It is in this joint alone that hyaline articular cartilage faces and moves against fibrocartilage. On the sacral side (Fig. 2.1), this hyaline cartilage is usually 1–3 mm in depth (Bowden & Cassidy 1981). As in other articular surfaces, the collagen fibers are aligned parallel to the joint surface only in the superficial zone. However, on the iliac cartilage side, which is thinner, the chondrocytes are arranged in palisades and clumped together between bundles of collagen fibers that are all oriented parallel to the joint surface. It gives the appearance of fibrocartilage although the collagen is type II, typical of hyaline cartilage (Bernard & Cassidy 1991).

In addition to the microscopic anatomy, it is apparent from gross anatomy that this joint is not designed for significant motion. Vleeming et al (1990a) pointed out that in the human dissections there was a consistent presence of ridges and depressions, creating an extremely rough surface.

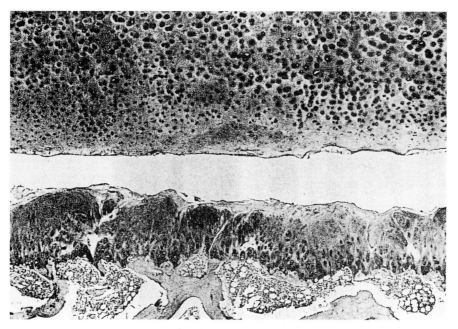

Fig. 2.1   Photomicrograph of the SIJ articular surfaces. The sacral hyaline cartilage faces the fibrocartilage on the ilium.

This study also noted that the amount of irregularity and coarseness was somewhat greater in males than in females. The authors pointed out that under abnormal loading conditions of the SIJ with these macroscopic irregularities, it is theoretically possible that an SIJ can be forced into a new position in which ridge and depression are no longer complementary. This unique characteristic of the joint would allow it to be set into a slightly subluxed 'locked position'. The amount of displacement, however, is so minimal that it has not been documented radiographically.

LIGAMENTOUS STRUCTURE

In that the SIJ is a relatively flat joint, loading stability cannot be achieved on the basis of skeletal orientation. The ligamentous structures must offer considerable resistance to shear. The ligamentous relationships between the posterior ilium and the sacrum are quite complex. The anterior sacroiliac (SI) ligament (Fig. 2.2) interfaces directly with the articular cavity and thus synovial fluid. The interosseous ligaments are quite short, but the posterior SI ligament is oriented obliquely to resist the loading of the sacrum relative to the ilium.

Superficial to these ligaments are two other significant ligamentous structures. First is the sacrotuberous ligament, which connects to the ischial tuberosity. Detailed dissections of anatomic material by Vleeming et al (1989) noted that, in all the sections, the gluteus maximus fascia was connected to the sacrotuberous ligament. In most dissections, a portion of the long head of the biceps femoris tendon is in continuity with the sacrotuberous ligament, traversing the ischium (Fig. 2.3). An additional discovery from these dissections noted that the fascia covering the posterior aspect of the piriformis muscle was continuous with the posterior SI ligament. The implication of these findings is that physical activity such as straight leg raising tests could stress the SIJ owing to the insertion from the bicep femoris muscle. Thus, injury-induced reactive inflammation of the SI ligament could affect the piriformis muscle and create resultant muscle spasm and its associated syndrome. Finally, all activity, such as walking and standing, which requires function of the powerful gluteus maximus muscle can affect the stability of the SIJ through its attachments to the posterior SI ligaments.

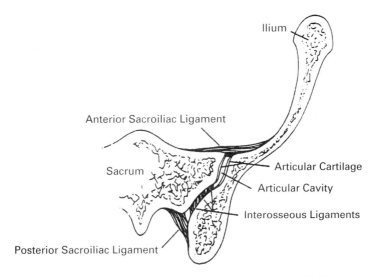

Fig. 2.2   The ligamentous relationships of the SIJ. The anterior SI ligament interfaces directly with the synovial lining of the joint.

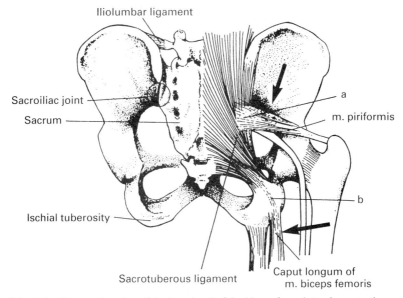

Fig. 2.3   The continuation of the long head of the biceps femoris tendon onto the sacrotuberous ligament is noted by the inferior arrow. The fascia of the piriformis muscle blends with the posterior SI ligament. Thus, muscle activity of the leg can influence and be influenced by the SI ligaments.

Another significant ligament attachment is the long dorsal SI ligament. This ligament becomes stretched when the sacrum is rotated in a posterior manner relative to the ilium. Thus, in situations where there is a decrease in lumbar lordosis, such as in the early stages of pregnancy or in aging,

this ligament may be stretched. It is the most superficial ligament and thus easily palpable just caudal to the posterior superior iliac spine (PSIS) (Fig. 2.4) (Vleeming et al 1996).

Another significant aspect of the anatomic structures related to the SIJ is the fascial layers,

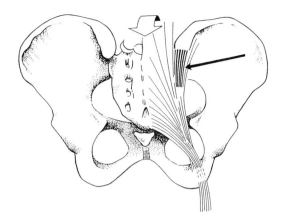

Fig. 2.4 The palpable long dorsal SI ligament is stressed in situations in which there is a decrease in lumbar lordosis, such as pregnancy, and may become tender.

superficial to the ligamentous structures. In anatomic dissections, it was clear that in all specimens, traction on the posterior layer of the thoracolumbar lumbar fascia transmitted force to the contralateral side, specifically into the fascia of the gluteus maximus (Vleeming et al 1995). This work on an anatomic level defined how an

interaction between thoracic and leg function, such as that concerning the latissimus dorsi related to the contralateral gluteus maximus, could affect the stability of the SIJ owing to traversing fascia. This study also reinforced the concept that dynamic activity, 'force closure', can achieve stability of the SIJs as much as can the 'form closure' based on anatomic orientation. Stability must be achieved by a combination of ligamentous and dynamic function from the associated muscles. Thus, the SIJ becomes stable with the combination of form and force closure (Fig. 2.5). If the form and the force closure is not sufficient owing to insufficient muscle action or insufficient ligamentous competence, functional and symptomatic instability can emerge. These concepts provide some insight into the clinical syndrome and possible therapeutic maneuvers.

INNERVATION

It has long been recognized that the SIJ is a pain-sensitive structure (Hirsch et al 1963). As in all

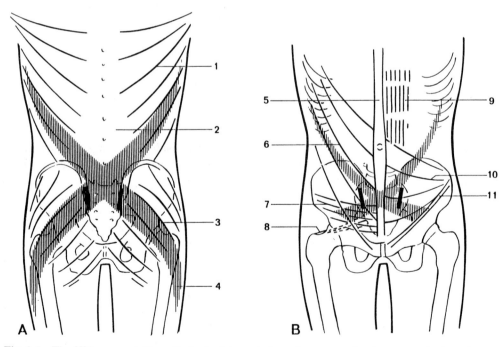

Fig. 2.5 The SIJ becomes stable on the basis of dynamic force closure as well as its structural orientation. The crossing musculature is noted. (A): 1-m. latissimus dorsi, 2-thoracolumbar fascia, 3-m. gluteus maximus, 4-tractus ilio tibialis. (B): 5-linea alba, 6-m. obliquus abdominis externus, 7-m. transversus abdominis, 8-m. piriformis, 9-m. rectus abdominis, 10-m. obliquus abdominis internus, 11-lig. inguinale.

joints, such as the posterior facet joint, the synovial capsule of the SIJ and overlying ligaments have many unmyelinated free nerve endings that transmit pain and temperature sensation. The SIJ capsule is also innervated by complex nerves providing pressure and position sense to the central nervous system (Lamb 1979). The posterior ligaments of the joint capsule are supplied by lateral branches of the posterior primary rami from L4 to S3. However, the anterior ligamentous structures are innervated from L2 through S2 (Solonen 1957).

This wide level of innervation is important in that it can be used to explain the extremely variable clinical presentation of pain complaints relative to the SIJ. The phenomenon of referred pain has long been recognized as part of the clinical presentation of back pain (Inman & Saunders 1994). The reproduction of referred pain has also been recognized as potentially arising from the SIJ (Steindler 1938). Given the wide distribution of innervation, it is, of course, quite possible that pain referred from the SIJ will not be associated with any motor, reflex, or sensory deficit on physical examination.

BIOMECHANICS

The postulated functions of the SIJ are to dissipate or attenuate the loads of the torso to the lower extremities and vice versa. As noted earlier, there are articular characteristics, ligamentous support, and muscular forces that are all useful in achieving the load transfer. In vitro, downward shear strength for both SIJs is about 4800 N (Gunterberg et al 1976). For comparison, the maximum compressive load in vitro to the L3 vertebra is estimated to be about 3500 N (Miller et al 1987).

With these calculated loads being necessary for function, some motion of the SIJ is inherent in transferring these forces. It seems, however, to be very difficult to analyse the motion. The problem is very complex in that the SI motion is effected by motion in the lumbar spine, hip joint, and symphysis pubis. It has not been established that there is a fixed axis about which the joint rotates. The joint is wedge shaped, both in an anterior to posterior perspective, as well as cranially to caudally. If there were a single axis, gapping would

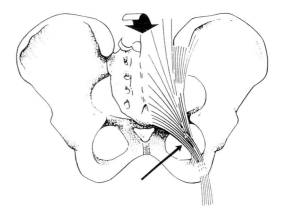

Fig. 2.6 The complex forward gliding motion of the sacrum upon the ilium is noted. Restraint is created dynamically by the extension of the biceps femoris attachment onto the sacrotuberous ligament.

occur during the flexion or extension motions. This has not been demonstrated radiographically. It is more likely that there is a complex gliding motion (Fig. 2.6).

Specific studies on the motion of the SIJ were initiated by the classic studies of Weisl (1954, 1955). These studies indicated that most movement occurred when the individual rose from a supine to a standing position. There was an average of 5 mm of motion wherein the sacrum moved anteriorly (ventrally) with a glide/rotation of the promontory of the first sacral segment being measured radiographically. In a cadaver study using more modern techniques, Vleeming et al (1990b) found similar mobility. This study noted a considerable range in motion from zero to about 4°, with an average of 2°. It was also noted that radiographic sclerosis was not a predictor of mobility in this anatomic study. There was even side-to-side variation in the same specimen.

A definitive in vivo study was carried out by Sturesson et al (1989). This is the most accurate study to date in that it used the Selvik (1974) technique to analyse motion in subjects and patients. In this technique, small metal balls are implanted in the appropriate skeletal structures under local anesthetic, and the relative motion between the metallic reference points of the ilium and the sacrum are evaluated in various positions by dual radiographic techniques. The stereoradiography is considered to be very accurate. In Sturesson et al's study of healthy young people, the posture change from standing normally to hyperextension produced the greatest degree of motion. This was slightly more than 2° on average, with a maximum of 4°. The amount of translation was extremely small, with an average of 0.5 mm and no value greater than 1.6 mm. The men were slightly less mobile than the women, but there was no decrease in mobility with advancing age. The study was also quite interesting in that it was also performed on individuals who had been classed as having SI dysfunction based on a consensus from two physiotherapists, an orthopedic surgeon, and a chiropractor. Seventeen patients had unilateral symptoms. The range of motion was no different on the involved side compared with the uninvolved side. In this study, too, there was no decrease in mobility with advancing age. There was also no difference in average joint motion between symptomatic individuals and normal subjects (Sturesson 1992).

All of these studies point to the recognition that a small amount of motion occurs at the joint, but it is so minimal that it would be difficult to assess from a physical examination standpoint.

A predisposition to SI strain has not been identified. Such abnormalities as leg length discrepancy, scoliosis, and hip joint disease with associated limited range have not been associated with a higher incidence of SI dysfunction. An earlier study of lumbar spinal fusions did not appear to affect SIJ mobility or hasten degenerative changes in the SIJ (Frymoyer et al 1978). This older study was accomplished when internal fixation was not commonly used for lumbar spinal fusions. A more recent study suggests that there may be some additional strain placed upon the SIJ with internal fixation (Jamich et al 1995). In this study, there were 389 patients who had low back pain after previous lumbar surgery, including fusion; 137 of these patients had a clinical picture similar to that of SI arthropathy, with tenderness over the posterior iliac spine, a positive Faber test, and a pain diagram with pain lateral to the midline, covering the buttock area, being typical of SI dysfunction. Using the two-injection technique for the evaluation of SI pain, 13 patients were found to have a positive response, suggesting SI dysfunction as their source of pain. All had had

previous fusions. The location of pain was unrelated to the site of bone graft. With greater experience within this new era of lumbar spine surgery, it is likely that additional causes of strain to the SIJ may occur.

CLINICAL DIAGNOSIS

What is the incidence of SI dysfunction in persons with low back pain? The incidence, of course, is variable depending upon the criteria on which the diagnosis is made and the population studied. Cibulka et al (1992) presented a study in which 81% of 88 patients with chronic low back pain demonstrated some evidence of SI dysfunction. This was in contrast to 112 patients who were evaluated for problems other than chronic low back pain, in whom there was only a 12% incidence of SI dysfunction. The main test in this study was evaluation of the PSIS on motion and variation in leg length after the subject changed position.

A larger study was reported by Bernard and Kirkaldy-Willis (1987). In this consecutive series of 1200 patients referred with chronic low back pain, the authors found SI dysfunction on a clinical basis as the major source of back pain in 22.5% of the patients. It was their view that SI syndrome was coexistent with other sources of pain in one-third of all the patients. Only history and physical examination were used to make this assessment.

In another study of chronic back pain patients with an average of over 30 months' symptoms, 86% were positive on at least two out of six SI dysfunctional tests (Greenman & Tate 1988). There is great variation in incidence depending upon the population being studied.

Bernard and Kirkaldy-Willis' study did try to display a clinical picture in a consecutive series of patients referred to a specialty clinic with chronic back pain. In this series of 250 patients, there were 160 women and 90 men with an average age in their early forties. The onset of symptoms was unrelated to significant trauma in 58% of the patients. The duration of symptoms averaged over 11 months, but some had symptoms lasting for many years. The pain was right sided in 45%, left sided in 35%, and bilateral in 20%. In only 10%

did the pain radiate below the knee. It could be referred to the buttocks groin, posterior thigh, and anterior thigh. There were rarely any associated neurologic symptoms or neurologic findings. The most common physical finding was tenderness over the sacral sulcus and in the posterior SIJ area. Ranging of the lumbar sacral spine did not necessarily increase pain, although hamstring tightness was occasionally present. Obviously, therefore, a blurred clinical picture emerges. What, then, are the possible clinical tests?

Although many tests have been advocated as being effective in delineating SIJ dysfunction, there have been few studies that have tried to evaluate the reproducibility of clinical examination. Potter and Rothstein (1985) identified 13 tests of SI dysfunction that were performed by experienced therapists on 17 patients. Only in the distraction and compression pain provocation tests did the reliability of the therapists' results exceed 70% agreement.

Among the clinical tests, there is a school of practice that relies on palpation to determine abnormal motion, compared with using pain reproduction as an endpoint for a definition of a positive test. There is considerable doubt concerning the reliability of palpation tests. In Gillet's test, in which posterior inferior iliac spine (PIIS) relationships are evaluated, a positive result has been found in 20% of asymptomatic individuals (Dreyfuss et al 1992). In another study, VanDuersen et al (1990) found that the interexaminer reliability of six commonly used palpation tests was only fair and was in some cases worse than would be expected by chance. Thus, it seems appropriate to consider pain provocation tests as potentially more reliable. Laslett and Williams (1994), using pain provocation tests that scored best in Potter and Rothstein's study, presented a reliability study using the following tests:

1. *Distraction.* Pressure is applied directly posteriorly and laterally to both anterior superior iliac spines (ASISs) with the patient in the supine position. The object is to stretch the anterior SI ligaments.

2. *Compression.* While the patient is lying on one side, pressure is applied to the uppermost iliac crest and directly toward the opposite iliac crest, theoretically compressing the pelvis.

3. *Posterior shear or thigh thrust test.* A posterior shearing stress is applied to the SIJ of a supine patient by a sudden downward force applied to a 90° flexed femur in a neutral position.

4. *Pelvic torsion test (Gaenslen's test).* With one hip fully flexed onto the abdomen, the other hip is extended past neutral with the pelvis displaced on the edge of the table to allow this maneuver.

5. *Sacral thrust.* Pressure is applied directly on the sacrum, the patient lying prone.

6. *Cranial shear test.* Pressure is applied to the coccyx and sacrum and directed cranially.

Only the cranial shear and the sacral thrust test had lower levels of agreement, with 90% agreement in the other tests. These tests were performed by two experienced physiotherapists on a group of 51 apparently symptomatic patients.

One other type of test has been advocated as demonstrating SI dysfunction. The leg length change test is reported by some experienced observers to be reliable (Don Tigny 1990). In this test, with the patient supine and leg length equal on examination, the leg on the symptomatic side, following forced full flexion of the hip and knee on that side, appears to move up, its malleolus lying higher than the malleolus of the uninvolved side. All these tests have to be compared with some sort of gold standard, and except for the reference noted above, the reproducibility and the correlation from examiner to examiner are difficult to assess.

A recent study has been reported evaluating the results of 38 patients who underwent SI arthrodesis and had positive confirmation by radiographic injection (Moore 1995). In this group of patients, who had such severe SI dysfunction that they had failed to respond to the usual conservative measures, there was no consistent clinical picture. The most common positive physical finding was that in 32 of the 38 patients there was a positive Faber test (flexion, abduction, external rotation; also known as the figure 4 test). Other physical examination maneuvers, such as Gillet's test, Gaenslen's test, and the forward bending test, did not show a consistent correlation. Plain X-rays were not helpful, nor was there a correlation with computerized tomography (CT) scans that showed significant anatomic variation between individuals. Pain frequently radiated into the groin and down either the front or the back of one leg. No patient presented with leg pain alone.

All patients underwent diagnostic injection with local anesthetic under radiographic control. All patients reported significant pain relief following injection and surgical care was undertaken. This study is valuable in that it confirmed the wide variation in clinical presentation and the relatively small incidence of SI dysfunction of such severity that surgical care was a consideration.

RADIOGRAPHIC EVALUATION

No studies, as confirmed by Moore, have documented abnormal radiographic abnormalities in SI dysfunction. This is in contrast to disease processes such as rheumatoid spondylitis where radiographic abnormalities of the SIJ may be diagnostic and positive bone scans may be expected. No study has reported positive bone scans as pathognomonic of SI dysfunction. Nonetheless, it is possible to document abnormal SI rotation in plain X-ray films, especially with the individual standing (Fig. 2.7).

The most definitive radiographic study is CT scanning. This can frequently document abnormal

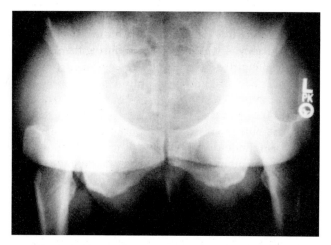

Fig. 2.7   Abnormal sacral rotation can often be noted on standing weight-bearing X-ray films. The relative elevation of one ischium compared with the other is notable.

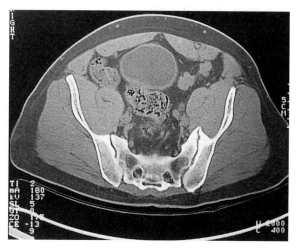

Fig. 2.8   CAT scan of the SIJ, noting reactive spurring suggestive of abnormal motion. The CAT scan provides the most accurate imaging study.

motion of the joint with reactive spurring or with significant gas in the joint. (Fig. 2.8).

The most precise method of evaluating SI dysfunction is by specific injection techniques, but even this is a complex issue. If it is assumed that SI pain is due to reactive inflammation in the ligamentous structures, the joint itself may be irrelevant in terms of pain reproduction. Injections into multiple levels of the SI ligaments may be necessary to determine a symptomatic area. This type of testing, however, lacks specificity.

The most specific and demanding test has recently been reported by Schwarzer et al (1995). In this study, in order to offer greatest specificity, an anatomically exact injection was accomplished. Recognizing the difficulty of placing the needle into the joint itself from a directly posterior position due to the overlying ilium, the authors used an inferior approach. By this maneuver, the skin entry is 1–3 cm below the inferior margin of the SIJ. A 22-gauge needle is introduced directly cephalad into the inferior aspect of the joint. The tip of the needle is manipulated until it enters the joint space. Entry can be confirmed by the distinct bend of the needle as it conforms to the irregular joint contour (Fig. 2.9). Following this, contrast is injected to confirm appropriate localization.

In addition to avoid the problem of a placebo effect, a double-injection technique was utilized. In these circumstances, the initial injection was

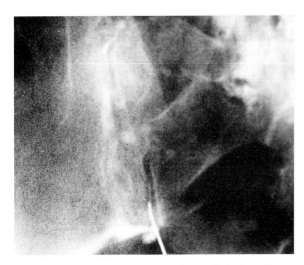

Fig. 2.9 Appropriate localization of a needle in the SIJ is confirmed by the slight needle bend as it conforms to the irregular joint contour.

performed with short-acting local anesthetic, and those who were positive on this part of the test were subsequently injected with long-acting anesthetic. A positive test was only achieved when, after the second injection, the individual reported a more prolonged relief of symptoms appropriate to the action of the longer-acting anesthetic.

Using this stringent procedure, 100 consecutive patients at two spine treatment centers were evaluated. All had chronic back pain and diagnoses undefineable by standard physical examination and radiographic procedures. In this group of 100 patients, 43 had pain below the L5–S1 level overlying the SIJ. In this group, the distribution between men and women was about equal, with an average pain duration of 14 months.

Following injection, which noted the reproduction of their usual pain, 30% of the patients (13% of the original consecutive 100 patients) responded with appropriate pain relief. The most consistent pain referral pattern was to the groin and was the only clinically distinguishing characteristic of pain referral in the SI patients compared with pain referral from facet injection or disc injection. No other pain distributions were found to be more common in one group of injections (discogram and facet) than in SI injections. There were no historical features in common in those with SI pain reproduction and relief compared with the

others. Tears of the ventral capsule of the joint were significantly associated with a positive test. This occurred in 85% of those testing positive for SI dysfunction.

To date, this is the most definitive study on the expected incidence of pure SI dysfunction in a group of chronic back pain patients without clear-cut diagnostic definition. Once again, it confirms that there is no pathognomonic clinical picture, although pain referred to the groin is suggestive. It also confirms that the incidences are relatively small (13% of preselected possible candidates). If the most stringent criteria are used (relief of pain and ventral capsular tear), as well as pain provocation after injection, the prevalence of possible candidates is perhaps 16% and 7% respectively in all chronic back pain patients without diagnostic criteria. Thus, we are left with a clinical syndrome of low incidence and no consistent clinical findings, and an invasive test as the basic gold standard on which to make a diagnosis.

SI PAIN IN PREGNANCY

Pregnancy offers an unique opportunity to evaluate SI dysfunction. It is well recognized that pregnancy is associated with relaxation of ligamentous structures. Also, the incidence of back pain is unusually high. In one study, wherein mothers were interviewed within several days following delivery, the incidence of back pain was 56% (Fast et al 1987). In another study, in which 855 pregnant women were followed starting with the 12th week of pregnancy, 49% had back pain during the pregnancy (Östgaard et al 1991). In this study, the individuals were divided into three groups based on the pain drawing localization of their pain. Over 50% of them localized the pain to the SI area. In this group, the pain became worse with increasing duration of pregnancy, while in the other groups the pain got somewhat better. Also, in this large group of women with back pain, only 1% had true sciatica with an appropriate dermatome distribution suggesting disc problems. This points out that disc disease may not be the primary source of back pain during pregnancy. In addition, the location suggests that the SI dysfunction may be a significant factor.

To reinforce the concept that ligamentous laxity may be a significant contributor to back pain associated with pregnancy, Kristiansson (1995) studied a group of 200 consecutive pregnant women during their pregnancy. Sixty-eight per cent of this population reported back pain during pregnancy. The incidence and severity of back pain was positively correlated to the level of relaxin.

Because of the inability to carry out a specific X-ray test during pregnancy, it is not possible to pinpoint the SIJ as the source of pain secondary to ligamentous relaxation. Because of this, Ostgaard has proposed the definition of the problem as that of posterior pelvic pain, which is to be separated from more common back ache. This pain definition requires a pain drawing to show the area of pain to be in the buttock below L5–S1 and that there be positive pelvic pain from a provocation test. This test is essentially the thigh thrust test described by Laslett and Williams (1994) (Fig. 2.10). An additional clinical feature of this syndrome is that the pain is increased on single-leg weight-bearing. In this group of patients, significant relief was achieved using an SI belt (Östgaard et al 1991). In another study concerning back pain in pregnancy, Mens et al (1992) found that 70% of 518 pregnant women who responded to a questionnaire had pain before or shortly after pregnancy. Only 5% of women in the study developed pain when the delivery position was in a half-sitting position, whereas those who had a delivery position of bilateral extreme hip flexion, typical of the use of stirrups, had a 70% incidence of pain at time of delivery or shortly thereafter. The stirrup position, which may place excessive SI strain on this occasion of high levels of relaxin, may thus be a source of additional injurious stress.

Of course, the aspect of stability of the SIJ is extremely difficult to assess. Recently, Mens et al (1995) have come up with a very simple test that offers some potential in identifying individuals with incompetent SI function. In this test women who had developed pelvic pain associated with or shortly after delivery were examined by a simple active straight leg raising test while in a supine position. All patients had asymmetric pain in which most of the pain localized to one side or the other. The active straight leg raising was achieved merely be elevating the heel from the table by about 5 cm and holding it for a short period of time. Various modifications to the conditions of the test were achieved, and the individual was asked whether the maneuvers created a sense of more or less strength or no change at all. One condition was severe flexion of the opposite hip. In all but one of the 15 patients examined, the individual felt the leg on the involved side to be weaker during active straight leg raising. However, by the addition of a pelvic belt, most of the participants felt their leg to be considerably stronger. Pressure from the examiner's hand on the ASIS in a medial and cranial direction increased the sense of strength in all patients, whereas pressure

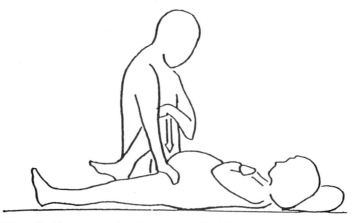

Fig. 2.10   Posterior pelvic pain created by the thigh thrust serves as a specific SI stress test.

on the opposite side decreased the sense of strength in all patients. All of these tests, therefore, point to the fact that a sense of instability or stability can be created in the pelvic girdle, probably in the SIJ.

There is concern, of course, as to the validity of a test defining the source of pain as the SIJ based purely on pain location as defined by pain drawings, pain reproduction, or a sense of stability. However, it would be unethical to carry out injection under fluoroscopy in pregnant females to confirm the SIJ as a pain source. Is there thus any evidence that pain localization is specific to the SIJ?

An interesting study was reported by Fortin et al (1994a) confirming the appropriate localization of pain as arising from the SIJ. In this study, 10 volunteers had their SIJ irritated by a radiographically controlled injection of contrast medium into the SIJ. The pain pattern described by the subjects was documented by pain drawings, and then all the pain drawings were correlated into a composite referral map illustrating the overall area of pain complaint in the 10 volunteers. In this group, there was no pain down the leg other than in the upper part of lateral thigh. However, in this group also, none of the subjects showed incompetence of the anterior ligament and there was no flow of contrast outside the SIJ. There was thus competency of the ligament, both anteriorly and posteriorly.

In a follow-up to this study; these SI pain referral patterns were used to define a group of 54 consecutive patients (Fortin et al 1994b). In this group, two clinicians, blinded to the examination of the individuals, picked from the pain drawings of the patients those which were thought to represent SI pain based on the pain distribution pattern noted in the earlier study. There was 100% agreement between the two clinicians as to the patients selected with SI pain. All 16 patients selected had a provocation-positive SIJ injection. In addition, 10 out of the 16 had lumbar discography and lumbar facet injections. These were negative. Only the SIJ injection created pain. The SIJ injection, in all cases, reproduced their pain. Thus, this study indicates that pain referral located laterally to the sacrum and below the iliac crest is a reasonable indication of SIJ dysfunction.

TREATMENT

Although incompetence of the SIJ seems to be a reasonable concept based on the information noted above, the rationale for treatment remains elusive. There are two divergent themes of treatment, one being mobilization and manipulation to realign the SIJ, and the other stabilization by dynamic or surgical maneuvers.

The theory behind joint manipulation is still not clear. One of the most experienced physical therapists in the treatment of SI dysfunction is DonTigny (1990), who feels that the abnormality based on physical examination is a forward rotation of the ilium on the sacrum. This, therefore, is corrected by a hyperflexion of the involved hip to reduce the forward displacement. Sometimes manipulation is necessary in addition to self-mobilization. Documentation of efficacy is noted by relative leg length change after correction of the position following manipulation. However, no comparative study has been presented establishing efficacy.

On the other hand, an equally experienced clinician, Cassidy (Cassidy et al 1985), recommends manipulation of the PSIS or ischial tuberosity with the patient side-lying, and a mobilization of the joint in various directions. In a series of 1293 consecutive low back pain patients, 22% were diagnosed as having SI syndrome. In these 336 patients, the Cassidy manipulation was accomplished in 258, with excellent results in all but 13. The other 66 patients were treated by injection (Bernard & Kirkaldy-Willis 1987). These manipulations were daily for a 2–3-week period and were apparently successful in about 90% of the patients (Bernard & Kirkaldy-Willis 1987). The authors suggested that this might result from the readjustment of muscle tone secondary to reflex inhibition of the gamma and alpha motor neurons owing to the strenuous stimulation of the articular mechanical receptors. At present, there seems to be no way of proving exactly what events occur with manipulation, although it appears to be successful in a large number of patients suffering from SI dysfunction. How this manipulation prevents recurrence is not explained by any of the advocates. This whole issue remains puzzling and, at this point, unmeasurable.

As noted above, the alternative to manipulation is stabilization. Stabilization can be achieved by orthotic devices, stimulation to ligamentous repair, dynamic stabilization due to enhanced motor muscle function, and finally stabilization with fusion.

The use of orthotic devices, such as an SI belt, has been demonstrated to be effective, especially in pregnancy (Vleeming et al 1992). This stabilization requires minimal force, and it has been demonstrated in cadavers that the motion of the SIJ can be reduced by an average of 30%. A more profound method of stabilization is the use of external fixation, as reported by Sturesson et al (1989). In this situation, an external Hoffman–Slatis frame was externally fixed to the iliac crests. This equipment was useful in reducing SIJ range from a maximum 2.4° down to 0.7°. It was a predictor for successful fusion in three out of four patients (Sturesson 1992).

A less drastic maneuver is the use of a stimulus to repair. In the Bernard and Cassidy study noted earlier, steroid injection offered relief for at least 9 months in 91% of cases. About 10% required repeat injections. The assumption, of course, is that there was reactive inflammation that was diminished by the steroids. No comparative studies exist, however, as to efficacy compared with other methods of care, specifically of the SIJ. It is recognized, however, that steroids have the adverse effect of reducing the potential for healing.

This concept has actually been proposed since the 1950s, when Hackett (1958) advocated the use of injections to strengthen tendons and ligaments. This treatment has gained various degrees of support by clinicians treating soft tissue pain. In a prospective double-blinded comparative series that did not break its code until 6 months after the conclusion of treatment, proliferant injections were found to be more effective than local anesthetic (Kline et al 1993). In a more specific study, which included both the injection of proliferant and flexion self-manipulation, a series of eight patients documented consistent pain improvement, as well as there being an objective definition of the maintenance of correct alignment. An inclinometer developed by Dorman compared the orientation of the ilium to the sacrum in the symptomatic side with that in the non-involved side. The accuracy of the inclinometer method had been previously documented in students (La Course et al 1990). The documentation of the efficacy of proliferant injections has presented with positive results both historically and biomechanically, when tested in rabbit medial collateral ligaments (Liu et al 1983). No adverse events have been reported from the injection of proliferants into ligamentous tissues.

A much more attractive approach to enhancing the competence of the SIJ is a progressive strengthening program. The reason for this is intuitively understandable and it has the potential for measurement. The rationale for muscle strengthening is based on the relationship of the latissimus dorsi and obliques on one side contrasted with the gluteus maximus on the other side by way of a posterior layer of the lumbodorsal fascia (Vleeming et al 1992). To document the reality of the anatomic relationship, recent myoelectric studies have been undertaken to demonstrate this in the normal individual. While walking, the reciprocal relationship can be easily demonstrated. However, when there is no rotation of the pelvis contrasted with the walking situation, one can still demonstrate the reciprocal relationship using specialized equipment that appropriately isolates torso rotation while the pelvis is fixed (MedX, Ocala, FL, USA). Using this equipment, myoelectric relationships can be demonstrated, once again confirming the reciprocal relationship (Mooney 1995). In an individual with proven SI dysfunction confirmed by physical examination, as well as by provocation and relief with radiographically controlled SI injections, hyperactivity of the gluteus musculature has been noted (Fig. 2.11). However, with strengthening and a progressive isotonic training, an associated reduction in pain occurs and decrease in myoelectric activity of the gluteus with increase in that of the latissimus dorsi is noted. On the basis of this, it is felt that a rational treatment program should be tried, to enhance the closure created by the reciprocal action of the latissimus dorsi on one side and the gluteus maximus on the other side, with enhanced activity of the oblique musculature. Strengthening of the torso rotator musculature is thus justified.

The definitive stabilization, of course, is SI fusion. Only recently has it re-emerged as a

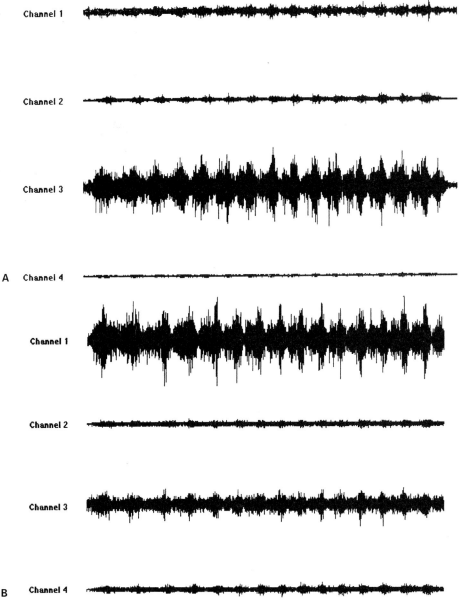

Fig. 2.11 (A) Channel 3 indicates myoelectric activity of the gluteus while in a fixed sitting position during right rotation for an individual with a painful SIJ on the right. Reciprocal activity of the left latissimus dorsi is noted in channel 1. (B) Reduced myoelectric activity of the gluteus maximus is noted after training (and reduction in pain), while the reciprocal left latissimus dorsi has now become hyperactive in its role as a stabilizer of the right SIJ.

potential treatment mode. For many years, it was ignored on the assumption that disc surgery and associated lumbar fusions would resolve the problem. There may actually even be some question of whether fusion to achieve symptomatic stabilization is necessary. Lippitt has presented a series of 23 patients with isolated SI dysfunction, of whom 48% obtained complete symptomatic relief by transfixing the SIJ with three percutaneous screws. In this series, only 3 out of the 23 patients had no relief at all (Lippitt 1995), and there was no incidence of infection, screw breakage, or screw

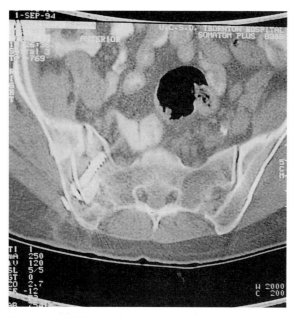

Fig. 2.12 CAT scan demonstration of screw fixation in the bone block technique of Smith-Peterson. This represents a solid SI fusion.

backing-out. This is a unique experience, and all other surgical approaches point to the need for a solid bony fusion.

The most extensive series reported so far is that of Moore (1995). In this study of 38 patients, 35 were available for follow-up of a median of 20 months. The workers' compensation patients reported on average improvement of 32%, while those not receiving compensation reported an average improvement of 61%. There were four pseudarthroses. This methodology used a threaded fuse fixation with a modification of the bone block technique first described by Smith-Peterson and Rogers (1926) in a series of 26 cases (Fig. 2.12). Another recent study by Waisbroad et al (1987) has a similar success rate in a similar number of patients.

CONCLUSIONS

1. The reality of pain emanating from the SIJ is now well established.
2. Physical tests are not consistently reliable. At present, the most significant diagnostic event is radiographically controlled injection into the SIJ.
3. Most individuals, even with this definition, will respond to non-surgical methods of care. Methods of care are, however, quite varied and cross several specialty boundaries.
4. Ultimately, however, a small number of patients will require fusion, which does not result in universal success, but gives a level of benefit equal to that of other spine fusion treatments for the painful spine.

REFERENCES

Albee F H 1909 A study of the anatomy and the clinical importance of the sacroiliac joint. Journal of the American Medical Association 53(16): 1273–1276

Bernard T N, Cassidy J D 1991 The sacroiliac joint syndrome: pathophysiology, diagnosis and management. In: Frymoyer J W (ed.) The adult spine, principles and practice. Raven Press, New York, pp 2107–2130

Bernard T N, Kirkaldy-Willis W H 1987 Recognizing specific characteristics of non specific low back pain. Clinical Orthopaedics 217: 266–280

Bowen V, Cassidy J D 1981 Macroscopic and microscopic anatomy of the sacroiliac joint from embryologic life until eighth decade. Spine 6: 620–628

Cassidy J B, Kirkaldy-Willis W H, MacGregor M 1985 Spinal manipulation for the treatment of chronic low back and leg pain: an observational study. In: Berger A A, Greenman P E (eds) Empirical approaches to the validation of spinal manipulation. Charles C Thomas, Springfield, IL, pp 119–148

Cibulka M T, Delitto A, Erhard R E 1992 Pain patterns in patients with and without sacroiliac joint dysfunction. In: Vleeming A, Mooney V, Snijders C J, Dorman T (eds) First interdisciplinary world congress on low back pain and its relation to the sacroiliac joint. San Diego, CA, 5–6 November, pp 110–112

DonTigny R L 1990 Anterior dysfunction of the sacroiliac joint as a major factor in the ideology of idiopathic low back pain. Physical Therapy 70: 250–265

Dreyfuss P, Dreyer S, Griffin J, et al 1992 Positive sacroiliac screening test in asymptomatic adults – a prospective blinded study. In: Vleeming A, Mooney V, Snijders C J, Dorman T (eds) First interdisciplinary congress on low back pain and its relation to the sacroiliac joint. San Diego, CA, 5–6 November, pp 190–192

Fast A, Shapiro D, Ducommune J, et al 1987 Low back pain in pregnancy. Spine 12: 368–371

Fortin J D, Dwyer A P, West S, Pier J 1994a Sacroiliac joint: pain referral maps upon applying a new injection/arthrography technique. Part I. Spine 19: 1475–1482

Fortin J D, Aprill C N, Ponthieux B, Pier J 1994b Sacroiliac joint: pain referral maps upon applying a new injection arthrography technique. Part II: Clinical evaluation. Spine 19: 1483–1489

Frymoyer J W, Howel G, Kuhlman D 1978 The long term effects of spinal fusion on the sacroiliac joints and ilium.

Clinical Orthopaedics 134: 196–201

Goldthwait J E, Osgood R B 1905 A consideration of the pelvic articulations from the anatomic and pathologic and clinical standpoint. Boston Medical and Surgical Journal 152: 293–601

Greenman P E, Tate B 1988 Structural diagnosis in chronic low back pain. Manual of Medicine 3: 114–117

Gunterberg B, Romanus B, Steiner B 1976 Pelvic strength after major amputation of the sacrum – an experimental study. Acta Orthopaedica Scandinavica 47: 635–642

Hackett G S 1958 Ligament and tendon relaxation treated by prolotherapy, 3rd edn. Charles C Thomas, Springfield, IL, pp 1–151

Hirsch C, Ingelmark B-E, Miller M 1963 The anatomic basis for low back pain. Acta Orthopaedica Scandinavica 33: 1–17

Inman V T, Saunders J C 1944 Referred pain from skeletal structures. Journal of Nervous and Mental Disorders 99: 660–667

Jamich E R, Moore M R, Odom J A 1995 Incidence of sacroiliac arthropathy in patients with previous lumbar spine surgery. Proceedings North American Spine Society, Washington DC p 76

Kline R G, Eek B C, DeLong W B, Mooney V 1993 A randomized double blind trial of dextrose–glycerine–phenol injections for chronic low back pain. Journal of Spinal Disorders 6: 23–33

Kristiansson P 1995 Relaxin – a marker for back pain during pregnancy. In: Vleeming A, Mooney V, Dorman T, Snijders C J (eds) Second interdisciplinary world congress on low back pain. San Diego, CA, 9–11 November, pp 203–208

LaCourse M, Moore C, Davis K, Fune M, Dorman T 1990 A report on the asymmetry of iliac inclinations. Journal of Orthopaedic Medicine 12: 69–72

Lamb D W 1979 The neurology of spinal pain. Physical Therapy 59: 971–973

Laslett M, Williams M 1994 The reliability of selected pain provocation tests for sacroiliac joint pathology. Spine 19: 1243–1249

Lippitt A B 1995 Percutaneous fixation of the sacroiliac joint. In: Vleeming A, Mooney V, Dorman T, Snijders C J (eds) Second interdisciplinary world congress on low back pain. San Diego, CA, 9–11 November, pp 369–392

Liu U K, Tipton C N, Mattes R D, et al 1983 An in situ study of the influence of an erosing solution in rabbit medial collateral ligaments and junction strength. Connective Tissue Research 11: 95–102

Mens J M A, Stam H J, Stoeckart R, Vleeming A, Snijders C J 1992 Peripartum pelvic pain: a report of the analysis of an inquiry among patients of a Dutch patients' society in low back pain and its relationship to sacroiliac joint. In: Vleeming A, Mooney V, Snijders C J, Dorman T (eds) First interdisciplinary world congress on low back pain and its relation to the sacroiliac joint. San Diego, CA, 5–6 November, pp 521–533

Mens J M A, Vleeming A, Snijders C J, Stam H J 1995 Active straight leg raising. A clinical approach to the load transfer function of the pelvic girdle. In: Vleeming A, Mooney V, Dorman T, Snijders C J (eds) Second interdisciplinary world congress on low back pain. San Diego, CA, 9–11 November, pp 205–208

Miller J A, Schultz A B, Andersson J B 1987 Load displacement behavior of the sacroiliac joints. Journal of Orthopaedic Research 5: 92–101

Mooney V 1995 Evaluation and treatment of sacroiliac

dysfunction in the integrated function of lumbosacral and lumbar spine and sacroiliac joint. In: Vleeming A, Mooney V, Dorman T, Snijders C J (eds) Second interdisciplinary world congress on low back pain. San Diego, CA, 9–11 November, pp 391–396

Mooney V, Robertson J 1976 The facet syndrome. Clinical Orthopaedics 115: 149–156

Moore M R 1995 Diagnosis and surgical treatment of chronic painful sacroiliac dysfunction. In: Vleeming A, Mooney V, Dorman T, Snijders C J (eds) Second interdisciplinary world congress on low back pain. San Diego, CA, 9–11 November, pp 339–345

Östgaard A C, Zetherstron G, Roos-Whansson E, Svanberg B 1990 Reduction of back pain and posterior pelvic pain in pregnancy. Spine 19: 894–900

Östgaard A C, Andersson G B J, Karlsson K 1991 Prevalence of back pain in pregnancy. Spine 16: 549–552

Potter N A, Rothstein J M 1985 Intertester reliability for selected clinical tests of the sacroiliac joint. Physical Therapy 65: 1671–1675

Quebec Task Force on Spinal Disorders 1987 Scientific approach to the assessment and management of activity related spinal disorders: a monograph for clinicians. Report of the Quebec Task Force on Spinal Disorders. Spine 12: S1–S59

Schwarzer A C, Aprill C N, Bogduk K 1995 The sacroiliac joint in chronic low back pain. Spine 20: 31–37

Selvik G 1974 A roentgen stereophotogrammetric method for the study of the kinematics of the skeletal system. AV-Centralen, Lund, Sweden

Smith-Peterson M N, Rogers W A 1926 End result of arthrodesis of sacroiliac joint for arthritis – traumatic and non traumatic. Journal of Joint and Bone Surgery (US) 8: 118–136

Solonen K A 1957 The sacroiliac joint in the light of anatomical roentgenological and clinical findings. Acta Orthopaedica Scandinavica Supplement 27: 1–127

Steindler A 1938 Differential diagnosis of pain low in the back: allocation by source of pain by procaine hydrochloride method. Journal of the American Medical Association 110: 106–113

Sturesson B 1992 Mobility of the pelvis measured in living persons. In: Vleeming A, Mooney V, Snijders C J, Dorman T (eds) First interdisciplinary world congress on low back pain and its relation to the sacroiliac joint. San Diego, CA, 5–6 November, pp 58–60

Sturesson B, Selvick G, Uden A 1989 Movements of the sacroiliac joints: a roentgonographic stereophotogrammetric study. Spine 14: 162–165

VanDuersen L L J M, Pitiji N, Ockhuysen L, Vortman B J 1990 The value of some clinical tests of the sacroiliac joint. Journal of Manual Medicine 5: 96–99

Vleeming A, Van Wingerden J P, Snijders C J et al 1989 Load application of the sacrotuberous ligament: influences on sacroiliac joint mechanics. Clinical Biomechanics 4: 203–205

Vleeming A, Stoeckart R, Volkers C W, Snijders C J 1990 Relation between form and function in the sacroiliac joint. Part I: Clinical anatomic aspects. Spine 15: 130–132

Vleeming A, Volkers A C, Snijders C J, Stoeckart R 1990 Relationship between form and function of the sacroiliac joint. Part II: Biomechanical aspects. Spine 15: 133–136

Vleeming A, Buyruk M, Stoeckart R 1992 A study of the biomechanical effects of pelvic belts. American Journal of Obstetrics and Gynecology 162: 535–543

Vleeming A, Pool-Goudzwaard A L, Stoeckart R, Van Wingerden J P, Snijders C J 1995 The posterior layer of the thoracic lumbar fascia – its function in load transfer from spine to legs. Spine 20: 753–758

Vleeming A, Pool-Goudzwaard A L, Hammudoghlu H D, Stoeckart R, Snijders C J, Mens J M A 1996 The function of the long dorsal sacroiliac ligament: its implications for understanding low back pain. Spine 21 (5): 556–562

Waisbroad H, Krainic J U, Gerbershagen H U 1987 Sacroiliac joint arthrodesis for chronic low back pain. Archives of Orthopaedic and Traumatic Surgery 106: 2–38

Weisl H 1954 The articular surfaces of the sacroiliac joint and the relationship to the movements of the sacrum. Acta Anatomica (Basel) 22: 1–14

Weisl H 1955 The movements of the sacroiliac joint. Acta Anatomica (Basel) 23: 80–91

3. The role of the sacroiliac joints in coupling between spine, pelvis, legs and arms

A. Vleeming   C. J. Snijders   R. Stoeckart   J. M. A. Mens

INTRODUCTION

Musculoskeletal disorders, particularly low back pain, are very expensive for modern society. The causes of low back pain are not well understood, and therapy frequently fails. Appropriate models to explain non-specific low back pain are not available.

In the 1970s we studied a group of pregnant women and noticed flattening of the lumbar spine in normal erect standing (Snijders et al 1976). This was surprising, since low back pain experienced during pregnancy was generally thought to be due to hollowing of the lumbar spine. Obviously, hollowing of the lumbar spine cannot explain the low back pain which is frequently experienced during pregnancy. Low back pain during pregnancy is categorized as non-specific low back pain, which simply means that its cause is unknown. In fact, this diagnosis holds for approximately 80% of all patients with low back pain! It seems justified to assert that in most low back pain patients, the etiology is obscure. We wondered whether a new approach, based on functional anatomy, could lead to a better understanding of the usual severe and enduring pains experienced by these patients.

When starting the research project, we were hampered by our knowledge, which was mainly based on topographic anatomy. This branch of anatomy has been developed to map the body, to answer the question of what structures our body consists of, and to categorize them. The use of topographic anatomy is not satisfactory for answering complex questions such as 'Why are there so many low back pain patients?' and 'How do the spine, pelvis, and legs function as an integrated system?' In fact, categories such as 'spine' and 'pelvis' are already confusing. 'Spine' muscles are strongly connected to the pelvis and to the ligaments around the sacroiliac joints (SIJs). The SIJs are the joints between the sacrum and left and right iliac bones, which are part of the pelvis. Officially, pelvic joints and ligaments are classified as belonging to the legs. Classifications such as 'legs', 'pelvis' and 'spine' may serve a didactic purpose, but they impede our understanding of the mechanisms operating in this region.

In scrutinizing the literature on spine and pelvis, our attention was triggered by the studies of the American therapist DonTigny, and of Bowen and Cassidy. DonTigny (1979) consistently reported that the SIJs are essential for understanding spinal function, while Bowen and Cassidy (1981) described a peculiar cartilage pattern of the human SIJ. However, the literature did not give additional clues to understanding the mechanisms that may lead to non-specific low back pain.

A commercial device used in painting ceilings helped us to conceive the concept of the SIJ

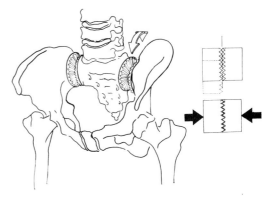

Fig. 3.1 Whimsical depiction of SIJs with friction device.

functioning as a friction joint (Fig. 3.1). This was, of course, scientific heresy since the main characteristic of a joint is its capacity to function smoothly. Twelve years later, however, there is ample evidence for the view that the SIJs function as friction joints. This concept initiated a fundamental change in our thinking about stabilizing mechanisms of the human body in rest and during movement. Now we are beginning to understand how stability of the pelvis is warranted by a coupled function of spine, pelvis, legs, and even arms. We will consider the implications for diverse situations such as standing, sitting, walking, and forceful trunk rotation. Finally, we will deal with the implications for low back pain.

GENERAL OUTLINE OF THE CONNECTIONS BETWEEN SPINE AND PELVIS

In all quadrupeds and bipeds, the pelvic girdle forms a firm connection between spine and lower extremity. To enhance stability, the sacral vertebrae have been fused into one bone, the sacral part of the SIJ. To allow bipedal gait in humans, specific adaptations of the pelvis are requested, for example a dramatically increased attachment site for the gluteus maximus muscle. Lovejoy (1988) states, 'The need to stabilize an upright torso dictated the most dramatic change in musculature that has come with the adoption of bipedality; the transformation of the gluteus maximus, a relatively minor muscle in the chimpanzee, into the largest muscle of the human body.'

Besides muscular connections, extensive fibrous connections exist between sacrum and pelvis (interosseous ligaments, surrounding an iliac protrusion fitting in a dorsal sacral cavity [Bakland & Hansen 1984], ventral and dorsal SIJ ligaments, sacrotuberous and sacrospinous ligaments) and between sacrum and lumbar spine (longitudinal ligaments). In addition, a direct fibrous connection, the iliolumbar ligament, exists between the iliac bone and L4 and L5. Owing to these connections, any movement of the sacrum with respect to the iliac bones also affects the joints between L5 and S1 and between the higher lumbar levels.

As a consequence of the tightness of the fibrous connections and the specific architecture

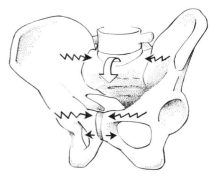

Fig. 3.2 Nutation in the SIJ. The iliac bones are pulled to each other due to ligament tension (among others) and compress the SIJs (upper black arrows). It can be expected that especially the upper (anterior) part of the pubic symphysis is compressed.

of the SIJ, mobility in the SIJ is normally very limited, but movement does occur (Egund et al 1978, Lavignolle et al 1983, Miller et al 1987, Solonen 1957, Sturesson et al 1989, Vleeming et al 1992a, Weisl 1955). The main movements are forward tilting of the sacrum relative to the iliac bones (nutation; Fig. 3.2) and backward tilting (counternutation). We could show that, even in old age (over 72 years), the combined movement of nutation and counternutation can amount to 4°. The SIJ with the lowest mobility showed radiologically marked arthrosis (Vleeming 1990). Ankylosis of the SIJ was found to be an exception, even at a great age. This is in agreement with studies of Stewart (1984) and Miller et al (1987).

In standing, nutation is increased, particularly in case of hollowing of the lower back (lordosis) (Egund et al 1978, Sturesson et al 1989, Weisl 1955). Counternutation occurs in unloaded situations such as lying down (supine or prone) and increases in situations when the lumbar spine is flattened. Counternutation in supine positions can be altered by maximal flexion in the hips, as in a labor position.

THE SELF-LOCKING MECHANISM OF THE SIJ

The SIJs are relatively flat, unlike ball and socket joints such as the hip. Flat articular surfaces are vulnerable for shear forces and therefore the presence of flat surfaces in the pelvis is surprising. Two questions arise: (1) why did nature·create relatively instable, flat SIJs and (2) what specific adaptations are available to prevent shear in these joints?

As far as the first question is concerned, a large transfer of forces is required in the human SIJ; indeed, flat joints are well suited to transfer large bending forces (Snijders et al 1993a, 1993b; see also Chapter 6 in this volume). An alternative for effective load transfer by these flat joints would be a fixed connection between sacrum and iliac bones, for example by ankylosis of the SIJ. In fact, such ankylosed joints do occur in light-weight bipeds such as birds (owls for instance). Obviously, the flat SIJ of humans serves a purpose: to economize gait, to allow shock absorption, and to alleviate the birth of – in evolutionary terms – abnormally large babies.

In relation to the second question, the SIJs are quite abnormal. The articular cartilage is already extraordinary before birth. In contrast to normal synovial joints, the cartilaginous surface is not smooth. Several authors have described cartilage changes, especially at the iliac side of the joint. They were interpreted as evidence for degenerative arthrosis (Bowen & Cassidy 1981, Sashin 1930). These modifications of the cartilage are more prominent in men than in women. The gender difference may be related to childbearing and possibly to another localization of the center of gravity in relation to the SIJ (Dijkstra et al 1992, Vleeming et al 1990a, 1990b). It should be expected that these 'arthrotic' changes cause pain or sacroiliac (SI) problems, especially in older men. This is not the case; we consider that these modifications reflect a functional adaptation. These features seem to be promoted by the increase in body weight during the pubertal growth spurt. They concern coarse cartilage texture (Fig. 3.3) and a wedge and propeller-like form of the joint surface (Fig. 3.4). By studying frontal slides of intact joints of embalmed specimens, we could furthermore show the presence of cartilage-covered bone extensions protruding into the joint. They seemed irregular, but are in fact complementary ridges and grooves. All these features are expected to increase friction, reflecting the adaptation to human bipedality. As a consequence, less muscle and ligament force is required to bear the upper part of the body.

To verify the idea of a friction joint, a device was developed to study friction in the SIJ (Vleeming et al 1990b). Indeed, joint samples taken from normal SIJ, with both coarse texture and complementary ridges and grooves, were characterized by the highest friction coefficients. Friction was considerably higher when compared with cartilage samples of the knee.

Form and force closure

To illustrate the importance of friction in the SIJ, we introduced the principles of form and force closure (Vleeming et al 1990b). Form closure refers to a stable situation with closely fitting joint surfaces, in which no extra forces are needed to maintain the state of the system, given the actual load situation. If the sacrum would fit in the pelvis with perfect form closure, no lateral forces would be needed. However, such a construction would make mobility practically impossible. With force closure, both a lateral force and friction are needed to withstand vertical load. Shear in the SIJ is prevented by the combination of the specific anatomic features (form closure) and the compression generated by muscles and ligaments that can be accommodated to the specific loading situation (force closure).

We termed this shear prevention system, characterized by the combination of form and force closure, the self-locking mechanism (Fig. 3.5). It might well be that the self-locking mechanism is not unique for the SIJ. Mechanisms comparable to self-locking may be present elsewhere in the body, for example in the calcaneocuboid connection (Bojsen–Møller & Lamoreux 1979).

Ligaments

In self-locking the pelvis, nutation of the SIJ is crucial. Nutation winds up most SIJ ligaments, among them the vast interosseous ligaments. They are located between sacrum and iliac bones, directly posterior to the main articular surfaces. Due to tension of the interosseous (and short dorsal SI) ligaments, the posterior parts of the iliac bones are pulled together. This heightens compression of the SIJ.

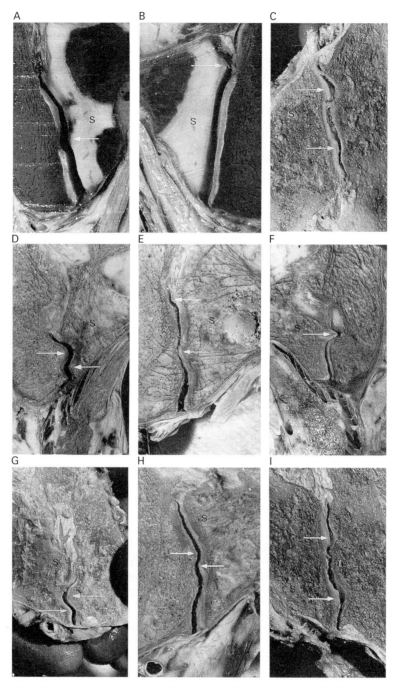

Fig. 3.3 Frontal sections of the SIJ of embalmed male specimens. S indicates the sacral side of the SIJ. (A) and (B) concern a 12-year-old boy. (C–I) concern specimens over 60 years of age. Arrows are directed at complementary ridges and depressions. They are covered by intact cartilage, as was confirmed by subsequently opening the joints.

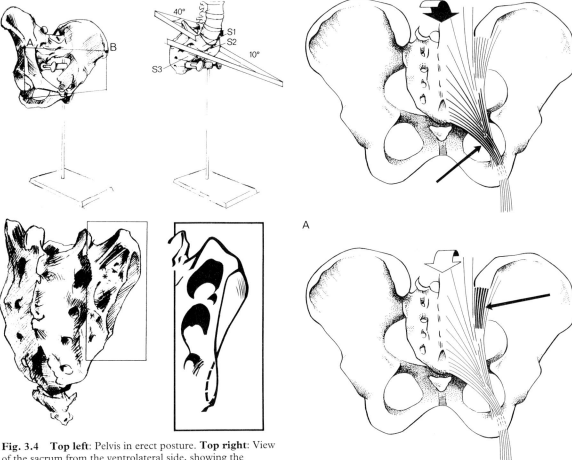

Fig. 3.4 **Top left**: Pelvis in erect posture. **Top right**: View of the sacrum from the ventrolateral side, showing the different angles between left and right sacral articular surface. **Bottom left**: Dorsolateral view of the sacrum. *indicates a cavity in the sacrum into which an iliac tubercle fits. **Bottom right**: Schema of the sacral articular surface at the right side. The different angles reflect the propeller-like shape of an adult SIJ.

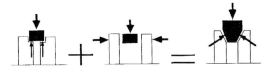

Fig. 3.5 Model of the self-locking mechanism: the combination of form closure and force closure establishes stability in the SIJ.

For several reasons, two sets of ligaments (Fig. 3.6) merit special attention in self-locking of the pelvis: the sacrotuberous ligaments (Vleeming et al 1989a, 1989b, van Wingerden et al 1993) and the long dorsal SI ligaments (Vleeming et al

Fig. 3.6 (A) Nutation winds up the sacrotuberous ligament. (B) Counternutation the long dorsal SI ligament.

1996). In the literature, specific data on the functional and clinical relevance of the long ligaments are not available. In several anatomic atlases and textbooks, the long ligament and the sacrotuberous ligament are portrayed as fully continuous ligaments. The drawings generally convey the impression that the ligaments have identical functions. As shown by the contrasting effects of nutation and contranutation on these ligaments (see below), this is not the case. Essentially, the long ligament connects the sacrum and posterior superior iliac spine (PSIS), whereas the main part of the sacrotuberous ligament connects the sacrum and ischial tuberosity. However, some of the fibers derived from the ischial tuberosity pass to the iliac bone. Generally, they are denoted as part of the sacrotuberous ligament, although 'tuberoiliac ligament' would be more appropriate. In the 'Nomina Anatomica', such a ligament does not exist. In fact, this also holds for the long (dorsal SI) ligament, reflecting one of the problems of topographical anatomy.

Sacrotuberous ligaments. In our embalmed human specimens, we could demonstrate a direct relation between nutation and tension of the sacrotuberous ligament (Fig. 3.6A). By straining this ligament, we found a decrease of nutation. This is particularly due to increasing the bone contact force and increasing the compression of the joint (Vleeming et al 1989a, 1989b). It can be expected that the opposite (diminished ligament tension) will increase nutation. Obviously, the sacrotuberous ligaments are well suited to restrict nutation.

Long dorsal SI ligaments. In view of the role of the sacrotuberous ligaments in restricting nutation, we wondered which ligament(s) could restrict counternutation. Because of its connection to the PSIS and to the lateral part of the sacrum (Fig. 3.6B), we expected that the long dorsal SI ligament could fulfill this function. The ligament can be easily palpated in the area directly caudal to the PSIS. This ligament is of special interest since women complaining of instability and lower back pain during pregnancy frequently experience pain within the boundaries of this ligament (Mens et al 1992, Njoo 1996). Men also regularly indicate pain in this area. Since, surprisingly, this ligament is not well known in medical practice, we will provide data obtained in an anatomic and biomechanic study (Vleeming et al 1996). The object of that study was to assess the function of the ligament by measuring its tension during incremental loading of biomechanically relevant structures.

For that purpose, the tension of the long dorsal SI ligament ($n = 12$) was tested under loading. Tension was measured with a buckle transducer. Several structures, including the erector spinae muscle, the posterior layer of the thoracolumbar fascia, the sacrotuberous ligament, and the sacrum, were incrementally loaded (with forces of 0–50 N). The sacrum was loaded in two directions, causing nutation (ventral rotation of the sacrum relative to the iliac bones) and counternutation (the reverse).

Anatomical aspects At the cranial side, the long ligament is attached to the PSIS and the adjacent part of the ilium, at the caudal side to the lateral crest of the third and fourth sacral segments. In some specimens, fibers also pass to the fifth sacral segment. From the sites of attachment on the sacrum, fibers pass to the coccyx. These are not considered to be part of the long ligament.

The lateral expansion of the long ligament directly caudal to the PSIS varies between 15 and 30 mm. The length, measured between the PSIS and the third and fourth sacral segments, varies between 42 and 75 mm. The lateral part of the long ligament is continuous with fibers passing between ischial tuberosity and iliac bone. The variation is wide. Medial fibers of the long ligament are connected to the deep lamina of the posterior layer of the thoracolumbar fascia and to the aponeurosis of the erector spinae muscle. After dissection of the erector spinae aponeurosis, the connections between ligament and fibers of the multifidus muscle become visible.

Biomechanical aspects Forced nutation in the SIJ diminished the tension, whereas forced counternutation increased the tension. Tension in the long dorsal SI ligament increased during loading of the ipsilateral sacrotuberous ligament and erector spinae muscle. The tension decreased during traction on the gluteus maximus muscle. Tension also decreased during traction on the ipsilateral and contralateral posterior layer of the thoracolumbar fascia in a direction simulating contraction of the latissimus dorsi muscle.

Obviously, the long dorsal SI ligament has close anatomic relations with the erector spinae muscle, the posterior layer of the thoracolumbar fascia, and a specific part of the sacrotuberous ligament (tuberoiliac ligament). Functionally, it is an important link between legs, spine, and arms. The ligament is tensed when the SIJs are counternutated and slackened when nutated. Slackening of the long dorsal SI ligament can be counterbalanced by both the sacrotuberous ligament and the erector spinae muscle.

Pain localized within the boundaries of the long ligament could indicate, among other things, a spinal condition with sustained counternutation of the SIJ. In diagnosing patients with a specific lower back pain or peripartum pelvic pain, the long dorsal SI ligament should not be neglected. Even in cases of arthrodesis of the SIJ, tension in the long ligament can still be altered by different structures.

This observation implies that the tension of the long ligament can be altered by displacement of the SIJ as well as by action of various muscles. Obviously, nutation in the SIJ induces relaxation of the long ligament, whereas counternutation increases tension. This is in contrast to the effect on the sacrotuberous ligament: nutation leads to increase of tension, counternutation to relaxation (Fig. 3.6). Increased tension in the sacrotuberous ligament during nutation can be due to SI movement itself as well as to increased tension of the biceps femoris and/or gluteus maximus muscle. This mechanism can help to *control nutation*. Since counternutation increases tension in the long ligament, this ligament can assist in *controlling counternutation* (Fig. 3.6).

Ligaments with opposite functions, such as the long and sacrotuberous ligaments, apparently do not interact in a simple way. After all, loading of the sacrotuberous ligament leads to increased tension of the long ligament. This effect will be due to the connections between long ligament and tuberoiliac ligament and possibly also to a counternutating force generated by the loading of the sacrotuberous ligament.

A comparable complex relation may hold for the long ligament and the erector spinae, or more specifically the multifidus muscle. Since the multifidus is connected to the sacrum (MacIntosh & Bogduk 1986, 1991; see also Chapter 1 in this volume), its action induces nutation. As a result, the long ligament will slacken. However, the present study shows an increase of tension in the long ligament after traction to the erector spinae muscle. This counterbalancing effect is due to the connections between the erector spinae muscle and the long ligament, and opposes the slackening. In vivo this effect may be smaller because the moment of force acting on the sacrum is raised by the pull of the erector spinae muscle and the resulting compression force on the spine (Snijders et al 1993b). This spinal compression was not applied in this study. Both antagonistic mechanisms – between long and sacrotuberous ligaments

and between the long ligament and the erector spinae muscle – may serve to preclude extensive slackening of the long ligament. Such mechanisms could be essential for a flat joint such as the SIJ, which is susceptible to shear forces (Snijders et al 1993a, 1993b). It can be safely assumed that impairment of a part of this interconnected ligament system will have serious implications for the joint since load transfer from spine to hips and vice versa is primarily transferred via the SIJ (Snijders et al 1993a, 1993b).

As also shown in that study, traction to the biceps femoris tendon hardly influences tension of the long ligament. This is in contrast to the effect of the biceps on the sacrotuberous ligament (Vleeming et al 1989a, 1989b, van Wingerden et al 1993). The observations may well be related to the spiraling of the sacrotuberous ligament. Most medial fibers of the ligament tend to attach to the cranial part of the sacrum, whereas most fibers arising from a lateral part of the ischial tuberosity tend to the caudal part of the sacrum (Fig. 3.6A). The fibers of the biceps tendon, which approach a relatively lateral part of the ischial tuberosity, mainly pass to the caudal part of the sacrum. As a consequence, the effect of traction to the biceps femoris on the tension of the long ligament can only be limited.

Obviously, the effect on the long ligament of loading the posterior layer of the thoracolumbar fascia depends on the direction of the forces applied. Traction to the fascia mimicking the action of the transverse abdominal muscle has no effect. Traction in a craniolateral direction, mimicking the action of the latissimus dorsi muscle, results in a significant decrease in tension of the ipsilateral and contralateral ligament. As shown in another study (Vleeming et al 1995), traction to the latissimus dorsi influences the tension in the posterior layer of the thoracolumbar fascia, ipsilaterally as well as contralaterally, especially below the level of L4. Thus slackening of the long ligament could be the result of increased tension in the posterior layer by the latissimus dorsi. This may itself lead to a slight nutation, which probably leads to more effective compression and force closure of the SIJ. As shown in this study, slackening of the long ligament can also occur due to action of the gluteus maximus muscle, which is ideally suited to compress the SIJ.

It is inviting to draw prompt conclusions when palpation of the long ligament directly caudal to the PSIS is painful. This must be avoided for the following reason. Pain in this area may be due to pain referred from the SIJ itself (Fortin et al 1994a, 1994b), but also to counternutation of the SIJ. Counternutation is part of a pattern of flattening the lumbar spine (Egund et al 1978, Lavignolle et al 1983, Sturesson et al 1989) that especially occurs late in pregnancy when women counterbalance the weight of the fetus (Snijders et al 1976). However, such a posture combined with counternutation could also result from a pain withdrawal reaction to impairment elsewhere in the system. Hence, even specific pain of the long ligament could be a side-effect. An example of such a condition could be the following. Pain of the pubic symphysis following delivery (Mens et al 1992) could preclude normal lumbar lordosis and hence nutation owing to pain of an irritated symphysis. After all, lumbar lordosis leads to nutation in the SIJ (Egund et al 1978, Lavignolle et al 1983, Sturesson et al 1989, Weisl 1955). Nutation implies that the left and right PSISs approach each other slightly while the pubic symphysis is caudally extended and cranially compressed (Lavignolle et al 1983, Walheim & Selvik 1984). In this example the patient will avoid nutation and flattens the lower spine, leading to sustained tension and pain in the long ligament. It seems justified to conclude that when palpation of the long ligament is painful, one must examine whether extension of the lower spine and nutation in the SIJ is possible.

In conclusion, the long ligament, which can be easily palpated in the area directly caudal to the PSIS, can be viewed anatomically, as a pelvic structure. However, the ligament has close relations with, among others, the erector spinae muscle, the posterior layer of the thoracolumbar fascia, and the sacrotuberous ligament. Therefore, it is functionally an important link between legs, spine, and arms. The long ligament is tensed when the SIJ are counternutated and slackened when they are nutated. During nutation, both the erector muscle and the sacrotuberous ligament can counterbalance the slackening of the long ligament. The anatomic connections between ligaments and muscles with opposing functions could serve as a mechanism to preclude excessive slackening of ligaments.

In dealing with lower back or peripartum pelvic pain, the long ligament should not be overlooked since localized pain within the boundaries of the long ligament could indicate a spinal condition with sustained counternutation of the SIJ. However, if pain is felt not exclusively in the long ligament but also in the medial buttock region, this could be part of a typical pain referral pattern of the SIJ itself (Fortin et al 1994a, 1994b).

Before focusing on the role of the muscles, we want to draw attention to some anatomic and biomechanic aspects of the thoracolumbar fascia (Vleeming et al 1995).

Thoracolumbar fascia

In 10 embalmed human specimens, the posterior layer of the thoracolumbar fascia was loaded by simulating the action of various muscles.

Anatomical aspects   The posterior layer of the thoracolumbar fascia covers the back muscles from the sacral region, through the thoracic region as far as the fascia nuchae. At the level of L4–5 and the sacrum, strong connections exist between the superficial and deep lamina. The transverse abdominal and internal oblique muscles are indirectly attached to the thoracolumbar fascia through a dense raphe formed by fusion of the middle layer (Bogduk & MacIntosh 1984) of the thoracolumbar fascia and both laminae of the posterior layer. This 'lateral raphe' (Bogduk & MacIntosh 1984, Bogduk & Twomey 1987) is localized lateral to the erector spinae and cranial to the iliac crest.

Superficial lamina (Fig. 3.7).   The superficial lamina of the posterior layer of the thoracolumbar fascia is continuous with the latissimus dorsi, gluteus maximus, and part of the external oblique muscle of the abdomen and the trapezius muscle. Cranial to the iliac crest, the lateral border of the superficial lamina is marked by its junction with the latissimus dorsi muscle. The fibers of the superficial lamina are orientated from craniolateral to caudomedial. Only a few fibers of the superficial lamina are continuous with the apo-

At sacral levels, the superficial lamina is continuous with the fascia of the gluteus maximus. These fibers are orientated from craniomedial to caudolateral. Most of these fibers attach to the median sacral crest. However, at the level of L4–5, and in some specimens even as caudally as S1–S2, fibers *partly or completely* cross the midline, attaching to the contralateral PSIS and iliac crest. Some of these fibers fuse with the lateral raphe and with fibers derived from the fascia of the latissimus dorsi. Owing to the different fibre directions of the latissimus dorsi and the gluteus maximus, the superficial lamina has a cross-hatched appearance at the level of L4–5, and in some preparations also at L5–S2.

Deep lamina (Fig. 3.8). At lower lumbar and sacral levels, the fibers of the deep lamina are oriented from craniomedial to caudolateral. At sacral levels, these fibers are fused with those of the superficial lamina. Since in this region fibers of the deep lamina are continuous with the sacrotuberous ligament, an indirect link exists between this ligament and the superficial lamina. There is also a direct connection with some fibers of the deep lamina. In the pelvic region, the deep lamina is connected to the PSIS, iliac crests, and long dorsal SI ligament. This ligament originates from the sacrum and attaches to the PSIS. In the lumbar region, fibers of the deep lamina derive from the interspinous ligaments. They attach to the iliac crest and more cranially to the lateral raphe, to which the internal oblique is attached. In some specimens, fibers of the deep lamina cross to the contralateral side between L5 and S1. In the depression between the median sacral crest and the posterior superior and inferior iliac spines, fibers of the deep lamina fuse with the fascia of the erector. More cranially, in the lumbar region, the deep lamina becomes thinner and freely mobile over the back muscles. In the lower thoracic region, fibers of the serratus posterior inferior muscle and its fascia fuse with fibers of the deep lamina.

Biomechanical aspects
Traction to the superficial lamina. Depending on the site of the traction, quite different results were obtained. Traction to the cranial fascia and muscle fibers of the latissimus dorsi muscle showed limited displacement of the

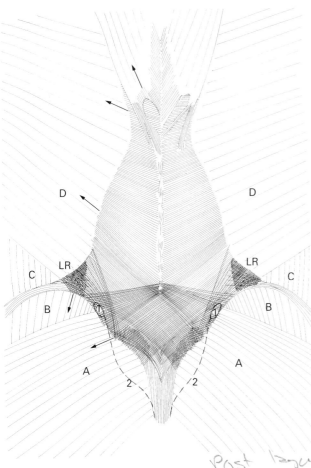

Fig. 3.7 The superficial lamina.
A, fascia of the gluteus maximus; B, fascia of the gluteus medius; C, fascia of external oblique; D, fascia of latissimus dorsi; 1, posterior superior iliac spine; 2, sacral crest; LR, part of lateral raphe. Arrows (at left) indicate, from cranial to caudal, the site and direction of the traction (50 N) given to trapezius, the cranial and caudal parts of the latissimus dorsi, gluteus medius, and gluteus maximus respectively.

neurosis of the external oblique and the trapezius. Most of the fibers of the superficial lamina derive from the aponeurosis of the latissimus dorsi and attach to the supraspinal ligaments and spinous processes cranial to L4. Caudal to L4–5, the superficial lamina is generally loosely (or not at all) attached to midline structures, such as supraspinal ligaments, spinous processes and median sacral crest. In fact, they cross to the contralateral side, where they attach to sacrum, PSIS, and iliac crest. The level at which this phenomenon occurs varies; it is generally caudal to L4 but in some preparations already occurs at L2–3.

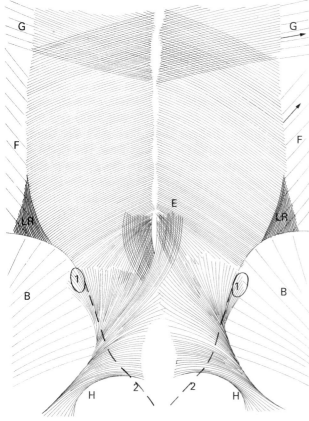

Fig. 3.8 The deep lamina.
B, fascia of the gluteus medius; E, connections between the deep lamina and the fascia of the erector spinae; F, fascia of the internal oblique; G, fascia of the serratus posterior inferior; H, sacrotuberous ligament; 1, posterior superior iliac spine; 2, sacral crest; LR, part of lateral raphe. Arrows (at right) indicate, from cranial to caudal, traction to serratus posterior inferior and internal oblique respectively.

superficial lamina (homolaterally up to 2–4 cm). Traction to the caudal part of the latissimus dorsi caused displacement up to the midline. This midline area is 8–10 cm removed from the site of traction. Between L4–5 and S1–2, displacement of the superficial lamina occurred even contra-laterally. Traction to the gluteus maximus also caused displacement up to the contralateral side. The distance between the site of traction and visible displacement varied from 4 to 7 cm. The effect of traction to the external oblique varied markedly between the different preparations. In all preparations, traction to the trapezius muscle resulted in a relatively small effect (up to 2 cm).

No effect of traction to the medial gluteal muscles was seen.

Traction to the deep lamina. Traction to the biceps femoris is tendon, applied in a lateral direction, resulted in displacement of the deep lamina up to the level L5–S1. Obviously, this load transfer is conducted by the sacrotuberous ligament. In two specimens, displacement occurred at the contralateral side, 1–2 cm away from the midline. Traction to the biceps tendon directed medially showed homolateral displacement in the deep lamina, up to the median sacral crest. Traction to the internal oblique did not result in visible displacement.

As shown by the traction tests, the tension of the posterior layer of the thoracolumbar fascia can be influenced by contraction or stretch of a variety of muscles. It is noteworthy that especially muscles such as the latissimus dorsi and gluteus maximus are able to exert a contralateral effect. This implies that the gluteus maximus muscle and contralateral latissimus dorsi muscle both tense the posterior layer. Hence, parts of these muscles provide a pathway for uninterrupted mechanical transmission between pelvis and trunk. One could argue that the lack of connection between the superficial lamina of the posterior layer and the supraspinous ligaments in the lumbar region is a disadvantage for stability. However, it would be disadvantageous only in case strength, coordination, and effective coupling of the gluteus maximus and the caudal part of the contralateral latissimus dorsi are diminished. It can be expected that an increase in strength of the mentioned muscles accomplished by torsional training could influence the quality of the posterior layer. In this theory, the posterior layer of the thoracolumbar fascia can play an integrating role in rotation of the trunk and in load transfer, and hence instability of the lower lumbar spine and pelvis.

Pelvic instability (and peripartum pain) can be relieved by application of a pelvic belt, a device that 'self-braces' the SIJ (Vleeming et al 1992b). By exerting compression on the lower lumbar spine and pelvis, the posterior layer of the thoracolumbar fascia can accomplish force closure physiologically. It is noteworthy that, as shown in this study, the coupled function of the gluteus maximus and the contralateral latissimus dorsi creates a force perpendicular to the SIJ.

Attention is drawn to a possible role of the erector muscle in load transfer. Between the lateral raphe and the interspinous ligament, the deep lamina encloses the erector muscle. It can be expected here that contraction of the erector muscle will longitudinally increase the tension in the deep lamina by pull. In addition, the whole posterior layer of the thoracolumbar fascia will be 'inflated' by contraction of the erector spinae (Vleeming et al 1995), comparable to pumping up a ball. Consequently, it can be assumed that the training of muscles such as the gluteus maximus, latissimus dorsi and erector spinae can assist in increasing force closure by strengthening the posterior layer of the thoracolumbar fascia.

In conclusion, in transferring forces between spine, pelvis, and legs, the posterior layer of the thoracolumbar fascia could play an important role, especially in rotation of the trunk and stabilization of lower lumbar spine and SIJ. The gluteus maximus and the latissimus dorsi merit special attention since they can conduct forces contralaterally, via the posterior layer. The effect of contraction of especially the latissimus dorsi will be large, since forces derived from its caudal part are fully transferred to the thoracolumbar fascia. Because of the coupling between the gluteus maximus and the contralateral latissimus dorsi muscle via the posterior layer of the thoracolumbar fascia, one must be very cautious in categorizing certain muscles as arm, spine, or leg muscles.

Muscles

Various muscles are involved in force closure of the SIJ. Four muscles are specifically important: the erector spinae, gluteus maximus, latissimus dorsi, and biceps femoris (Fig. 3.9). In 'Self-

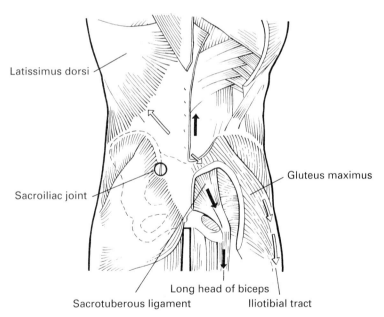

Fig. 3.9 Schematic dorsal view of the lower back. The right side shows a part of the longitudinal muscle–tendon–fascia sling. Below is the continuation between biceps femoris tendon and sacrotuberous ligament, above a continuation of biceps femoris tendon to the aponeurosis of the erector spinae. To show the right erector spinae, a part of the thoracolumbar fascia has been removed. The left side shows the sacroiliac joint (◯) and the cranial part of the oblique dorsal muscle–fascia–tendon sling: latissimus dorsi muscle and thoracolumbar fascia. In this drawing, the left part of the thoracolumbar fascia is tensed by the left latissimus dorsi and the right gluteus maximus. (Reproduced with permission from Spine)

Latissimus dorsi

Sacroiliac joint

Sacrotuberous ligament

Long head of biceps

Gluteus maximus

Iliotibial tract

locking in unconstrained positions', we will deal with the abdominal muscles.

The erector spinae is the pivotal muscle that loads and extends spine and pelvis. The sacral connection of the muscle pulls the sacrum forward, inducing nutation in the SIJ and tensing ligaments such as the interosseous, sacrotuberous and sacrospinal. The muscle has a double function since its iliac connection pulls the posterior sides of the iliac bones towards each other, constraining nutation. This implies that during nutation, due to action of the erector spinae, the cranial side of the SIJ tends to be compressed whereas the caudal side has a tendency to widen. The latter is restricted by the sacrotuberous ligament, which has direct connections with the erector spinae. A comparable process will occur in the pubic symphysis where the largest symphyseal ligament runs inferior to the joint (see Fig. 3.2).

Owing to its perpendicular orientation to the SIJ, the gluteus maximus can compress the joints directly, and also indirectly by its firm connections with the sacrotuberous ligament. We noted in a study on the thoracolumbar fascia that compression of the SIJ can be established by coupling of the gluteus maximus with the contralateral latissimus dorsi via this fascia (Fig. 3.9; see also Chapter 6 in this volume). This oblique system, whose collagenous fibers cross the spine, will be of value during rotational activities such as walking and running, and in forced rotation, as in swinging a club. Owing to the connections, the thoracolumbar fascia can be tensed directly by the erector spinae muscle and indirectly by contraction of the underlying erector muscle, 'inflating' the fascia.

In contrast to common belief, it could be shown that tension of the sacrotuberous ligament is increased by traction to the long head of the biceps femoris (in the direction of the knee). This can happen since not all fibers of the long head of the biceps attach to the ischial tuberosity: partly, and often completely, its proximal tendon is continuous with the sacrotuberous ligament (Fig. 3.9). It turned out that this tension mechanism of the biceps femoris depends on body position (van Wingerden et al 1993). In most specimens, a higher percentage of force was transferred from the biceps to the sacrotuberous ligament in a

flexed, stooped position than in an erect stance. This could be expected since the flexion torque on the lumbar spine increases when changing from an erect to a flexed stance. Consequently, in stooped positions, larger compression forces are needed to prevent the sacrum from tilting forward. This force can be derived in part from the biceps femoris muscle but also from other muscles attached to the sacrotuberous ligament (the sacral part of the erector spinae and gluteus maximus).

The biceps femoris is part of the hamstring muscles. Comparable to the erector muscle, a double function of the hamstrings can be described (see Chapter 15 in this volume). Particularly in stooped positions and in sitting with straight legs, sitting upright, the hamstrings as a group are well positioned to rotate the iliac bones backwards relative to the sacrum. This nutating effect (Sturesson et al 1989) can be constrained by the biceps femoris with its connections to the sacrotuberous ligament. Nutation in stooped positions can help to avoid excessive loading of the posterior part of the lumbar discs.

Self-locking during forward bending

The sacrum assumes a more or less horizontal position in a stooped position. When lifting objects in this posture, the vertical force from the upper part of the body and the object acts almost perpendicularly to the longitudinal axis of the sacrum. In this situation, the joint also becomes loaded in the transverse plane and stability will now depend on effective compression of the transverse diameter of the SIJ. This diameter is small in comparison with the longitudinal diameter, so additional forces are needed to protect the SIJ. In an EMG study, it was found that during lifting the activity of the gluteus maximus paralleled that of latissimus dorsi and erector spinae (Noe et al 1992). These observations may indicate that, in this position, self-locking of the pelvis can be established by contraction of these muscles.

Self-locking in unconstrained positions

The question of how the SIJ can be stabilized in unconstrained sitting and standing led to the following experiment. We expected that during unconstrained sitting, the oblique abdominal muscles particularly would be active to self-lock the pelvis. Using electromyography (EMG), the abdominal muscle activity was recorded in different positions (supine, unconstrained standing, and sitting with and without crossed legs on an office chair with the use of a backrest and armrests). For both the external and internal obliques, the activity was significantly higher in standing than in sitting. The activity of particularly the internal obliques turned out to be significantly higher in sitting than in a supine position (Fig. 3.10). Surprisingly, the activity of the oblique abdominals was lowered by crossing the legs (Snijders et al 1995; cross-legged or ankle on knee as preferred by the individual; see Fig. 3.10 above). In contrast, the activity of the rectus abdominus was not altered by leg-crossing. We concluded that to stabilize the pelvis: (1) unconstrained sitting and standing initiates an oblique ventral muscle–tendon sling (see Chapter 6 in this volume); and (2) leg-crossing is a functional habit. Crossing the legs causes rotation in the pelvis and possibly tenses the thoracolumbar fascia. Due to creep of tissues (elongation), leg-crossing is only temporarily functional; then the legs are crossed to the other side (Snijders et al 1995).

Failed self-locking

The different mechanisms that warrant stability of the SIJ can become less effective owing to decline of muscle performance and/or increased laxity of ligaments. This occurs in people withdrawing from sports, undertaking sedentary work, etc. A characteristic case could be a girl who at young age performed top level gymnastics. Through excessive training, the mobility of spine and pelvis is markedly enhanced and the girl will develop extremely strong muscles. Thus the mobile pelvis can be adequately constrained with force closure. If such an athlete abruptly terminates high-level training, the muscles rapidly decline. The muscles are no longer strong enough to effect adequate force closure, and form closure will be limited because of enlarged mobility and laxity.

Laxity of pelvic ligaments especially occurs during pregnancy. We assume that the serious impairments of patients suffering from peripartum pain are caused mainly by hypermobility of the SIJ (Mens et al 1996, Vleeming et al 1992b; see also Chapter 35 in this volume). In addition, a patient with a painful pubic symphysis will avoid nutation since nutation strains the symphysis. Consequently women will 'choose' a counter-nutated position.

One method to facilitate pelvic stability and reduce pain is the use of a pelvic belt (Mens et al 1996). In a loading experiment on embalmed human preparations, nutation of the sacrum decreased by about 20% when applying a belt force of only 50 N. Based on the biomechanical model presented here, such a belt must be applied with a small force, like the laces of a shoe. This will be sufficient to generate a self-locking effect in the SIJ under heavy load (Snijders et al 1993a, 1993b, Vleeming et al 1992a). The model indicates that the belt must be positioned just cranial to the greater trochanters; it then crosses the SIJ.

We like to emphasize that, according to our model, weakening of the erector spinae (insufficient nutation) and the gluteus maximus (insufficient ligament pull and SIJ compression) will lead to diminished straining of the sacrotuberous ligament. Weakness of these muscles also has implications for the strength of the thoracolumbar fascia, especially if combined with a weak latissimus dorsi. All lead to diminished force closure of the SIJ. With deficient force closure, the body can be expected to implement other strategies, for example tensing the sacrotuberous ligament through activation of the biceps femoris. Although experimental data are still lacking, we presume that tension of the biceps and other hamstring muscles can be increased over an extended period. Higher tension of the hamstrings will force the pelvis to rotate backwards, leading to a flattening of the lumbar spine. The biceps femoris especially will strain the sacrotuberous ligament, diminishing nutation. Both processes will be harmful if hamstring tension is continuously increased, since in this relatively counternutated position, load will be unnaturally distributed to the lower lumbar discs. In our opinion, it is of key importance to realize that counternutation in the SIJ disengages the self-locking of the pelvis.

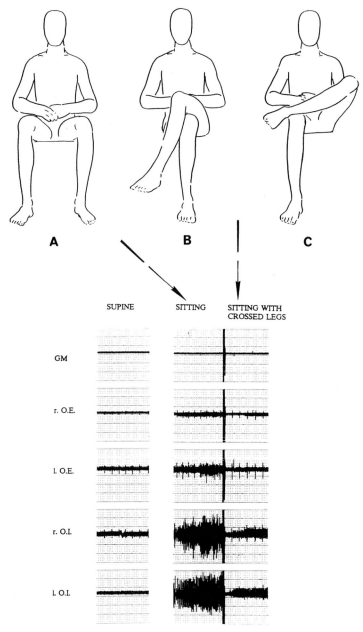

Fig. 3.10   The EMG data show a remarkable increase of the internal obliques during sitting with uncrossed legs (A). The activity diminishes when the legs are crossed (B and C). gm = gluteus maximus, rOE – right external oblique, lOE – left external oblique, rOI – right internal oblique, lOI – left internal oblique.

Hence, the lower spine can become unstable and prone to infringement, leading to low back pain.

We tried to define a simple exercise that could help to prevent low back pain and counteract the detrimental effects of modern life. The exercise shown in Fig. 3.11 nutates the SIJ and couples the action of biceps femoris, erector spinae, and gluteus maximus. We suppose this to be an effective and natural way to stretch the hamstring. To

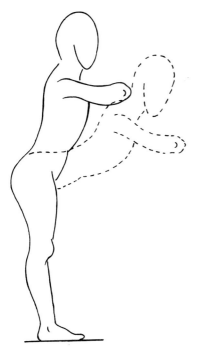

Fig. 3.11 A suggested exercise with lordosis of the lumbar spine and nutation of the SIJ. The biceps femoris, gluteus maximus, and erector muscle are simultaneously activated.

evaluate its effectiveness, the exercise needs further practical study.

GAIT

After birth, the general orientation of the human SIJ is similar to that in quadrupeds. The articular surfaces are orientated in the sagittal plane as the synovial joints of the vertebral arches of most lumbar vertebrae. Change begins when the child starts to walk. The sacrum enlarges laterally and the orientation of the articular surfaces transforms into the adult curvatures (Fig. 3.4, bottom right). These changes are brought about by mechanical factors such as body weight, load on the femur, and strain on the pubic symphysis (Schunke 1938, Solonen 1957). We wondered what stabilizing mechanisms operate during gait, when muscle function has to be adjusted to the various stages of walking.

Swing phase

During the swing of the right leg forwards, the cranial part of the right iliac bone tends to

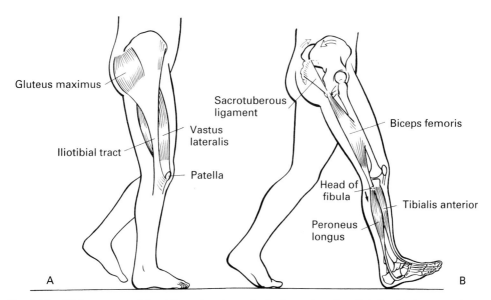

Fig. 3.12 (A) Lower part of the oblique dorsal muscle–fascia–tendon sling. Relationship between gluteus maximus muscle, iliotibial tract, vastus lateralis muscle, and knee in the single support phase. The iliotibial tract can be tensed by action of the dorsally located gluteus maximus and ventrolaterally located tensor fascia latae muscle. The tract can also be tensed by contraction of the vastus lateralis. (B) The longitudinal muscle–tendon–fascia sling. Relationships at the end of the swing phase.

rotate dorsally with respect to the sacrum (Greenman 1992; see also Chapter 19 in this volume) (Fig. 3.12B). Stated otherwise, at the right side, the top of the sacrum inclines forward relative to the iliac bones. Nutation increases, enlarging ligament tension and SIJ compression, whereas at the left the opposite transpires. These movements are normally very small. Increased nutation at the end of the swing phase will prepare the joint for the impact of heel strike. At this moment, the leg and the ipsilateral SIJ become weight-bearing. Gait analysis shows that the hamstrings become active just before heel strike (Weil & Weil 1966). As a consequence, knee extension is limited at the right side, and tension of the sacrotuberous ligament increases, due to biceps femoris activation and nutation.

What would be the effect of activation of the biceps femoris on its distal connection? The biceps is connected to the head of the fibula (Fig. 3.12B) and also to the strong fascia of the peroneus muscles. To answer the question, we loaded the biceps femoris in embalmed specimens and measured tension in the peroneus fascia. Approximately 18% of the applied load was transferred to the fascia (van Wingerden, in preparation). We questioned what would happen with the fibula during the impact. Fortunately, this was already described by Weinert et al (1973). In contrast to what is commonly believed, they showed a downward movement of the fibula during heel strike. This fits in nicely with the concept of a spine–leg mechanism. The downward movement of the fibula will further 'load' the already tensed biceps muscle and sacrotuberous ligament.

Is the mechanism described confined to the lateral part of the leg? An important muscle attached to the medial part of the foot is the tibialis anterior. To keep the point of the foot raised during the swing phase (dorsiflexion of the foot), this muscle contracts prior to heel strike. What a smart trick of nature that this muscle is attached to the plantar side of the large first metatarsal bone where it blends with the peroneus longus muscle that crosses the foot underneath. Together they form a long longitudinal muscle–tendon–fascia sling (Fig. 3.12B). The action of tibialis anterior and biceps femoris are smartly coupled to load the longitudinal sling, which could serve to store energy.

Single support phase

Heel strike is followed by the single support phase. The action of the biceps femoris diminishes. The ipsilateral iliac bone gradually starts to rotate forward with respect to the sacrum (nutation) and subsequently compression diminishes. The gluteus maximus gradually replaces biceps activity. To compress the SIJ, the gluteus is better positioned than the biceps since it compresses the SIJ both directly and indirectly (by straining the sacrotuberous ligament).

As in quadrupeds, the arms and legs of bipeds move rhythmically. Before right-sided heel strike, the trunk already shows counter-rotation (left arm forwards). This is distinct in energetic movements such as jumping. As mentioned above, the gluteus maximus and contralateral latissimus dorsi are coupled via the thoracolumbar fascia. The counter-rotation of the trunk and anteflexion of the arm assist in tensing the latissimus dorsi and consequently the thoracolumbar fascia. In combination with the action of the gluteus maximus, an oblique dorsal muscle–fascia–tendon sling is active, which crosses the spine (Fig. 3.12A; see also Chapter 6 in this volume).

The tension of the gluteus maximus is partly transferred downwards in the vast iliotibial tract (Fig. 3.12A). Like the thoracolumbar fascia, this is a strong and large sheath of connective tissue, tensed by the gluteus maximus and tensor fasciae latae muscle. In addition, the iliotibial tract can be tensed by expansion of the huge vastus lataralis muscle during its contraction. The vastus is an important part of the extensor muscle of the knee (the quadriceps). During the single support phase, this extensor muscle is active to counteract flexion in the knee. As a result, the iliotibial tract is pushed aside (to lateral) and further stretched. In contrast to what is described in many textbooks, the distal end of the tract in reality participates in the outer lateral capsule of the knee (Fig. 3.12A). The direction of the collagenous fibers is perpendicular to the patella tendon, the distal part of the quadriceps muscle that is attached to the tibial bone. In the single support phase, when the knee is fully loaded by body weight, forward shear of the femur (S Y Gracovetsky, 1994, personal communication) in the knee joint can be precluded by the tension through the thoracolumbar fascia, gluteus maximus, and iliotibial tract.

This system, involving left and right parts of the body, could also function as a smart spring. It is based on trunk torsion, action of the latissimus dorsi and gluteus maximus, and expansion of the vastus lateralis. Because of its length it is suited to store ample energy and can assist among others in unwinding the trunk.

Energy storage as a concept was raised by Margaria (1968) and needs explanation. According to Margaria, energy is accumulated during gait. He describes that the work done by muscles in active tension is partly stored as elastic energy. This energy can be utilized if the muscle is allowed to shorten immediately afterwords. Dorman compares this mechanism with maximally extending a finger and releasing it (Dorman 1992). McNeil Alexander (1984; see also Chapter 17) raised the question of where energy is stored during gait. He supposes that the elastic strain is stored in tendons, and that the extensor muscles of knee and ankle, particularly, could serve as springs. Dorman (see Chapter 40) expects that the fasciae are the main structures to store energy. However, it can be questioned whether the topographic division between muscle, tendon, and fascia is functional. By functional coupling of these seemingly separate structures, the longitudinal sling might be an effective energy storage system. The energy stored can be used to minimize muscle action.

All slings, the longitudinal, and both obliques overcome the shortcoming of relatively small individual tendons and muscle fibers, which only can conserve limited amounts of energy. The slings are coupled to the function of the SIJ. We assume that these slings reflect our capacity to use our legs and trunk for energizing the body. According to Dorman (1992), defects in this system may lead to a higher oxygen demand. We assume also that, without defects, activities such as sluggish strolling inadequately energize the

slings. This could be the reason why shopping is such a hardship for many people.

The single support phase is followed by the double support phase. In this, the SIJs are less loaded since both legs carry the weight. The gluteus maximus becomes less active. At the start of the new swing phase, nutation in the SIJ is diminished and the leg can freely swing forward.

CONCLUSIONS

1. We emphasize that functional anatomic models are requested to attack a complex puzzle such as non-specific low back pain. Such an approach can help to understand that seemingly different structures are functionally related. In this respect, we like to quote Radin (1990). He perceptively remarked, 'Functional analysis, be it biological, mechanical or both, of a single tissue will fail to give a realistic functional analysis as, in all complex constructs, the interaction between the various components is a critical part of their behavior.'

2. The intervertebral discs are loaded by compression, bending and torsion. As a result of body weight and force moments, the largest force acts perpendicularly to the discs. In contrast, this force is almost parallel to the surfaces of the practically flat SIJ. As a result, there is considerable shear loading in the SIJ and a risk of damaging the ligaments. In general, the ligamentous structures surrounding the SIJ are assumed to be sufficient to prevent shear and stabilize the joints. We do not agree with that view. We put forward evidence that the ligaments alone are not capable of transferring lumbosacral load effectively to the iliac bones. This holds especially for heavy loading situations and for conditions with sustained load resulting in creep, such as standing and sitting.

3. According to the self-locking mechanism described above, resistance against shear results from the specific properties of the articular surfaces of the SIJ (form closure) and from the compression produced by body weight, muscle action and ligament force (force closure). Different aspects of this mechanism are operating in standing, sitting, and walking and during actions such as forceful rotation and lifting in a stooped

posture. The study reveals a functional relation between the biceps femoris, gluteus maximus, latissimus dorsi, and erector spinae muscles. In understanding their coupled function, the SIJ plays a central role.

4. We conclude that knowledge of the coupling mechanisms between spine, pelvis, legs, and arms is essential to understand dysfunction of the human locomotor system, particularly the lower back. It has led us to describe three muscle slings (one longitudinal and two oblique) that can be energized.

5. We have provided evidence that unstable pelvic connections can be a main cause of complaints in patients with low back pain. Diminished and/or unbalanced muscle function can lead to sustained counternutation in the SIJ. According to the model, the SIJ becomes especially prone to shear forces if loaded in counternutation. Counternutation, which is coupled to a supine position and to flattening of the spine in standing

and sitting, can lead to abnormal loading of the lumbar discs and, in the end, herniation. Based on the data presented, disc herniation is not necessarily a separate syndrome but can be the result of failed stabilization of the pelvis and lower spine.

6. As a consequence, non-specific low back pain can be prevented and treated by modifying posture and by specific training methods. On the basis of the model presented above, advice is to treat and prevent low back pain by appropriately strengthening and coordinating trunk and leg muscles.

Acknowledgement

We would like to extend our gratitude to Cees de Vries, Annemarie van Randen, Jan-Paul van Wingerden, Annelies Pool, Ria van Kruining, Eddy Dalm, Jan Velkers, and Cees Entius.

REFERENCES

Alexander R McN 1984 Walking and running. American Scientist 72: 348–354

Bakland O, Hansen J H 1984 The axial sacroiliac joint. Anatomica Clinica 6: 29–36

Bojsen-Møller F, Lamoreux L 1979 Significance of free dorsiflexion of the toes in walking. Acta Orthopaedica Scandinavica 50: 471–479

Bogduk N, MacIntosh J E 1984 The applied anatomy of the thoracolumbar fascia. Spine 9(2): 164–170

Bogduk N, Twomey L T 1987 Clinical anatomy of the lumbar spine. Churchill Livingstone, Melbourne

Bowen V, Cassidy J D 1981 Macroscopic and microscopic anatomy of the sacro-iliac joints from embryonic life until the eighth decade. Spine 6: 620

Dijkstra P F, Vleeming A, Stoeckart R 1992 Complex motion tomography of the sacroiliac joint: an anatomical and roentgenological study. In: Vleeming A, Mooney V, Snijders C J, Dorman T (eds) First interdisciplinary world congress on low back pain and its relation to the sacroiliac joint. San Diego, CA, 5–6 November, pp 301–309

DonTigny R L 1979 Dysfunction of the sacroiliac joint and its treatment. Journal of Orthopedics and Sports Physical Therapy 1: 23–35

Dorman T A 1992 Storage and release of elastic energy in the pelvis: dysfunction, diagnosis and treatment. In: Vleeming A, Mooney V, Snijders C J, Dorman T (eds) First interdisciplinary world congress on low back pain and its relation to the sacroiliac joint. San Diego, CA, 5–6 November, pp 585–600

Egund N, Ollson T H, Schmid H, Selvik G 1978 Movements in the sacroiliac joints demonstrated with roentgen stereofotogrammetry. Acta Radiologica, Diagnosis 19: 833

Fortin J D, Dwyer A P, West S, Pier J 1994a Sacroiliac joint: pain referral maps upon applying a new injection/

arthrography technique. 1: Asymptomatic volunteers. Spine 19: 1475–1482

Fortin J D, Aprill C N, Ponthieux B, Pier J 1994b Sacroiliac joint: pain referral maps upon applying a new injection/ arthrography technique. 2: Clinical evaluation. Spine 19: 1483–1489

Greenman P E 1992 Clinical aspects of sacroiliac function in human walking. In: Vleeming A, Mooney V, Snijders C J, Dorman T (eds) First interdisciplinary world congress on low back pain and its relation to the sacroiliac joint. San Diego, CA, 5–6 November, pp 353–359

Lavignolle B, Vital J M, Senegas J et al 1983 An approach to the functional anatomy of the sacroiliac joints in vivo. Anatomica Clinica 5: 169

Lovejoy C O 1988 Evolution of human walking. Scientific American 259: 118–125

MacIntosh J E, Bogduk N 1986 The biomechanics of the lumbar multifidus. Clinical Biomechanics 1: 205–213

MacIntosch J E, Bogduk N 1991 The attachments of the lumbar erector. Spine 16: 783–792

Margaria R 1968 Positive and negative work performances and their efficiencies in human locomotion. Internationale Zeitschrift für angewandte Physiologie einschliesslich Arbeitsphysiologie 25: 339–351

Mens J M A, Stam H J, Stoeckart R, Vleeming A, Snijders C J 1992 Peripartum pelvic pain: a report of the analysis of an inquiry among patients of a Dutch patient society. In: Vleeming A, Mooney V, Snijders C J, Dorman T (eds) First interdisciplinary world congress on low back pain and its relation to the sacroiliac joint. San Diego, CA, 5–6 November, pp 521–533

Mens J M A, Vleeming A, Stoeckart R, Stam H J, Snijders C J 1996 Understanding peripartum pelvic pain: implications of a patient survey. Spine 21(11): 1303–1369

Miller J A, Schultz A B, Andersson G B 1987 Load displacement behavior of sacroiliac joint. Journal of

Orthopaedic Research 5: 92

Njoo K H 1996 Nonspecific low back pain in general practice: a delicate point. Thesis, Erasmus University, Rotterdam

Noe D A, Mostardi R A, Jackson M E, Portersfield J A, Askew M J 1992 Myoelectric activity and sequencing of selected trunk muscles during isokinetic lifting. Spine 17(2): 225

Radin E L 1990 The joint as an organ: physiology and biomechanics. Abstracts of the first world congress on biomechanics, La Jolla, September, 2:1

Sashin D 1930 A critical analysis of the anatomy and the pathological changes of the sacroiliac joints. Journal of Bone and Joint Surgery 12: 891

Schuncke G B 1938 The anatomy and development of the sacroiliac joint in man. Anatomical Record 72: 313–331

Snijders C J, Seroo J M, Snijder J G N, Hoedt H T 1976 Change in form of the spine as a consequence of pregnancy. Digest of the 11th international conference on medical and biological engineering, Ottawa, May, pp 670–671

Snijders C J, Vleeming A, Stoeckart R 1993a Transfer of lumbosacral load to iliac bones and legs. 1: Biomechanics of self-bracing of the sacroiliac joints and its significance for treatment and exercise. Clinical Biomechanics 8: 285–294

Snijders C J, Vleeming A, Stoeckart R 1993b Transfer of lumbosacral load to iliac bones and legs. 2: Loading of the sacroiliac joints when lifting in a stooped posture. Clinical Biomechanics 8: 295–301

Snijders C J, Slagter A H E, Strik R van, Vleeming A, stoeckart R, Stam H J 1995 Why leg-crossing? The influence of common postures on abdominal muscle activity. Spine 20(18): 1989–1993

Solonen K A 1957 The sacroiliac joint in the light of anatomical, roentgenological and clinical studies. Acta Orthopaedica Scandinavica 27: 1–127

Stewart T D 1984 Pathologic changes in aging sacroiliac joints. Clinical Orthopaedics and Related Research 183: 188

Sturesson B, Selvik G, Udén A 1989 Movements of the sacroiliac joints. A roentgen stereophotogrammetric analysis. Spine 14: 162–165

Vleeming A 1990 The sacroiliac joint. A clinical-anatomical, biomechanical and radiological study. Thesis, Erasmus University, Rotterdam

Vleeming A, Stoeckart R, Snijders C J 1989a The sacrotuberous ligament: a conceptual approach to its dynamic role in stabilizing the sacroiliac joint. Clinical

Biomechanics 4: 201–203

Vleeming A, Wingerden J P van, Snijders C J, Stoeckart R, Stijnen T 1989b Load application to the sacrotuberous ligament: influences on sacroiliac joint mechanics. Clinical Biomechanics 4: 204–209

Vleeming A, Stoeckart R, Volkers A C W, Snijders C J 1990a Relation between form and function in the sacroiliac joint. 1: Clinical anatomical aspects. Spine 15: 130–132

Vleeming A, Volkers A C W, Snijders C J, Stoeckart R 1990b Relation between form and function in the sacroiliac joint. 2: Biomechanical aspects. Spine 15(2): 133–136

Vleeming A, Wingerden J P van, Dijkstra P F, Stoeckart R, Snijders C J, Stijnen T 1992a Mobility in the SI-joints in old people: a kinematic and radiologic study. Clinical Biomechanics 7: 170–176

Vleeming A, Buyruk H M, Stoeckart R, Karamursel S, Snijders C J 1992b Towards an integrated therapy for peripartum pelvic instability. American Journal of Obstetrics and Gynecology 166(4): 1243–1247

Vleeming A, Pool-Goudzwaard A L, Stoeckart R, Wingerden J P van, Snijders C J 1995 The posterior layer of the thoracolumbar fascia: its function in load transfer from spine to legs. Spine 20: 753–758

Vleeming A, Pool-Goudzwaard A L, Hammudoghlu D, Stoeckart R, Snijders C J, Mens J M A 1996 The function of the long dorsal sacroiliac ligament: its implication for understanding low back pain. Spine 21(5): 556–562

Walheim G G, Selvik G 1984 Mobility of the pubic symphysis. In vivo measurements with an electromechanic method and a roentgen stereophotogrammetric method. Clinical Orthopaedics and Related Research 191: 129–135

Weil S, Weil U H 1966 Mechanik des Gehens. Georg Thieme Verlag, Stuttgart

Weinert C R, MacMaster J H, Ferguson R J 1973 Dynamic function of the human fibula. American Journal of Anatomy 138: 145–150

Weisl H 1955 The movements of the sacroiliac joints. Acta Anatomica 23: 80

Wingerden J P van, Vleeming A, Snijders C J, Stoeckart R 1993 A functional-anatomical approach to the spine–pelvis mechanism: interaction between the biceps femoris muscle and the sacrotuberous ligament. European Spine Journal 2: 140–144

Wingerden J P van, Vleeming A, Stoeckart R, Raissadad K, Snijders C J 1996 Force transfer between biceps femoris and peroneus muscle; a proposal for a longitudinal spring mechanism in the leg (in preparation)

4. The role of the sacroiliac joints in low back pain: basic aspects of pathophysiology, and management

T. N. Bernard

INTRODUCTION

At the beginning of the twentieth century, the sacroiliac joint (SIJ) was well recognized as a cause of low back pain in postpartum females and even as a source of unexplained low back and leg pain (Goldthwait & Osgood 1905). Over the next 75 years, however, interest in the SIJ waned as the lumbar disc became the major focus of attention as a primary source of low back pain. In the past 25 years, there has been a resurgence of interest in the SIJ as a potential source of low back pain.

In spite of this interest, the SIJ remains to be proven as a cause of low back pain. Because of its anatomical location, it is a difficult structure to examine. Many of the pain-provoking stress tests also stress the lumbar spine and the hip joint, thereby lessening the accuracy of these tests. In addition, many of the SIJ stress tests lack inter-examiner reliability, which further limits their usefulness (DonTigny 1989, Dreyfuss et al 1994, Hobbs 1988, Potter & Rothstein 1985). Also, there are other, well-recognized syndromes, such as posterior facet joint syndrome, herniated nucleus pulposus, and lateral recess spinal stenosis, that can refer pain to the SIJ region. Furthermore, the imaging of the SIJ in conditions other than infection, inflammation, or trauma adds little evidence to support the SIJ as a primary source of pain. These problems have led many to dismiss the SIJ as a clinical source of pain. Thus, at present, the evidence supporting SIJ syndrome is only empirical.

The objectives of this chapter are to review the pertinent developmental, anatomic, and patho-physiologic information that supports the hypo-thesis that the SIJ is a potential source of low back pain. This foundation of knowledge will afford the reader with additional insight into the interaction between the SIJ, the lumbar spine, and the pelvis to provide a rational basis for treating patients with this condition.

DEVELOPMENTAL ANATOMY

Birth and infancy

The development of the SIJ has several features that are unique and not shared by other synovial joints. The SIJ develops slowly; cavitation is delayed until the 10th week of intrauterine life and is not well established until the second trimester (Walker 1986). Most human synovial joints cavitate by 8 weeks of gestation.

Normally, opposing surfaces of synovial joints develop between two cartilage anlagen. As the joint matures, the cartilage anlagen ossify, form-ing the primary centers of ossification, and leaving a cap of cartilage to form the articular surfaces of the joint. By the time the SIJ has cavitated, the adjacent ilium has already ossified, so the newly formed SIJ develops between a hyaline cartilage anlage and the newly ossified ilium instead of the iliac cartilage anlage. Since the ilium is the first bone to ossify in the pelvis and the SIJ is late in developing, the possibility of unequal chondro-genesis exists where a joint cavity forms between cartilage and bone instead of normally cavitating between two cartilage anlagen (Cassidy 1994).

During the second trimester, another unique event occurs in SIJ development. A thin layer of fibrocartilage, which is derived from the iliac periosteum or from the remaining undifferentiated mesenchyme at the joint interzone, forms at the iliac surface. Thus the iliac fibrocartilage is actually secondary cartilage, which develops after cavitation, unlike the sacral cartilage, which is derived from a primary center of chondrogenesis (Fig. 4.1).

Unlike other synovial joints in humans, there are distinct microscopic differences between the sacral and iliac sides of the joint (Fig. 4.2). By the third trimester, the chondrocytes on the sacral side are evenly dispersed in a proteoglycan-rich matrix, which is characteristic of hyaline cartilage. On the iliac side, the cartilage layer is composed of a thin layer of stacked chondrocytes adjacent to the iliac trabeculae and an overlying layer of undifferentiated spindle cells in a collagenous proteoglycan-depleted matrix. The iliac fibrocartilage is thin, and nearly transparent; it has a bluish color due to the underlying bone. The sacral surface appears white, resembling other hyaline cartilage joint surfaces.

With weight-bearing, there is a gradual change in the contour and orientation of the SIJ. By puberty, a small ridge develops on the iliac surface, allowing interdigitation with a corresponding depression on the sacral side.

Adult sacroiliac joint

The adult SIJ is auricular or C-shaped, with the convexity oriented anteriorly and inferiorly. The longer arm of the joint surface is directed posteriorly and caudally, and the shorter arm faces posteriorly and cranially. The vertically oriented articular surface twists obliquely at an angle to the sagittal plane. SIJs can vary widely with respect to size, shape, and surface contour between individuals and from side to side in the same individual. The articular compartment of the SIJ always includes the second sacral segment and rarely includes the L4, L5, or S4 segments. In man, the most common combination of segments is S1, S2, and the midportion of S3 (Solonen 1957). In comparative vertebrate anatomy, more sacral segments participate in the sacroiliac (SI) articulation when more weight-bearing is required of the hind limbs. Amphibians usually have only two sacral segments in the SIJ, whereas mammals commonly have three or four (Bellamy et al 1983).

Age-related changes in the SIJ

The SIJ undergoes unique age-related changes (Bowen & Cassidy 1981, Brooke 1923–1924,

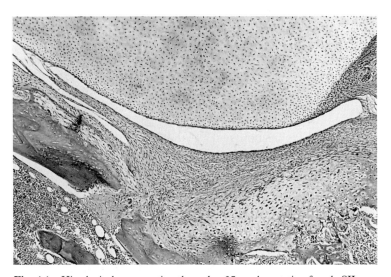

Fig. 4.1 Histological cross-section through a 25-week gestation female SIJ. The sacral cartilage anlage (above) has the appearance of fetal hyaline cartilage. Below the newly formed joint space, there is a layer of undifferentiated mesenchymal cells overlying a small nest of developing chondrocytes. These chondrocytes are arranged in stacks or rows, parallel to the iliac bone below (×23, Safranin O staining). (Reproduced with permission from Bernard & Cassidy 1991.)

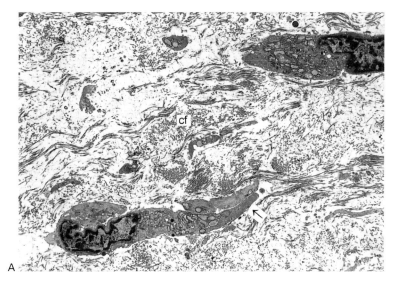

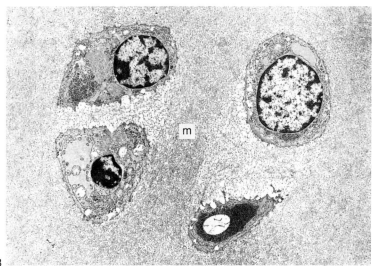

Fig. 4.2 (A) Transmission electron microscopy through the iliac fibrocartilage of a 32-week gestation female reveals a matrix full of collagen fibrils (cf) and deplete of proteoglycan aggregates. The cells have long processes (arrow) similar to fibroblasts (×2925). (B) Transmission electron microscopy through the sacral hyaline cartilage of the same specimen reveals a matrix (m) full of electron-dense dots, which represent proteoglycan aggregates. Collagen fibrils are not prominent in the matrix. The chondrocytes are more round with very short cell processes (×2925). (Reproduced with permission from Bernard & Cassidy 1997.)

Sashin 1930, Solonen 1957). Prior to puberty, the iliac side is rough in texture and looks bluish in color, reflecting the friable nature of the fibrocartilaginous surface and the bluish color of the underlying trabecular bone (Fig. 4.3). The sacral surface appears smooth, glistening and creamy-white in color, typical of hyaline cartilage.

These differences in gross appearance are maintained throughout life. By the second decade of life, a crescent-shaped ridge develops along the iliac surface that interdigitates with a corresponding depression on the sacral side of the joint. By the third decade, this interdigitation is more pronounced, which further limits SIJ motion.

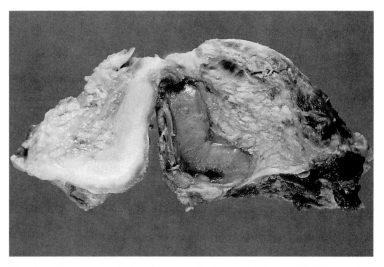

Fig. 4.3   Gross anatomical appearance of a 6-year-old female SIJ. The sacral surface (left) has a creamy-white smooth appearance, while the iliac surface has a dark-blue roughened appearance. (Reproduced with permission from Bernard & Cassidy 1991.)

Degenerative changes occur on the iliac side of the SIJ as early as the third decade of life in males. Macroscopically, these changes appear as fibrillation of the joint cartilage, crevice formation, and joint irregularity. Microscopically, the iliac chondrocytes appear clumped together (Fig. 4.4). Similar changes do not affect the sacral side until the fourth or fifth decade of life. With aging, these degenerative changes occur at an accelerated rate. By the fourth and fifth decades, fibrous ankylosis further limits joint motion, which gives the SIJ the appearance of an amphiarthrosis. Degenerative changes occur at a younger age in men than in women, but these changes have the

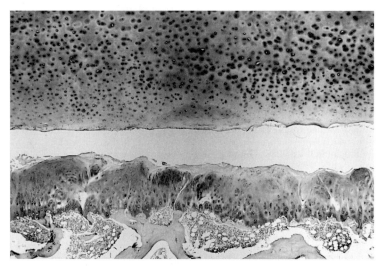

Fig. 4.4   Histological cross-section through a 20-year-old male SIJ. The sacral surface (above) has the typical appearance of hyaline cartilage. The iliac surface (below) is much thinner and has the appearance of fibrocartilage (×23, Safranin O staining). (Reproduced with permission from Bernard & Cassidy 1991.)

same macroscopic and microscopic appearance of degenerative changes occurring in other synovial joints.

Similar age-related changes have been described in equine and canine SIJ (Cassidy 1994, Cassidy & Townsend 1985, Gregory et al 1986). Whether or not these degenerative changes predispose humans toward developing symptomatic SIJ syndrome is not known, and their occurrence may only be a manifestation of the normal process of aging.

Accessory SIJ articulations

Accessory SIJ articulations are acquired fibrocartilaginous joints that develop between the second sacral vertebra and the ilium (Ehara et al 1988, Hadley 1952, Solonen 1957). These articulations may have a joint capsule, and can occur singly, doubly, unilaterally, or bilaterally. They are thought to occur secondary to the stress of weight-bearing, and their incidence is estimated at between 8% and 35.8% in the general population (Trotter 1937, 1940). In men, the incidence of these accessory articulations increases with age, but they are rarely seen before the fourth decade of life. Their presence is not known to contribute toward the development of pain in the SIJ.

SIJ LIGAMENTS

The primary SI ligaments are the anterior, posterior, and interosseous ligaments (Fig. 4.5).

The anterior SI ligament is represented by a thickening in the anterior joint capsule. The posterior portion of the SIJ has no true joint capsule, and the interosseous ligament forms the border of the posterior joint space. The interosseous ligament is the strongest of the SI ligaments, and when the SIJ is forced apart, the interosseous ligament usually avulses bone rather than failing in midsubstance.

The accessory SI ligaments are the iliolumbar, sacrotuberous, and sacrospinous ligaments (Fig. 4.6). The long dorsal SI ligament, which connects the posterior superior iliac spine (PSIS) to the lateral aspect of the third and fourth sacral segments, has a close anatomic relationship with the erector spinae muscles, posterior layer of the thoracolumbar fascia, and a specific part of the sacrotuberous ligament (Vleeming et al 1995, Willard 1995). The SI ligament complex immobilizes the sacrum between the two ilia, limiting motion. After puberty, there is considerable difference between the SIJ of men and women. In men, these ligaments remain well developed and strong. In women, the SIJ ligaments are not as well developed, thereby allowing the mobility required during parturition.

INNERVATION OF THE SIJ

The SIJ, like other synovial joints, has a nerve supply (Bogduk 1983, Bogduk et al 1982, Hirsch et al 1963, Jackson et al 1966). The joint capsule

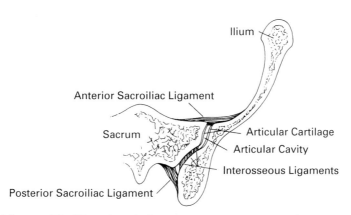

Fig. 4.5 The SIJ consists of a ligamentous compartment posteriorly and an articular compartment anteriorly. (Reproduced with permission from Bernard & Cassidy 1991.)

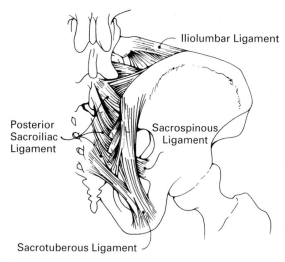

Fig. 4.6 Posterior accessory SIJ ligaments. (Reproduced with permission from Bernard & Cassidy 1991.)

and overlying ligaments have unmyelinated free nerve endings terminating in these structures. The joint capsule contains complex encapsulated and unencapsulated nerve endings capable of providing position sense and pressure information. The presence of these nerve endings in the SIJ capsule and ligaments gives further indirect evidence of its potential role as a pain-sensitive structure.

The posterior innervation to the SIJ is from the posterior primary rami of L4 through S3. The anterior innervation arises from branches of the anterior primary rami from L2 through S2 (Solonen 1957; see also Chapters 1 and 12). The contribution from the posterior and anterior rami is variable and accounts for the inconsistent pain referral pattern seen with SIJ syndrome.

Wyke (1967) recognized two types of articular nerve supplying a joint. There are independent branches of peripheral nerves crossing a joint that innervate the underlying joint, and there are non-specific articular branches derived from the muscles overlying a joint. This observation led to the hypothesis of the arthrokinetic reflex: articular nerves have a unique feedback mechanism from the overlying muscles that receive the same innervation. This arthrokinetic reflex exists because articular mechanoreceptors regulate muscle tone. This reflex mechanism is postulated to play a role in pain syndromes involving the SIJ.

BIOMECHANICS

From a biomechanical perspective, the two primary functions of the SIJ are to dissipate the load of the upper trunk to the lower extremities and to facilitate childbearing by ligamentous relaxation during pregnancy. Recently, it has been recognized that to fully understand the function of the SIJ from a kinesiologic standpoint, it is necessary to consider how the SIJ interacts with the pelvis, the lumbar spine, and the musculoligamentous complex that surrounds this joint. The ligamentous structures of the lumbar spine and sacrum and the overlying muscles are believed to play a key role in the self-bracing mechanism of the pelvis. This allows stability of the pelvis and lumbar spine during energy transfer from the spine to the lower extremities (Vleeming et al 1989a, 1989b).

Although the SIJ is surrounded by some of the most powerful muscles of the body, none of these muscles directly influences SIJ motion. Contractions of the erector spinae, psoas, quadratus lumborum, and gluteal muscles places shear and moment loads across the SIJ in proportion to their contraction forces (Miller et al 1987). The long head of the biceps femoris, piriformis, and gluteus maximus muscles often have direct attachments to the sacrotuberous ligament (Vleeming et al 1989a). It has been hypothesized that these muscles, interacting with the sacrotuberous ligament, have a role in SIJ mobility and stability (Vleeming et al 1989b, 1995).

There has been considerable debate surrounding the existence and degree of any motion occurring in the SIJ. Both in vivo and in vitro kinematic studies have demonstrated various types of motion in the SIJ, including rotation, gliding, tilting, nutation, and translation (Colachis et al 1963, Frigerio et al 1974, Grieve 1983, Kim 1984, Vleeming et al 1992). The precise nature of this motion in both the normal SIJ and dysfunctional states is unclear. It has been determined that SIJ mobility is affected by motions in the hip joints, the lumbar spine, and the symphysis pubis.

There has been considerable research interest in whether or not any motion occurring in the SIJ does so around a fixed axis (Bakland & Hansen

1984). Various plain radiographic and stereo-radiographic techniques have been devised for in vitro and in vivo investigations to determine the extent and nature of SIJ motion (Chamberlain 1930, Colachis et al 1963, Egund et al 1978, Weisl 1955). The results of these studies are inconclusive, and it seems that whatever motion is present in the SIJ, it is small and involves complexed coupled motions that do not occur around a fixed axis (but see also the opinions given by Sturesson, and Kissling and Jacobs in Chapters 11 and 12 respectively). The predominant motion appears to be a combination of X-axis rotation and Z-axis translation. It remains unclear whether any departure from normal motion contributes to painful conditions in the SIJ.

PATHOLOGIC CONDITIONS AFFECTING THE SIJ

The most commonly recognized conditions that affect the SIJ are infection, inflammation, degenerative arthritis, and trauma. Treatments for these commonly occurring conditions are well described. The SIJ as a primary source of low back pain is proposed to be a frequently occurring but not well-recognized entity. The following discussion will concentrate on the historical and physical findings that support the diagnosis of SIJ syndrome.

SIJ syndrome

The concept of the SIJ as a primary source of low back pain is gaining recognition but lacks universal acceptance. The evidence supporting this hypothesis is only empiric, and it is derived from the successful treatment of patients whose clinical symptoms and physical findings fit the description of SIJ syndrome.

Adding to the difficulty in establishing the diagnosis is the similar pain referral patterns that this condition shares with other well-recognized causes of low back pain, such as herniated nucleus pulposus, posterior facet joint syndrome, and lateral recess spinal stenosis. In addition, SIJ may exist alone or in combination with other syndromes causing low back pain. It is proposed that the diagnosis of SIJ can be established by obtaining the appropriate clinical history and by eliciting confirmatory SIJ stress tests (Bernard & Cassidy 1991, 1997; see also Chapters 2, 34, 35 and 38).

History and physical examination

The quality of pain that patients with SIJ syndrome describe can be sharp, dull, or aching. The pain can refer to the groin, buttocks, posterior thigh, and occasionally below the knee. Symptoms are usually unilateral, are aggravated by sitting and are relieved by standing or walking. It is rare to have associated neurologic symptoms, such as paresthesia, dysesthesia, or weakness, unless there is a coexisting nerve root entrapment syndrome.

The physical findings common to SIJ syndrome include tenderness over the posterior sacral sulcus and the posterior joint line (see also Chapter 3, especially the section on the long dorsal SI ligament). Ranging the lumbar spine in flexion and extension may elicit low back pain, but lateral bending does not, unless there is a concomitant posterior facet joint syndrome. In the absence of primary hip joint disease but in the presence of SIJ syndrome, flexion, abduction, and adduction of the hip joints are painless, but extremes of internal and external rotation of the hip joints may elicit groin pain or pain along the posterior joint line of the SIJ. Hamstring tightness is frequently present in SIJ syndrome.

SIJ stress maneuvers

Since there is no direct way to isolate the SIJ during physical examination, the examiner must rely upon various tests that seem to be specific to this joint. A positive stress test is only significant when the clinical history and remaining physical findings support the diagnosis of SIJ syndrome and at the same time rule out other conditions.

There are many physical tests or maneuvers that have been described to detect dysfunction in the SIJ. Although commonly used by practitioners of chiropractic or manual medicine, many of these tests are difficult to perform and interpret (Bemis & Daniel 1987, Bernard & Cassidy 1991, 1997, DonTigny 1979, 1989, Hobbs 1988, Macnab 1977, Potter & Rothstein 1985, Russel

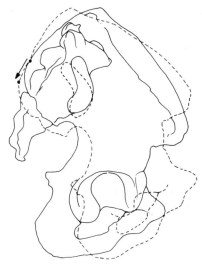

Fig. 4.7 The physiologic motion in the SIJ is amplified at the level of the PSIS. This allows this structure to be used as a reference point to detect subtle changes in joint motion. (Reproduced with permission from Bernard & Cassidy 1991.)

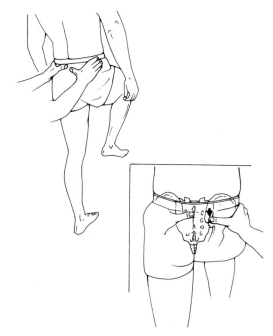

Fig. 4.8 Gillet's test is designed to detect normal and dysfunctional SIJ motion. With normal SIJ function, when raising the right leg, the PSIS moves inferior relative to the sacrum. (Reproduced with permission from Bernard & Cassidy 1991.)

et al 1981). Some of these tests lack reproducible interexaminer reliability (Laslett & Williams 1994). The following tests are selected because they are easily learned and have a high degree of interexaminer correlation.

Gillet's test presumes that SIJ motion occurs along the X-axis of rotation through the joint. Any motion in the SIJ can, therefore, be detected by noting a change in the relative positions of the second sacral spinous process and the PSIS with maximal hip flexion. Because the PSIS is located posterior to the presumed axis of rotation, any rotary component of SIJ motion is amplified and therefore more easily detected during this examination (Fig. 4.7).

Gillet's test is performed while the patient is standing, with one of the examiner's thumbs on the second sacral spinous process and the other thumb on the PSIS. With normal SIJ mobility, as the patient maximally flexes the hip joint, the PSIS moves inferiorly relative to the second sacral spinous process (Fig. 4.8). With a dysfunctional SIJ, the PSIS remains at the level of the second sacral spinous process or paradoxically elevates because the patient compensates by tilting the pelvis at terminal hip flexion (Fig. 4.9). In symptomatic patients, Gillet's test is usually

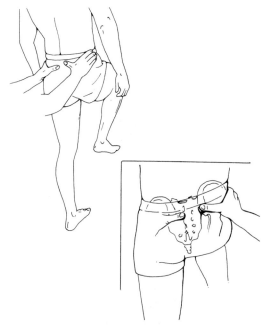

Fig. 4.9 With dysfunctional motion, patients will tend to compensate by tilting the pelvis. This will cause the PSIS to move superiorly with reference to the sacrum. (Reproduced with permission from Bernard & Cassidy 1991.)

painful. This test assumes that there is no intrinsic hip disease and that the patient has no leg length inequality or lumbar scoliosis. Since palpable bony landmarks are required, Gillet's test may be difficult to perform in obese patients.

Patrick's test is performed by flexing, abducting, and externally rotating the hip (Fig. 4.10). This test distracts the anterior part of the SIJ and compresses the posterior portion. The hip joint is also stressed during this test. Patrick's test is positive when familiar back, buttock, or groin pain is reproduced. Both SIJs should be tested for comparison in all SIJ stress testing.

Yeoman's test stresses the SIJ by extending the hip and rotating the ilium on the fixed sacrum (Fig. 4.11). This test also stresses the hip joint, extends the lumbar spine, and stretches the femoral nerve. Yeoman's test is positive when pain is produced over the posterior SIJ line.

Gaenslen's test is performed with the patient supine but with one leg hanging free off the edge of the examining table (Fig. 4.12). The hip joint is maximally flexed and stabilized while the opposite hip is extended. This maneuver stresses the hip joints and both SIJs by counter-rotation at the extremes of motion. The femoral nerve is placed under tension on the side of hip extension. In the absence of hip joint disease or femoral nerve neuropathy, a positive test with Gaenslen's maneuver reproduces familiar groin and posterior SIJ line pain.

The *SIJ shear test* is conducted with the patient prone. The palms of the examiner's hands are placed over the posterior iliac wing, and an inferiorly directed thrust is applied, causing a shearing force across the SIJ (Fig. 4.13). A positive test reproduces familiar pain over the SIJ with the shearing maneuver.

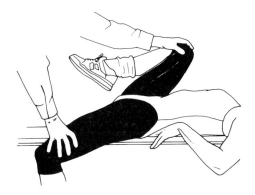

Fig. 4.12 Gaenslen's test. (Reproduced with permission from Bernard & Cassidy 1991.)

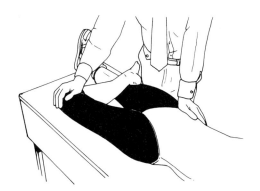

Fig. 4.10 Patrick's test. (Reproduced with permission from Bernard & Cassidy 1991.)

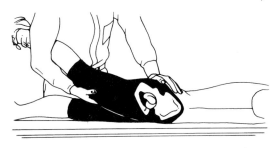

Fig. 4.11 Yeoman's test. (Reproduced with permission from Bernard & Cassidy 1991.)

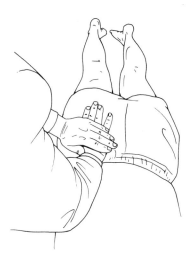

Fig. 4.13 Sacroiliac joint shear test. (Reproduced with permission from Bernard & Cassidy 1991.)

The *hip rotation test* provides an indirect assessment of SIJ function by allowing the examiner to compare relative lengthening and shortening of the lower extremities with maximal hip internal and external rotation. The test assumes no intrinsic hip disease, leg length inequality, pelvic obliquity, or lumbar scoliosis. With the patient lying supine, the levels of the medial malleoli of both legs are noted and marked on the skin (Fig. 4.14A). The extremity on the side to be tested is abducted, externally rotated, and adducted (Fig. 4.14B). With normal SIJ function, there is apparent leg lengthening (Fig. 4.14C). Next, the same leg is abducted, internally rotated, and then adducted (Fig. 4.14D). Normally, there is apparent shortening of the extremity (Fig. 4.14E). The same maneuvers are performed on the opposite extremity for comparison. Lack of apparent lengthening or shortening of the extremity implies SIJ dysfunction. This test is frequently painful on the affected side. A positive test is felt to be indicative of an imbalance in the arthrokinetic reflex. This imbalance leads to dysfunction in those muscles crossing the SIJ whose innervation is similar to that of the SIJ (see also Chapter 34).

IMAGING THE SIJ

(See also the chapters on visualization.)

The most useful plain radiographic view of the SIJ is a 30° cephalad tilt view, which projects the radiographic beam at a right angle to the sacrum (Fig. 4.15). This view allows good visualization of both the anterior and posterior SIJ lines. Since SIJ syndrome is a clinical diagnosis, plain X-rays, computerized tomography, radionuclide scanning, and magnetic resonance imaging rarely add any useful diagnostic information to support this diagnosis. The value of these imaging modalities is in establishing the presence of other syndromes that are contributing to low back pain.

TREATMENT

The goals in treating symptomatic SIJ syndrome are directed toward restoring or rebalancing the arthrokinetic reflex, which becomes imbalanced in SIJ syndrome (Fig. 4.16). This imbalance leads to nociception, and the patient enters the painful cycle. Exercise, joint mobilization, joint manipulation, and joint injection seem to re-establish the normal arthrokinetic reflex by restoring normal muscle tone and joint kinematics. It should be noted that, with the exception of manipulation, there are no randomized, controlled, and prospective clinical trials on the efficacy of any other commonly used treatment modalities, such as supports, medications, injections, exercise or SIJ fusion.

Exercise

Range of motion and flexibility exercises for the trunk, hip, and hamstring muscles can restore and maintain normal SIJ kinematics. It is believed that by restoring normal stretch length in muscles, the Golgi stretch mechanism is reset, which leads to central inhibition of pain (see also Chapter 38).

Manipulation

Although SIJ subluxation has never been proven in vivo or in vitro, one unproven theory to support the claims of success from manipulation is that small degrees of displacement in the SIJ can be painful (Bourdillon 1982, Grieve 1988). Since it has been demonstrated that whatever motion is present in the SIJ, it is quite small, it remains to be proven whether variations in normal motion can lead to pain emanating from the SIJ.

It is hypothesized that high-velocity, short-amplitude manipulation forcefully stretches hypertonic muscles against their muscle spindles, thereby leading to a release of afferent impulses to the central nervous system. This afferent information causes reflex inhibition of gamma and alpha motor neurons, which, in theory, leads to readjustment of muscle tone and muscle relaxation (Cassidy & Kirkaldy-Willis 1988). By this mechanism, the arthrokinetic reflex is rebalanced.

SIJ injection

Periarticular or intra-articular injections of a local anesthetic and cortisone solution is another effec-

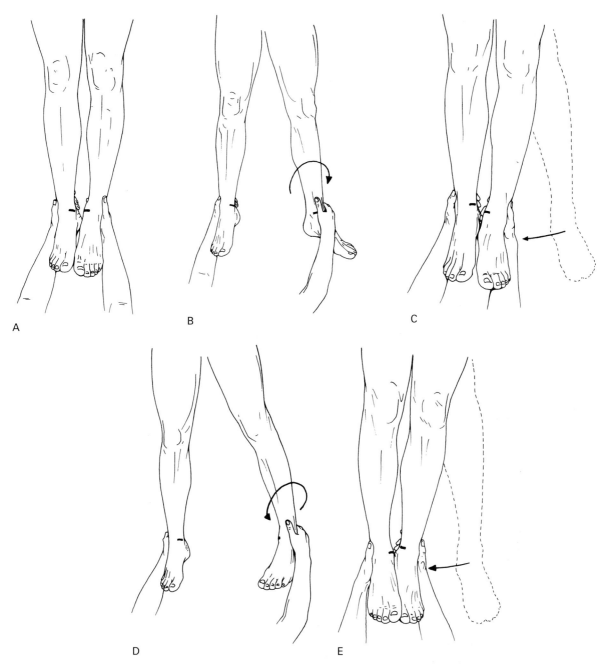

Fig. 4.14 The hip rotation test (A) is performed with the patient supine. The level of the medial malleoli is noted and marked on the patient's skin. (B) To test the left SIJ, the left leg is abducted and externally rotated. (C) The left leg is then brought back to the neutral position. With normal joint mechanics, the level of the medial malleolus will appear to have moved distally with respect to the right side. (D) The extremity is next abducted and internally rotated and brought back to the neutral position. (E) With normal joint mechanics, the level of the medial malleolus will appear to have moved proximally with respect to the right side. (Reproduced with permission from Bernard & Cassidy 1991.)

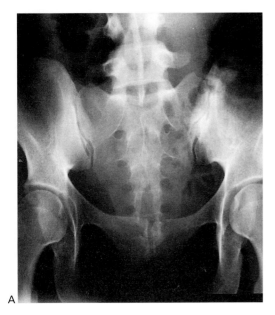

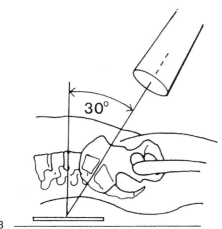

Fig. 4.15 (A and B) Thirty degree cephalad tilt view demonstrating both the anterior and posterior SIJ margins. (Reproduced with permission from Bernard & Cassidy 1991.)

tive treatment for SIJ syndrome (Aprill 1992, Haggart 1938, Haldeman & Soto-Hall 1938, Hendrix et al 1982, Kim 1984, LaBan et al 1978, Schuchmann & Cannon 1986, Shealy 1976, Solonen 1957). The diagnostic and therapeutic merits of joint injection are based upon the historical observations of Steindler and Luck (Steindler 1938, 1940). They recognized that if familiar pain is reproduced during the initial stages of injection of a local anesthetic agent into a structure, and if this pain is alleviated following the injection, this structure must be a source of the patient's pain.

There are two ways to inject the SIJ: the direct injection route and the subligamentous route (to block the posterior primary ramus innervation of the SIJ). Each injection should be performed with either conventional overhead fluoroscopy or C-arm image intensification. Patients should be examined before and after the injection by SIJ stress manuevers. For both injection techniques, the patient is laid prone on the fluoroscopy table, and the region over the SIJ is sterilely prepared. A 3.5 in, 22- or 25-gauge needle can be used for either injection technique. For the direct joint injection, the needle entry point into the articular compartment begins at the caudal one-third of the joint and is directed cephalad. Water-soluble contrast may be injected to reproduce pain and to determine whether there are any capsular leaks. Following this, 1–2 cm^3 of a combined solution of 0.25% bupivacaine and a water-soluble corticosteroid solution is injected. If familiar pain is reproduced during the injection and is alleviated by the anesthetic solution, this confirms the source of pain. Postarthrogram SIJ computerized tomography in the axial and coronal planes has been used to define pathologic distribution of contrast material (Aprill 1992, Fortin et al 1994a).

Because of the irregular topography of the SIJ, a direct injection technique may not be feasible. An equally effective injection method is to block the posterior primary ramus innervation to the SIJ by positioning needles at the superior, middle, and inferior subligamentous portions of the posterior aspect of the SIJ. Radiographic contrast is not required for this method. Once the needles are in position, 1 cm^3 of the anesthetic and steroid preparation are injected into both the superficial and deep ligamentous portions of the joint. When the injection reproduces familiar pain over the SIJ region and causes its referral into the extremity, the source of the patient's pain is confirmed. The pain reproduced by either joint injection technique may be referred to the groin, buttocks, posterior thigh, and distally into the extremity as far as the foot. This referral pattern is similar to other well-known causes of low back pain, such as herniated nucleus pulposus, posterior

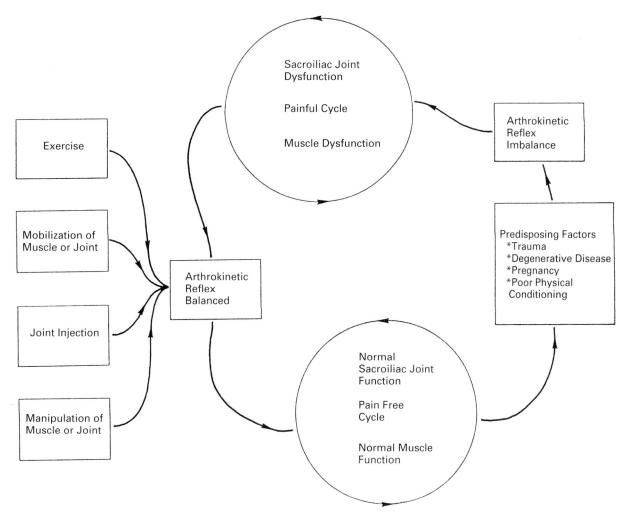

Fig. 4.16 The arthrokinetic reflex influences normal SIJ function and dysfunction. (Reproduced with permission from Bernard & Cassidy 1991.)

facet joint syndrome, and later recess spinal stenosis. After injection, patients are advised to continue with exercise or joint manipulation.

SIJ injections are not the primary mode of treatment for SIJ syndrome and should be considered when patients have failed a course of exercise, joint mobilization, and joint manipulation. As a rule, when a patient responds favorably to an injection by experiencing at least 3 months of pain relief, a repeat injection can be considered. No more than four injections are given in a 12-month period. The reported success rate from SIJ injection is 60–81% (Bernard & Cassidy 1991, Fortin 1995, Fortin et al 1994a,

1994b, Haldeman & Soto-Hall 1938, Norman 1968). The efficacy of SIJ injection has not been evaluated by a randomized, double-blinded, controlled study (see also Chapter 22).

SIJ arthrodesis

SIJ fusion has not been established as a therapeutic option for SIJ syndrome. The first reported series of SIJ fusions include small numbers of patients (Gaenslen 1927, Smith-Petersen & Rogers 1926, Solonen 1957, Waisbrod et al 1987). With current methods of internal fixation, anterior and posterior SIJ arthrodesis can be successfully accomplished (Moore 1995). Selecting a patient for SIJ fusion would require conclusively establishing the SIJ as the anatomic source of the patient's pain. A successful response to SIJ injection may aid in the selection process when considering a fusion. Even when a positive response to fluoroscopically controlled injections is used as a selection criterion for posterior screw fixation fusions of the SIJ, the good results have been mixed, ranging from 46% to 70% (Keating et al 1995, Lippitt 1995, Moore 1995). SIJ fusion is a well-established procedure following a major fracture or dislocation involving the SIJ (see also Chapters 45, 46 and 48).

CONCLUSIONS

1. The SIJ is a frequently overlooked source of primary low back pain. The basis for this conclusion comes from the anatomic similarities that this joint shares with other synovial joints, as well as empiric evidence from treating patients with this condition.

2. The diagnosis of SIJ syndrome is made by a careful clinical history and physical examination, and by ruling out other causes of low back pain. It should be noted that many patients have more than one ongoing cause of low back pain. A favorable response to joint mobilization, manipulation, or injection also helps to confirm the diagnosis, and these modalities are effective means of treatment.

3. Exercise and good physical conditioning seem to reduce the recurrence of symptoms.

4. At this time, SIJ fusion has a very limited role in treating SIJ syndrome.

5. To fully understand and appreciate the role that the SIJ has in low back pain syndromes, it is necessary to accept the broader view of the interaction that the SIJ has with the pelvis and the lumbar spine.

Acknowledgement

Photomicrographs for Fig 4.1–4.4 are courtesy of J. D. Cassidy, DC, PhD, FCCS(C), Royal University Hospital, Saskatoon, Saskatchewan.

REFERENCES

Aprill C N 1992 The role of anatomically specific injections into the sacroiliac joint. In: Vleeming A, Mooney V, Snijders C J, Dorman T (eds) First interdisciplinary world congress on low back pain and its relation to the sacroiliac joint. San Diego, CA, 5–6 November, pp 373–380

Bakland O, Hansen J H 1984 The 'axial sacroiliac joint'. Anatomica Clinica 6: 29–36

Bellamy N, Park W, Rooney P J 1983 What do we know about the sacroiliac joint? Seminars in Arthritis and Rheumatism 12(3): 282–313

Bemis T, Daniel M 1987 Validation of the long sitting test on subjects with iliosacral dysfunction. Journal of Orthopaedic and Sports Physical Therapy 8(7): 336–345

Bernard T N Jr, Cassidy J D 1991 Sacroiliac joint syndrome. Pathophysiology, diagnosis and management. In: Frymoyer J W (ed.) The adult spine: principles and practice. Raven Press, New York, pp 2107–2130

Bernard T N Jr, Cassidy J D 1997 Sacroiliac joint syndrome. Pathophysiology, diagnosis and management. In: Frymoyer J W (ed.) The adult spine: principles and practice, 2nd edition. Raven Press, New York, pp 2343–2366

Bogduk N 1983 The innervation of the lumbar spine. Spine 8(3): 286–293

Bogduk N, Wilson A S, Tynan W 1982 The human lumbar dorsal rami. Journal of Anatomy 134: 383–397

Bourdillon J F 1982 Treatment of the joints of the pelvis. In: Spinal manipulation. William Heinemann, London/Appleton-Century-Crofts, New York, pp 105–117

Bowen V, Cassidy J D 1981 Macroscopic and microscopic anatomy of the sacroiliac joint from embryonic life until the eighth decade. Spine 6(6): 620–628

Brooke R 1923–1924 The sacro-iliac joint. Journal of Anatomy 58: 299–305

Cassidy J D, Kirkaldy-Willis W H 1988 Manipulation. In: Kirkaldy-Willis W H (ed.) Managing low back pain, 2nd edition. Churchill Livingstone, New York, pp 287–296

Cassidy J D 1994 A study of the gross, microscopic, ultrastructural and comparative anatomy and development of the articular surfaces of the human sacroiliac joint. PhD thesis, University of Saskatchewan

Cassidy J D, Townsend H G G 1985 Sacroiliac joint strain as a cause of back and leg pain in man – implications for the horse. In: Proceedings of the 31st annual convention of the American Association of Equine Practitioners, pp 317–334

Chamberlain W E 1930 The symphysis pubis in the roentgen examination of the sacroiliac joint. American Journal of Roentgenology and Radium Therapy 24: 621–625

Colachis S C Jr, Worden R E, Bechtol C O, Strohm B R 1963 Movement of the sacroiliac joint in the adult male: a preliminary report. Archives of Physical Medicine and Rehabilitation 44: 490–498

DonTigny R L 1979 Dysfunction of the sacroiliac joint and its treatment. Journal of Orthopaedic and Sports Physical Therapy 1(1): 23–35

DonTigny R L 1989 Dialogue on the sacroiliac joint. Physical Therapy 69(2): 164–165

Dreyfuss P, Dreyer S, Griffin J, Hoffman J, Walsh N 1994 Positive sacroiliac screening tests in asymptomatic adults. Spine 19(10): 1138–1143

Egund N, Olsson T H, Schmid H M, Selvik G 1978 Movements in the sacroiliac joints demonstrated with roentgen stereophotogrammetry. Acta Radiologica Diagnosis (Stockholm) 19: 833–846

Ehara S, El-Khoury G Y, Bergman R A 1988 The accessory

sacroiliac joint: a common anatomic variant. American Journal of Roentgenology 150: 857–859

Fortin J D 1995 Sacroiliac joint injection and arthrography with imaging correlation. In: Vleeming A, Mooney V, Dorman T, Snijders C (eds) Second interdisciplinary world congress on low back pain. San Diego, CA, 9–11 November, pp 531–544

Fortin J D, Dwyer A P, West S, Pier J 1994a Sacroiliac joint: pain referral maps upon applying a new injection/arthrography technique. Part I: Asymptomatic volunteers. Spine 19(13): 1475–1482

Fortin J D, Aprill C N, Ponthieux B, Pier J 1994b Sacroiliac joint: pain referral maps upon applying a new injection/arthrography technique. Part II: Clinical evaluation. Spine 19(13): 1483–1489

Frigerio N A, Stowe R R, Howe J W 1974 Movements of the sacroiliac joint. Clinical Orthopaedics and Related Research 100: 370–377

Gaenslen F J 1927 Sacro-iliac joint arthrodesis; indications, author's technic and end-results. Journal of the American Medical Association 89(24): 2031–2035

Goldthwaite J E, Osgood R B 1905 A consideration of the pelvic articulations from an anatomical, pathological and clinical standpoint. Boston Medical and Surgical Journal 152: 593–601

Gregory C R, Cullen J M, Pool R, Vasseur P B 1986 The canine sacroiliac joint. Preliminary study of anatomy, histopathology and biomechanics. Spine 11(10): 1044–1048

Grieve E F J 1983 Mechanical dysfunction of the sacroiliac joint. International Rehabilitation Medicine 5: 46–52

Grieve G P 1988 Common vertebral joint problems, 2nd edn. Churchill Livingstone, New York

Hadley L A 1952 Accessory sacro-iliac articulations. Journal of Bone and Joint Surgery (US) 34: 149–155

Haggart G E 1938 Sciatic pain of unknown origin; effective method of treatment. Journal of Bone and Joint Surgery (US) 20(4): 851–859

Haldeman K O, Soto-Hall R 1938 The diagnosis and treatment of sacro-iliac conditions by the injection of procaine (novocain). Journal of Bone and Joint Surgery (US) 20(3): 675–685

Hendrix R W, Lin P J, Kane W J 1982 Simplified aspiration or injection technique for the sacro-iliac joint. Journal of Bone and Joint Surgery (US) 64: 1249–1252

Hirsch C, Ingelmark B-E, Miller M 1963 The anatomical basis for low back pain. Acta Orthopaedica Scandinavica 33: 1–17

Hobbs D 1988 Inter- and intra-examiner reliability of palpation for sacroiliac joint dysfunction. Journal of Manipulative and Physiological Therapeutics 11(4): 336–337 (letter)

Jackson H C II, Winkelmann R K, Bickel W H 1966 Nerve endings in the human lumbar spinal column and related structures. Journal of Bone and Joint Surgery (US) 48: 1272–1281

Keating J, Sims V, Avillar M 1995 Sacroiliac joint fusion in chronic low back pain population. In: Vleeming A, Mooney V, Dorman T, Snijders C J (eds) Second interdisciplinary world congress on low back pain. San Diego, CA, 9–11 November, pp 359–365

Kim L Y S 1984 Pelvic torsion: a common cause of low back pain. Orthopedic Review 13(4): 206–211

LaBan M M, Meerschaert J R, Taylor R S, Tabor H D 1978 Symphyseal and sacroiliac joint pain associated with pubic symphysis instability. Archives of Physical Medicine and Rehabilitation 59: 470–472

Laslett M, Williams M 1994 The reliability of selected pain provocation tests for sacroiliac joint pathology. Spine 19(11): 1243–1249

Lippitt A 1995 Percutaneous fixation of the sacroiliac joint. In: Vleeming A, Mooney V, Dorman T, Snijders C (eds) Second interdisciplinary world congress on low back pain. San Diego, CA, 9–11 November, pp 369–390

Macnab I 1977 Lesions of the sacroiliac joint. In: Backache. Williams & Wilkins, Baltimore, pp 64–79

Miller J A, Schultz A B, Andersson G B 1987 Load-displacement behavior of sacroiliac joints. Journal of Orthopaedic Research 5: 92–101

Moore M R 1995 Diagnosis and surgical treatment of chronic painful sacroiliac dysfunction. In: Vleeming A, Mooney V, Dorman T, Snijders C (eds) The second interdisciplinary world congress on low back pain. San Diego, CA, 9–11 November, pp 339–354

Norman G F 1968 Sacroiliac disease and its relationship to lower abdominal pain. American Journal of Surgery 116: 54–56

Potter N A, Rothstein J M 1985 Intertester reliability for selected clinical tests of the sacroiliac joint. Physical Therapy 65(11): 1671–1675

Russell A S, Maksymowych W, LeClercq S 1981 Clinical examination of the sacroiliac joints: a prospective study. Arthritis and Rheumatism 24(12): 1575–1577

Sashin D 1930 A critical analysis of the anatomy and the pathologic changes in sacroiliac joints. Journal of Bone and Joint Surgery (US) 12: 891–910

Schuchmann J A, Cannon C L 1986 Sacroiliac strain syndrome: diagnosis and treatment. Texas Medicine 82: 33–36

Shealy C N 1976 Facet denervation in the management of back and sciatic pain. Clinical Orthopaedics and Related Research 115: 157–164

Smith-Petersen M, Rogers W 1926 End-result study of arthrodesis of the sacro-iliac joint for arthritis – traumatic and non-traumatic. Journal of Bone and Joint Surgery (US) 8: 118–136

Solonen K A 1957 The sacroiliac joint in the light of anatomical, roentgenological and clinical studies. Acta Orthopaedica Scandinavica (supplement) 27: 1–127

Steindler A 1938 Differential diagnosis of pain low in the back; allocation of source of pain by procaine hydrochloride method. Journal of the American Medical Association 110: 106–113

Steindler A 1940 The interpretation of sciatic radiation and the syndrome of low-back pain. Journal of Bone and Joint Surgery (UK) 22(1): 28–34

Trotter M 1937 Accessory sacro-iliac articulations. American Journal of Physical Anthropology 22(2): 247–261

Trotter M 1940 A common anatomical variation in the sacro-iliac region. Journal of Bone and Joint Surgery (US) 22(2): 293–299

Vleeming A, Stoeckart R, Snijders C J 1989a The sacrotuberous ligament: a conceptual approach to its dynamic role in stabilizing the sacroiliac joint. Clinical Biomechanics 4: 201–203

Vleeming A, Van Wingerden J P, Snijders C J, Stoeckart R, Stijnen T 1989b Load application to the sacrotuberous ligament: influence on the sacroiliac joint mechanics. Clinical Biomechanics 4: 204–209

Vleeming A, Van Wingerden J P, Dijkstra P F, Stoeckart R,

Snijders C J, Stijnen T 1992 Mobility in the sacroiliac joints of the elderly: a kinematic and radiological study. Clinical Biomechanics 7: 170–176

Vleeming A, Pool-Goudzwaard A L, Hammudoghlu D, Stoeckart R, Snijders C J, Mens J 1995 The function of the long dorsal sacroiliac ligament: its implication for understanding low back pain. In: Vleeming A, Mooney V, Dorman T, Snijders C J (eds) Second interdisciplinary world congress on low back pain. San Diego, CA, 9–11 November, pp 123–137

Waisbrod H, Krainick J U, Gerbershagen H U 1987 Sacroiliac joint arthrodesis for chronic lower back pain. Archives of Orthopedic and Trauma Surgery 106: 238–240

Walker J M 1986 Age-related differences in the human sacroiliac joint: a histological study: implications for therapy. Journal of Orthopaedic and Sports Physical Therapy 7(6): 325–334

Weisl H 1955 The movements of the sacro-iliac joint. Acta Anatomica (Basel) 23(1): 80–91

Willard F 1995 The lumbosacral connection: the ligamentous structure of the low back and its relation to pain. In: Vleeming A, Mooney V, Dorman T, Snijders C J (eds) Second interdisciplinary world congress on low back pain. San Diego, CA, 9–11 November, pp 29–58

Wyke B 1967 The neurology of joints. Annals of the Royal College of Surgeons of England 41: 25–50

Biomechanics

5. Biomechanics of the human pelvic bone

M. Dalstra

INTRODUCTION

In the skeleton, the pelvic bones form the intermediary between the spinal column and the lower extremities, and as such they play a crucial role in the load transfer mechanism from the trunk to the legs and vice versa. A single pelvic bone interacts directly with the rest of the skeleton through three joints: (1) the sacroiliac joint (SIJ), which connects the pelvic bone to the spine; (2) the hip joint, which connects it to the leg; and (3) the pubic symphysis, which connects it to the contralateral pelvic bone. It is between these three joints that the major part of the load transfer across the pelvic bone takes place.

It is well known that for normal everyday activities, such as walking, the hip joint force can easily reach values of up to four times the body weight; for jumping and running, it is even higher. This means that the pelvic bone is subject to relatively high loads. In the first part of this chapter, we will take a closer look at the structure of the pelvic bone to see how it is able to deal with these high loads. In the second part, we will examine the actual load transfer across the pelvic bone. This is done by making use of the so-called finite element method to calculate stress distributions throughout the pelvic bone generated by certain external loading conditions. The normal pelvic load transfer may be affected by trauma or disease, as far as these alter the mechanical circumstances in the pelvic bone. One of the most striking examples of this is the placement of a total hip arthroplasty. The reconstruction of the acetabulum with an acetabular cup clearly alters the pelvic mechanics. In the final part of the chapter, we will then look briefly at how the normal load transfer mechanism will be affected by this latter circumstance.

THE STRUCTURE OF THE PELVIC BONE

The shape of the mature pelvic bone is the result of an evolutionary process to allow for efficient attachment sites for the powerful musculature, needed to control and propel the legs, and to provide a protective containment for the organs of the lower abdomen.

The stability and strength needed for the pelvic bone to function are provided both on an internal and an external level. Starting with the latter, the pelvic ring, a closed chain formed by both pelvic bones and the sacral bone, is of major importance. Normally, external loading of this ring will result in these three bones being pressed together, whereby in the SIJs a self-locking mechanism is activated. The relative position in which the bones interlock depends on the type of loading, for example walking or sitting (Vleeming et al 1995). Being part of this pelvic ring, a single pelvic bone thus receives both support and stability from the other constituents. This interaction will be discussed in depth in other chapters, and we will consider here the internal strength and stability of the pelvic bone.

From its very structure, consisting of a core of low-density trabecular bone covered by a thin shell of high-strength cortical bone, the pelvic bone derives its own inherent strength. An engineering analogy of this structure would be a so-called sandwich construction, which is used in particular to combine high bending stiffness with low weight. For example, a simple engineering calculation for the deflection of a beam shows that a 10 mm

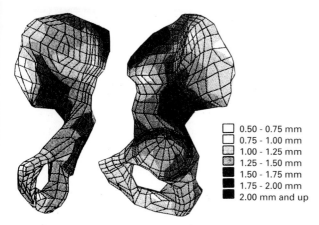

Fig. 5.1 Cortical thickness distribution in a pelvic bone of an 87-year-old man.

thick plate of trabecular bone with two 0.5 mm thick cortical shells on either side would have the same resistance against bending as a plate of solid cortical bone with a thickness of 7.3 mm. Thus only a 50% increase in thickness is needed to cause a 75% decrease in weight.

This is an idealized example, and in the adult pelvic bone the situation is a little more complex. In the first place, the thickness of the pelvic cortical shell is not uniform, but varies from less than 0.5 mm up to around 3 mm. Figure 5.1 shows a thickness distribution of the cortical shell

measured from computerized tomography (CT) scans of a pelvic bone of an 87-year-old man. This distribution data are then projected onto a computer model of a pelvic bone. Cortical thicknesses of 2–3 mm are found around the incisura ischiadaca major region, extending up the iliac bone. The iliac crest also has a relatively thick cortex. At the articular surfaces of the SIJ and the pubic symphysis, cortical thickness is less than 1 mm.

Furthermore, the bone in the trabecular core is not homogeneous. In a series of six pelvic bones, which were CT scanned using dual-energy quantitative CT, the average Calcium-equivalent (Ca-equivalent) density was measured for each scan level (Dalstra 1993, Dalstra et al 1993). Figure 5.2 shows these measurements together with four specific regions, each with an average Ca-equivalent statistically different from the corresponding values in neighboring regions, these being (1) the ala of the iliac bone (with an average Ca-equivalent density and standard deviation of 0.09 ± 0.02 g/cm^3); (2) the superior part of the acetabulum and the corpus of the iliac bone (0.17 ± 0.03 g/cm^3); (3) the inferior part of the acetabulum, the ischial bone and the pubic-ischial junction (0.10 ± 0.04 g/cm^3); and (4) the crista and superior ramus of the pubic bone (0.14

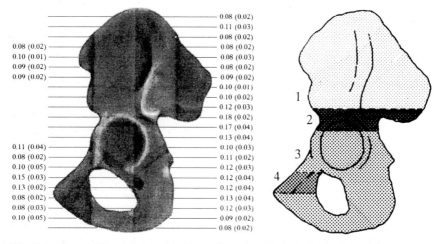

Fig. 5.2 Average Ca-equivalent densities and standard deviations (g/cm^3) at each scan level (left) and the identification of the areas between which the average Ca-equivalent densities are significantly different, based on six pelvic bones (right; see text for further explanation). Those levels for which Ca-equivalents are also indicated on the left had such a thin (or even no) connection between the anterior and posterior trabecular bone masses that separate anterior and posterior measurements were made.

± 0.03 g/cm³). These density values are comparable to bone densities found in vertebral bodies and are significantly lower than trabecular bone densities in, for example, the femoral head or proximal tibia.

In general, trabecular bone is known to have a very varied appearance, depending on its location and mechanical function in the skeleton. Ever since Julius Wolff in the second half of the nineteenth century observed the relation between form and function of bone (Wolff 1892), bone has been looked upon as a self-optimizing material, which adapts its shape and form to the mechanical circumstances to which it is subjected. Using experimentally determined relations between the Ca-equivalent density and the Young's modulus (stiffness) of pelvic trabecular bone (Dalstra 1993, Dalstra et al 1993), a distribution of the Young's modulus of bone in the trabecular core could be made based on the density measurements (Fig. 5.3). This is only an approximate distribution as trabecular bone is in reality anisotropic, meaning that it has different Young's moduli in different directions. Unlike the trabecular bone in the proximal tibia, for example, the degree of anisotropy in the pelvic bone is relatively low, but the bone is not entirely isotropic. It often features a plate-like structure, with the trabecular plates oriented perpendicularly to the cortical shells. From a mechanical point of view, this is quite understandable, because, as core material in a sandwich construction, pelvic trabecular bone

will predominantly have to withstand shear loading modes, against which a plate-like structure forms the best resistance.

LOADING AND LOAD TRANSFER

Loading of the pelvic bone is usually due to movement of the lower extremities and/or stabilization of the upper body. The magnitudes of the individual muscle forces and joint reaction forces involved in this are often in the order of body weight. We have already seen how the structure of the pelvic bone is well adapted to these high loads. In this section, we will look at how the load transfer across the pelvic bone takes place: which parts will be heavily loaded, which parts loaded only in a minor way.

For this purpose, we will examine internal stress distributions that occur in the pelvic bone for given external loading conditions. Because of its irregular form, the best way to do this for the pelvic bone is to use the finite element method (FEM). The FEM is a computer simulation technique that allows the calculation of internal stresses and strains for a structure when the external loads are known. Since its introduction into the field of biomechanics in the early 1970s, the FEM has become a well-established tool to study the mechanics of bone and bone/prosthesis configurations. It is basically a mathematical approach, whereby a structure is divided into small geometrical entities, the elements. For each of these elements there exists an analytical relation between force, deformation, strain, and stress, given their geometry, material properties, and boundary conditions. Owing to the large number of elements, handling of input and output data and the actual calculation of the stresses and strains are performed using special computer software.

The pelvic finite element model

The pelvic FE model, which will be described below to study the pelvic load transfer mechanism (Dalstra & Huiskes 1995), was originally developed to study the full three-dimensional stress situation around acetabular implants (Dalstra 1993, Dalstra et al 1995). The outer geometry of this model was based on a series of subsequent contours,

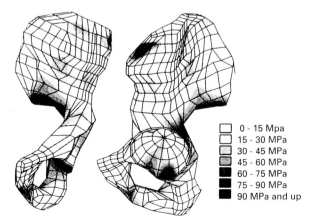

☐ 0 - 15 Mpa
☐ 15 - 30 MPa
▨ 30 - 45 MPa
▨ 45 - 60 MPa
■ 60 - 75 MPa
■ 75 - 90 MPa
■ 90 MPa and up

Fig. 5.3 Young's modulus (stiffness) distribution in the pelvic trabecular core.

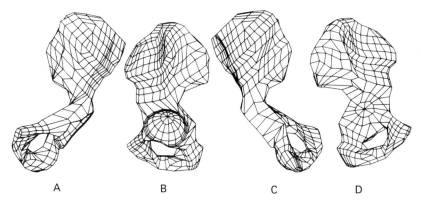

A   B   C   D

Fig. 5.4 Geometry of a pelvic finite element model seen from an anterior (A), lateral (B), posterior (C), and medial (D) viewpoint.

obtained from digitizing cross-sectional cuts of a pelvic bone submerged in polyester resin. The body defined by these contours was divided into three-dimensional brick elements to represent the trabecular core, and finally the free outer surface was covered with membrane elements to represent the thin cortical shell. This model is shown from various viewpoints in Fig. 5.4. Initially, material properties like the Young's modulus of the trabecular core and the thickness of the cortical shell were assumed to be constant, but this was later refined by using CT scanning data. Local distributions of the apparent density of the trabecular core and the thickness of the cortical shell were measured directly from these CT scans

and attributed (the apparent densities first being calculated into Young's moduli) to the appropriate elements in the model (Fig. 5.5). The outcome of this exercise has been shown above in Figs 5.1 and 5.3.

External loading of the model included the hip joint force and 22 muscle forces, and was meant to represent eight characteristic phases in a normal walking cycle. These phases are summarized in Table 5.1. The directions and the magnitudes of the hip joint force for these phases were based on data obtained with a telemetrized hip prosthesis by Bergmann et al (1990). These showed a maximum of nearly 350% body weight on one-legged stance, which then decreased to 15% body weight

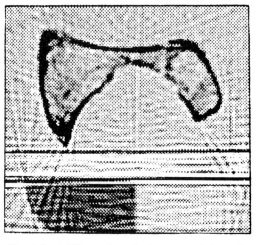
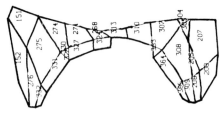

Fig. 5.5 A CT-scan from the lower acetabular region with the accompanying section through the FE model.

Table 5.1 Description of the eight considered phases in a gait cycle

Load case	Description	% Walking cycle
1	Double support, beginning of left stance phase	2
2	Beginning of left single support phase	13
3	Halfway in left single support phase	35
4	End of left single support phase	48
5	Double support, end of left stance phase	52
6	Beginning of left swing phase	63
7	Halfway in left swing phase	85
8	End of left swing phase	98

during the swing phase. For an assumed body weight of 650 N, these and the other values of the hip joint force are given in Table 5.2.

To ensure a smooth introduction of the hip joint force onto the acetabular surface, the femoral head was modeled as a half-sphere, and the hip joint force was applied as a distributed load to the flat back side of this. Contact between the femoral head and the acetabulum was then described by so-called gap elements, which only allow the transfer of compressive forces. Furthermore, this contact was assumed to be frictionless to simulate the presence of articular cartilage in the acetabulum. The directions of the muscle forces were found by subtracting the coordinates of the distal and proximal insertion points, as given by Dostal and Andrews (1981), and making corrections for the flexion/extension position of the leg relative to the trunk during the walking cycle. The magnitudes of the muscle forces were based on data reported by Crowninshield and Brand (1981). These values are also given in Table 5.2. The table shows that some muscles, for example the gluteus group, are more active during the stance phase whereas other muscles, for example the adductor and obturator groups, are more active during the swing phase. The single highest value in this array of muscle forces was the force in the gluteus medius at the end of the one-legged stance phase, which was approximately 1500 N. A mapping of the insertion areas of each of the muscles was made on the FE model (Fig. 5.6), and the muscle forces were applied as distributed loads on the surfaces of those elements, which were located in these respective areas. For the

Table 5.2 Magnitudes (N) of the hip joint force and the muscle forces for the considered eight load cases (see also Table 5.1)

	Load cases							
	1	2	3	4	5	6	7	8
Hip joint force	426	2158	1876	1651	1180	187	87	379
Gluteus maximus	842	930	167	377	456	491	114	482
Gluteus medius	1018	1053	1474	1509	1412	982	105	421
Gluteus minimus	228	140	263	228	175	123	114	219
Tensor fascia lata	0	132	88	158	149	88	70	96
Iliacus	0	0	0	228	307	272	0	0
Psoas	149	0	316	175	88	175	105	140
Gracilis	0	0	0	0	88	158	70	140
Sartorius	0	88	0	0	35	158	88	88
Semimembranosus	579	368	333	368	421	298	61	421
Semitendinosus	0	140	105	246	316	368	105	0
Biceps femoris longus	298	202	88	70	123	114	79	377
Adductor longus	0	88	0	0	88	158	70	140
Adductor magnus	0	0	0	0	132	263	0	0
Adductor brevis	0	114	0	0	0	202	0	114
Obturator externus	0	0	0	0	123	167	132	123
Obturator internus	167	123	0	61	61	149	123	0
Pectineus	0	0	175	96	0	149	0	0
Piriformis	202	175	0	0	0	0	123	228
Quadratus femoris	61	96	0	0	88	184	0	0
Superior gemellus	140	88	123	79	0	0	158	202
Inferior gemellus	0	0	0	0	0	140	79	149
Rectus femoris	0	123	0	0	0	175	105	96

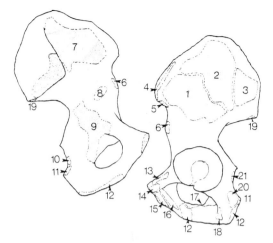

Fig. 5.6 Insertion areas of the muscles considered in the FE model. (1) gluteus minimus, (2) gluteus medius, (3) gluteus maximus, (4) tensor fascia lata, (5) sartorius, (6) rectus femoris, (7) iliacus, (8) psoas, (9) obturator internus, (10) gemellus inferior, (11) semitendinosus, (12) adductor magnus, (13) pectineus, (14) adductor longus, (15) gracilis, (16) adductor brevis, (17) obturator externus, (18) quadratus femoris, (19) piriformis, (20) semimembranosus, (21) gemellus superior.

boundary conditions, it was assumed that the pelvic model was supported at the SIJ. Furthermore, a dummy model of the contralateral pelvic bone was added by mirroring the initial model in the sagittal plane. This was done to provide a more natural support for the actual model at the pubic symphysis.

The pelvic load transfer mechanism

To achieve a good insight in the pelvic load transfer mechanism, the results of the FE analyses are represented in the following as stress distributions. Looking at the stress intensity in the cortical shell (Fig. 5.7), we see that the highest stresses occur during the stance phase of the leg and are located in the insertion area of the gluteus major and around the incisura ischiadaca major region. At the beginning of the swing phase, the pubic ramus is also highly stressed.

When we think of the cortical shell being 'peeled off' and look at the stresses in the underlying trabecular core (Fig. 5.8), two differences can immediately be noticed. First, the magnitude of the stresses in the trabecular core is about 50 times lower. This is the result of the sandwich

construction of the pelvic bone: the stiff cortex draws more load to itself than does the less stiff trabecular core. Second, the areas of high stress do not coincide with those in the cortex. It is still during the stance phase that the highest stress values are found, but here the stress peaks occur in the center of the iliac wing. The trabecular bone stresses are also relatively high at the antero-superior acetabular rim and the bottom of the acetabulum. In fact, it is at these locations that the sandwich construction analogy plays a lesser role: in the center of the iliac wing because the medial and the lateral cortical shell almost merge into one (in many cases they actually do), and in the acetabulum because the principal loading mode is direct compressive load-bearing rather than bending.

When we look in more detail at the contact in the acetabulum between the femoral head and the pelvic bone, it becomes clear that this is far from uniform. Even under the assumption of a perfect fit between the femoral head and the acetabular socket, and despite the fact that under physiologic loading the femoral head is always pushed into the acetabulum, there are parts of the articular surface of the acetabulum that remain unloaded. During the eight considered load phases, there is constant contact along most of the acetabular rim, in the central part of the antero-superior quadrant of the acetabulum, and at the bottom of the posteroinferior quadrant. However, a large part of the posterosuperior quadrant of the acetabulum is not in contact with the femoral head at all (Fig. 5.9). Pauwels (1973) argued that, for a normal configuration of the hip joint, the stress distribution in the acetabulum should be uniform. This idea, however, is based on the assumption that the acetabulum can transfer loads in all directions. The present results, however, indicate that loads are mainly transferred from the acetabulum through the lateral cortical shell to the SIJ and the pubic symphysis. The actual stress distribution in the acetabulum is therefore somewhat affected by this load transfer mechanism, and the deeper parts of the acetabulum are stressed much less. The high stresses at the superior acetabular wall demonstrate its importance in the natural load transfer mechanism of the hip joint.

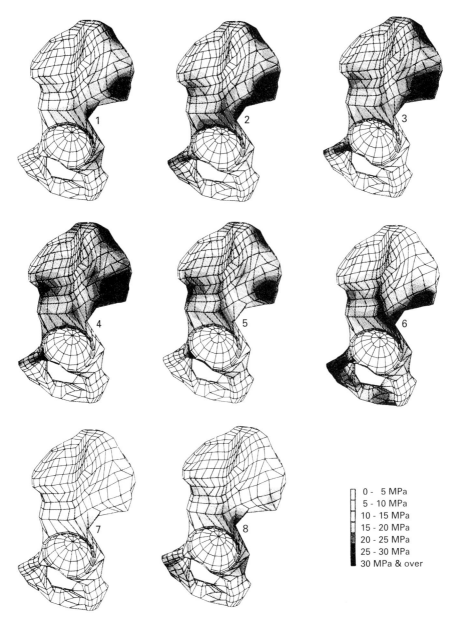

Fig. 5.7   Lateral views of the stress intensity (von Mises stresses) distribution in the cortical shell of the left pelvic bone for the eight phases in a walking cycle (see also Table 5.1).

In dysplastic acetabula, this part of the wall is underdeveloped or sometimes even missing. An alternative load transfer mechanism, with higher stresses in the remaining wall to compensate for this, will result. This is shown by Schüller et al (1993) in a case of reconstructed acetabula. Therefore, a dysplastic acetabulum can definitely be considered to be a consider-

able risk factor for progressive wear of the hip joint.

In conclusion, we can say that the pelvic load transfer mechanism is centered around the acetabulum. During normal walking, the hip joint force remains directed towards a relatively small area in the anterosuperior quadrant of the acetabulum. Its line of action does not intersect the

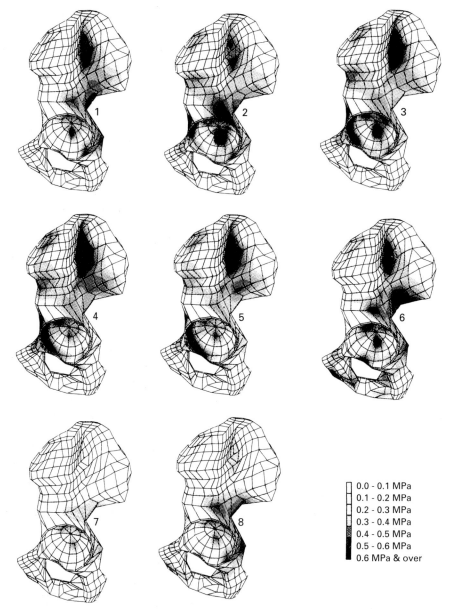

Fig. 5.8 Lateral views of the stress intensity distribution in the trabecular core of the left pelvic bone for the eight phases in a walking cycle (see also Table 5.1.).

line between the iliac and the pubic support areas, and the hip joint force therefore tends to tilt the acetabulum upwards. This tilting is to a large extent counteracted by the muscle forces acting on the iliac and the ischial bones. Owing to the muscle forces, the stress distributions in the bone remain fairly constant during a walking cycle, even though the hip joint force varies consider-

ably (from almost 200 N to 2200 N). Thus the muscle forces apparently help to keep changes in the stress distribution to a minimum, which is supposedly favorable with regard to fatigue failure of the bone. In and closely around the acetabulum, the highest stresses occur in the superior acetabular wall, and from there they are transferred to both the SIJ and the pubic

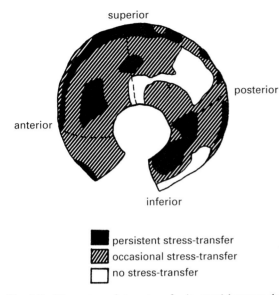

persistent stress-transfer
occasional stress-transfer
no stress-transfer

Fig. 5.9 The nature of stress transfer (contact) between the femoral head and the acetabulum (projected onto the latter) during a full gait cycle.

symphysis. The ratio between the reaction forces at these two joints for the considered load cases lies between 4 and 6. At the beginning of the swing phase of the leg, for example, the joint reaction force at the pubic symphysis reaches its maximal value of 115% of body weight. At the same time, however, the reaction force at the SIJ has a value of nearly 500% of body weight. Owing to the large surface area of the SIJ, the stresses here are, however, much lower than at the pubic symphysis.

CONSEQUENCES FOR ACETABULAR RECONSTRUCTION

The reconstruction of a hip joint with a total hip arthroplasty is primarily meant to relieve pain and restore function of the joint. However, at the same time, it creates a rather unnatural situation from a mechanical point of view. At the femoral side, a metal stem is inserted into the medullary canal. Owing to the high stiffness of this stem compared with that of the bone shaft, the surrounding cortex will become stress-shielded (it does not transfer as much load as it did preoperatively). This phenomenon carries the potential danger of a local reduction of bone mass

(Wolff's Law: bone in disuse will gradually disappear), which may eventually lead to loosening of the implant due to the lack of supporting bone stock.

At the pelvic side, the acetabulum is reamed to allow the placement of an acetabular implant. In general, these may differ in shape (hemispherical or conical), type of fixation (cemented or noncemented), or the presence of a metal backing. The insertion of such a cup also creates an unnatural situation, but its consequences are not as directly apparent as on the femoral side.

In the last part of this chapter, we will take a brief look at how the mechanical situation in the pelvic bone changes owing to the presence of an acetabular implant. The same FE model as described earlier will be used to illustrate the differences in load transfer before and after insertion of an acetabular implant.

Figure 5.10 shows a comparison between the stresses in the cortical shell of both a normal pelvic bone and a pelvic bone reconstructed with a traditional hemispherically shaped cemented cup. Differences between both stress distributions are only marginal and seem to be restricted only to the immediate vicinity of the acetabulum. In the superior acetabular rim, the load transfer has shifted slightly posteriorly after reconstruction. For both the subchondral and the trabecular bone in the acetabular region, the changes are, however, more substantial. In the normal case, the highest stress in the subchondral bone occurs in the

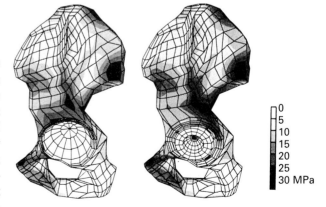

0
5
10
15
20
25
30 MPa

Fig. 5.10 Comparison between the stress intensity in the cortical shell of a normal pelvic bone (left) and a pelvic bone reconstructed with a conventional cemented cup (right).

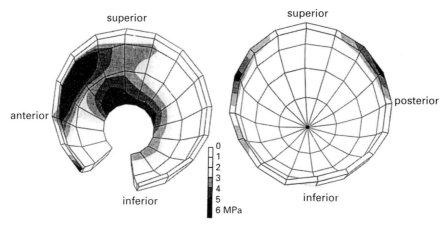

superior

superior

posterior

anterior

0
1
2
3
4
5
6 MPa

inferior

inferior

Fig. 5.11   Comparison between the stress intensity in the subchondral bone layer of a normal pelvic bone (left) and a reconstructed pelvic bone (right) during one-legged stance.

anterosuperior quadrant of the acetabulum. In the reconstructed case, stresses have not only reduced considerably, but have also shifted from the dome area towards the edges (the posterosuperior edge in particular), as can be seen in Fig. 5.11. This leaves the deeper areas in the acetabulum stress-shielded.

Two separate effects seem to play a role in this phenomenon. First, the addition of material in the acetabulum makes the pelvic bone stiffer. This leads to a general stress reduction in those locations, where the deformations used to be highest. This is the stiffening effect. Second, the transfer of the anterosuperiorly directed hip joint force to the posterosuperiorly directed support area (the SIJ) no longer occurs in the subchondral bone layer and the lower ilium. Instead, it takes place within the cup and the cement mantle. This can be seen as the load-diverting effect.

We have seen that the changes caused by the presence of an acetabular cup occur only locally in the acetabular region of the pelvic bone. It is therefore perhaps not surprising that the effect of a change in the design of an acetabular implant is also only seen locally. Yet these local changes may be important for a good understanding of the mechanics of acetabular prostheses. This is best illustrated by looking at stresses in the subchondral layer. Figure 5.12 shows the stress intensity patterns for four different types of acetabular cups (cemented/cementless and metal-backed/non-backed). In all four cases, stresses are highest

at the anterosuperior rim. The principal effect of adding a cement layer is a shift of the stresses from the anterosuperior rim to both the posterosuperior and anteroinferior rims. This phenomenon is comparable to the load-diverting effect mentioned above. The main effect of a metal backing is, on the other hand, more comparable to the above-mentioned stiffening effect and causes a shift of load transfer from the deeper areas of the acetabulum to the acetabular rim.

The clinical consequences of this may be detrimental in two ways: the reduction of the stresses underneath the cup might lead to unwanted local bone resorption, and the increase of the stresses around the rim may lead to earlier disruption of the prosthesis–bone interface in this area. Schmalzried et al (1992) have actually demonstrated that the prosthesis–bone interface of cemented, metal-backed cups starts to fail along this acetabular rim. The reduction of the stresses underneath the cup in case of metal backing was also observed in earlier pelvic FE models (Carter et al 1982, Pedersen et al 1982), but it was then seen as a positive aspect of metal-backed acetabular cups. In fact, the results of these studies were to some extent used to promote metal backing for acetabular cups. Clinically, however, metal-backed cups have not quite lived up to their expectation (e.g. Ritter et al 1990). This shows the importance of interpreting the results from FE analyses. Particularly, as in the 'real life' situation, additional effects, such as wear particles (Schmalzried

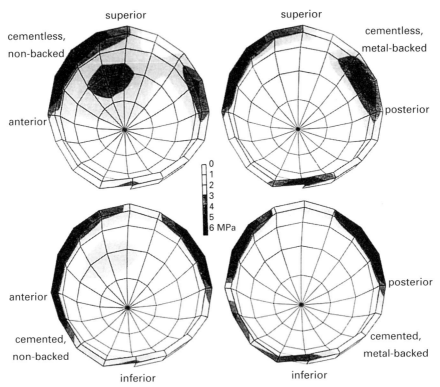

Fig. 5.12   Comparison betwen the stress intensity in the subchondral bone layer of pelvic bones reconstructed with a cementless full-polyethylene cup (top left), a cementless titanium-backed cup (top right), a cemented full-polyethylene cup (bottom left), and a cemented titanium-backed cup (bottom right).

et al 1992), play an important role in the failure mechanism of acetabular implants.

CONCLUSIONS

1. With its structure consisting of a trabecular core covered by a thin cortical shell, the pelvic bone resembles a sandwich construction.

2. This sandwich construction allows relatively high loading (up to a couple of times body weight) for a bone that mainly consists of low-strength and low-stiffness trabecular bone.

3. The main load transfer across the pelvic bone takes place between the acetabulum and the SIJ; a minor part is directed towards the pubic symphysis.

4. Areas with stress peaks in the cortical shell and the trabecular core of the pelvic bone do not coincide.

5. The overall load transfer is not much changed by the reconstruction of the acetabulum by an acetabular implant.

6. Changes in the stresses in the bone after such a reconstruction occur only in the immediate vicinity of the acetabulum.

7. Despite this local effect, however, some of these changes, such as stress-shielding of the bone in the dome of the acetabulum, may be of great importance in determining the ultimate success of such an implant.

REFERENCES

Bergmann G, Graichen F, Rohlmann A 1990 Instrumentation of a hip prosthesis. In: Bergmann G, Graichen F, Rohlmann A (eds) Implantable telemetry in orthopaedics. Freie Universität, Berlin, pp 35–63

Carter D R, Vasu R, Harris W H 1982 Stress distributions in the acetabular region. II: Effects of cement thickness and metal backing of the total hip acetabular component. Journal of Biomechanics 15: 165–170

Crowninshield R D, Brand R A 1981 A physiologically based criterion of muscle force prediction in locomotion. Journal of Biomechanics 14: 793–801

Dalstra M 1993 Biomechanical aspects of the pelvic bone and design criteria for acetabular prostheses. Doctoral thesis, University of Nijmegen, The Netherlands

Dalstra M, Huiskes R 1995 Load transfer across the pelvic bone. Journal of Biomechanics 28: 715–724

Dalstra M, Huiskes R, Odgaard A, van Erning L 1993 Mechanical and textural properties of pelvic trabecular bone. Journal of Biomechanics 26: 523–535

Dalstra M, Huiskes R, van Erning L 1995 Development and validation of a three-dimensional finite element model of the pelvic bone. Journal of Biomechanical Engineering 117: 272–278

Dostal W F, Andrews J G 1981 A three-dimensional biomechanical model of hip musculature. Journal of Biomechanics 14: 802–812

Pauwels F 1973 Atlas zur Biomechanik der gesunden und kranken Hüfte. Springer Verlag, Berlin

Pedersen D R, Crowninshield R D, Brand R A, Johnston R C 1982 An axisymmetric model of acetabular components in total hip arthroplasty. Journal of Biomechanics 15: 305–315

Ritter M A, Keating, E M, Faris P M, Brugo G 1990 Metal-backed acetabular cups in total hip arthroplasty. Journal of Bone and Joint Surgery (US) 72: 672–677

Schmalzried T P, Kwong L M, Jasty M et al 1992 The mechanism of loosening of cemented acetabular components in total hip arthroplasty. Clinical Orthopaedics and Related Research 274: 60–78

Schüller H M, Dalstra M, Huiskes R, Marti R K 1993 Total hip reconstruction in acetabular dysplasia: a finite element study. Journal of Bone and Joint Surgery (UK) 75: 468–478

Vleeming A, Snijders C J, Stoeckart R, Mens J M A 1995 A new light on low back pain – the selflocking mechanism of the sacroiliac joints and its implications for sitting, standing and walking. In: Vleeming A, Mooney V, Dorman T, Snijders C J (eds) Second interdisciplinary world congress on low back pain. San Diego, CA, 9–11 November, pp 95–108

Wolff J 1892 Das Gesetz der Transformation der Knochen. Verlag von August Hirschwald, Berlin

6. Biomechanics of the interface between spine and pelvis in different postures

C. J. Snijders   A. Vleeming   R. Stoeckart   J. M. A. Mens
G. J. Kleinrensink

INTRODUCTION

Low back pain during pregnancy has often been ascribed to postural adaptation, resulting in a pronounced lumbar lordosis. However, we and others have found that, in general, the curvature of the lumbar spine is less before than after childbirth (Snijders et al 1976). Thus, the prime cause of pain during pregnancy must be related to something other than hollowing of the lumbar curvature. Because mechanical problems in the pelvis seem to be a probable alternative cause, a logical step was the introduction in 1977 of a pelvic belt for treatment of peripartum pelvic pain; most patients reported a positive effect (Snijders et al 1984). Although many factors may play a role, the belt was expected to have a direct mechanical effect on the stability of the sacroiliac joints (SIJs). This initiated the development of a biomechanical model by the Musculoskeletal Research Group, which consists of anatomists, physicists, engineers, and clinicians in Rotterdam. The description of this model begins with aspects of the mechanical vulnerability of the SIJ.

Mechanical solutions to protect the joints against dislocation are presented, along with electromyographic (EMG) and other findings that validate the underlying model.

MECHANICAL VULNERABILITY OF THE SIJ

The risk of dislocation can be traced to (a) shearing of flat SIJ surfaces (translation/rotation), (b) large sagittal loads parallel to the SIJ surfaces, and (c) the lumbopelvic click-clack phenomenon.

Figure 6.1a illustrates that flat joint surfaces are not protected against dislocation, in contrast to the closed form of a ball and socket joint (Snijders et al 1995a). However, compared with a spherical joint, a flat joint shape provides better capacity for the transfer of bending moments. Figure 6.2 shows that the longitudinal forces on the spine are always greater than transverse forces (Snijders et al 1993). This schematic model is used for the assessment of postural load imposed by working conditions (Van Riel et al 1995). The

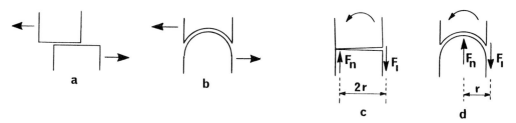

Fig. 6.1   (a) Subjecting a bone to a transverse force near the joint leads to a shift with respect to the adjacent bone before it is stopped by ligaments. The bones do not 'stay in line', which points to vulnerability to (sub)luxation by this loading mode. (b) This disadvantage does not occur with a ball and socket joint. (c, d) Because of a greater lever arm, a flat joint is more appropriate than a ball and socket joint to transfer a pure bending moment (Reproduced from Snijders et al 1995a.)

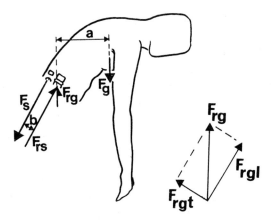

Fig. 6.2 Longitudinal forces on the spine (F_{rs} + F_{rgl}) are always greater than transverse forces (F_{rgt}) because the lever arm of the weight force (a) in a stooped posture is greater than the lever arm of the counteracting dorsal muscles (b) (Reproduced from Snijders et al 1995a.)

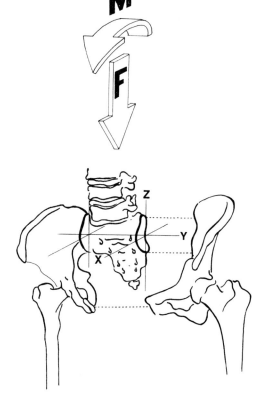

Fig. 6.3 Flat joints, such as the SIJ, are vulnerable to shear (rotation/translation) when loaded in the plane of the joint surfaces. M, moment; F, force. (Reproduced with permission from Snijders et al 1995c.)

reaction force in the spine due to gravity (F_{rg}) has a transverse component (F_{rgt}) that is maximal when the trunk is in horizontal position, and is equal to the weight of the upper body plus the weight in the hands. However, the longitudinal force on the spine is greater than the transverse force because of the unfavorable ratio between the lever arms of muscle force (F_s) and gravitational force (F_g) in relation to the intervertebral discs. The position of the intervertebral discs is optimal, because they are perpendicular to the longitudinal orientation of the spine. In contrast, the flat SIJ surfaces are almost parallel to the plane of maximal load (lumbosacral forces, F, and moments, M, in the sagittal plain) (Fig. 6.3) (Snijders et al 1992, 1995c). When the resultant lumbosacral force (F) acts lateral to the midsagittal plane, the load on one of the SIJ can be doubled. Thus, vulnerability especially exists in asymmetric loading. Lifting with torsion of the trunk can serve as an example, because it is associated with an unequal distribution of the load on the legs. Furthermore, Granata and Marras (1994) developed an EMG-assisted model to predict spinal loads during free-dynamic lifting exertions, which indicated that spinal load increases with asymmetry.

The clinical significance of the present biomechanical model covers both dynamic and static loading situations. Because of the creep of collagenous tissue exposed to prolonged loading,

as in sitting, the gravity-loaded SIJs are vulnerable to dislocation. The SIJs seem to be the only flat joints that sustain gravity load in the plane of the joint surfaces. The phenomenon of spinal shrinkage has been well documented (Looze et al 1994); it is related to lowering of the intervertebral discs and is not connected to joint dislocation in the direction of loading.

A significant change of load in the lumbopelvic region can be experienced when one sits upright on the edge of a straight chair (Fig. 6.4). Slow forward translation of the trunk increases lumbar lordosis, whereas backward translation moves the center of gravity above the ischial tuberosities into an unstable position. Further backward translation results in backward tilt of the pelvis and lumbar kyphosis. We call this a click-clack phenomenon because of the unstable intermediate

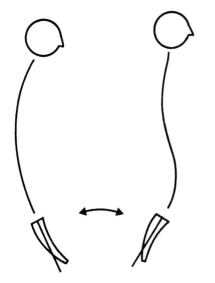

Fig. 6.4 Translation of the trunk from a forward position to a backward position involves transition from one stable position to another in sitting. The intermediate posture with the center of gravity above the ischial tuberosities is an unstable position. This transition from lumbar lordosis to lumbar kyphosis is called the lumbopelvic click-clack phenomenon. (Reproduced with permission from Snijders et al 1995d.)

position and the sudden reversion of loading (Snijders 1970).

PROTECTION AGAINST DISLOCATION

In mechanical engineering a distinction is made between form and force closure (Snijders et al 1992). With form closure, construction elements remain in place independent of external load (Fig. 6.5A). Force closure is essential when form closure is absent (Fig. 6.5B) or insufficient (Fig. 6.5C). The construction elements remain in place by friction forces between, and tangential to, the contact surfaces; these forces are exclusively generated by compression. With respect to the SIJ, we can identify a combination of form and force closure (Fig. 6.5C). Aspects of form closure that resist gliding are symmetric ridges and grooves in the joint surfaces (Vleeming et al 1990a), the undulated shape of the surfaces, which resemble the form of a propeller (Vleeming et al 1990a), and the wedge shape of the sacrum in between the hip bones.

Essential in the biomechanical model of SIJ stability is the introduction of force closure (Snijders et al 1984). In several reports, it is assumed that ligament structures ensure stability of the SIJ and that muscle forces are of no significance (Bernard & Cassidy 1992, Grieve 1983). In contrast, we assume that the ligament structures surrounding the SIJ are not capable of transferring lumbosacral load to the iliac bones in heavy loading situations or in conditions such as standing and sitting with prolonged load (because of creep). According to our model, additional compressive forces are needed to resist shearing of the SIJ surfaces. Compression can be produced by muscle forces, in combination with forces in ligaments and

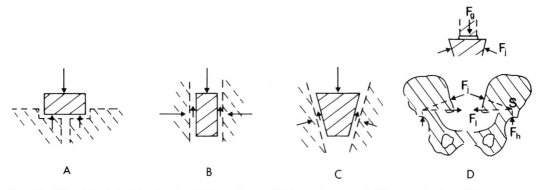

Fig. 6.5 The object is held in place by (A) form closure, (B) force closure, and (C) a combination of form and force closure, less friction – and thus less compression – being needed than in (B). (D) shows the mechanism of an arch. Force F_l may be raised by ligaments, muscles, or a pelvic belt just cranial to the greater trochanter and caudal to the SIJ. This force prevents lateral movement of the hip bones to secure the form of an arch.

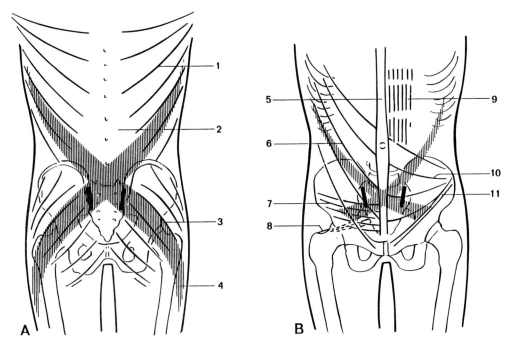

Fig. 6.6 Trunk, arm, and leg muscles that can compress the SIJ. The cross-like configuration indicates treatment and prevention of low back pain with strengthening and coordination of trunk, arm, and leg muscles in torsion and extension rather than flexion. (A) (1), latissimus dorsi; (2) thoracolumbar fascia; (3), gluteus maximus; (4), iliotibial tract. (B) (5), linea alba; (6), external abdominal obliques; (7), transverse abdominals; (8), piriformis; (9), rectus abdominis; (10), internal abdominal obliques; (11), ilioinguinal ligament. (Reproduced with permission from Snijders 1995d.)

fascia that cross the SIJ surfaces. This protective system requires the concerted action of muscles in the back, pelvis and legs. Muscles with an appropriate direction are indicated in Fig. 6.6. A special effect of the oblique and transverse abdominal muscles is shown in Fig. 6.7. The abdominal muscle force (F_o) results in a larger SIJ compression force because of the different lever arms of muscle force and the force in the dorsal SI ligaments in relation to the SIJ. This magnification of the abdominal force resembles the mechanism of a nutcracker. Optimal function is obtained with stiff interosseous SI ligaments. Data from Miller et al (1987) indicate that this requirement is met.

SIJ surfaces can also be protected against shearing by a loading mode that avoids shear. This interesting mechanical solution is created by the architecture of the pelvis, which resembles the mechanical principle of a Roman arch (see Fig. 6.5D above). The arch mechanism depends

on the firm connection between the two ends. In the foot, this function is ascribed to the plantar

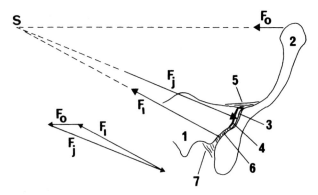

Fig. 6.7 Cross-section of the pelvis at the level of the SIJ. Force application by the oblique abdominal muscles (F_o), in combination with stiff dorsal sacroiliac ligaments (F_i), compresses the SIJ (F_j). Because the lever arms of muscle and ligament force are different, the joint reaction force is much greater than the muscle force. (1), sacrum; (2), iliac bone; (3), joint cartilage; (4), joint space; (5), ventral SI ligament; (6), interosseus SI ligaments; (7), dorsal SI ligaments. (Reproduced with permission from Snijders 1995d.)

aponeurosis (among other structures), whereas in the pelvis such action can be ascribed to the sacrotuberous and sacrospinal ligaments as well as the coccygeus and piriformis muscle, which can contribute to the force F_l (Snijders et al 1992, Vleeming et al 1990b). This force can also represent the action of a pelvic belt at the distal side of the SIJ. The pelvic arch receives bilateral support from the hip joints. When one sits on the ischial tuberosities, the support of forces is below the SIJ and the mechanism of the arch is absent.

CLICK-CLACK PHENOMENON

One of the assumptions in the biomechanical model on SIJ stability is that lack of control of the lumbopelvic click-clack phenomenon plays a role in the origin of low back pain. Of interest are typical loading modes (prolonged loading with creep of ligaments and abrupt reverse of loading) and typical positions of the sacrum with respect to the iliac bones (nutation, counternutation, and intermediate position). Movement into nutation or counternutation (related to lumbar extension and lumbar flexion respectively) is primarily connected with the inclination of the trunk in the gravity field. In principle, every force generated by back muscles, pelvic muscles, and leg muscles that acts directly or indirectly on the spine and iliac bones participates in these loading modes. In addition to the abrupt reverse of loading about the SIJ, the click-clack phenomenon may be related to other joint axes as well.

Control of the click-clack phenomenon depends on the rate of muscle action: the muscle forces must be generated at precisely the right time. This process may be viewed as a 'joint protecting' or 'arthrokinetic' reflex (Cohen & Cohen 1956). Impairment of elements in reflex chains may cause delayed muscle reaction and impair the functional stability of joints. This instability may be of short duration (the velocity of load application is once-only greater than the reaction time of the muscles) or becomes chronic. A permanent injury of one of the elements of the reflex chain may involve a permanent discrepancy between the velocity of load application and the reaction time of the muscles. Kleinrensink et al (1994) showed a relationship between inversion trauma

and impaired function of the peroneal nerve, which transmits both afferent and efferent information in the arthrokinetic reflex chain of the ankle. This relation may explain recurrences. In the arthrokinetic reflex chain, craniocaudal reflexes due to flexion or extension of the head may also play a role in loading and stability of the lumbopelvic region.

Some muscles that are directly attached to the spine are of special interest. Nutation of the sacrum can be supported by dorsal muscle force that acts on the sacrum (F_m in Fig. 6.8). In combination with its reaction force (F_{rm}) in the spine, a couple is produced that acts as a flexion moment on the sacrum (Snijders et al 1993). Here we think of the action of the sacral part of the multifidus muscle. Trunk muscles attached to the sacrum and trunk muscles attached to the iliac bones create a bifurcation in lumbosacral load. Muscles attached to the iliac bones induce shear loading of the SIJ and possibly counternutation in certain postures. Nutation of the sacrum may also be supported by the vertebral part of the iliopsoas muscle. This muscle, however, produces shear loading as well, because its orientation is almost parallel to the SIJ surfaces. For support of counternutation by muscle force acting directly on the sacrum, the levator ani and coccygeus muscles can be mentioned. The long head of the biceps femoris muscle can in some persons

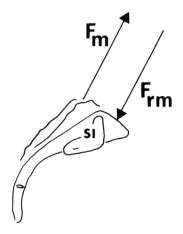

Fig. 6.8 The multifidus and part of the erector spinae muscle are attached to the sacrum. Muscle force (F_m) and its reaction force in the spine (F_{rm}) form a couple with a moment of force that tends to move the sacrum into nutation (Reproduced from Snijders et al 1995a.)

influence the tension in the sacrotuberous ligament (Vleeming et al 1990a).

VALIDATION OF THE BIOMECHANICAL MODEL

Validation can be searched for in biomechanical studies and in clinical evidence. First it can be seen that in vitro, loading tests showed SIJ mobility up to old age (Vleeming et al 1992a), and there was creep of ligaments during prolonged loading (Vleeming et al 1992b).

The concept of protection of the SIJ by muscle force agrees with reports that strenuous flexion–extension exercises and lifting involve coordinated action of the hamstrings, gluteus maximus, erector spinae, and latissimus dorsi muscles (Noe et al 1992 Oddsson & Thorstensson 1987).

Further validation was provided by EMG studies of muscle activity in unconstrained postures. As

expected, we found that in unconstrained standing and in sitting with firm support of the trunk by a backrest, the activity of hamstring, erector spinae, and gluteus maximus muscles was low (comparable to levels in the supine position). If the biomechanical model of SIJ stability is correct, other muscles should act to compress the SIJ. Indeed, in both unconstrained standing and sitting, the activity of the oblique abdominal muscles, especially the internal obliques, was significant (Fig. 6.9) (Snijders et al 1995b, 1995c). Because the continuous activity of the oblique abdominal muscles may be fatiguing, we looked for other mechanical solutions to stabilize the SIJ. Subjects sat on an office chair with a firm seat, backrest, and armrests. First we found that leg crossing (upper legs crossed or ankle on the knee, Fig. 6.10) correlates with a significant decrease in activity of the internal obliques (see Fig. 6.9 below) (Snijders et al 1995c). Another study focused on the pelvic

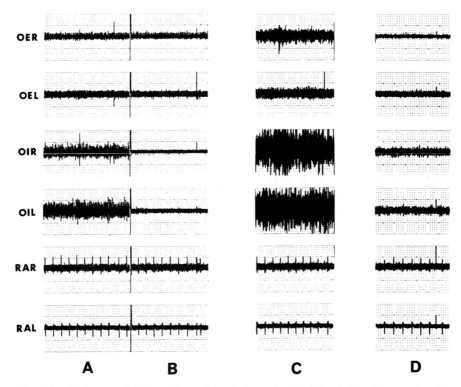

Fig. 6.9   (A) In normal sitting, oblique abdominal muscles left (L) and right (R) are active. (B) Leg-crossing (upper legs crossed or the ankle on the knee, see Fig. 6.10) leads to a significant decrease in internal oblique activity. (C) Oblique abdominal muscles are also active in unconstrained standing. Activity of erector spinae, gluteus maximus, and hamstring muscles, however, is absent. (D) Supine position. OE, external oblique; OI, internal oblique; RA, rectus abdominis. (Reproduced from Snijders et al 1995d.)

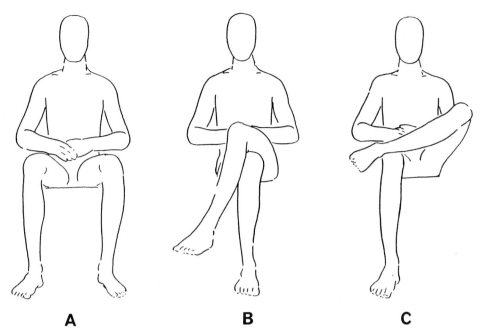

Fig. 6.10   (A) Sitting on an office chair with a firm seat using backrest and armrests. (B) Upper legs crossed. (C) Ankle on the knee. EMG recordings related to these postures are given in Fig. 6.9. (Reproduced with permission from Snijders 1995c.)

arch. Geometry indicates that sitting on the ischial tuberosities will not stabilize the SIJs, which are located above the tuberosities. The model predicts, however, that making a provision for a lateral support of the innominates restores the configuration of the pelvic arch. We therefore, measured EMG activity of subjects sitting on a soft seat of an old car. Indeed, the decrease in internal oblique activity compared with sitting on a hard seat was considerable: levels were as low as in the supine posture (Snijders et al 1995b).

It must be noted that the abdominal EMG activity levels in the sitting positions are low, in the order of magnitude of 3% of maximal voluntary contraction. In this respect, EMG levels obtained in different postures must be considered with caution. Change in posture can induce a shift of electrodes with respect to the muscle. The muscle configuration can change, which changes the moment arm of muscle force. However, a statistically significant difference could be determined between the postures mentioned. In seven men and eight women, oblique abdominal muscle activity was on average in the sitting position 450% that of supine, in the standing position

250% that of sitting on a firm seat, and in the sitting position 200% of that sitting with the upper legs crossed or the ankle on the knee (Snijders et al 1995c). These values have limited accuracy because of large inter- and intra-individual variations. Whether the pelvic floor and transverse abdominal muscles are active in standing and sitting positions is not known to us, since their electrical activity cannot be determined with surface electrodes (see also Chapter 37 in this volume). The recordings of oblique abdominal muscle activity may be influenced by the adjacent transverse abdominal muscles. However, all these muscles have significance in the compression of the SIJ.

CLINICAL EVIDENCE

We have had positive experience with the use of a pelvic belt in patients with peripartum pelvic pain (Fig. 6.11) (Snijders et al 1984). Although this effect may be related to unknown factors (for example proprioception), we believe that the mechanical effect also plays a role. The belt is often applied below the level of the SIJ, just

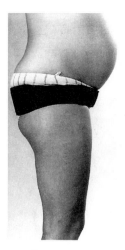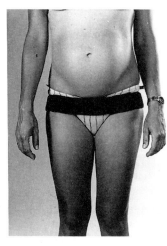

Fig. 6.11 A pelvic belt often reduces pain in the lower back and pelvis during pregnancy and after childbirth. A small force is sufficient. (Reproduced with permission from Snijders et al 1995d.)

above the level of the greater trochanters. Other patients profit more from a belt just below the anterior superior iliac spine (ASIS) or at the level of the pubic symphysis; elastic pants also may be effective and are often more convenient. It is not necessary to pull the belt forcefully. Forces of approximately 50 N are sufficient (Mens et al 1995, Vleeming et al 1992a). However, if after 15 min no effect is observed, the belt must not be pulled tighter; another solution must be sought. Pelvic belts are also beneficial in non-pregnant women and in men.

Physicians can simulate the action of a pelvic belt as well as of the oblique abdominal muscles (see Fig. 6.7 above) by applying medially directed manual forces to one or both hip bones. Patients with peripartum pelvic pain and instability severe enough to inhibit lifting their leg(s) while lying supine found that dysfunction could be restored by a manually applied adducting force across the pelvis through the iliac bones (see Chapter 35 in this volume). The applied force is approximately 50 N. This clinical test introduced by Mens may be interpreted as a strong validation experiment for the biomechanical model of the SIJ. This also seems to hold for the finding of Buyruk et al (see Chapter 24 on this volume) that a difference in stiffness levels between left and right, rather than hypo- or hypermobility of SIJ, is connected to

peripartum pain problems. In this study, SIJ stiffness levels were determined by vibration excitation of the hip bone at the ASIS, combined with measurement of the difference in vibration intensity between both sides of the ipsilateral SIJ (see Chapter 24). The finding of asymmetry in patients with peripartum pain meets with the previously mentioned vulnerability related to asymmetric lumbosacral loading.

With respect to the click-clack phenomenon, it is assumed that the intermediate position is unfavorable because of instability, and that counternutation is unfavorable because of loading of the long dorsal sacroiliac ligaments (see Chapter 3 in this volume). This ligament was reported to be painful in 42% of patients with peripartum pelvic pain (Mens et al 1995) and 46% with non-specific low back pain (Njoo 1996). This observation, together with literature on the mechanics of the lumbar spine, indicates that lumbar kyphosis, including counternutation of the sacrum, should be counteracted. This points to, for example, the importance of a proper lumbar support in prolonged, unconstrained sitting. Avoidance of counternutation of the sacrum can be observed in standing posture.

Instead of standing upright, patients with low back pain often adopt a slightly forward-bent position (Fig. 6.12B). This position supports nutation of the sacrum for two reasons:

1. The component of gravitational force that acts on the top of the sacrum in the transverse direction becomes larger.

2. The back extensor muscle (see Fig. 6.8 above) becomes significantly active in a slightly stooped posture (Snijders et al 1995b). Furthermore, this posture may relax the iliopsoas muscle and unload the SIJ.

The psoas muscles are continuously active in erect postures (Basmajian & De Luca 1985), as in Fig. 6.12A, and release of tension may correlate with reduction of lumbar lordosis, as in Fig. 6.12B. In the slightly forward-bent position, the erector spinae muscles may load painful structures, for example through its connection with the long dorsal SI ligaments. In a pilot EMG study, we demonstrated that addition of weight in a small rucksack decreased the erector

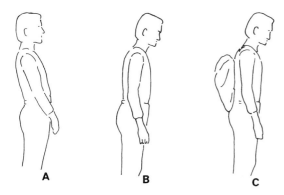

Fig. 6.12 (A) In unconstrained standing posture, iliopsoas muscles are always active, whereas erector spinae activity is absent. (B) Patients with low back pain often adopt a slightly stooped posture. Absence of iliopsoas activity means less load on the SIJ, whereas gravity load and erector spinae activity tend to move the sacrum into nutation, which is assumed to be favorable. (C) Application of a small rucksack diminishes erector spinae activity and may unload painful dorsal structures at the lumbopelvic level. The favorable slightly stooped posture can, however, be maintained. (Reproduced with permission from Snijders 1995d.)

is that in patients erector spinae and multifidus activity is persistent to secure nutation of the sacrum.

In the biomechanical model of SIJ stability, the pubic symphysis has no specific role. Thus the concept of the 'pelvic ring' is not required for the modeling of transfer of large lumbosacral loads to the legs. Supporting evidence may be found in the observation that after resection of the pubic bone because of osteosarcoma, the mechanical function can remain normal (Snijders et al 1992). Symphysiolysis may be associated with hypermobility of the SIJ. Therefore, isolated surgical symphysiodesis can be questioned; it interferes with the proper function of SI load transfer and does not resolve the problem of SIJ instability.

CONCLUSIONS

From the biomechanical model as described above we can derive the following conclusions.

1. Both the shape and the orientation of the SIJ point to mechanical vulnerability in situations of heavy loading, such as lifting, as well as in unconstrained postures such as sitting.
2. In addition to the strong ligamentous structures surrounding the SIJ, resistance against shearing can be produced by compression, which increases friction between the joint surfaces and presses the ridges and grooves.
3. Compression can be generated by muscles that cross the SIJ, by ligaments that are strained by muscle force, and by bending moments acting on the joint.
4. Muscles and fascia that contribute to self-bracing or self-locking of the SIJ have a cross-like configuration. Dorsally, this is formed by latissimus dorsi, the thoracolumbar fascia, gluteus maximus, and the iliotibial tract. Ventrally lie the external abdominal obliques, the linea alba, the internal abdominal obliques, and the transverse abdominals.
5. The oblique and transverse abdominal muscles are favorably situated for stabilization of the SIJ by means of jamming. Because the lever arms of ventral muscle force and dorsal SI ligament force are different, the joint reaction force is much greater than the muscle force, resembling the mechanism of a nutcracker.

spinae activity (Fig. 6.12C). Although this test involved subjects without low back pain, the results may explain the resolution of pain and the improved mobility after application of a small rucksack (3 kg) in the treatment of peripartum pelvic pain (J. M. A. Mens, unpublished data). We observed similar improvements in male patients with low back pain.

Although such observations are promising, they are preliminary. In a study on healthy subjects we observed that during static stooped postures up to 40°, the erector spinae demonstrated a strong increase in activity in all subjects. Within the range of 40–70°, activity fell to almost equal or lower levels than those measured during unconstrained standing (Snijders et al 1995b): the flexion–relaxation phenomenon. With respect to the role of the sacral part of the erector spinae and the multifidus muscle (see Fig. 6.8 above) in the nutation of the sacrum, the study of Shirado et al (1994) may be of interest. They compared the flexion–relaxation phenomenon of back muscles in the normal and in patients with chronic low back pain. The flexion–relaxation phenomenon was observed in all the healthy subjects. In contrast, no patients with chronic low back pain revealed the flexion–relaxation phenomenon. Our speculation

6. The architecture of the pelvis resembles a Roman arch. The sacrum remains in place when ligament or muscle forces distal to the SIJ prevent lateral movement of the hip bones.

7. The sacrotuberous and sacrospinal ligaments, as well as the coccygeus and piriformis muscles, support the mechanism of the pelvic arch. The effect of a pelvic belt distal to the SIJ has a similar effect.

8. The click-clack phenomenon implies unfavorable loading of the lumbosacral and SI region. Control of this phenomenon requires the concerted action of muscle groups which are part of a joint-protecting or arthrokinetic reflex mechanism.

9. Treatment and prevention of low back pain should be based on strengthening and coordination of trunk muscles, arm muscles, and leg muscles in torsion and extension rather than flexion.

10. Overload of, among others, the long dorsal SI ligaments may result from forcing the sacrum into counternutation. Such forcing may be related to an abrupt transition from lumbar lordosis to lumbar kyphosis, but may also be related to prolonged sitting without proper lumbar support.

11. In asymmetric postures, such as one-leg stance, transfer of the lumbosacral load is concentrated on one SIJ. Thus lifting with torsion of the trunk involves risk of injury, because it is associated with unequal distribution of the load on the legs.

12. While standing and sitting, compared with the supine position, the oblique abdominal muscles are significantly active.

13. Leg-crossing and sitting on a soft car seat result in a significant decrease of oblique abdominal muscle activity.

14. Application of a pelvic belt for peripartum pain, introduced in our clinic in 1977, has given positive results. This experience can serve as a validation of the biomechanical model of SIJ stability.

15. In the model of transfer of large lumbosacral forces to the iliac bones and legs, the pubic symphysis does not have a role. The pubic symphysis, however, must be deformable to allow small SIJ movement. Therefore, symphysiodesis may be questioned.

16. A small rucksack may relieve pain and improve mobility in some patients with low back pain. Although the initial results are promising, further clinical experiments are needed before definite conclusions can be drawn.

Acknowledgements

The authors thank J. V. de Bakker, C. A. C. Entius, G. A. Hoek van Dijke, M. G. van Kruining, R. Niesing, M. T. L. M. Ribbers, A. H. E. Slagter, J. G. Velkers, and A. de Vries for their valuable contributions.

REFERENCES

Basmajian F V, De Luca C J 1985 Muscles alive, their functions revealed by electromyography. Williams & Wilkins, Baltimore

Bernard T N Jr, Cassidy J D 1992 The sacroiliac joint syndrome, pathophysiology, diagnosis and management. In: Vleeming A, Mooney V, Snijders C J, Dorman T (eds) First interdisciplinary world congress on low back pain and its relation to the sacroiliac joint. San Diego, CA, 5–6 November, pp 119–144

Buyruk H M, Stam H J, Snijders C J, Vleeming A, Laméris J S, Holland W P J (1996) The measurement of sacroiliac joint stiffness in peripartum pelvic pain patients with colour doppler imaging (submitted for publication)

Cohen L A, Cohen M L 1956 Arthrokinetic reflex of the knee. American Journal of Physiology 184: 433–437

Granata K P, Marras W S 1994 EMG-assisted model of trunk loading during free-dynamic lifting exertions. Second World Congress of Biomechanics, Amsterdam, 10–15 July, pp 313

Grieve E F J 1983 Mechanical dysfunction of the sacroiliac joint. International Rehabilitation Medicine 5: 46–52

Kleinrensink G J, Stoeckart R, Meulstee J et al 1994 Lowered motor conduction velocity of the peroneal nerve after inversion trauma. Medicine and Science in Sports and Exercise 26: 877–883

Looze M P de, Dieën J H van, Visser B, Toussaint H M, Faessen H G M 1994 Spinal compression and spinal shrinkage in a brick laying activity. Second World Congress of Biomechanics, Amsterdam, pp 321

Mens J M A, Vleeming A, Snijders C J, Stam H J 1995 Active straight leg raising; a clinical approach to the load transfer function of the pelvic girdle. In: Vleeming A, Mooney V, Dorman T, Snijders C J (eds) Second interdisciplinary world congress on low back pain. San Diego, CA, 9–11 November, part I, pp 207–220

Miller J A A, Schultz A B, Andersson G B J 1987 Load-displacement behavior of sacroiliac joints. Journal of Orthopaedic Research 5: 92–101

Njoo K H 1996 Regional pain syndromes in patients with low back pain. PhD thesis, Erasmus University, Rotterdam, the Netherlands

Noe D A, Mostardi R A, Jackson M E, Portersfield J A, Askew M J 1992 Myoelectric activity and sequencing of selected trunk muscles during isokinetic lifting. Spine 17(2): 225–229

Oddsson L, Thorstensson A 1987 Fast voluntary trunk flexion movements in standing: motor patterns. Acta Physiologica Scandinavica 129: 93–106

Riel M P J M van, Derksen J C M, Burdorf A, Snijders C J 1995 Simultaneous measurements of posture and movements of head and trunk by continuous three-dimensional registration. Ergonomics 38(12): 2563–2575

Shirado O, Kaneda K, Toshikazu Ito 1994 An electromyographic analysis on flexion–relaxation phenomenon of back muscles. Second World Congress of Biomechanics, Amsterdam, pp 315

Snijders C J 1970 On the form of the human thoraco-lumbar spine and some aspects of its mechanical behaviour. PhD thesis, Eindhoven University, the Netherlands

Snijders C J, Seroo J M, Snijder J G N, Hoedt H T 1976 Change in form of the spine as a consequence of pregnancy. Digest of the 11th International Conference on Medical and Biological Engineering, Ottawa, 2–6 August, pp 670–671

Snijders C J, Snijder J G N, Hoedt H T E 1984 Biomechanische modellen in het bestek van rugklachten tijdens de zwangerschap. Tijdschrift voor Sociale Gezondheidszorg 62: 141–147

Snijders C J, Vleeming A, Stoeckart R 1992 Transfer of lumbosacral load to iliac bones and legs. Part I: Biomechanics of self-bracing of the sacroiliac joints and its significance for treatment and exercise. In: Vleeming A, Mooney V, Snijders C J, Dorman T (eds) First interdisciplinary world congress on low back pain and its relation to the sacroiliac joint. San Diego, CA, 5–6 November, pp 233–254

Snijders C J, Vleeming A, Stoeckart R 1993 Transfer of lumbosacral load to iliac bones and legs. Part II: Loading of the sacroiliac joints when lifting in a stooped posture. Clinical Biomechanics 8: 295–301

Snijders C J, Nordin M, Frankel V H 1995a Biomechanica van het spier-skeletstelsel; grondslagen en toepassingen. Lemma, Utrecht

Snijders C J, Bakker M P, Vleeming A, Stoeckart R, Stam H J 1995b Oblique abdominal muscle activity in standing and in sitting on hard and soft seats. Clinical Biomechanics 10(2): 73–78

Snijders C J, Slagter A H E, van Strik R, Vleeming A, Stam H J, Stoeckart R 1995c Why leg-crossing? The influence of common postures on abdominal muscle activity. Spine 20(18): 1989–1993

Snijders C J, Vleeming A, Stoeckart R, Mens J M A, Kleinrensink G J 1995d Biomechanical modeling of sacroiliac joint stability in different postures. In: Dorman T A (ed) Spine: prolotherapy in the lumbar spine and pelvis. State of the art reviews 9(2): 419–432

Vleeming A, Stoeckart R, Volkers A C W, Snijders C J 1990a Relation between form and function in the sacroiliac joint. Part I: Clinical anatomical aspects. Spine 15(2): 130–132

Vleeming A, Volkers A C W, Snijders C J, Stoeckart R 1990b Relation between form and function in the sacroiliac joint. Part II: Biomechanical aspects. Spine 15(2): 133–136

Vleeming A, Buyruk H M, Stoeckart R, Karamursel S, Snijders C J 1992a An integrated therapy for peripartum pelvic instability: a study of the biomechanical effects of pelvic belts. American Journal of Obstetrics and Gynecology 166(4): 1243–1247

Vleeming A, van Wingerden J P, Dijkstra P F, Stoeckart R, Snijders C J, Stijnen T 1992b Mobility in the sacroiliac joints in the elderly: a kinematic and radiological study. Clinical Biomechanics 7: 170–176

7. Coupled motion of contralateral latissimus dorsi and gluteus maximus: its role in sacroiliac stabilization

V. Mooney   R. Pozos   A. Vleeming   J. Gulick   D. Swenski

INTRODUCTION

The posterior layer of the thoracolumbar fascia has been defined as a mechanism of load transfer from the latissimus dorsi on one side to the gluteus maximus on the other side. This has been identified in dissections by Vleeming et al (1995). It had been hypothesized that a load transfer across the sacroiliac joint (SIJ) would require specific action of a variety of muscles, leading to sufficient compression of the SIJ to prevent shear (Snijders et al 1993). In this concept, the posterior layer of the thoracolumbar fascia plays an integrating role in rotation of the trunk and load transfer, and thus stability of the lower lumbar spine and pelvis.

These biomechanical concepts were confirmed by specific anatomic dissections described in these articles. Indeed, these dissections noted a direct fascial connection between the latissimus dorsi on one side and the gluteus maximus fascia on the other side. The mechanical relationship between these two muscles was confirmed by mechanical tests on cadavers, which noted a mechanical displacement greatest with traction on the latissimus dorsi on one side and the gluteus maximus on the other side. There was limited displacement of the fascia on the homolateral side of latissimus versus gluteus. The excursion was between 4 and 7 cm. There was no effect of traction on the gluteus medius muscle.

In our current study, therefore, we would like to verify whether muscles such as the gluteus maximus and contralateral latissimus dorsi are indeed active during trunk rotation. To confirm these anatomic observations in living individuals, it is necessary to test the electromyographic (EMG) activity in healthy subjects, as well as in patients, to evaluate the relationship between contralateral muscle activities during active function such as walking and torso rotation. This should be especially significant in individuals with an 'incompetent' SIJ. It would be helpful if one could document load transfer across the joint.

MATERIALS AND METHOD

To test this stabilization hypothesis, it is necessary to rotate the trunk without allowing any pelvic motion, as well as to evaluate natural rotation during gait. If the actions of the muscles noted above during rotation were confirmed, this would confirm the theory developed from the dissections noted above.

Fifteen normal healthy subjects (12 female and 3 male) without any complaints of back or leg pain were recruited to be evaluated for surface myoelectric activity of their latissimus and gluteus musculature. The EMGs were recorded on the ME 300P (Mega Electronics Inc., Finland). All subjects and patients had electrodes placed in the same locations. Both right and left gluteus and latissimus were recorded. The electrodes on the gluteus were located 10 cm medial and parallel to greater trochanter. The latissimus electrodes were 1 cm medial to the inferior lateral border of the scapula. Two test performances were carried out. In the first test, the surface myoelectric activity was tested during gait using a treadmill at constant speed. The subjects were also placed in a MedX torso rotation machine (MedX, Ocala, FL, USA). This device evaluates strength during torso rotation while the subject is sitting with hip and leg restraints that stabilize the pelvis but

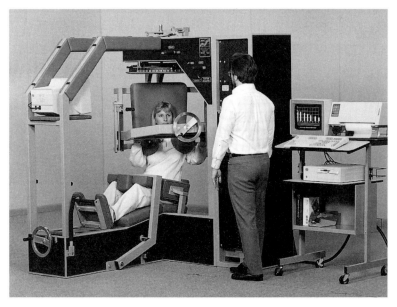

Fig. 7.1   MedX Torso machine.

allow rotation in a neutral sitting position. Isometric strength at equal points in the range of rotation motion is tested. The same equipment is used for dynamic isotonic eccentric and concentric exercise of torso rotating musculature (Carpenter et al 1991) (Fig. 7.1).

This same equipment has been used to treat individuals with symptomatic SIJ. It has been the most effective exercise regime for people with this diagnosis (Mooney 1995). Therefore, five patients with painful sacroiliac (SI) dysfunction, documented by radiographically controlled injections into the SIJ, were tested for strength and myo-electric activity in the latissimus and gluteus. All patients presented with unilateral buttock pain with a history of sudden onset. The duration of the complaint averaged 8 months. All were female.

RESULTS

Subjects walking on a treadmill at a constant rate confirmed the reciprocal relationship between the latissimus on one side and the gluteus maximus on the other (Fig. 7.2). The raw EMGs demonstrated no significant difference between males and females. When the root mean square (RMS) of all 15 subjects was graphically displayed, it was

apparent that the signal amplitude of the latissimus was far less than that of the gluteus. Of interest was that the right gluteus usually had a lower RMS than the left (Fig. 7.3). Twelve of the 15 subjects were right-handed. This reciprocal relationship of muscles correlates nicely with normal reverse rotation of the shoulders versus pelvis in normal gait.

When the subjects exercised on the torso rotation machine, the reciprocal relationship between the latissimus on one side and the gluteus on the other was again evident. A typical example of the raw EMG data is presented in Fig. 7.4. With right rotation of the trunk, the right latissimus dorsi is significantly more active than the left, but the left gluteus is more active than the right gluteus, although less so than the latissimus. In the torso rotation machine, very limited motion is occurring at the pelvis. The torso goes through an arc of 72° of right to left rotation and reverse. There was no significant difference in the EMG amplitude between rotation to the left or to the right (Fig. 7.5). When the mean RMS was displayed for all 15 subjects, it was apparent that all subjects reflected the findings of the raw EMG patterns. In the sitting pelvis-fixed posture, the latissimus was much more active than the gluteus, but the gluteus contralateral to the active latissimus was

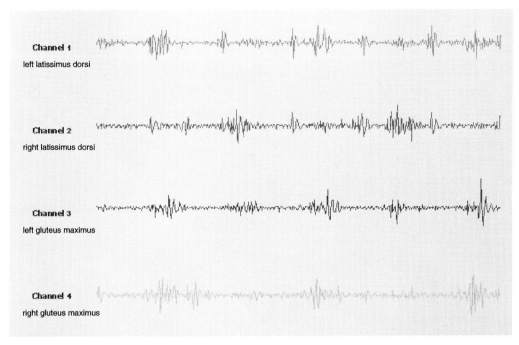

Fig. 7.2   EMG pattern of a female walking at a constant speed on a treadmill. This shows that, during ambulation, there is a reciprocal function between the latissimus dorsi on one side and the gluteus on the other.

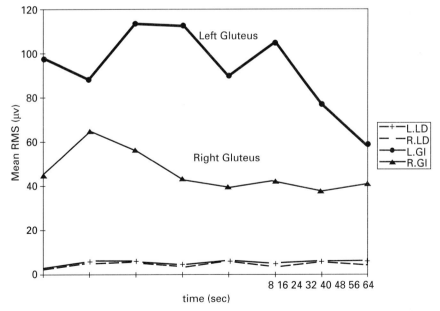

Fig. 7.3   This is a summary of myoelectric activity depicted as an average RMS (amplitude) of the gluteus versus the latissimus in all subjects. The right gluteus consistently showed less amplitude than the left. The amplitude of the left and right latissimi while walking was minimal but equal.

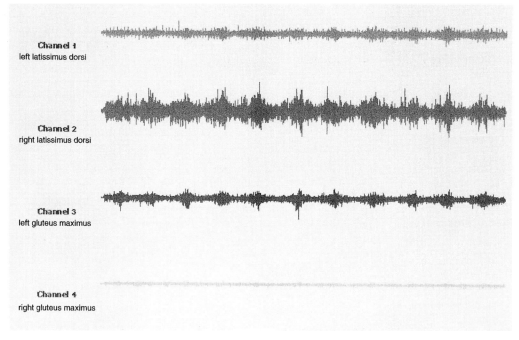

Fig. 7.4 Raw EMG pattern of a normal female subject carrying out rotation on the torso rotation machine, showing a greater degree of right latissimus activity contrasted to reciprocal left gluteus activity.

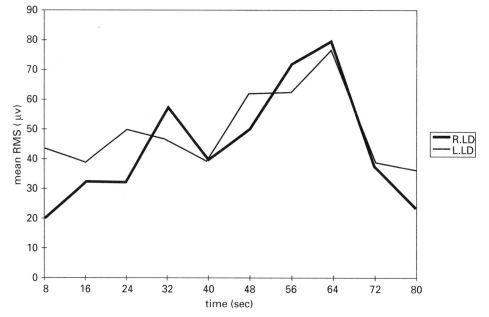

Fig. 7.5 In the torso rotation machine, the mean amplitude (all healthy subjects) of left and right latissimus dorsi is about the same.

more active than the homolateral gluteus maximus (Figs 7.6 and 7.7).

The patients demonstrated a strikingly different pattern. On initial evaluation, the gluteus on the symptomatic side was far more active than that demonstrated by the healthy subjects (Fig. 7.8). The reciprocal relationship between latissimus and gluteus was, however, still present. The patients

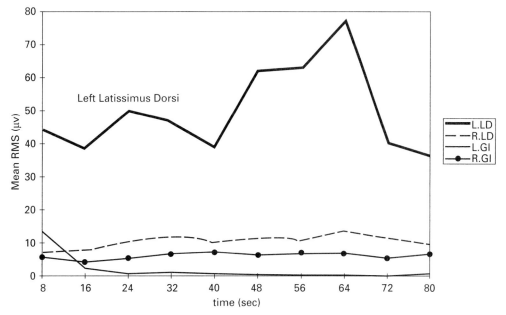

Fig. 7.6 This shows the normal activity of the latissimus dorsi (all healthy subjects) in the torso rotation machine as being strongest in the direction of rotation; the contralateral gluteus is more active than the homolateral.

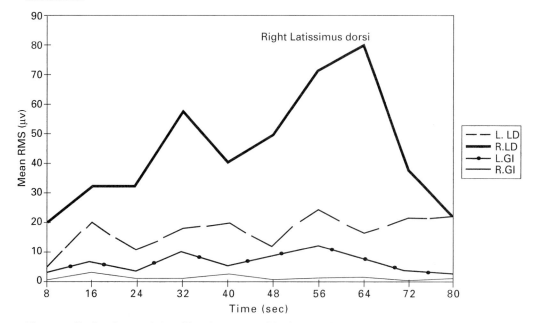

Fig. 7.7 Similar characteristics of function are noted in right rotation, the right latissimus being more active than the left; the contralateral gluteus (left) is more active than the homolateral.

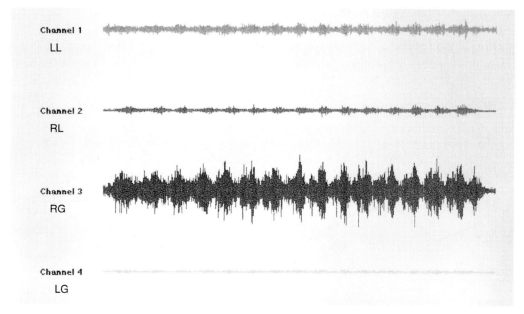

Fig. 7.8   Raw EMG recording of a patient with a painful right SIJ going through left torso rotation. Channel 1 is the left latissimus (LL) and channel 3 the right gluteus (RG). Hyperactivity of the gluteus on the painful side is demonstrated.

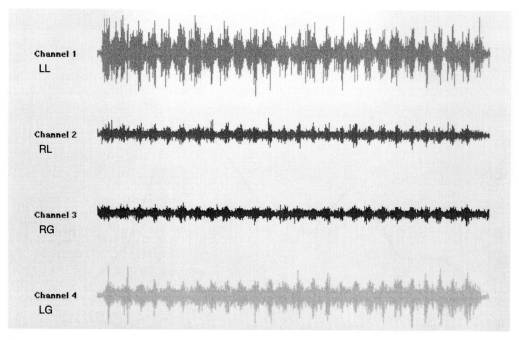

Fig. 7.9   Raw EMG from the same patient documenting that with improvement in strength and reduction of pain, the EMGs during left torso rotation are returning more to the normal status of high latissimus activity, contrasted with low gluteus activity. Channel 1 is the left latissimus (LL), and channel 3 the right gluteus (RG). Channel 4 (left gluteus, LG) has now become more active to substitute for the right gluteus.

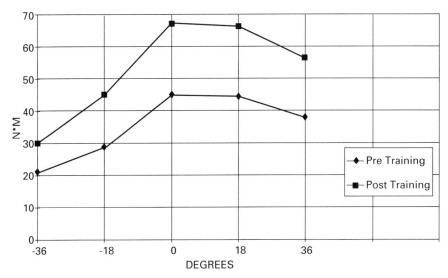

Fig. 7.10 This graph depicts the average increase for all patients in strength of rotation from the beginning to the end of an exercise program lasting approximately 2.5 months. This shows initially diminished strength compared with normal, especially at full external rotation.

were placed through a training program that set resistance at 50% of maximum isometric strength and progressed 5% after 20 repetitions could be completed. After 2 months of training, twice per week, there was a 25% increase in isometric strength of the patient whose raw data are presented in Figs 7.8 and 7.9. Myoelectric activity had also changed. With improvement in strength, as demonstrated by increased latissimus activity, there was a diminished activity of the gluteus on the reciprocal side (Fig. 7.9). The EMG still had not returned to the low levels typical of the asymptomatic subjects, but there was a reduction in the amount of myoelectric activity. This change corresponded with a significant reduction in pain of this typical patient. The change in strength is depicted in Fig. 7.10.

DISCUSSION

These myoelectric findings confirm the interrelationship between the latissimus on one side and the gluteus maximus on the other, as demonstrated by the anatomic findings of Vleeming et al (1995). This was demonstrated both in walking and measured torso rotation. The finding that the right gluteus maximus during gait consistently showed less amplitude than the left cannot

yet be explained. It should be noted, however, that in a large series of patients diagnosed as having primary SI pain, 45% had the pain on the right, 35% on the left, and 20% bilaterally (Bernard & Cassidy 1991). The small number of patients and lack of clear definition of leg dominance in this small group of normal subjects is not sufficient enough to draw important conclusions.

This reciprocal gluteus–latissimus relationship has also been suggested by Gracovetsky (1995) from mathematical analysis of the biomechanics of gait. This relationship, however, has seldom been described in articles on gait analysis (Gauge et al 1995).

The importance of these findings, from a therapeutic sense, is that it offers an opportunity for a rational treatment program for dysfunction of the SIJ. Stabilization of an incompetent joint is certainly theoretically possible by simultaneously activating these two muscles whose fascial connection traverses the SIJ.

An incompetent SIJ is a most difficult diagnosis to define and is thus difficult to treat rationally. There are few clinical tests that are thought to be reliable. In a very specific study carried out by Schwarzer et al (1995) in which the SIJ was carefully injected to evaluate pain production and relief, no specific physical examination test correlated with all of the positive responders. It has also been determined that there is no difference in the amount of motion at the SIJ in symptomatic versus non-symptomatic individuals (Sturesson et al 1989). Nonetheless, it has been determined that stabilization of the SIJ with external mechanical forces is of benefit. Pelvic belts have been useful to control back pain, especially in peripartum individuals (Vleeming et al 1992). It has also been demonstrated that abdominal musculature can carry out a self-bracing effect on the SIJ, both in standing and sitting (Snijders et al 1995).

The finding in this study of healthy subjects without pain is that the latissimus dorsi in the torso rotation movement has significantly greater EMG activity than does the gluteus maximus in a sitting posture with the pelvis stabilized. This would be expected based on the biomechanics of the situation. In the sitting position, the hip is not moving. However, the finding that, in this test situation, the gluteus maximus EMG activity is significantly greater in patients with painful SI dysfunction than in healthy subjects, indicates

that the effort of the gluteus maximus is to try and stabilize the SI dysfunction. The diminished EMG activity of the gluteus, corresponding with increased strength and decreased pain, supports the view that stabilization by the musculature can achieve symptomatic benefit in patients with SI dysfunction.

The comparison of myoelectric patterns in symptomatic individuals with those of normal subjects forms the basis of this study. In that individuals are quite varied in their habitual and non-conscious strategies in myoelectric activity, no sharp statistical differences can be made. The differences in patterns are apparent, however, from the various descriptions noted above. The most important finding was the significant hyperactivity of the gluteus on the painful side when stress was applied to the SIJ during strengthening of the torso-rotating muscles. The assistive role of the reciprocal latissimus dorsi is also important and thus forms a rational and justified goal for rehabilitative exercise programs.

REFERENCES

Bernard T N Jr, Cassidy J D 1991 The sacroiliac joint syndrome – pathophysiology, diagnosis and management. In: Frymoyen J (ed.) The adult spine: principles and practice. Raven Press, New York, pp 2107–2130

Carpenter D J, Graves M, Pollock S et al 1991 Quantitative assessment of isometric torso rotation net muscular torque. Archives of Physical Medicine and Rehabilitation 72: 804–808

Gauge J R, Deluca P A, Rinshaw T S 1995 Gait analysis: principles and applications. Journal of Bone and Joint Surgery (US) 77: 1607–1623

Gracovetsky S A 1995 Locomotion – linking the spinal engine with the leg. In: Vleeming A, Mooney V, Dorman T, Snijders C J (eds) Second interdisciplinary world congress on low back pain. San Diego, CA, 9–11 November, pp 171–174

Mooney V 1995 Evaluation and treatment of sacroiliac dysfunction. In: Vleeming A, Mooney V, Dorman T, Snijders C J (eds) Second interdisciplinary world congress on low back pain. San Diego, CA, 9–11 November, pp 393–407

Schwarzer A C, Aprill C N, Bogduk N 1995 The sacroiliac joint in low back pain. Spine 20: 31–37

Snijders C J, Vleeming A, Stoeckart R 1993 Transfer of lumbosacral load to iliac bones and legs. II: Loading of the sacroiliac joints when lifting in stooped posture. Clinical Biomechanics 8: 295–301

Snijders C J, Bakker M P, Vleeming A, Stoeckart R 1995 Oblique abdominal muscle activity on standing and sitting on hard and soft seats. Clinical Biomechanics 10: 1073–1078

Sturesson B T, Selvik G, Uden A 1989 Movements of the sacroiliac joints; a roentgen stereophotogrammetric analysis. Spine 14: 162–165

Vleeming A, Buyruk H M, Stoeckart R, Karamürsel S, Snijders C J 1992 Towards an integrated therapy for peripartum pelvic instability: a study of the biomechanical effects of pelvic belts. American Journal of Obstetrics and Gynecology 166: 1243–1247

Vleeming A, Pool-Goudzwaard A L, Stoeckart R, van Wingerden J P, Snijders C J 1995 The posterior layer of the thoracolumbar fascia: its function in load transfer from spine to legs. Spine 20(7): 753–758

8. Kinematic models and the human pelvis

A. Huson

INTRODUCTION

This chapter deals with kinematic models in relation to the human pelvis. It is mainly based on the ideas concerning modeling of the human locomotor apparatus that we have developed in our research group (Benink 1985, Huson et al 1989, Morrenhof 1989, Ottevanger et al 1989, Schreppers et al 1990, Spoor et al 1989, 1990, Van Langelaan 1983, Van Leeuwen et al 1990, Wismans et al 1980). Although most of our work focused on the lower extremity and did not pay particular attention to the sacroiliac joint (SIJ), there is still a clear link with the approach and ideas of Snijders' and Vleeming's work (e.g. Snijders et al 1993a, Vleeming et al 1995b). Therefore the line of thought unfolded in this chapter has an obvious relevance for the theme of this book.

In biomechanics, the human musculoskeletal system is often represented by a so-called multi-body system comprising (1) a number of rigid bodies (bones), which are connected to each other by (2) movable linkages (joints) and (3) force generators (muscles). This is of course an abstraction, a reduction of the complex reality, and as such is subject to all the restrictions inherent in abstractions. However, such an approach may enable us to unravel the complexity of particular mechanical relationships. An elegant example is Snijders' and Vleeming's explanation of the self-locking effect in the construction of the pelvis (Vleeming et al 1995b). Their model gives us an idea of the roles played by friction, the position of contact surfaces between the bones, and certain pelvic dimensions as parameters of pelvic shape in the functional task to keep the pelvic assembly together under a vertical static load. Snijders and

Vleeming arrived at this solution by treating the pelvic bones as so-called free bodies, virtually isolated from their real context (the pelvic ring), while a number of forces act under certain conditions on these bones. In this way, descriptive anatomy acquires in their hands a quantitative and measurable aspect and at once the description becomes explanatory.

The sacrum and the pelvic bones, connected to each other by the SIJ and the pubic symphysis, form what is described as a closed kinematic chain. This chain contains only three links connected by three linkages. Had these linkages been simple hinges, the chain would have been in kinematic terms a rigid structure. However, due to the nature of the pelvis and its linkages, this is in kinematic as well as in static terms not the case, and the ring has instead a certain mobility or deformability. Not only the pelvic ring, but, as has been said before, many if not all of the sub-systems of the musculoskeletal system can also be described as kinematic chains, either closed or open. While the pelvis is a structurally closed chain, many of the other chains are open and can be closed voluntarily. The general effect of such a closure leads to an increase of its kinematic constraints, in other words it is a reduction of the chain's kinematic degrees of freedom of motion (DFOM). Said in more general terms, closure leads to a reduction of the chain's mobility, or a gain in stability. Let us consider this effect in more detail.

CLOSED KINEMATIC CHAINS

Figure 8.1 shows a very simple model of the lower part of the human body, consisting of only

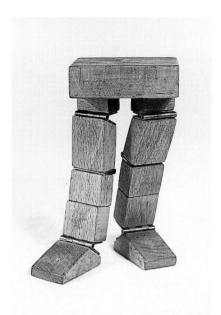

Fig. 8.1 A simple model of the lower part of the human body comprising the pelvis (the upper block as one of its six links), the thighs (two other links), the legs (again two links), and both feet (the feet, together with the floor, representing the sixth link). The purpose of the horizontal cleft dividing the legs into two parts will be clarified by Fig. 8.9 below. See text for further explanation.

the pelvis with the lower extremities and standing on a supporting base. In this case, the pelvis is conceived of as a single rigid piece. The pelvis, the thighs, the legs, and both feet, which are supposed to be firmly connected to the supporting floor by the combined effects of gravity and friction, together form a closed kinematic chain, containing six links. The linkages or joints in this model have been considerably simplified for modeling purposes. In this model, all the joints are reduced to simple hinge joints. For the time being, we are assuming that the muscles running in different directions around these joints are capable of imposing this reduction on the joints. Furthermore, in this model the feet are slightly abducted by exorotation of both legs at the hip joints. Notice that, in this position, the model can keep itself in an upright position while standing on a flat supporting surface without any external support, keeping its hips and ankles still in a mid-position between full extension and flexion. Only the knees are locked in full extension. Apparently, no muscles are needed to stabilize these

joints other than those supposed to change the hips and knees kinematically into hinges. It seems that we are confronted with another example of a self-locking effect. We have called this self-locking effect a muscle-saving principle because the chain can kinematically be stabilized with less muscular effort than would be expected from the total number of joints involved (Huson 1983). In this case, the self-locking effect is a consequence of the particular combination of joints in this closed kinematic chain. The next figures will explain this typical effect in more detail.

TWO-DIMENSIONAL SIMPLE CHAINS

Figure 8.2 shows an open kinematic chain comprising four links. It has one fixed or base link, indicated by the number 1 and recognizable by its hatching, and two arms, one of them containing two links (the right arm with the numbers 3 and 4) and the other one having only one link (number 2 at the left-hand side). All of the linkages – A (between links 4 and 1), B (between links 2 and 1), and D (between links 3 and 4) – are simple hinges. Because the hinge axes are parallel to each other and perpendicular to the plane of the drawing, this is called a two-dimensional or planar chain.

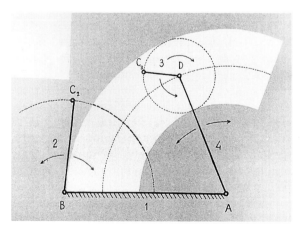

Fig. 8.2 A two-dimensional or planar four-bar chain. The chain has been opened at its linkage C. Now both arms can be moved independently with respect to the hatched reference link (1). In the depicted position of the arms, points C_2, C_3, and D can move along the circular paths depicted by the broken lines. The segment in bold of the circular path about rotation center B defines the only path along which C can move after closure of the chain.

Its motions occur in a single plane or in a set of parallel planes, in which case the motions can be projected on a single plane. Point C_2 of the one-link arm can move along the circular path about B; likewise point D can move along a circular path with A as its center of rotation, whereas in the position of link 4 depicted, point C_3 can move along the circular path with D as its rotation center. However, as soon as link 4 is set free to rotate about A, point C_3 can move freely within the boundaries of the curved lightly shaded area. Consequently, links 2 and 4 have only one DFOM each, whereas link 3 has two.

After assembling the two arms by joining the points C_3 and C_2 into a new hinge, i.e. after closure of the chain, the kinematic conditions within the chain have changed dramatically: the newly formed hinge C can move only along the common circular path of both formerly open arms. Thus link 3 also now has a limited freedom of one DFOM. It must be noted that in its closed configuration, the chain is provided with four hinges, one more than in its open condition. Together they are good for four DFOM. Yet the actual kinematic freedom of all its links allows only one DFOM because after closure both points C and D can move only along the circular paths about A and B in a particular combination, prescribed by the length of the connecting link 3. Apparently, three DFOM have disappeared after closure of the chain (see also the upper part of Fig. 8.4 below). Let us see what happens if we add one more link to the chain.

The upper part of Fig. 8.3 shows again an open chain, but now consisting of five links. This chain too has one fixed, or base link, number 1 (again recognizable by its hatching). Now, however, the two arms have two links each: numbers 2 and 3 at the left, and numbers 4 and 5 at the right. In this chain, both end links – 3 and 4 – can move with two DFOM within the boundaries of the two curved hatched and lightly shaded areas.

As soon as the two arms are connected with each other, by assembling D_3 and D_4 into a new hinge, the mobility of D in the now-closed chain is limited to the overlapping area only: the lightly shaded area without hatching. Yet it means that links 3 and 4 still have two DFOM each. How-

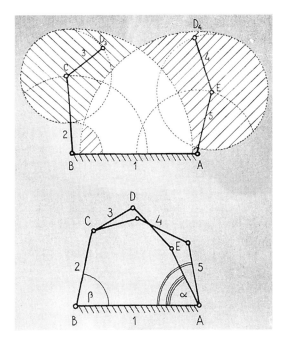

Fig. 8.3 The upper part shows a two-dimensional, five-bar chain in an open condition similar to the chain in Fig. 8.2. The lower part depicts a closed five-bar chain with two DFOM for point D. The position of the chain can be defined unequivocally by defining two variables, the angles α and β.

ever, in its closed configuration (the lower part of Fig. 8.3), the chain is provided with five hinges, representing in total five DFOM. Apparently again, *three* DFOM have disappeared after closure of the chain. A similar reduction of three DFOM would occur if we added another link to the chain, resulting in a six-bar chain that has one link having three DFOM with respect to its reference link.

COMPOUND CLOSED CHAINS

It is important to note that the four-bar chain, having only one DFOM, can be stabilized (immobilized) by stabilizing just one of its four hinges. Thus stabilizing one of the four joints has an immobilizing effect on all the other joints too. On the other hand, if we add one more link to the chain, turning it into a five-bar chain, two joints have to be stabilized in order also to immobilize all the other joints. However, as soon as we loosen one of these two stabilized joints, the chain has regained one DFOM, which means that, apart from the other as yet still immobilized joint, the other three joints can immediately move freely again. This transition can be described in another way by saying that stabilizing one joint of the five-bar chain changes this chain into a four-bar chain (see the lower part of Fig. 8.3).

Such an effect will also be seen under similar conditions if similar but longer chains are considered. The longer such a chain, the more joints will be included in the sudden increase of instability when one of its joints becomes disconnected or one of its links is broken. In other words, the muscle-saving principle suddenly loses its effect if the chain changes from the kinematic condition of zero DFOM to one or more DFOM.

If we consider the chain comprising the pelvis and both legs under the conditions of human walking, such sudden changes in its state of kinematic constraints occur physiologically at heel strike and toe-off. During each step cycle, the chain is alternately closed and opened twice, and it is exactly at these critical events that the main bursts of muscle activity occur (Morrenhof 1989).

Figure 8.4 shows two examples of a closed kinematic chain, the upper having only four links, the lower having six links, but now in two different configurations. The upper one is a simple-closed chain, like our four- and five-bar chains depicted in Figs 8.2 and 8.3 above. The lower chain, however, is a so-called compound-closed chain, having one link (number 6) as a cross-link between the two opposite triangular links 2 and 5. The simple chain has four hinges and its resulting kinematic freedom is one DFOM, a reduction, as we have seen, of three DFOM as a consequence of closure in a planar system. The compound chain, however, has seven hinges, yet a mobility of only one DFOM. It will move only according to a single prescribed and reproducible motion mode. Thus, reduction after closure in a *compound* configuration goes much further, since in this example apparently *six* DFOM have disappeared. Very long chains constructed as coupled compound configurations can effect even greater reductions. The example shown in Fig. 8.5 will result in a reduction of as many as 33 DFOM.

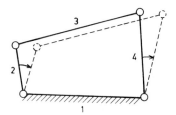
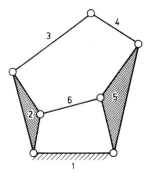

Fig. 8.4 Two different configurations of a closed, two-dimensional chain. The upper one has four links yielding one DFOM and is a simple chain. The lower one is a compound-closed chain and also has only one DFOM, even though it has seven linkages.

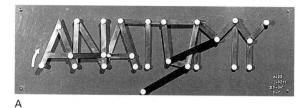
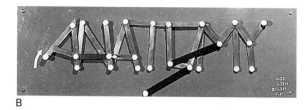

Fig. 8.5 A very long planar, compound-closed kinematic chain photographed in two positions. Despite its great number of linkages, it has only one DFOM. Note that the chain is essentially an assemblage of many coupled four-bar chains.

THREE-DIMENSIONAL CLOSED KINEMATIC CHAINS

Apart from a configuration characteristic such as compound closure, there can be still another

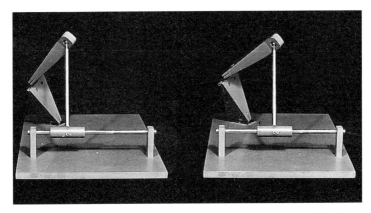

Fig. 8.6 Two different positions of a three-dimensional or spatial four-bar chain. The chain has only one DFOM, although its joints together represent seven DFOM: $(2 \times 1) + 3 + 2 = 7$. The four joints comprise two hinges (the two lower joints of the long arm, visible in the background, each having one DFOM), one ball and socket joint (the upper joint of the long arm having three DFOM: three rotational modes), and one cylindrical joint (the joint in the foreground having two DFOM: one rotational and one translational mode).

boundary condition that determines the extent to which the mobility of a particular kinematic chain will be reduced. If a simple closed chain is not a two-dimensional or planar chain but a three-dimensional or spatial chain instead, closure of the chain in a simple configuration will produce a reduction of *six* DFOM, twice the reduction occurring after closure of a planar chain. In a spatial chain, hinge-like linkages have no parallel axes and these chains may even have ball and socket joints; in more general terms, they may have joints with more DFOM than simple hinges have. Their motions do not occur in single plane only but in space, which is three-dimensional. Therefore they have to be described with respect to three orthogonal references axes. Figure 8.6 shows such a three-dimensional chain in two different positions.

In spatial configurations of closed kinematic chains, the reduction of its DFOM will also increase considerably when the chain has a compound configuration. Such three-dimensional, compound-closed kinematic chains occur in the complex skeletoligamentous system of the human body. A typical example of such a three-dimensional, compound-closed kinematic chain is the carpal complex of the human wrist. Figure 8.7 shows a schematic representation of this

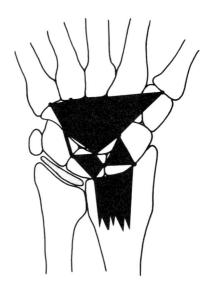

Fig. 8.7 Schematic representation of the carpus as a spatial, compound-closed kinematic chain. This example comprises only the following linkages: the radio-scaphoid joint, the radio-lunatum joint, the lunato-scaphoid joint, the lunato-triquetrum joint, the hamato-scaphoid joint, the hamato-lunatum joint, and the hamato-triquetrum joint.

complex. An estimation of the kinematic reduction incorporated in this system yields 20–30 DFOM, depending on certain assumptions concerning its kinematic features. This may illustrate why rupture of a single small ligament (e.g. an injury of the fibrous connection between lunatum and scaphoid, which is so hard to detect on a standard X-ray), or fracture of only one bone (e.g. the notorious scaphoid fracture), is such a fatal occurrence for the normal function of the carpal mechanism.

TIBIAL TORSION: A KINEMATIC CONSTRAINT?

We will now return to our model consisting of pelvis, lower extremities, and floor because it demonstrates so well another interesting kinematic feature. Figure 8.8 shows a schematic representation of the model. The left-hand part of this figure illustrates that the model can be seen as an open box with six sides. These sides are connected to each other by a set of six hinges comprising two subsets of three parallel hinges. It is obvious that the upper side can move vertically up and down, stretching or folding the sides of the box. Thus the upper lid of the box has one DFOM.

In the central figure, the box has been translated into our pelvis-with-lower-limbs model, showing similar kinematic features. According to our foregoing reasoning, this is a spatial, simple-closed kinematic chain with six hinges, and for this reason it should be subject to a reduction of six DFOM. This actually means that its kinematic condition should have yielded a mobility of zero DFOM: it should have been immobile! However, its actual kinematic condition produces, as we have seen from the example of the six-sided box, one DFOM. This is due to its particular kinematic

feature of having two sets of three parallel hinge axes.

The figure at the right shows our pelvis-legs-and-feet model again, but in contrast to the central model this one is not able to move up and down: it does indeed have zero DFOM. The difference has to be sought in the torsion of the two bars that represent the lower legs. This torsion disturbs the parallel position of the hinge axes of knee and ankle. The chain has apparently acquired the kinematic features of a spatial chain, and this is sufficient to give a further reduction of the mobility of the closed chain. It is a well-established fact that tibial (external) torsion is a real anatomical characteristic of the human lower limb that develops during the first 10 years after birth (Lang & Wachsmuth 1972).

A physical representation of the model (Fig. 8.9) demonstrates this special kinematic effect. The model can stand upright as did the model in Fig. 8.1 above, but now it is even able to do so with flexed knees while the hips and ankles are still in the midpositions of their motion ranges. Owing to the external torsion of the lower links (the tibial parts) of the legs, these joints apparently need no external stabilizing support to maintain their positions, like the situation demonstrated in Fig. 8.1 above.

However, this configuration of the limbs and joints leads to another complication. In order to obtain full flat contact between the supporting surface and the feet, the model has to lean backwards. To prevent it falling down backwards, the feet have to be fixed by external forces to the floor, as can be seen in the photograph. As soon

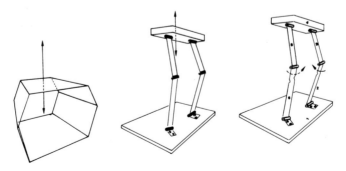

Fig. 8.8   Drawings of two different configurations of the model shown in Fig. 8.1 above (central and right figure), together with their basic kinematic model (left figure).

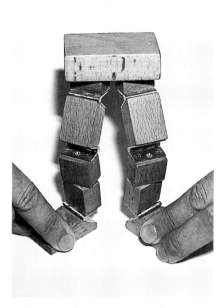

Fig. 8.9   The model from Fig. 8.8 in a physical representation.

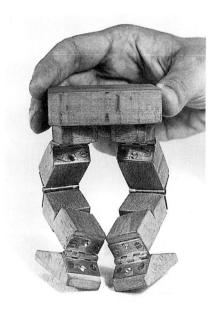

Fig. 8.10   The same model as in Fig. 8.9, but in this position the feet are everted. See text for further explanation.

as one hand is removed, the model collapses. After undoing the tibial torsion the demonstrator not only has to keep the feet in contact with the floor, but also has to stabilize one of the joints. Again, removing this external stabilization leads to a collapse of the model in spite of its feet being kept fixed to the floor. Thus under certain kinematic conditions, a particular *anatomic* feature such as a tibial torsion produces a kinematic boundary condition with a functional effect that concerns all the joints within the closed kinematic chain of pelvis and legs.

Apart from this contribution to 'self-locking', the tibial torsion has yet another functional effect. This effect became already apparent by the backward leaning posture that the model assumed when both feet were placed in flat contact with the floor (Fig. 8.9). If we want to avoid this backward leaning posture by holding the pelvic piece of the model vertically in line with its feet, the model assumes a posture as shown in Fig. 8.10. In this photograph, the model is brought into a vertical alignment of the pelvis and feet while its knees are slightly abducted and flexed. As can now be seen, the tibial torsion forces both feet into an everted, or pronated, position with respect

to the floor. An additional abduction of the flexed knees to improve bilateral stabilization will further increase this effect. In order to bring the feet into firm contact with the ground, both feet must invert. Thus inversion seems to be an indispensable mechanism in the normal functional range of the lower extremities and not only a useful capability of the foot to adapt its position to an uneven underground.

A KINEMATIC MODEL FOR THE TARSAL MOTIONS

Inversion is effected by the tarsal mechanism of the foot, which again has the configuration of a spatial, closed kinematic chain with only one DFOM. As will be apparent from Fig. 8.11, showing a kinematic model of the foot in two positions, inversion of the tarsus is a complex combination of different motions of the bones involved in the tarsal mechanism. When the foot is inverted by tilting over its lateral border, the accompanying adduction of the foot is blocked and has to be compensated for by an external rotation of the leg. The ankle mortice compels the talus into a similar and concurrent abduction,

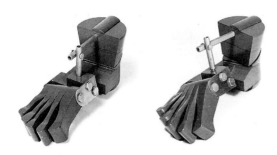

Fig. 8.11 A physical model of the foot comprising the tarsus and metatarsus. The tarsal part is represented as a spatial, closed kinematic, four-bar chain. At the left is the neutral position, at the right, the inversion position.

and the calcaneus follows this motion with a less extensive abduction and a slight inversion tilt. The abducting talar head forces the navicular together with the cuboid into an inversion added to the calcaneal inversion. Thus the forefoot supinates with respect to the hindfoot. This becomes visible as a heightening of the medial foot arch. In certain postures, as we have seen in Fig. 8.9, inversion is an indispensable mechanism. Thus if the legs are used with flexed knees, the knee joints must provide for the possibility of meeting this requirement by allowing external and internal rotation in their flexed position in order to make the feet free for a compensating inversion (Huson 1991).

FINAL REMARKS AND DISCUSSION

All the examples shown point to the fact that the human body comprises a great number of kinematic chains. Therefore mobility and stability of the human body in terms of their kinematic DFOM is determined by the kinematic constraints of these chains. Such constraints can be imposed by muscles (active elements) and ligaments (passive elements). However, apart from these easily recognizable elements, there are, as we have seen, other determinants that are less self-evident. Such

structural and/or configuration-dependent determinants are:

- the actual state of the chain – closed versus open
- the composition of the chain – compound versus simple
- the dimensionality of the chain – two- versus three-dimensional
- the axial angularity, i.e. this special relationship between the axes of motion of the joints in the chain, such as parallelism or co-axiality.

So far we have dealt only with the kinematic approach to modeling, forces have not been taken into consideration. It is obvious that a more complete picture of the conditions that determine mobility and stability requires a more comprehensive model, including the acting forces (Vleeming et al 1995b). However, in such a more comprehensive approach we can also observe within the locomotor system mechanical effects acting at a distance in a musculoskeletal system, such as we have seen in our kinematic models (Bobbert & Van Ingen Schenau 1988). The ideas presented by Snijders, Stoeckart and Vleeming concerning the force streams and their anatomical findings give clear support to this point (e.g. Vleeming et al 1995a, 1995b).

CONCLUSIONS

1. Changes in the kinematic condition of a particular closed articular chain in the human body has immediate effects on the kinematics of other joints.
2. These effects can be observed even at a great distance, thus affecting the kinematic behaviour of the whole chain.
3. The model predicts that reduction of the stability of the SIJ (loosening of the joint) must lead to instability of other joints.
4. This is especially relevant since it is difficult to stabilize the loosened SIJ effectively and directly with the help of local muscles.

REFERENCES

Benink R J 1985 A biomechanical study of the constraint mechanism of the human tarsus. Acta Orthopaedica Scandinavica 56 (supplement) 215: 1–135

Bobbert M F, Van Ingen Schenau G J 1988 Co-ordination in vertical jumping. Journal of Biomechanics 21: 249–262

Huson A 1983 Morphology and technology. Acta Morphologica Neerlando-Scandinavica 21: 69–81

Huson A 1991 Functional anatomy of the foot. In: Jahss M J (ed) Disorders of the foot. Medical and surgical management, 2nd edn, vol. I, part II. WB Saunders, Philadelphia, pp 409–431

Huson A, Spoor C W, Verbout A J 1989 A model of the human knee, derived from kinematic principles and its relevance for endoprosthesis design. Acta Morphologica Neerlando-Scandinavica 27: 45–62

Lang J, Wachsmuth W 1972 Praktische Anatomie, vol. I, part IV. Springer, Berlin, p 282

Morrenhof J W 1989 Stabilisation of the human hip-joint. A kinematical study. PhD thesis, Medical Faculty, University of Leiden

Ottevanger E J C, Spoor C W, Van Leeuwen J L, Sauren A A H J, Janssen J D, Huson A 1989 An experimental set-up for the measurements of forces on a human cadaveric foot during inversion. Journal of Biomechanics 22: 957–962

Schreppers G J M A, Sauren A A H J, Huson A 1990 A numerical model of the load transmission in the tibio-femoral contact area. Proceedings of the Institution of Mechanical Engineers 204: 53–59

Snijders C J, Vleeming A, Stoeckart R 1993a Transfer of lumbosacral load to iliac bones and legs. Part 1: Biomechanics of self-bracing of the sacro-iliac joints and its significance for treatment and exercise. Clinical Biomechanics 8: 285–294

Snijders C J, Vleeming A, Stoeckart R 1993b Transfer of lumbosacral load to iliac bones and legs. Part 2: Loading of the sacro-iliac joints when lifting in a stooped posture. Clinical Biomechanics 8: 295–301

Spoor C W, Van Leeuwen J L, De Windt F H J, Huson A 1989 A model study of muscle forces and joint-force direction in normal and dysplastic neonatal hips. Journal of Biomechanics 22: 873–884

Spoor C W, Van Leeuwen J L, Meskers C G M, Titulaer A F, Huson A 1990 Estimation of instantaneous moment arms of lower-leg muscles. Journal of Biomechanics 23: 1247–1259

Van Langelaan E J 1983 A kinematical analysis of the tarsal joints. Acta Orthopaedica Scandinavica 54 (supplement) 204: 1–267

Van Leeuwen J L, Speth L A W M, Daanen H A M 1990 Shock absorption of below-knee prostheses: a comparison between the SACH and the Multiflex foot. Journal of Biomechanics 23: 441–446

Vleeming A, Pool-Goudzwaard A L, Hammudoghlu D, Stoeckart R, Snijders C J, Mens J M A 1995a The function of the long dorsal sacroiliac ligament: its implication for understanding low back pain. In: Vleeming A, Mooney V, Dorman T, Snijders C (eds) Second interdisciplinary world congress on low back pain. San Diego, CA, 9–11 November, pp 125–137

Vleeming A, Snijders C J, Stoeckart R, Mens J M A 1995b A new light on low back pain. In: Vleeming A, Mooney V, Dorman T, Snijders C (eds) Second interdisciplinary world congress on low back pain. San Diego, CA, 9–11 November, pp 149–168

Wismans J, Veldpaus F, Janssen J, Huson A, Struben P 1980 A three-dimensional mathematical model of the knee-joint. Journal of Biomechanics 13: 677–685

9. Suboptimal posture: the origin of the majority of idiopathic pain of the musculoskeletal system

Alleviation of the majority of pain of the musculoskeletal system without known cause by use of orthotics and manual manipulation to optimize normal posture towards an ideal configuration

R. E. Irvin

INTRODUCTION

Herein, a postural model is presented to explain prevalent and idiopathic musculoskeletal pain as an outcome of less than ideal posture, albeit normal. Although the problem is well studied, prevalent pain of the musculoskeletal system (MS) is idiopathic. In recent years, it has become apparent that abnormality of neither anatomy (Boden et al 1990, Jensen et al 1994) nor posture (Dieck et al 1985) is reliably predictive of pain (Fig. 9.1). This lack of correlation is surprising because abnormality has been successful as a criterion by which to identify cause of other diseases and disorders.

There are several possibilities to explain this paucity of cause by the criterion of abnormality. For one, an abnormal factor (or factors) could exist, not yet identified, that is causal for back pain. Another possibility is that the concept of abnormality alone is inadequate to provide a true picture of the origin of common pain of the MS. If so, a different criterion with better predictive value than biologic abnormality could exist.

To contemplate a standard other than abnormality for identification of disease and disorder comes precariously close to reconsideration of our contemporary paradigm with respect to back pain. If redefinition were necessary and feasible, a shift of this paradigm could ensue, and for this picture criteria for identifying and testing the need for a shift of paradigm are relevant. Kuhn gives the following three criteria for an impending shift of a paradigm in his writing 'The structure of scientific revolutions' (Kuhn 1970):

1. an existing paradigm has ceased to function adequately in the exploration of an aspect of nature to which that paradigm itself had previously led the way;
2. observed anomalies whose characteristic feature is a stubborn refusal to be assimilated into existing paradigms; and
3. a successful new theory which permits predictions that are different from those derived from its predecessor.

The inadequacy of biologic abnormality to indicate the cause of prevalent back pain meets the first of these three criteria.

An observed anomaly not assimilable into the contemporary paradigm prompted the inception of this study in 1980, and satisfied the second criterion for an impending shift of the contemporary paradigm. Two advanced students of dance enrolled at Texas Christian University complained of difficulty in maintaining balance while performing turns *en pointe* (Fig. 9.2). They also reported a variety of regional discomforts for which there might or might not have been a memorable stress associated with the onset of each discomfort. The incidence and distribution

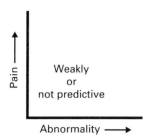

Fig. 9.1 Abnormality of neither anatomy nor physiology is reliably predictive of pain.

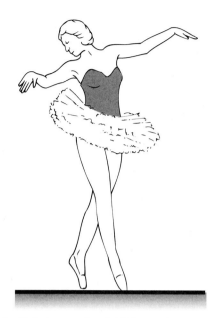

Fig. 9.2 Ballerina *en pointe*. Initially, two dancers complained of difficulty in performing turns *en pointe*, or on the tips of the toes, that was inconsistent with their advanced level of training.

of these discomforts was not uncommon for dancers: aches and/or cramps of the lower extremity and back. Physical examination revealed minor asymmetry of alignment of joint segments with restricted freedom of motion local to the pains. Treatment by manual manipulation was often followed by a period of improved comfort, but without any effect on their chief complaint, which was difficulty with turns.

Factors that might bear on postural balance were sought. The lumbopelvis was radiographed in the anatomic stance. For both dancers, the lumbopelvis was anatomically normal. A slight unlevelness of the sacral base, well within the range of normal variation, was detected in both dancers. As this mild unlevelness was the only aspect detected that might conceivably bear on balance of weight-bearing, it was leveled by placement of a 3 mm lift beneath the heel on the low side of the first dancer, a 5 mm lift being used for the other dancer. A level sacral base was confirmed by radiography with the lifts in place. These lifts were worn routinely outside class.

Over the next month, subsequent to this leveling of the base of the sacrum, the two dancers reported:

- an increase in the quantity and quality of turns and, more surprisingly,
- a marked reduction of multiple and chronic regional discomforts from foot to head.

This report was a surprise for several reasons and raised several questions. How could a lift worn in a shoe while not dancing positively affect the dancer's performance while turning on one leg? How could this single change within the range of normal variation result in alleviation of chronic discomforts throughout the body? One would normally expect that:

- a lift worn in a shoe while outside the dance studio would not affect the ease of turns while in dance class
- reduction of a normal extent of unlevelness would not have any substantial effect on chronic musculoskeletal pain
- if there did occur a reduction of pain, this reduction would occur primarily at the level of the low back where the lift most directly affected the picture; instead, relief was reported throughout the body.

These observed anomalies could not be assimilated into the contemporary paradigm and agreed with Kuhn's second criterion for an impending shift of paradigm. Yet, confidence in the generality of this phenomenon was low given the few subjects involved.

Using two different populations of subjects, a clinical trial followed that affirmed the phenomenon. Both populations studied had chronic pain of the MS but were without degenerative changes of the lumbopelvis discernible by plain radiography. One population ($n = 42$) comprised ambulatory adults with chronic, multiregional pain. The other population ($n > 100$) was college freshmen enrolled in classes of modern and ballet dance. For both populations, the sacral base was gradually leveled with a heel lift, while manual manipulation was used to reduce articular restriction. Like the two dancers who initially complained of difficulty with balance, both the dancer and adult subjects reported marked, pancorporeal and enduring reduction of pain. This affirmation of an anomalous observation, not assimilable into a paradigm that relies on abnormality as a discriminant, met Kuhn's second criterion for an impending shift of paradigm.

To explain these anomalous observations, it is necessary to reconsider what is presupposed of back pain. One presupposition is that the typical patient has a singular pain (such as of the low back) for which there exists a particular cause that often is proximate to the painful site. Instead, those persons with chronic pain of the low back more commonly have discomfort in multiple regions, namely the neck, thorax, pelvis, and extremities. These pains are commonly spontaneous in onset and are not attributable to any unusual event or anatomic abnormalities (if present) that are proximal to the sites of pain. In accord with the principle of parsimony, for people who are otherwise normal, it is more likely that these multiple sites of pain have a common origin than that there exist numerous, independent and respective causes for multiple pains.

It would not be surprising for the majority of pain of the MS to relate directly to the principle stress the MS endures: gravitation. What is both surprising and a paradox – in the context of our present paradigm – is that modification of normal posture towards ideal configuration had such a strong and broad effect on the MS that had not been achieved otherwise. The history of this study is one of a strong and unexplained effect in need of a paradigm that is sufficiently broad to admit this observed effect.

It seems a contradiction that abnormal posture is not predictive of pain, yet improvement of even normal posture is followed by significant relief of pain. This apparent contradiction is resolved by a close look at the forms of causality recognized by operational philosophy which regards every statement about causality as a hypothesis to be tested (Rapoport 1954). The operations performed in the test give meaning to the assertion that event A is the cause of event B. When we look at those operations, we find that at least three different kinds of causality must be distinguished:

a. *Observational causality* means simply 'Watch for the occurrence of the event A, and you will observe the occurrence of the event B'. For instance, watch for the event 'sufficient radiation' and one can observe a significant occurrence of

'neoplasia'. Contradistinctively, watch for 'abnormality of the musculoskeletal system' and one does not reliably see 'pain'. Thus observational causality is not evidenced between abnormal anatomy or posture of the musculoskeletal system and pain.

b. *Postulational causality* means that given a rule that 'A causes B', then where we see 'A' we are surprised not to see 'B'. Consider the second law of thermodynamics. *The entropy of an isolated system always increases.* In most cases of increasing entropy in the real world, the system is not isolated. With respect to gravitation, the human system is not very isolated and some actions of gravitation can be damaging to the body.

Given that entropy is a measure of disorder in a system, a breakdown of structure would be an increase in entropy. Certain degenerative changes of joints that bear weight are known to be due to mechanical stress (osteoarthrosis), but if not excessive are considered 'normal aging'. When we see an 'aged human' we are not surprised to see 'degenerate joints'. Thus postulational causality is evidenced between advancing age and the likelihood of degenerated joints. This relation does not preclude the possibility that reduction of normal stress by optimization of normal posture can reduce pain of joints, aged or not.

c. *Manipulable causality* means that 'change A and B changes'. An example is that the use of orthotics to optimize posture is followed by alleviation or reduction of chronic or recurrent pain. Restated, 'optimize posture and pain is reduced'. Thus manipulable causality is evidenced between improved posture and reduced pain.

The fact that abnormal posture is not predictive of pain relates to only one of these three forms of causality, i.e. observational, and does not contradict the presence of manipulable causality. The conclusion by investigators that lack of predictive value of abnormal posture for pain proves lack of causal relation between posture and pain is overly broad because reduction of pain following optimization of posture evidences causality of the manipulable kind (Irvin 1995).

POSTURE AS AN ORIGIN OF ARTHRALGIA

Posture can be defined as the size, shape, and

attitude of the MS with respect to gravitation. Subtle departure from ideal posture, which is normally the case, entails routine, eccentric, and increased mechanical stress throughout the body (Kappler 1982) (Fig. 9.3).

For a person in the upright stance, posture is directly dependent on the size, shape, and attitude of three cardinal bases of support:

1. the surface on which one stands
2. the feet, as they are the lowermost support of the MS
3. the base of the sacrum, as it is both the approximate center of the structure of the MS and the lowermost support of the vertebral column.

In modern times, the prevalent surface on which we stand has been artificially configured from a natural one that is irregular in shape and attitude to one that typically is flattened and horizontal. Whatever the stress of weight-bearing, this stress is more consistent given a flat and horizontal surface of support than otherwise. Plausibly, the artificial levelness of the ground in modern times may contribute to the tendency towards pain of the MS owing to a more consistent focus of postural stress.

The feet are composed of three cardinal arches:

1. transverse, which spans the medial-to-lateral margins of the forefoot
2. lateral longitudinal, which spans the lateral portion of the foot
3. medial longitudinal, which spans the medial portion of the foot.

Hypothetically, each of these arches has an ideal amplitude, under which condition the arch function of supporting and transferring weight during the upright stance and gait is optimal. Also hypothetically, the ideal alignment of the foot with the lower leg is for the ankle to be straight and vertical in the coronal plane. Importantly, the alignment of the ankle and the superincumbent MS is partly dependent on the amplitude of the cardinal arches of the feet.

The sacrum has three joint surfaces:

1. lumbosacral
2. right sacroiliac
3. left sacroiliac.

The size and shape of the sacroiliac (SI) surfaces do not form a fully stable joint under posturally loaded conditions, necessitating complementary support from ligaments, fascia, and musculature (Vleeming et al 1990). Greatest stability of the SI joint (SIJ) depends in part on there being a perpendicular intersection between the vector of

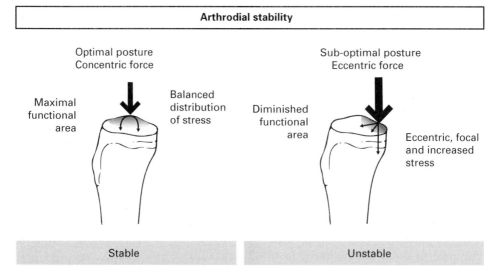

Fig. 9.3 Arthrodial stability exists where there is balanced distribution of stress acting through the joint. Suboptimal posture results in eccentric load across a diminished surface that bears weight. Torque results, with decreased arthrodial stability.

load that passes through the SIJ, and the plane of the SIJ (Snijders et al 1992). The right–left symmetry of the magnitude and direction of the vectors of load through the SIJ depends on a level base of the sacrum which receives the load from the superincumbent vertebral column. Balanced support of superincumbent structures, as well as concentric load-ing of dependent structures, is partly dependent on sacral levelness. Thereby, greatest stability of the SI and superincumbent and dependent joints depends, in part, on levelness of the sacral base.

Optimization of posture in the upright stance can be achieved by use of four modes of physical manipulation:

1. contoured orthotics worn in the shoes and precisely configured so as to optimize the amplitude of the arches of the feet (Irvin 1995)
2. a flat orthotic (heel lift) of thickness sufficient to level the sacral base while standing (Irvin 1991)
3. manual manipulation directed to restore resilience of soft tissues and alignment of joint segments
4. for the duration of the course of treatment, practice of a therapeutic posture for 20 min daily to counter the bias of soft tissues reflective of the initial posture.

With optimization of posture alone, or where combined with current treatments for chronic and idiopathic pain, results are far greater and more enduring than otherwise.

This strategy for treatment of idiopathic and chronic pain of the MS by the use of orthotics in combination with manual manipulation is distinct from the preferred treatment for idiopathic and acute pain, which treatment is the combined use of a brief period of rest, non-steroidal anti-inflammatory medication, and manual manipulation.

This model, admittedly not complete, has by straightforward application alleviated the chronic pain of 70% of regions and markedly reduced discomfort for the remaining 30% (Irvin 1986, 1995). A pilot study by independent investigators (Hoffman & Hoffman 1994) shows that leveling the sacral base is followed by a marked reduction of pain of the low back. Use of a Levitor orthotic device to reduce excessive sacral tilt in the sagittal plane (Kuchera & Jungman 1986) reduces pain of the low back in patients otherwise not responsive to treatment. Idiopathic pain of the MS that is relieved subsequent to optimization of posture can be termed postural arthralgia, rather than pain without known cause.

This model of postural arthralgia permits predictions that are different from those derived from its predecessor. For those persons with idiopathic pain of the MS, improvement of their posture from normal towards ideal can be expected markedly to reduce eccentric weight-bearing, arthrodial stress, and related pain throughout the MS. This improved predictive value satisfies Kuhn's third criterion for there being a need for a shift of paradigm and warrants a novel approach to an old problem.

ARCHETYPES THAT REGULATE PERCEPTION OF CAUSALITY

A close look at how we perceive causality in medical science has led to a novel application of a concept which has been successful in physics but which I have not previously encountered in medical science.

Past failure to identify the cause of prevalent pain permits the possibility that there is some inadequacy in what we presuppose that is sufficient to preclude our discovery of this cause. Early Greeks, the founders of science, frequently organized their thoughts in terms of dyads or pairs of related terms. A dyad is an example of a fundamental pattern of conceptual order, or archetype (Jung), which has great value as an organizer of what we observe. An example of a dyadic association presupposed in science is that of (1) cause with (2) effect.

It is evidenced below that the origin of prevalent and idiopathic pain cannot be adequately characterized in dyadic constructs alone. Instead, the archetypic frame must be broadened to a triadic one that admits origin as a perceivable and manipulable aspect that can bear on subsequent cause and eventual effect. Important to understanding idiopathic pain of the MS, this cognitive model does not necessitate that there be a particular cause for each effect, which is often the picture of prevalent pain of the MS.

A bias towards dyadic patterns of order prevails in biologic science. When dyadic order is looked for, dyadic relations can be found. An example of a natural dyad of opposing aspects is the DNA molecule, which is something like a very long table of opposite-matching base pairs (Rucker 1987). The molecule consists of two intertwining 'back bones' held together by a long series of dyads.

The grouping of observables into dyads, triads, etc. presupposes that in nature there exist archetypes or corresponding patterns of order. As is explained in the material that follows, two principles that prevail in medical science – namely identity and relativity – can be contrasted archetypally according to particular relata: (1) the number of aspects that comprise the relationship regulated by the principle, (2) the quality of these aspects that is emphasized, and (3) the relational 'orientation' of these aspects (Fig. 9.4).

We shall consider these two principles in terms of their relata and provide examples of how these relata are reflected in the anatomy of the MS, yet have not resolved the origin of prevalent pain of the MS. Then a third concept, 'complementarity', is introduced in the context of its original application in quantum physics. Certain adjustments of this concept follow that are sufficient to establish a principle of complementarity by which the origin of prevalent pain of the MS can be resolved as being a feature of suboptimal posture.

The principle of identity pertains abstractly to a monadic (singular) class of entities that correspond to real situations that can be identified according to aspect(s) that are unique, inverse, or isomorphic. Each of these three abstract forms can be found in the MS.

With respect to the human being, a unique identity is not similar to any other structure or event. An example of a unique structure within the human body is the heart. Comparatively, an early and successful application of the concept of a unique identity was by Aristotle in the systematic classification of living organisms according to five predicates: genus, species, property, differentia, and accidents. Accidents were untoward events in the development of an organism that resulted in effects that were not characteristic of the identity reflected by the first four predicates. Examination of the body for a unique structure or event that causes prevalent pain of the back has not been successful.

A second variant of identity is to have a symmetry with aspects that are mutually inverse, or reciprocal, yet which jointly complete the identity. For the human being, an example of anatomy having inverse symmetry is the genitalia. The invagination of the pelvic floor is a feminine aspect and the exvagination is a masculine aspect. These two configurations are mutually inverse and jointly complete the identity of genitalia. While this inverse symmetry has meaning with respect to reproduction of the MS, these differences do not seem to bear directly on prevalent pain.

A third form of identity comprises isomorphic aspects that are similar in shape but mutually different in size, region, and orientation. Each region of the body has an isomorphic aspect, 180° different in orientation respectively. Examples of isomorphic symmetry are the occiput, sternum, sacrum, patella, and calcaneus.

When applied to anatomy, the principle of relativity pertains to a dyad of aspects which may be grouped according to whether they are the same (equivalent), opposite, or proportionate.

Archetypes		Relata	
Principles	Quantity	Quality	Mutual orientation
Identity	Monad	Unique,	●
		inverse, or	◐
		isomorphic	⊽ ◖
Relativity	Dyad	Same,	A = B
		opposite, or	A ●——● B
		proportionate	A ●—— B
Complimentarity	Triad	Mutually exclusive, jointly complete, & operationally linked	B╲ C / A ; C/ B

Fig. 9.4 Table of archetypes (fundamental patterns of order) that abstractly contrasts three principles in terms of the quantity, quality, and orientation of the related aspect(s) (relata) to which the principle applies.

Equivalence is sameness of a measurable aspect of two or more aspects. A biologic example of near-equivalence is the lengths of legs. Normally, however, legs are not equal in length. Abnormal disparity of leg lengths is considered a possible cause of pain of the low back, and is treatable by use of a heel lift to reduce the disparity in length. Normal inequality of leg length is not predictive of pain of the low back (Grundy & Roberts 1984). As there is no other opposing pair of structures that could reasonably affect back pain, this picture evidences the limited applicability of the principle of relativity to resolve the cause of prevalent pain of the MS.

Opposition is having a position at either end of an axis. An example of opposition is the right and left aspects of the upper extremity positioned at either end of a transverse axis.

Proportion is a portion in relation to the whole. A proportion called the Golden Section was discovered by the Pythagoreans around the sixth century BC and was found to agree with measurable extents of neighboring aspects of living systems. The Golden Section is the uniquely reciprocal relationship between two unequal parts of the whole, in which the small part stands to the large part as the large part stands to the whole (Fig. 9.5). The Golden Section was later used by the classical Greeks to regulate the proportionality of some statues and buildings to effect especially beautiful and life-like forms that were harmonious with the natural surroundings. While the Golden Section has been highly useful in nature, art and architecture (Doczi 1994), this proportionality has not yet shown usefulness with respect to enabling a better understanding of back pain.

The 'complementarity principle' is the organization of one's thoughts and information with respect to a situation or system by seeing that it is composed of three aspects that (1) are sufficiently distinct from each other that they can be viewed as mutually exclusive, (2) 'complement' each other in that they are 'jointly complete' (Bohr 1934), and (3) are operationally linked, such that by manipulation of one property the remaining two can be correspondingly affected (Irvin 1995).

In a two-dimensional picture, an example of complementary symmetry is the Pythagorean

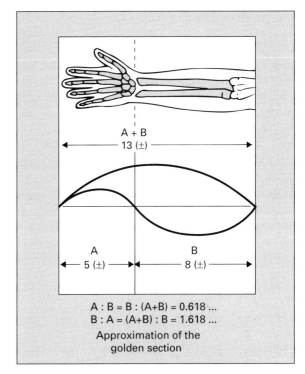

Fig. 9.5   The Golden Section is a proportionality of longitudinal extents of neighboring regions of natural systems stated, 'The smaller extent (A) is to the larger extent (B) as the larger extent is to the sum of them both (A + B).'

triangle comprising two legs of unequal length that form a right angle, and a hypotenuse that subtends the right angle. A change of the length of one side correspondingly changes the length of the other two sides. An anatomic example of a complementary triad is the three layers of musculature that comprise the abdominal wall. The rectus abdominis forms one leg of this triangular relation, the transversus abdominis intersects with the rectus to form a right angle, and the obliquus abdominis subtends this right angle.

The abdominal muscles are often ascribed an important role in the treatment of back pain. Recent study shows that for those who had never experienced back pain, contraction of the transversus abdominis precedes that of the other two muscle groups of the abdominal wall, and that a delay in contracture of the transversus is a feature of chronic sufferers of pain of the low back. Abstractly, this situation can be characterized as a functional discord among this complementary triad of muscles. Training of subjects to enable isolation and intentional activation of the transversus abdominis prior to initiation of activity of the MS restores the operational integrity of this complementary triad of abdominal muscles and reduces chronic pain of the low back (Richardson & Jull 1995).

In a three-dimensional picture, an example of complementary order of the MS is the three cardinal planes of anatomy that are mutually exclusive in their orientation, jointly complete, and operationally linked such that a change of anatomy in one cardinal plane necessarily affects the anatomy in the other two cardinal planes.

THE ORIGINAL APPLICATION OF THE CONCEPT OF COMPLEMENTARITY IN QUANTUM MECHANICS

The introduction of a new principle for better understanding of the MS warrants a close inspection of the history of the principle.

The original conception of complementarity was applied by Bohr with considerable success to explain particle–wave duality as being a complementary rather than a contradictory relationship (Bohr 1934, Held 1994, Petruccioli 1993). The particle–wave duality is the strange behavior of small entities such as protons, electrons, and even atoms. These entities, which we are accustomed to calling particles, sometimes behave like particles in that they are localized inside a very small volume (for the electron it seems to be a mathematical point), but at other times their behavior has only been explained as that of a wave. The wave, to be a wave, occupies a tremendous amount of space compared with a particle. The argument for contradiction is based on the assertion that no physical object can be both localized at one point in space and also spread over space. A weakness of this objection is that a given experimental design yields either a particle or a wave picture, but not both at the same time. Instead of being a contradiction, Bohr asserts that this duality is a sum of two complementary events that jointly complete the atomic object. As stated by Bohr:

evidence obtained under different experimental conditions cannot be comprehended within a single picture, but must be regarded as complementary in the sense that only the totality of the phenomenon *exhausts the possible information* about the objects.

While Bohr argues ably for the admission of both particle and wave natures as a relation that is mutually complementary rather than contradictory, the concept in its present form is not sufficient adequately to explain how particle–wave duality occurs.

ADJUSTMENT FROM A CONCEPT OF COMPLEMENTARITY TO A PRINCIPLE

Several adjustments of the concept of complementarity lead to a principle of complementarity that can be applied to better understand any natural system, including both that of particle–wave duality in the microcosm and the structure–function duality of the MS.

One adjustment is needed for reason that the dyadic quantity of the archetypic frame of reference for particle–wave duality does not exhaust all of the observable aspects of the picture. Bohr's definition of complementarity presupposes that we are directly observing dual natures of an atomic object (meaning small objects such as molecule, electron, proton, etc.). In a stricter sense, what is observed is not the object itself. Instead, what we observe is a picture of the object. The aspect of the object that is seen is determined in part by the method of observation.

Abstractly, this third aspect can be described as the boundary condition within which the particle and wave aspects of the atomic object correspondingly take form. Thereby, the archetypic frame of reference for particle–wave natures is a triadic quantity that includes the interacting environment as a third aspect of the situation.

A second adjustment concerns the presupposition that 'atomic' necessarily refers solely to a small body in the quantum domain. Instead of a small body in the quantum domain, the entity that is atomic can be any system – regardless of size – that is comprised of complementary aspects that are not mutually separable without sacrificing the integrity of the system.

A third and final adjustment of the concept of complementarity is to infer that, by virtue of joint completeness, the mutually exclusive aspects are also correspondently linked, such that manipulation of one aspect correspondingly effects the other two. The addition of correspondent linkage as a cardinal aspect of complementarity forms a triad of complementary characteristics that is distinct from the original dyadic conception of (1) mutual exclusivity and (2) joint completeness asserted by Bohr.

Importantly for the MS, the generality of this adjusted concept of complementarity constitutes a principle that applies to all systems without consideration of their size. In these terms, the human system is atomic, comprising triads of complementary aspects such as anatomy and physiology that perform within and are manipulable by modification of the postural boundaries.

REGULATION OF THE SCHEME OF THE MS TO A MANIPULABLE SCHEME OF COMPLEMENTARITY

Complementarity can be represented abstractly in a geometric way. Three mutually exclusive aspects suggest three perpendicular directions, since two such directions can be no further apart. Three crossed lines on a sheet of paper suggests that the three aspects are jointly complete and operationally linked (Fig. 9.6). To represent the complementarity of a system, one can group triads of mutually exclusive aspects into a composite scheme.

As a point of departure towards fitting our contemporary model of the MS into a complementary scheme, let us begin with the statement that 'Patients are aware of pain in their musculoskeletal frame'. Examination of this picture for complementarity reveals a triad of aspects that are mutually exclusive and jointly complete:

• awareness
• of pain
• in their MS frame.

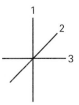

Triad of mutually exclusive aspects that are jointly complete and operationally linked

Fig. 9.6 An abstract image of the principle of complementarity.

To regulate this picture in terms of complementarity, these aspects are assigned to broad categories that are mutually exclusive, jointly complete, and operationally linked. *Awareness* has a sufficiently broad identity to be a category in itself. Pain can be assigned to a more general category called *feeling*. The MS frame can be abstracted as an expression of fundamental *freedoms* of statics and kinetics that form within the boundaries of posture. With this beginning, we can extend this scheme to include a myriad of known anatomic and physiologic components of the MS, grouped into complementary triads that are mutually linked, such that alteration of one or more aspects of one triad correspondingly alters other triads (Fig. 9.7).

Correspondingly, disorder within one triad can affect disorder throughout the system. For example, other than symmetric alignment of joint segments can correspondingly affect receptors by virtue of operational linkage. Idiopathic pain can be our experience of imperfection within the complementary scheme of the MS. Conversely, coherent manipulation of the six categories of awareness (placebo response), statics, kinetics, receptors, expressers, and conditions of boundary can correspondingly result in a more ideal structure, more optimal function, and reduction of related pain throughout the system.

Complementary aspects can be either solely intrinsic to the system or can include the gravitational context of the system as one complementary aspect. The two non-gravitational aspects do *not* form an independent dyad since gravitation enters into their interaction. An example is the

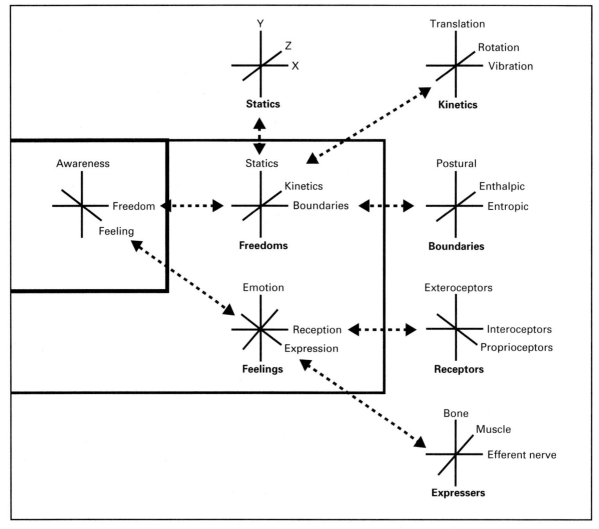

Fig. 9.7   An abstract scheme of complementary triads of familiar aspects that comprise the MS.

triad of 1) structure, and 2) function performing within 3) postural boundaries. The complementary triads of systems form a correspondent continuum from the very small to the very large frames of reference (Fig. 9.8).

That there is complementarity between structure, function, and posture agrees with the osteopathic objective for manipulative treatment of somatic dysfunction, which treatment is directed to promote symmetry of structure and restore physiologic function of the MS in postural balance.

Kappler (1982) defined perfect postural balance as that state in which the body mass is

distributed so that the muscles are in a state of normal tonus and ligamentous tension is balanced against compressive forces. This reasonable thought is in the direction of a practical definition of perfect postural balance, yet there are four shortcomings to this definition. One shortcoming is that electromyographic (EMG) activity (and tonus, proportionately) of paravertebral musculature in the lumbar region is normally imbalanced, right-to-left, while in the anatomic and upright stance (Barker & Irvin 1986). This imbalance is largely due to normal unlevelness of the sacral base, which usually features some degree of lateral bend of the

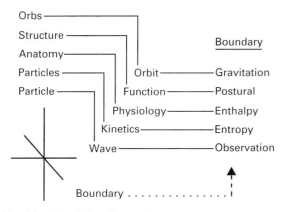

Increasing dimension

Fig. 9.8 Boundaries of natural systems.

lumbar spine in the sagittal plane mediated by paralumbar musculature. In contrast, reduction of sacral unlevelness markedly reduces both intensity and right-to-left asymmetry of EMG activity, with increased economy. Economy that is less than optimal is short of perfect, so normal tonus is not a feature of perfect postural balance.

A second shortcoming of this definition of perfect postural balance is that the distribution of body mass is not easily measurable, whereas skeletal symmetry is far more so. Certainly, mass matters; where mass is not measurable, the shape of the mass matters more.

Third, compressive forces within the body also are not easily measurable and are thereby not a practical feature of postural balance. Necessarily, balance depends upon 1) symmetry of superincumbent structures, and 2) condition of postural boundaries. Contradistinctive to compressive forces, both structural symmetry and postural boundaries are easily observable and manipulable, whereas compressive forces are not.

Fourthly, in the anatomic and upright stance in perfect postural balance, weight-bearing joints would be positioned at the approximate midpoint of articular range. Ligaments are usually not engaged within the midrange of a weight-bearing joint. Instead, they secure the limits of articular range. Thus, ligamentous tension is not a feature that is characteristic of perfect postural balance.

These shortcomings of this definition of perfect postural balance, on which the objective for treat-

ment of somatic dysfunction depends, are corrected by change of this objective from 'Treatment is directed to promote symmetry of structure and physiologic function of the MS in postural balance' to 'Treatment is directed to promote ideal symmetry, function and postural boundaries of the MS'. For this therapeutic objective, the terms of mass and force need not be introduced, and thus the difficulty of measurement of distribution of mass and force is avoided.

For the reason that perfection is not achievable in reality, this standard of ideal is not a practical objective but is rather a practical direction towards which the operator can aim, with diminishing return once comfort is achieved. Beyond comfort, still greater economy and power can reasonably be achieved by further correction of posture. For the MS that is normally less than ideal in posture, this correction cannot be achieved by manual manipulation alone. For broad and enduring alleviation of postural arthralgia, it is necessary to identify and correct the boundaries on which posture depends.

IDENTIFICATION OF POSTURAL BOUNDARIES

For the MS in the upright stance, the dependent conditions for posture can be identified in terms of the condition of three boundaries (Fig. 9.9):

1. supportive: the ground on which the MS stands
2. dependent: the feet, which are the lowermost support of the superincumbent MS
3. central to the MS: the base of the sacrum, which is approximately central to the circumference from toes of the extended feet to the tips of the extended fingers.

Under conditions in which the attitude of postural boundaries are perpendicular to gravitation and the mass is centrally supported, the stress of compression is without torque. Otherwise, torque results in pressure away from ideal structure and optimal function, and this torque must be balanced by opposing muscular action. This departure from a standard (in this case, an ideal) of structure and function can be termed 'somatic difformity' (Fig. 9.10).

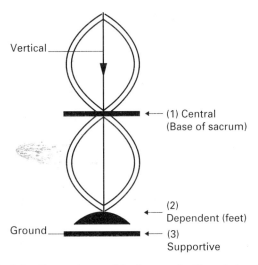

Fig. 9.9   Abstract image of the three cardinal boundaries of posture and symmetric superincumbent MS.

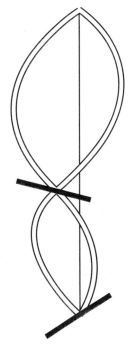

Fig. 9.10   Abstract image of suboptimal conditions of postural boundaries and correspondent difformity of MS.

Somatic **dif**formity is distinct from **de**formity, or abnormality, in several ways. One way is that the measure of difformity is the extent of displacement from the ideal rather than normal, and the range extends from ideal to the deviation

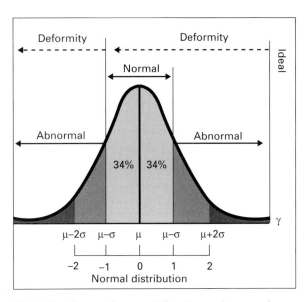

Fig. 9.11   Contrast between difformity as a departure from ideal and deformity as a 2nd and 3rd standard deviation from the side of the median of normal distribution opposite to ideal.

beyond which the part is considered deformed (Fig. 9.11).

Somatic difformity is distinct from somatic dysfunction in that the suffix 'form' can refer to the component aspects of both structure and function. Although 'dysfunction' is defined as including both structural and functional aspects, where the root term is 'function' the structural aspect is implicitly de-emphasized.

CORRECTION OF POSTURAL BOUNDARIES TOWARDS IDEAL

In the context of modern civilization and for the three boundaries of posture, the shape and attitude of the ground are essentially flat and horizontal. The shape and attitude of the feet are manipulable by contoured orthotics worn within the shoes, and the attitude of the pelvis is manipulable both by contoured and flat (heel lift) orthotics. For most people, there is an extent of flatness of the arches (pes planus), angularity of the ankles (pes valgus), and unlevelness of the sacral base. These deformities can be symmetrized by the proper use of orthotics (Irvin 1995). This chapter focuses on methods for correction of the attitude of the sacral base and correspondent deformity of the MS.

CORRECTION OF THE CENTRAL BOUNDARY OF POSTURE

Measurement of the attitude of the base of the sacrum is by radiography, performed with the patient standing in the anatomic position. The objective is to delineate unlevelness of the sacral base in the coronal plane, excessive anterior tilt of the sacral base in the sagittal plane, and anterior or posterior displacement of the superincumbent load from the lumbar spine with respect to the sacral base of support. Where these factors are present, treatment is directed to leveling the sacral base, minimizing the excessive tilt, and positioning the superincumbent load over the sacral base.

RADIOGRAPHY OF THE LUMBOPELVIS

On a minimum of two occasions, the lumbar spine and pelvis are radiographed with the patient in the upright stance. This examination, termed a postural survey (Denslow et al 1955, Loyd 1934), is initially performed without shoes. For those subjects with contoured orthotics, these are in place beneath the feet for radiography. On completion of the initial course of treatment, the patient is reradiographed, with lift and contoured orthotic in place, to evaluate response to treatment and measure residual unlevelness and tilt for further correction.

To position the patient for the anteroposterior view, the feet are parallel, positioned directly beneath the acetabula, with the buttocks in direct contact with the plane of the cassette. This contact minimizes pelvic rotation with respect to the vertical axis. For both views, the participant folds the arms across the chest in order to remove them from the visualized field.

Rectangular film is supported on a base horizontally controlled via a bubble level. A Quanta III intensifying screen is used with constant kilovoltage (kVp) technique. The focal-spot-to-film distance is 1.016 m, with the ray centered at the level of L5. For each subject, approximately 0.12 rad is delivered to the midplane at 80 kVp and 40 mAs.

For the lateral view of the lumbopelvis, the feet are parallel, positioned directly beneath the acetabula, with the lateral margin of the pelvis in direct contact with the plane of the cassette at the level of the greater trochanter. This technique minimizes lateral pelvic shift from the anatomic position.

DELINEATION OF THE ATTITUDE OF THE SACRAL BASE IN THE CORONAL PLANE

For most adults, the base of the sacrum as viewed in the coronal plane is not level. For the average adult, unlevelness of the sacral base delineated by the method described below is 6.7 $\pm$ 1.0 mm, with unlevelness $\geq$ 2 mm present for 98% (Irvin 1991). An effect of this unlevelness is that the lumbar spine tends to bend laterally towards the high side of the sacral base in order to maintain balance in the upright stance (Greenman 1979).

By the following method and for the coronal plane, the weight-bearing plane of the sacral base is delineated and its unlevelness measured relative to the lateral position of the femora (Fig. 9.12). The developed film is supported in a film holder with its lower margin level (Fig. 9.12, Line D). A line (line A) is drawn on the film parallel to the transverse stratum of eburnation within the sacral base (Irvin 1991).

This stratum of eburnation (Fig. 9.13) is thought to be a physiologic response to the compressive stress of weight-bearing in accord with Wolff's Law, and thereby truly to delineate the weight-bearing plane of the sacral base (F. M. Wilkins 1980, personal communication). Often, immediately below the most superior stratum having the greatest radio-opacity, one can discern multiple and parallel strata immediately neighboring each other. These strata are thought to represent laminar depositions of calcium within the trabecular matrix of the first sacral segment consequent to the compressive stress of weight-bearing.

Line A is extended laterally to intersect the vertical line segments B, drawn from the lower

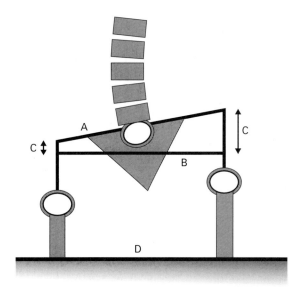

Fig. 9.12 A diagram of measurement of unlevelness of the base of the sacrum radiographed while in the upright and anatomic stance.

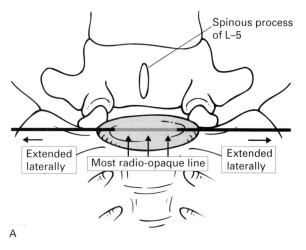

A

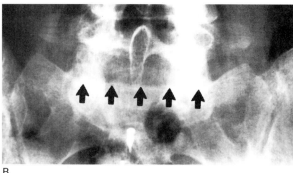

B

Fig. 9.13 (A) Line drawing of the radiographic reference for delineation of the base of the sacrum that directly bears the load of the lumbar spine. (B) Radiograph of the base of the sacrum with arrows that emphasize the transverse stratum of greatest radio-opacity that directly bears the load of the lumbar spine.

margin of the film and extended vertically through the vertex of each femora to intersect line A. The vertical line spans from the right and left points of intersection to the lower margin of the film are compared and the difference (line segment C) is recorded as millimeters of unlevelness of the sacral base with respect to the femora.

The margin of error of unlevelness of the sacral base measured radiographically is ±0.75 mm (Greenman 1979). For most subjects, the measurement of the unlevelness of the transverse plane of the sacral base is easily made. In approximately 20% of subjects, a clear delineation of this reference plane is somewhat difficult but measurable.

The operator is cautioned against the use of any reference other than the transverse stratum of eburnation for delineation of the weight-bearing plane of the sacral base. There can be significant disagreement in unlevelness where measured by the stratum of eburnation, when compared to unlevelness measured using as reference the alar notches, heights of the femoral heads, or heights of the iliac crests (Dott et al 1994). This stratum of eburnation is recommended as reference for the plane of weight-bearing for the reason that other references do not actually bear the weight and do not mutually agree (Irvin 1991).

DELINEATION OF THE ATTITUDE OF THE SACRAL BASE IN THE SAGITTAL PLANE

This measurement is an indication of the attitude of the sacral base with respect to horizontal and as viewed in the sagittal plane. From this view, the lordotic curve of the lumbar spine is usually in accord with the attitude of the sacral base. The clinical significance of the angle of tilt of the sacral base with respect to the curvilinearity of the lumbar spine is at least two fold:

1. Where the sacral angle is greater than normal, the functional area of the sacral base that is available for support of the lumbar spine is reduced. As mechanical stress is equal to force

per area across which the force is distributed, reduction of functional area increases the stress of the remaining area of the sacral base.

2. Where the sacral angle is less than normal, there typically occurs flatness of the lordotic curve of the lumbar spine. Elastic recoil of the lumbar spine during gait is reduced as the lumbar spine more closely approximates a column rather than a coil, with a resultant increase of compressive stress of the intervertebral discs at heel strike.

Measurement of the attitude of the sacral base in the sagittal plane (sacral angle) is by the method of Ferguson, who studied pelvic tilt in cadavers radiographed in the lateral recumbent position. Ferguson reported that the normal angle of pelvic tilt for cadavers is 30–40° (Ferguson 1939). Greenman observes that, for living subjects filmed in the upright stance, the normal angle is closer to 40 ± 2° (Greenman 1979). This angle measured in living subjects in the upright stance is known as the modified method of Ferguson for measurement of the sacral angle.

Reduction of too great a sacral angle (≥ 40°) can usually be achieved by this method for correction of posture. Increase of too small a sacral angle towards normal following correction of posture is far less reliable.

To measure the sacral angle (Fig. 9.14):

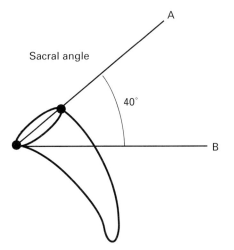

Fig. 9.14 Line drawing to depict the attitude of the sacral base relative to horizontal in the sagittal plane (sacral angle).

1. Dots are placed at the anterior and posterior margins of the sacral base.

2. A line (A) is drawn to connect these dots, and is extended posteriorly for a span of 75–100 mm.

3. A horizontal line of reference (B) is drawn from the sacral promontory and extended posteriorly for 75–100 mm.

4. The angle between lines A and B is measured; this is referred to as the modified angle of Ferguson.

For reasons that are obscure to this investigator, for those with a sacral angle of over 41°, as the sacral angle is reduced towards 41° there appears an unlevelness of the base of the sacrum additional to that apparent in the initial study. Typically, such persons end up with a heel lift significantly thicker than the amount of unlevelness initially measured. For example, a sacral base that initially is 5 mm unlevel with a sacral angle of 46° can end up with an unlevelness of 2 mm, a sacral angle of 42°, and a lift 8 mm thick. Perhaps this phenomenon is an illustration of the correspondent linkage between the mutually exclusive situations of the base of the sacrum as viewed in the coronal and sagittal planes.

DELINEATION OF THE SUPERINCUMBENT LOAD OF THE SACRAL BASE IN THE SAGITTAL PLANE

This measurement is an indication of where the load through the lumbar spine passes with respect to the sacral base. For the ideal posture in the sagittal plane, there is vertical alignment of the following points: the external meatus of the ear, the acromioclavicular joint, the midpoint of the body of L3, the anterior third of the sacral base, and the fibular heads. Load of the sacral base can be represented by extension of an imaginary line from the midpoint of the vertebral body of L3 downward through the level of the sacral base (Fig. 9.15).

Under less than ideal conditions, these anatomic references are not vertically aligned. Displacement of alignment of superincumbent regions displaces their load. Displacement of the load

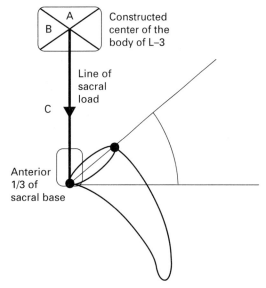

Fig. 9.15 From the sagittal view, a delineation of the superincumbent load transmitted by the lumbar spine to the sacral base. Ideally, the line of this load passes through the anterior third of the sacral base.

anterior to the base of the sacrum results in increased shear at the lumbosacral junction as well as an anterior-ward torque about the transverse axis. Countertorque is generated by the rectus abdominis and psoas muscles.

Posterior displacement shifts the load from the vertebral bodies and base of the sacrum to the pedicles and intervertebral facets. These structures are less suitable for bearing load than are the bodies of the vertebrae and the first sacral segment.

The method for delineation of the sacral load is as follows:

1. One dot is placed at each of the corners of the vertebral body of L3.
2. Two diagonal lines (A and B) are drawn to connect the four dots, intersecting at approximately the midpoint of the body of L3.
3. A vertical line (C) is drawn extended downward from the midpoint of L3 to the level of the anterior margin of the sacral base; this line indicates the placement of sacral load.

Ideally in this sagittal view the load represented by this line passes through the anterior third of the sacral base. Under other conditions, the load

is displaced anteriorly or posteriorly. Anterior displacement can be measured as millimeters of horizontal span from the vertical line of load to the promontory of the sacral base. Where there is posterior displacement, the line passes through the middle or posterior third of the sacral base. Displacement posterior to the sacral base can be measured as millimeters of horizontal span extending from the posterior margin of the sacral base to the vertical line of sacral load.

CORRECTION OF ATTITUDE OF THE SACRAL BASE

In the coronal plane

Unlevelness can be corrected by placement of a lift inside the shoe and beneath the heel. The lift is composed of material that is not compressible under the stress of normal weight, such as cork or rubber. For those patients with unlevelness of 2 mm, incorporate a 2 mm lift. For those patients with unlevelness $\geq$ 3 mm, the thickness of the initial lift recommended by this author is 3 mm. An initial lift of thickness greater than 3 mm can be followed by transient discomfort of the MS.

Biweekly, the heel lift can safely be augmented in thickness by 2 mm. After the initial lift of 3 mm, subsequent augmentation of thickness of the lift by extents of over 2 mm can be followed by transient discomfort and for this reason is also not recommended.

At the time of the introduction of the lift, and with each augmentation of thickness, the soft tissues and joints of the subjects are examined for restriction of physiologic freedom of motion. Where such resistance is identified, the restricted soft and articular tissues are taken through the physiologic range of motion to reduce resistance to a possible increase in postural symmetry. This activity is performed for an average of 20 min per session. This cycle is repeated biweekly until the thickness of the lift is equal to the number of millimeters of sacral unlevelness initially measured.

Two weeks after the final increase in lift thickness, the patient is radiographed a second time, with the lift inside shoes routinely worn by the subject (Fig. 9.16). From this second film, initial measurements are repeated and compared for improvement, and residual unlevelness/tilt/displacement is identified for further correction. On completion of this second course of treatment, a final film is taken, both to assess for residua and to assure that overcorrection has not occurred.

A clinical example of excessive 'dose' of lift was the case of a 52-year-old patient with chronic and idiopathic pain of the low back. Postural radiography revealed an 11 mm unlevelness of the sacral base, with 13° of lateral bend of the lumbar spine. She was told of this unlevelness and initially given a 3 mm lift. Later that same day she increased her lift to the full 11 mm. Ten days later she reported that her low back pain was presently much better but that she was experiencing new discomforts in other multiple regions of the MS. Repeat of the postural radiography showed a level sacral base and reduction of the lateral bend of the lumbar spine from 13° to 2°. The new discomforts were attributed to the stress of abrupt reduction of the lumbopelvic obliquity. Pleased with her radiographic improvement, she opted to continue with the lift at the full thickness and to ride out the subsequent discomforts.

The multiregional discomforts gradually worsened over the next several weeks such that by the third week after the introduction of the lift she was unable to stand and required a wheelchair for transportation. It was 5 weeks after the introduction of the lift before she fully recovered her level of function and comfort that was typical prior to the lift, and by the end of the sixth week she reported an overall and marked improvement of her original pains as well as alleviation of the pain that developed after the lift. While this case is extreme, it demonstrates that a risk of abrupt and full leveling of the sacral base from 11 mm of

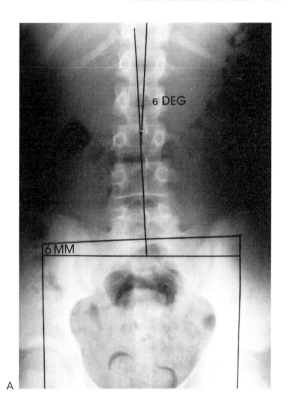

A

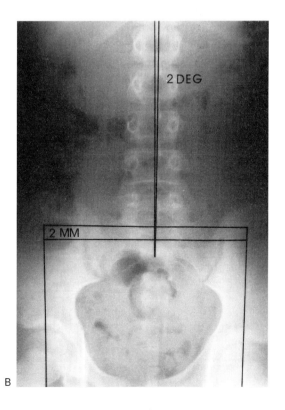

B

Fig. 9.16 Effect of incorporation of a heel lift and contoured orthotics on unlevelness of the base of the sacrum and lateral bend of the lumbar spine. (A) shows 6 mm of unlevelness with 6° of lateral bend of the lumbar spine. (B) is an X-ray performed with a 6 mm lift beneath the heel on the low side, and shows reduction of initial unlevelness of the sacral base to 2 mm, and of lateral bend of the lumbar spine to 2°.

unlevelness is iatrogenic and possibly debilitating pain, albeit temporary.

In the sagittal plane

Throughout the course of postural correction, a therapeutic posture (Fig. 9.17) is practiced daily at home to reduce resistance to postural correction, accelerate relief of pain, reduce excess sacral tilt and anterior displacement of sacral load, and minimize possible transitional discomforts consequent to the stress of postural correction. Patients recline daily for 20 min in a supine position on a carpeted floor with a towel rolled tightly and placed lengthwise along the posterior midline of the thorax. For patients with excessive anterior tilt of the sacral base ($\geqslant$ 42°), a paperback book, 25 mm thick, is placed directly beneath the sacrum. This posture reduces the concavity of the anterior aspect of the femoral–pelvic junction, lordosis of the lumbopelvis, and kyphosis of the thorax. The rolled towel is recommended for all undergoing postural correction, and the book is recommended only for those with tilt $\geqslant$ 42°. Use of the book by those with a tilt $\leqslant$ 41° can exert pressure at the physiologic limit and result in transient pain of the low back without therapeutic advantage.

ADJUSTMENT OF SHOE

If the thickness of the lift exceeds the available space within the shoe, either the excess lift was added to the outer heel (by an orthotist or cobbler) or the vertical span of the contralateral heel reduced. For subjects with an augmentation of the heel greater than 8 mm, the thickness of the sole also was augmented so the difference between the thickness of the heel and sole did not exceed 8 mm. This increase in thickness of the sole is intended to minimize the difference in pitch between the right and left shoes and thereby avoid secondary torsion of the pelvis about the vertical axis.

A practical limit to this rule is that the tensile strength of the sole is commensurate with thickness. A sole that has been augmented more than 10 mm can be noticeably stiff during gait. For benefit within the tolerance of comfort, a minimal augmentation is 5 mm and a maximum approximately 10 mm.

EFFECT OF OPTIMIZATION OF POSTURE ON PAIN WITHOUT KNOWN CAUSE

There is no apparent relation between the initial extent of sacral unlevelness and the intensity or multiplicity of sites of recurrent pain. For the central boundary, increase in comfort is proportional to correction of sacral attitude and load. Due to the incremental augmentation, those with less unlevelness completed their course of treatment and achieved comparable relief more rapidly than did those who were initially more unlevel.

Reduction of discomforts tend to occur in an ascending pattern, with initial relief reported in the lowermost regions, and the uppermost

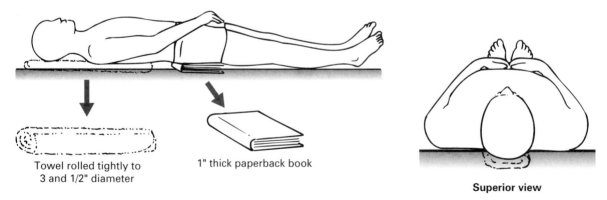

Towel rolled tightly to 3 and 1/2" diameter

1" thick paperback book

Superior view

Fig. 9.17   A therapeutic posture practiced for 20 min daily to reduce resistance to postural correction, accelerated relief of discomfort, and reduce increased sacral tilt and anterior displacement of sacral load.

regions being the last to respond. An exception to this trend was the complaint of headache, which tended to resolve during the first half of the course of correction.

Pretreatment, patients with pain of non-specific cause reported recurrent discomfort in, on average, 43% of eight regions. Post treatment, subjects reported recurrent discomfort in 13% of the eight regions. For 7 out of 8 regions, the number of patients for whom previously recurrent discomforts were absent was statistically significant ($p < 0.01$ for each) (Fig. 9.18). Of those regions where discomfort was not absent after treatment, subjects routinely reported a marked reduction in both the frequency and intensity of the discomfort(s). Overall, recurrent pain without specific cause is alleviated for 70% of the regions and markedly reduced for the remaining 30%.

There is no apparent relationship between the age of the subject and the outcome. Also, there is no apparent relation between weight of the subject and outcome. Certainly, mass matters, but it appears that the shape of the body mass with respect to gravitation matters far more.

Incidentally, subjects typically report a reduction or alleviation of three visceral discomforts without specific cause: dysphagia, dyspepsia, and constipation that is not cathartic dependent.

Approximately one-third of patients reported a brief (1–7 day) and mild increase of discomfort as the final 20% of the unlevelness was corrected. These discomforts included myalgia, malaise, occasional slight nausea, and dizziness, and occurred more commonly in those subjects with initially greater degrees of lateral bend of the lumbar spine.

SUMMARY

Presented above is a model sufficient to explain the majority of prevalent pain of the MS as our experience of non-ideal, albeit normal, posture. Posture is characterized as being dependent on boundary conditions within which structure and function take form and to which sensory receptors are correspondingly linked. This model makes reasonable the otherwise surprising finding that correction of normal posture towards an ideal form is followed by alleviation of the majority of such pain, with marked reduction of pain for those regions with residual discomfort. Idiopathic pain of the MS that is relieved subsequent to optimization of posture can be termed postural arthralgia, rather than pain without known cause.

Let us compare the present model of posture with several contemporary and leading concepts of the MS. This model agrees with the concepts of form and force closure that Vleeming and Snijders applied to characterize two scenarios for joint stability (Snijders et al 1992, Vleeming et al

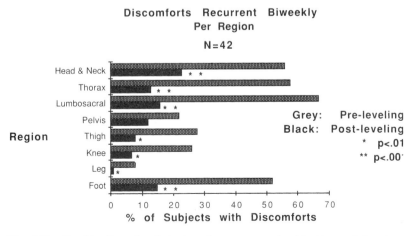

Fig. 9.18 Graphic effect of optimization of posture on regional incidence of chronic and otherwise idiopathic pain.

> Form closure + Force closure = Unity
>
> Where:
>
> [Form closure]$^{\to\,max.}$, [Force closure]$^{\to\,min.}$

Fig. 9.19 This states the relation of form closure, force closure, and unity of the MS with respect to arthrodial stability. Where form closure is maximized, the need for additional force closure is minimized.

1995). Form closure refers to a stable situation with closely fitted joint surfaces, in which no extra force is needed to maintain the state of the system, given the actual load situation (Fig. 9.19). (See also Chapters 3 and 6.) A condition for form closure is proper size, shape, and attitude of postural boundaries, on which the load is dependent. In this situation, the joint is self-acting and stable.

Postural scoliosis that is compensatory to unlevelness of the sacral base illustrates inverse correspondence of form-to-force closure. To counter torque that results from sacral unlevelness, muscular force is necessary to stabilize the picture by formation of scoliosis. For adults, use of a heel lift to level a normal extent of unlevelness of the sacral base results in reduction of degrees of lumbar scoliosis, otherwise idiopathic, by about one-third (Irvin 1991).

This model also agrees with Gracovetsky's model of the pelvis–shoulder–spine system as a mechanical oscillator resonating within the field of gravity (Gracovetsky 1965). A condition for resonance is proper phase relation of oscillations. Because proper phase relations are dependent on ideal conditions of boundary, the later are necessary for resonance. To the extent that the skeletal system functions as a mechanical oscillator, ideal boundaries are a condition for maximal transfer of energy from potential to kinetic.

Denslow and Korr associated the theory of the facilitated spinal segment with somatic dysfunction (Denslow et al 1947) with component hyper-reflexia of the sympathetic nervous system. Hyper-reflexic sympathetic tone is credited with organization of disease (Korr 1976). The motor reflexes, from moment to moment, adjust the muscular forces around each joint, the parts of the body to each other and to the body as a whole, and of the body to the forces of gravity (Korr 1979). Because sympathetic tone corresponds to gravitation, boundary conditions of posture can relate to disease mediated by sympathetic hyper-reflexia. This argument agrees with the report that correction of posture is followed by reduction of dyspepsia, functional dysphagia, and constipation.

Risks

There is risk of experiencing a brief crescendo of discomfort as the final 20% of unlevelness is corrected. Both central and peripheral discomfort can be a feature of symmetrization of posture, particularly for those with greater degrees of bend of the spinal column. A possible cause of this discomfort is resistance of tissue to spinal straightening. Such discomfort passes spontaneously or can be reduced more rapidly by physical manipulation.

The only contraindication to postural correction pertains to the earlier stage of pregnancy, as this method includes radiography of the pelvis and thereby incurs a risk for the fetus in early development.

Benefits

This coherent scheme for the MS, based on a novel definition and application of the principle of complementarity, provides a sound philosophic basis and scientific method with results that far exceed that obtained from conventional treatment based on other principles alone.

Low back pain can be prevented and treated by modifying posture, and specific training of the musculature can enhance the ability to resist postural stress (Vleeming et al 1995). A limitation of this strategy is the fact that gravity is inexhaustible, but we are not. Perhaps this difference accounts for the modest effect on stability derived from muscle strengthening. It can be anticipated that postural symmetrization, performed in combination with strengthening of deconditioned musculature, would greatly enhance the outcome over that achieved by strengthening alone.

Physical manipulation directed to reduce arthrodial malrotation, restriction, and altered sensitivity of soft tissue cannot be expected to have lasting effect where the pressure towards derangement persists. Such manipulation, in concert with optimization of normal posture, has far better results than can otherwise be obtained. This finding agrees with evidence that manual manipulation can improve acute pain but has a weak effect on recurrence.

Surgery to relieve pain previously attributed to a herniated intervertebral disc, stenosis of the vertebral foramen, facet osteoarthropathy, or painful irregularity of the stress-bearing surface of the knee or patella can be expected to have better results where the difforming pressure as well as the deformed tissue is corrected. In some cases, correction of postural stress can preclude surgery, which is otherwise needed.

By this method for the alleviation of prevalent pain, the therapeutic relation can often be converted from maintenance to one that yields marked reduction or removal of the need for periodic treatment. Also, the proportion of the population who are candidates for a course of treatment is greatly increased from the minority who are abnormal to the great majority who are posturally imperfect.

Cost

Cost of optimization of posture is proportionate to the initial extent of flatness of the arches of the feet, angularity of the ankles, unlevelness of the sacral base, and degree of lumbopelvic lordosis. For the typical patient with mild pes planovalgus, sacral unlevelness of 6 mm, and without lumbo-pelvic lordosis, optimization can be completed within 3–4 months, with 6–8 treatments at a net cost of $1300–1500. This one-time cost can be favorably compared with the much greater cost from chronic reliance on medication, physical therapy, or surgical intervention, none of which reduces the principle pressure towards chronic and progressive disorder.

Future study

It is mysterious why most adults are posturally asymmetric but only some have pain. One possibility is that we are seeing the effect of biologic variance in the capacity to compensate for stress, sensitivity to noxious stimuli, or both. This leaves room for other possible effects.

Although the majority of discomfort was alleviated, discomfort did remain for some. Subsequent to this clinical study, the criteria for intervention and technique for correction of the feet have improved considerably (Irvin 1995). Future study can measure the effect of full correction of the feet, in combination with complete leveling of the sacral base. Anecdotally, results are better in this case. Yet, for subjects with more full correction, some discomfort can persist. This fact indicates that one or more factors (cofactors), in addition to attitude of the feet and sacral base when standing, have bearing on the reducibility of chronic, idiopathic discomfort.

The possibility exists, and is likely, that postural correction for those with chronic pain from specific cause known to have a postural component can also result in reduction of discomfort. Particular examples include post-polio syndrome, tension cephalgia, double-crush syndrome, primary fibromyalgia, and osteoarthritis.

Finally, the reported reduction of dysphagia, dyspepsia, and constipation warrants further investigation. This report was especially interesting, as there was nothing in the design of this study that would lead the subject to expect improvement of visceral discomforts. In accordance with Beckwith (1935), Korr (1979), Kappler (1982), Kuchera and Jungman (1986), and others, it is possible that visceral dysfunction is significantly mediated by normal posture, and is further correctable by optimization of posture.

CONCLUSIONS

1. The majority of idiopathic and chronic pain of the musculoskeletal system is alleviated by sufficient improvement of normal posture towards ideal configuration.

2. This outcome can be understood as an effect derived by a complementary relationship between structure, function and postural boundaries, such that manipulation of postural boundaries results in modification of structure and function.

3. Further research is merited to test the effect of postural correction on chronic pain attributed to known disease, disorder or dysfunction, both visceral and somatic.

Acknowledgements

Special appreciation is extended to the following: Ellen Page Garrison, MFA and Associate Professor of Ballet and Modern Dance, who initially challenged this investigator with the possibility that the standard of perfect motion pertains practically to the comfort of normal movers; Jason Ellis, PhD and Associate Professor of Physics, who for 10 years has provided this investigator the invaluable service of answering the question, 'Can it be that . . .' with 'No, it cannot . . .', until finally it could; Paul Stern, DO and Professor of Anesthesiology, for his insistence on a testable model of somatic dysfunction. David J. Barker, PhD and Associate Professor of Neurophysiology; for grantsmanship; research grants and awards, including funding from AOA Grant # 85–11–190 and 86–11–190.

REFERENCES

Barker D J, Irvin R E 1986 Electromyographic responses to osteopathic manipulative treatment and structural balancing. Journal of the American Osteopathic Association 9: 608/122

Beckwith C G 1935 Postural studies and the influence of feet. Journal of the American Osteopathic Association 35: 117

Boden S D, Davis D O, Dina T S, Patronas N J, Wiesel S W 1990 Abnormal magnetic-resonance scans of the lumbar spine in asymptomatic patients: a prospective investigation. Journal of Bone and Joint Surgery (US) 72: 403–408

Bohr N 1934 Atomic theory and the description of nature. Cambridge University Press, Cambridge

Denslow J, Korr I, Krems A 1947 Quantitative studies of chronic facilitation in human motorneuron pools. American Journal of Physiology 150: 229–238

Denslow J S, Chase J A, Gutensohn O R, Kumm M G 1955 Methods in taking and interpreting weightbearing x-ray films. Journal of the American Osteopathic Association 54: 663–670

Dieck G, Kelsey J L, Goel V K et al 1985 An epidemiologic study of the relationship between postural asymmetry in the teen years and subsequent back and neck pain. Spine 10: 872–877

Doczi G 1994 The power of limits: proportional harmonies in nature, art, and architecture. Shambala, Boston

Dott G A, Hart C L, McKay C 1994 Predictability of sacral base unlevelness based on iliac crest measurements. Journal of the American Osteopathic Association 5: 383

Dvorak J, Dvorak V 1984 Manual medicine therapy. Thieme-Stratton, New York

Ferguson A B 1939 Roentgen diagnosis of the extremities and spine. Paul Hoeber, New York

Gracovetsky S 1965 A hypothesis for the role of the spine in human locomotion: a challenge to current thinking. Journal of Biomedical Engineering 7: 205–216

Greenman P E 1979 Lift therapy: use and abuse. Journal of the American Osteopathic Association 79: 238–250

Grundy P F, Roberts C J 1984 Does unequal leg length cause back pain? Lancet 2: 256–258

Held C 1994 The meaning of complimentarity. Studies in the History and Philosophy of Science 25(6): 871–893

Hoffman K, Hoffman L 1994 Effects of adding sacral base leveling to osteopathic manipulative treatment of back pain: a pilot study. Journal of the American Osteopathic Association 3: 217–226

Irvin R E 1986 Postural balancing: a protocol for routine reversal of chronic somatic dysfunction, abstracted. Journal of the American Osteopathic Association 86: 608

Irvin R E 1991 Reduction of lumbar scoliosis by use of a heel lift to level the sacral base. Journal of the American Osteopathic Association 1: 33–44

Irvin R E 1995 Is normal posture a correctable origin of common, chronic, and otherwise idiopathic discomfort of the musculoskeletal system? In: Vleeming A, Mooney V, Dorman T, Snijders C J (eds) Second interdisciplinary world congress on low back pain. San Diego, CA, 9–11 November, pp 425–460

Jensen M C, Brant-Zawadzki M N, Obuchowski N, Modic M T, Malka S D, Ross J S 1994 Magnetic resonance imaging of the lumbar spine in people without back pain. New England Journal of Medicine 331(2): 69–73

Kappler R E 1982 Postural balance and motion patterns. Journal of the American Osteopathic Association 81: 598–606

Korr I 1976 The spinal cord as organizer of disease process: some preliminary perspectives. The peripheral autonomic nervous system. Journal of the American Osteopathic Association 9: 35–45

Korr I 1979 The spinal cord as organizer of disease process. II: The peripheral autonomic nervous system. Journal of the American Osteopathic Association 2: 82–90

Kourany J A 1987 Scientific knowledge: basic issues in the philosophy of science. Wadsworth, Belmont

Kuchera M L, Jungman M 1986 Inclusion of a Levitor orthotic device in management of refractive low back pain patients. Journal of the American Osteopathic Association 10: 673

Kuhn T 1970 The structure of scientific revolutions. University of Chicago, pp 92–110

Loyd P 1934 Roentgenographic postural examination of the lumbar spine and pelvis. Read before the College of Osteopathic Surgeons

Petruccioli S 1993 Atoms, metaphors, and paradoxes: Neils Bohr and the construction of a new physics. Cambridge University Press, Cambridge

Richardson C A, Jull G A 1995 Muscle control – pain control. What exercises would you prescribe? Manual Therapy 1: 2–19

Rucker R 1987 Mind tools: the five levels of mathematical reality. Houghton Mifflin, Boston

Snijders C J, Vleeming A, Stoeckart R 1992 Transfer of lumbosacral load to iliac bones and legs. I: Biomechanics of self-bracing of the sacroiliac joints and its significance for treatment and exercise. In: Vleeming A, Mooney V, Snijders C J, Dorman T (eds) First interdisciplinary world congress on low back pain and its relation to the sacroiliac joint. San Diego, CA, 5–6 November, pp 233–254

Vleeming A, Volkers A C W, Snijders C J, Stoeckart R 1990 Relation between form and function in the sacroiliac joint.

2: Biomechanical aspects. Spine 15: 130–132

Vleeming A, Snijders C J, Stoeckart R, Mens J M A 1995 A new light on low back pain, part I. In: Vleeming A, Mooney V, Dorman T, Snijders C J (eds) Second interdisciplinary world congress on low back pain. San Diego, CA, 9–11 November, pp 149–168

10. A different approach to the mechanics of the human pelvis: tensegrity

S. M. Levin

INTRODUCTION

The paradigm

According to conventional wisdom, the human spine behaves as an architectural column or pillar and transfers the superincumbent weight through the sacrum, to the ilium, through the hips and down the lower extremities. The pillar holds the base in place with the pressing weight of gravity. In this model, the sacrum, as the base, locks into the pelvis, either as a wedge or by some other gravity-dependent closure.

The anomalies

Architectural pillars orient vertically and function only in a gravity field and are rigid, immobile, base-heavy, and unidirectional. Pillars and columns resist compression forces well but need reinforcement when stressed by bending moments and shear. Stressed by internal shear, they are high energy consuming structures. Rigid Newtonian mechanical laws such as Hooke's law, Euler's formula, Galileo's square-cube law, and Poisson's ratio govern conventional columns (Box 10.1). Yet, if biologic systems conformed to these laws, the human bony spine would bend with less than the weight of the head on top of it (Morris & Lucas 1964) and the vertebral bodies would crush under the leverage of a fly rod held in a hand. Animals larger than a lion would continually break their bones, and dinosaurs and mastodons larger than a present-day elephant would have crushed under their own weight. Urinary bladders and pregnant uteri would burst when full and, with each heartbeat, arteries would lengthen enough to crowd the brain out of the skull (Gordon 1978).

While it is a teleological conceit that the human spine acts as a column, phylogenetic and ontogenetic development of the human spine was not in the form of a column, but as some form of a beam. It would not be an ordinary beam, a rigid bar, but an extraordinary beam composed of rigid body segments connected by flexible connective tissue elements that floated the segments in space (Fielding et al 1976). During human gestational development and during the first year or so of life, the human spine does not function as a column but as such a beam.

It must be recognized that in many postures the adult human spine does not function as a column or even a simple beam. When the spine is horizontal, the sacrum is not a base of a column but the connecting element that ties the beam to the pelvic ring. Even when upright, the vertebral blocks are not fixed by the weight of the load above, as they must be in an architectural pillar. S-shaped curves can create intolerable loads and instability in a column, particularly if it is an articulated column that has flexible, frictionless joints, as the spine does. With each breath, the interconnected bodies translate, some forward, some backward. While architectural columns bear loads from above, the human spine can accept loads from any direction with arms and legs cantilevered out in any way. The hallmark of a pillar is stability, but the hallmark of a spine is flexibility and movement. Movement of an articulated column, even along a horizontal, is more challenging than moving an upright Titan missile to its launch pad. The spine can bend forward so a person can touch his toes and bend backward almost equally well. It can twist and bend simultaneously. It can perform intricately controlled

Box 10.1   Laws of mechanics

Hooke's law   For any given material that obeys Hooke's law, the slope of the graph or the ratio of stress to strain will be constant. Biologic materials are non-Hookian and get stiffer and stronger as they load. The strength and stiffness of bone is about the same in all animals. Their brittleness is such that they fracture easily once the animal reaches the size of a human or a lion. Since larger animals exist, it is obvious that either the calculations are wrong or the calculated loads are wrong.

Euler's formula $P = \pi^2 E/L^2$
where P = load at which the column will buckle, E = Young's modulus of the material.
   The taller the column, the weaker and less stable it is. Very tall columns will bend of their own weight. If the Empire State Building were as slender as a stalk of wheat, it would be less than 2 m wide at the base. The ligamentous spine will buckle under a load of only 2.2 kg.

Galileo's square-cube law   As the surface area of a structure squares, its volume cubes. Eventually, it will crush from its own weight. The maximum size of a land-based animal can, by calculation, be no more than a modern elephant. Larger animals cannot exist. Many dinosaurs exceeded the calculated breaking point of biologic tissue. The assumption was that they lived half buried in swamp water to support their weight. We now know that that was not true. Biologic constructs exhibit non-Newtonian behavior and do not conform to Galileo's Law.

Poisson's ratio   If one stretches a rubber band, it gets thinner. If one shortens a material by compressing it, it bulges out. The ratio of these changes in a material is Poisson's ratio. For engineering materials, the ratio lies between 0.25 and 0.5 and cannot exceed 0.5. However, biologic materials usually have a ratio greater than 0.5, and it may approach unity. This is another example of the non-Newtonian behavior of biologic structures.

movements in space, as in gymnastics, dance, aquatic diving, or basketball. The spine is flexible, mobile, functionally independent of gravity, and has property behavior inconsistent with an architectural column or beam.

In all studies, the spine, unlike columns and beams, is a low energy consumer. The individual components of the spine, and the structure as a whole, behave non-linearly and do not conform to the standard linear Newtonian mechanical laws that govern columns and beams (Fox 1988, White & Panjabi 1978). Yet, in an attempt to make complex problems simple, bioengineers have converted non-linear complexities to linear mathematics models. The new science of non-linear dynamic systems (such as the weather) has shown the fallacy of that process (Gleick 1988).

The alternative

If, instead of a column, the spine is considered to be a series of rigid bodies tied together by the discs and soft tissues, with the sacrum as the con-

necting link to the pelvis, what locks the sacrum in place so that the spine is supported in all its functions? An omnidirectional mechanical system exists that can function in any posture and be capable of transferring considerable loads, coming from any direction, through the pelvis and to the lower extremities. Such a system must be consistent with evolutionary theory. It must also be structurally hierarchical so that in any instant in its ontological development it is mechanically functional and stable. (Embryos and fetuses do not fall apart either in or out of the womb.)

KINEMATICS

The kinematics of the pelvis must take into account mechanical laws that affect a free body in space. Until the work of White and Panjabi (1978), movements of anatomic structures were usually described in anatomic, rather than mechanical, terms such as forward bending or side-bending. Planes of movement were also described in anatomic terms, such as 'coronal' or

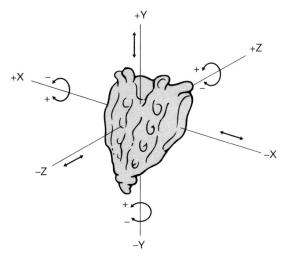

Fig. 10.1 The sacrum in a three-dimensional Cartesian coordinate system. A body can be described as rotating around the three axes, X, Y and Z, in one direction, positively (+), or the other, negatively (–). It also can be described as translating (+) or (–) in the XY, XZ, or YZ planes. A body free to move in any direction is characterized as having 12 degrees of freedom.

'sagittal'. This terminology worked as a barrier to the precise description of movements in biologic systems. For example, forward bending is more precisely described in terms of rotations and translations of vertebral bodies in space and in relation to each other, which would be difficult to describe in anatomic terminology (Fryette 1954). In mechanical terminology, a rigid body in space is described as having six degrees of freedom of movement in a three-dimensional Cartesian coordinate system. White and Panjabi (1978) adapted the Cartesian coordinate system to the biomechanical description of the spine (Fig. 10.1). Cartesian coordinates are now widely used in the biomechanical literature to describe joint move-

ments. Although in classical mechanics there are six degrees of freedom, others have considered that describing 12 degrees of freedom – six positive and six negative – may be more useful. It is easy to plot these coordinates and generate computer graphics. This system seems suitable for describing the complex movements of the sacrum. However, before we can discuss the dynamics of the sacrum or any other structure, we should understand the statics of that structure. How is the sacrum stabilized in its position in the body?

STATICS

To fix in space a body that has 12 degrees of freedom, it seems logical that there need to be 12 restraints. Fuller (1975) proves this. One restraint will allow pendulum movement, two restraints will allow the body to move in a plane around an axis, and three restraints fix the body but allow movement in a line along an axis. Four restraints, configured as corresponding to the vertices of a tetrahedron, are the minimum required to fix a point in space (Fig. 10.2). However, this would still allow turbining positively and negatively on three axes. According to Fuller's proof, to be rigidly fixed a total of 12 restraints would be necessary.

This principle is demonstrated in a wire-spoked bicycle wheel. A minimum of 12 tension spokes rigidly fixes the hub in space (anything more than 12 is a fail safe mechanism) (Fig. 10.3). In a bicycle wheel, tension-loaded spokes transmit compressive loads from the frame and the ground. The hub remains suspended in its tension network, and the compression loads distribute around the rim. The compression elements are discontinuous and behave in a counterintuitive way. Rather than

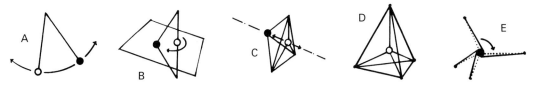

Fig. 10.2 Fixing a point in space. Four vectors of restraint define a minimum system in which a point is fixed in space (D). However, turbining is still possible (E). An additional eight restraints are needed to rigidly fix a point. (Adapted from Fuller 1975.)

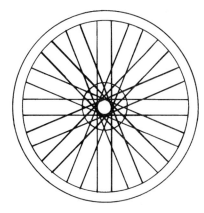

Fig. 10.3   A wire-spoked cycle wheel. The hub is rigidly fixed in a tension network. The compressive load applied to the hub by the weight of the load is transferred to the rim solely through tension. The load distributes evenly around the rim. The bicycle frame and its load hang from the hubs like a hammock between trees.

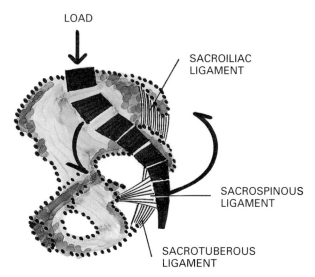

Fig. 10.4   The sacrum suspends in the pelvic ring by its many ligaments. Motion is restricted by the balanced tension of these ligaments.

becoming the primary support elements of the system, as they would be in a pillar or wagon wheel model, the compression elements become secondary to the tension support network. Fuller (1975) calls these structures 'tensegrity' structures, a contraction of 'tension integrity'. Other familiar tensegrity structures are tennis rackets, which transmit the compression force of the racket frame to the ball through the strings, snow shoes and Buckminster Fuller geodesic domes (which are high-frequency icosahedrons). Tensegrity structures transmit loads through tension and compression only. Because they are fully triangulated, there are no bending moments in these structures, nor is there shear. By linking the hubs of front and rear wire bicycle wheels by its frame, we create a hierarchical system in which the load on the bicycle suspends in a tension network. This network works even when the bike is doing 'wheelies' (rearing-up on one wheel) and transfers all the load to one wheel.

It is generally accepted that the sacrum hangs from the ilia by its ligaments (Grant 1952, Kapandji 1974). A ligamentous tension system for support and stability is consistent with the known anatomy. If we use a bicycle wheel tensegrity structure as our model for the pelvis, the pelvic ring would be the rim and the sacrum would be the hub of the pelvis. The many tension elements of ligaments and muscles attached to

the sacrum stabilize it (Fig. 10.4). The sacrum suspends as a compression element within the musculoligamentous envelope and transfers its loads through that tension network. Even when a person stands on one leg, the sacrum sits within its tension network, just as does the bicycle hub when doing wheelies. This tension network provides omnidirectional structural stability, independent of gravity and hierarchical. The rim could distribute its load, rather than locally loading the forces at a point.

In a compressive loading pelvis system, as exists in the column model, the heads of the femurs would, with each step, smash into the soft cancellous bone of the acetabulum. In a tensegrity system, the forces generated at the hip would not concentrate in the acetabulum but be efficiently distributed throughout the pelvic bones and soft tissue. The sacrum would remain suspended in its soft tissue envelope (Willard 1995; see also Chapter 1 in this volume) and transmit the loads above and the forces below through the pelvic ligaments and muscles. Suspended in its tension network, it does not require gravity to hold it in place, as does a keystone model. The tensegrity-modeled sacrum functions right side up, upside down or sideways. A tension-fixed sacrum works equally well for the upright or space-walking human, the horizontal horse, the flying bat, or the swimming otter. It is the most widely adaptable, and therefore the most likely, pelvic model.

DYNAMICS

As a hub suspended by its spokes, the tension system must have a dynamic balance of the tension structures. A load on the wheel hub does not change its relative position within the rim. If the tension of the spokes remains constant and the spokes do not distort, the hub does not move at all. Ligaments of the body, likewise, have a high tensile strength and do not distort much when loaded. Assuming a minimum of 12 properly vectored restraints, as with the bicycle model, the sacrum cannot translate or rotate in any direction. It is fixed in position as is the hub of a wheel. Some of the restraints would have to be altered to allow pistoning or rotation to occur. However, if the sacrum moves in tandem with the other bones of the pelvis, so that the ligaments remain at the same length, tension-coupled movement patterns occur.

The body does have this coupled movement option available. It is present in the double tie bar hinge mechanism that is the model for the dynamics of knee movement (Dye 1987, Mueller 1983). This type of movement occurs in the 'Jacob's ladder' (Fig. 10.5), a 2000-year-old children's toy, which is itself a tensegrity structure. It is a series of tiles connected by crossed ribbons under tension. Flipping one of the tiles creates a controlled tumble. If the end tiles are held apart so that the entire structure is held in tension, the coupled tumbling can occur from top to bottom, bottom to top or sideways. This crossed ligament pattern, clearly evident in the knee, also exists in the spine, at the disc, ligament, and muscle level (Gracovetsky 1988, Kapandji 1974). It explains the coupled motion observed in the spine (White & Panjabi 1978). It is also evident in other joints, such as the capsular ligaments of the hip and the crossed patterns of ligaments and muscles of the back. This crossed tie bar pattern is present at the sacroiliac joints (SIJs) with the crossing patterns of the sacrospinous and sacrotuberous ligaments, the iliolumbar ligaments, the ventral, interosseous, and long and short dorsal sacroiliac ligaments,

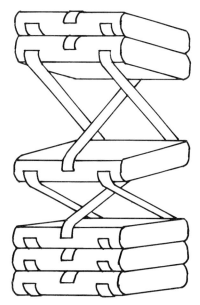

Fig. 10.5 Jacob's Ladder. Tilting a rigid tile at one end creates a controlled tumble of the other tiles by a crossed tie bar mechanism. The ties remain of the same length and tension throughout the movement.

piriformis, iliopsoas, coccygeus, and other muscles and soft tissues of the pelvis–spine–hip complex (Kapandji 1974). The crossed tie bar mechanism at the SIJ would account for the 'click-clack' phenomenon of the sacrum recognized by Snijders et al (see Chapter 6 in this volume). By rotating the ilia, as we do when we walk, the sacrum is forced to tumble and the movement transmits, Jacob's ladder-like, up the spine and to the limbs. Both the static and the dynamic mechanics of the pelvic structures are explained with tensegrity modeling.

THE EVOLUTION OF THE STRUCTURE

To fully understand pelvic mechanics and its integration in body mechanisms, it must be placed in its proper context. The tensegrity pelvic system is not creationist in design but is created by the physics of evolution (Fox 1988, Levin 1982, 1986, Prigogine & Stengers 1984). For biologic structures to exist as entities, they must be inherently stable and self-contained, not only when fully developed, but also at each instant of their existence. Only triangulated structures are inherently stable (Pearce

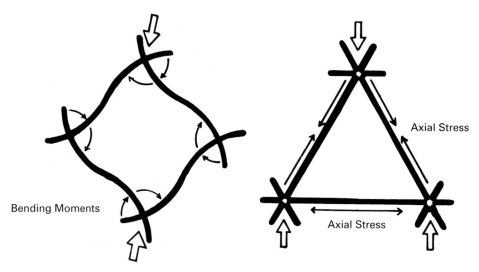

Fig. 10.6   Square frame structures are unstable and must have rigid joints to prevent collapse. Torque is created around these joints. Triangular frames are inherently stable, even with frictionless joints. The elements are under either tension or compression without any torque at the joints. (Adapted from Pearce 1978.)

1978). Structures that are not fully triangulated have joints that must be rigidly fixed to keep from collapsing. These joints generate torque and bending moments and have high energy requirements. Triangles are stable with flexible joints and have no torque or bending moments at the joints (Fig. 10.6). There are only tension and compression members in a triangle, so triangulated structures are low energy consumers. Truss systems made from triangles are used by engineers for constructing buildings and bridges because of their load distribution and high strength-to-weight ratios. Engineers will frequently build structures that mix triangulated and non-triangulated components, but to take maximum advantage of the construction properties of triangles, the trusses must be constructed only of triangles. The only fully triangulated, three-dimensional trusses are the polyhedra the tetrahedron, octahedron, and icosahedron (Fig. 10.7). All three-dimensional, fully triangulated trusses are some combination or permutation of these polyhedra. Thompson (1965), and later Gordon (1978), used truss systems to model biologic structures. Since only trusses are stable when their joints are flexible, it follows that if a structure has flexible joints and is stable, it must be triangulated. Thus biologic structures, stuck together by surface tension at

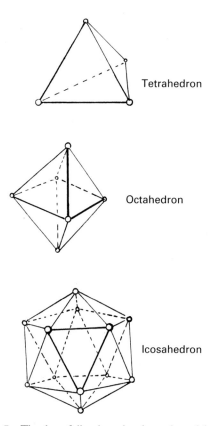

Fig. 10.7   The three fully triangulated, regular polyhedra, the tetrahedron with 4, the octahedron with 8, and the icosahedron with 12 triangular faces.

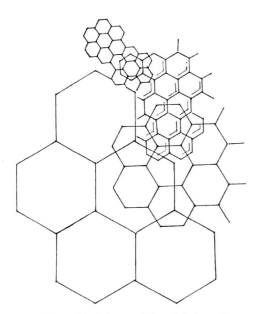

Fig. 10.8 Hierarchical close-packing of circles to hexagons.

the cellular level and freely jointed at the organism level, must be hierarchical, fully triangulated constructs composed of tetrahedrons, octahedrons, or icosahedrons.

Intimately related to the laws of triangulation are the laws of close-packing (Pearce 1978). In a planar arrangement of structures, the space- and energy-efficient configuration is hexagonal close-packing, as in a beehive (Fig. 10.8). Graphite is a hexagonal close-packed array of carbon atoms in sheets and is the first structural form of carbon. The laws of close-packing are independent of scale and apply to the molecular level as well as to plate tectonics.

In three-dimensional packing, the close-packed structure would also have to be a fully triangulated polyhedron. Diamonds, the hardest known materials, are a close-packed array of carbon atoms in a tetrahedral form and the second known structural form of carbon. Methane and water molecules are configured as tetrahedrons. A pile of oranges stacks as a tetrahedron. So do grains of sand and boulders to form mountains. Any oranges, sand grains, or boulders sticking out of the tetrahedron are unstable appendages and will fall if not held by friction or other force. Spherical forms of close-packed structures would have to be icosahedrons, which are mathematically the

most spherical and symmetric polyhedra as well as being fully triangulated. Carbon atoms' third molecular structural arrangement is as icosahedral-shaped fullerenes that are the roundest of all round molecules. Proteins lumped together to form viruses are icosahedral in shape. So are the silica shells of radiolaria (which are minute marine organisms), pollen grains, and blowfish.

Of the three triangulated polyhedra, the icosahedron has several attributes that are advantageous for biologic structures. It is the most spherical and has the largest volume for its surface area. In a planar arrangement, icosahedra pack as neatly as billiard balls. In spherical close packing, 12 icosahedra will close-pack around a central icosahedron-shaped space and form a stable icosahedron in a hierarchical construction (Fig. 10.9). Icosahedra also can be parts of fractals (Mandelbrot 1983), polymerizing and combining with other icosahedra. (A fractal dimension is a dimension greater than one and less than two, or greater than two and less than three, etc. It is the structural equivalent of conjoined twins, where one cannot exist on its own but must be part of another, each having components contributing to the whole.) Since it packs in stable arrays, it is self-generating (Kroto 1988). Tetrahedral- and octahedral-based trusses are not omnidirectional in form and function. They have a smaller volume for their surface area than do icosahedra, are not

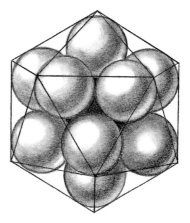

Fig. 10.9 Close-packing of 12 spheres to form a stable icosahedral array. Higher-frequency arrays that are stable conform to the formula $10(n-1)^2 + 2$, where n is the number of spheres along each edge of the icosahedron. Any other spherical array is structurally unstable.

fractal generators and do not close-pack. They would be less suitable for biologic structures, most of which require these properties (Barnesley et al 1987).

The mechanical laws of close-packing and triangulation apply to the multicelled embryo. Four cells will array as a tetrahedron, with four triangular faces. Eight cells will form an octahedron. Close-packing of cells will tend toward a spherical organization, the morula. The sphere is considered to be the optimum convex shape as it encloses the largest volume for its surface area. Composed of close-packed blastomeres, they could not be a perfect sphere but a convex polyhedron that is the most spherical, an icosahedron, with 20 triangular faces. Mathematically, it is impossible to create a convex polyhedron with more than 20 equilateral triangles (Pearce 1978). All higher-level stable spherical structures are just higher-frequency icosahedra.

The icosahedron is a regular solid with 20 triangular faces and 30 edges. Twelve vertices are created where 3 edges meet. Pressure on any point transmits along the 30 edges, some under tension, others under compression. It is possible to transfer all compression away from the outer edges by connecting opposite vertices of the icosahedron by compression rods. These rods do not pass through the center of the icosahedron but are eccentric and oddly angled; they hold the opposite corners away from each other. The outer shell of 30 edges is now entirely under tension, and the compression rods float within this tension shell like an endoskeleton (Fig. 10.10). A load applied to this structure causes a uniform increase in tension around all the edges and this distributes compression loads evenly to the six compression members. The mechanical properties of a tensegrity icosahedron are that they are omnidirectional structures, with the compression members and tension elements always maintaining their respective properties regardless of the direction of applied load, just as the wire spokes of a bicycle wheel are always under tension and the hub is always

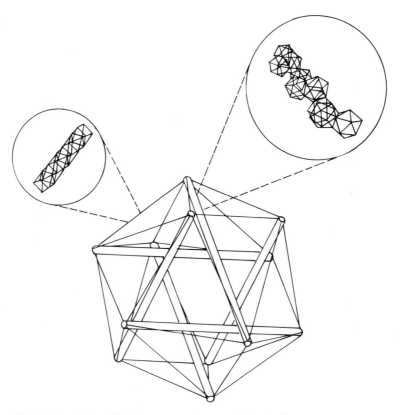

Fig. 10.10   A hierarchically constructed tensegrity icosahedron.

being compressed. Like the bike wheel, they can exist independent of gravity and are local load-distributing. They have a unique structural property of behaving non-linearly, as does the spine and its components, and most biologic tissue (Gordon 1988).

Fuller (1975) has shown that tensegrity icosahedra can link in an infinite array with any external form, as shown in Fig. 10.11. When linked, these structures can function as a single icosahedron in a hierarchical system. This model has been used to model endoskeletal structures, such as an upper extremity and cervical spine (Levin 1990), with the bones functioning as the compression rods and the soft tissues as the tension elements.

If we apply these evolutionary structural concepts to the sacrum, we can see how the tensegrity sacropelvic model develops. The sacrum, fixed in space by the tension of its ligaments and fascial envelope, functions as the connecting link between the spine and upper (or forequarter) extremities,

and the pelvis and lower (hindquarter) extremities. It evolved ontogenetically, directed not only by phylogenetic forces, but also by the physical forces of embryologic development. Wolff (1892) and Thompson (1965) state that the structure of the body is essentially a blueprint of the forces applied to these structures. Carter (1991) theorizes that the mechanical forces in utero are the determinants of embryologic structure that, in turn, evolves to fetal and then newborn structure. From the physicalist and biomechanics viewpoint, as well as from Darwinian theory, the evolution of structure is an optimization problem (Fox 1988, Hildebrandt and Tromba 1984). At each step of development, the evolving structure optimizes so that it exists with the least amount of energy expenditure. At the cellular level, the internal structure of the cells, the microtubules, together with the cell wall, must resist the crushing forces of the surrounding *milieu* and the exploding forces of its internal metabolism. Following Wolff's law, the internal skeleton of the cell aligns itself in the most efficient way to resist those forces. Ingber and colleagues (Ingber & Jamieson 1985, Wang et al 1993) have shown that the internal microtubular skeletal structure of a cell is a tensegrity icosahedron. Other subcellular structures, such as viruses, cletherins, and endocysts, are icosahedra (de Duve 1984, Wildy & Home 1963). A hierarchical construction of an organism would use the same mechanical laws that build the most basic biologic structure and use it to generate the more complex organism. Not only is the beehive an icosahedron, but so also is the bee's eye. Many other organelles and organisms look like and/or function as icosahedra (Levin 1982, 1986, 1990).

Following the concepts of Carter (1991), Wolff (1892), and Thompson (1965), a tensegrity-structured pelvis will build itself. Since the fetus develops upside down in a gravity-independent environment, as do fish eggs in water, the pelvis develops as a tensegrity ring, which is the most efficient structure to do that job. It does not develop as a structure to resist superincumbent weight-bearing. If it did, it would not function during its initial role in life of resisting in utero forces. It would also crush during delivery. Ontogeny recapitulates phylogeny. The one-celled

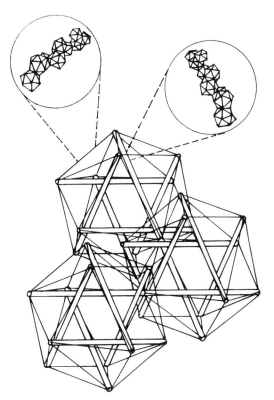

Fig. 10.11 An infinite array of tensegrity icosahedra. (Adapted from Fuller 1975.)

organism evolves as a series of stepwise mechanical accidents that are the most energy efficient and most adaptable, into a complex, energy efficient, symbiotic, multicelled organism. The different phyla get off the evolutionary ladder at different steps. To believe otherwise is to be a 'creationist' rather than a believer in Darwinian evolution. The development of a pelvis is not a 'design' but an evolutionary accident that worked in creating an energy-efficient, ambulating creature that could survive better in a gravity environment on land and could take advantage of the already evolved lungs that allowed breathing beyond the confines of the sea. It is the marvel of tensegrity structures that they are remarkably adaptable and can resist loads in a gravity-oriented environment equally well as they do when not affected by gravity (perhaps adding a few more trabeculae and ossifying some cartilage in accordance to Wolff's 'law'). The pelvis is cancellous bone because the distributed loads require nothing more, nothing less. Evolved to resist crushing forces from any direction, or exploding forces from within, the pelvis can adapt to unidirectional forces that are applied at two, three, or more points and distribute the load through the tension network of soft tissues and compression network of bones.

Icosahedral tensegrity structures are self-organizing space frames that are hierarchical and evolutionary (Kroto 1988). They will build them-selves, conforming to the laws of triangulation, close-packing, and, in biologic constructs, Wolff's Law. The pelvic wheel is a self-organizing structure that is part of a larger, fractal, space-frame, tensegrity construct with each part integrated into the whole. Simplicity and complexity intertwine in what Pearce (1978) calls 'minimum inventory, maximum diversity'.

CONCLUSIONS

1. This alternative approach to pelvic mechanics considers the pelvis part to be an integrated mechanical system based on the tensegrity icosahedron as its finite element.

2. This system can be used to model static one-legged or two-legged stance, or the dynamic mechanical functions of the pelvis.

3. Because of its ability to withstand omni-directional forces, the tensegrity icosahedron is appropriate for modeling pelvic mechanics, from weight-bearing to childbearing.

4. Tensegrity structures are low energy requiring structures and, as such, are favored by natural selection.

5. Since they are so adaptable and energy efficient, icosahedral mechanics may also be appropriate for modeling all biologic systems and subsystems at each stage of their development and whatever their eventual function.

REFERENCES

Barnesley M F, Massopust P, Strickland H, Sloan A D 1987 Fractal modeling of biologic structures. Annals of the New York Academy of Science 504: 179–194
Carter D R 1991 Musculoskeletal otogeny, phylogeny, and functional adaptation. Journal of Biomechanics 24 (supplement 1): 3–16
Duve C de 1984 A guided tour of the living cell. Scientific American Books, New York
Dye S F 1987 An evolutionary perspective of the knee. Journal of Bone and Joint Surgery (US) 69: 976–983
Fielding W J, Burstein A H, Frankel V H 1976 The nuchal ligament. Spine 1(1): 3–14
Fox R F 1988 Energy and the evolution of life. Freeman, New York
Fryette H H 1954 Principles of osteopathic technique. American Academy of Osteopathy, Carmel
Fuller R B 1975 Synergetics. Macmillan, New York
Gleick J 1988 Chaos. Penguin Books, New York
Gordon J E 1978 Structures: or why things don't fall down. De Capa, New York
Gordon J E 1988 The science of structures and materials. Freeman, New York
Gracovetsky S 1988 The spinal engine. Springer-Verlag, Vienna
Grant J C B 1952 A method of anatomy. Williams & Wilkins, Baltimore
Hildebrandt S, Tromba A 1984 Mathematics and optimal form. Scientific American Books, New York
Ingber D E, Jamieson J 1985 Cells as tensegrity structures. Architectural regulation of histodifferentiation by physical forces transduced over basement membrane. In: Andersonn L L, Gahmberg C G, Kblom P E (eds) Gene expression during normal and malignant differentiation. Academic Press, New York, pp 13–32
Kapandji I A 1974 The physiology of the joints, vol. 3, 2nd edn. Churchill Livingstone, Edinburgh
Kroto H 1988 Space, stars, C60, and soot. Science 242: 1139–1145
Levin S M 1982 Continuous tension, discontinuous compression, a model for biomechanical support of the body. Bulletin of Structural Integration, Rolf Institute, Bolder, pp 31–33
Levin S M 1986 The icosahedron as the three-dimensional finite element in biomechanical support. In: Proceedings of

the society of general systems research symposium on
mental images, values and reality G14–26. Society of
General Systems Research, St Louis

Levin S M 1990 The space truss as a model for cervical spine
mechanics – a systems science concept. In: Paterson J K,
Burn L (eds) Back pain – an international review. Kluwer
Academic, Lancaster, pp 231–238

Mandelbrot B 1983 The fractal geometry of nature. Freeman,
San Francisco

Morris J M, Lucas D B 1964 Biomechanics of spinal bracing.
Arizona Medicine 21: 170–176

Mueller W 1983 The Knee. Form, function and ligament
reconstruction. Springer, New York

Pearce P 1978 Structure in nature as a strategy for design.
MIT Press, Cambridge

Prigogine I, Stengers I 1984 Order out of chaos: man's new
dialogue with nature. Bantam Books, London

Thompson D 1965 On growth and form. Cambridge
University Press, London

Wang N, Butler J P, Ingber D E 1993 Microtransduction
across the cell surface and through the cytoskeleton.
Science 260: 1124–1127

White A A, Panjabi M M 1978 Clinical biomechanics of the
spine. JB Lippincott, Philadelphia

Wildy P, Home R W 1963 Structure of animal virus particles.
Progressive Medical Virology 5: 1–42

Willard F 1995 The lumbosacral connection: the ligamentous
structure of the low back and its relation to back pain. In:
Vleeming A, Mooney V, Dorman T, Snijders C (eds)
Second interdisciplinary world congress on low back pain.
San Diego, CA, 9–11 November, pp 31–58

Wolff J 1892 Das Gesetz der Transformation der Knochen.
Hirschwald, Berlin

Mobility of the sacroiliac joints

11. Movement of the sacroiliac joint: a fresh look

B. Sturesson

INTRODUCTION

To analyse movement in the sacroiliac joints (SIJs), several post mortem studies have been performed since the middle of the nineteenth century, and during the past decade, Miller et al (1987) and Vleeming et al (1992) have demonstrated load displacement behavior on cadavers. Studies on the movements of living subjects were performed by Weisl (1955) with lateral X-rays. He noted a 6 mm displacement between endpoints, but the error of measurement was calculated to be 3 mm. Colachis et al (1963) performed a study with rods in the iliac bones and reported 5 mm of translation but no other results.

Selvik, in 1974, described a roentgen stereophotogrammetric analysis (RSA) by which it was possible to measure movements in all three dimensions. Using this technique, Egund et al (1978) demonstrated a maximal rotation of 2°. In 1983 Grieve used a stereophotogrammetric method analysing movements of skin markers positioned on the posterior superior iliac spines and sacrum. She calculated the difference in millimeters of movement between standing and standing with one leg in flexion, the average movement being estimated to be about 10 mm between the two positions. The error of measurement was not calculated, but it was stated that 'skin is not totally adherent to the underlying structures'.

RECENT STUDIES

Over the past decade, three studies have been performed in vivo, and three different techniques for analysing movements have been used. Sturesson et al (1989) used the RSA technique described by Selvik (1974) and showed a mostly normally distributed range of motion and no differences between symptomatic and asymptomatic joints. These investigations are ongoing and will be discussed below.

Kissling and Jacob (1995) performed a study with Kirschner rods in both ilia and sacrum on healthy volunteers. Measurements were made in standing, and anteflexion and retroflexion of the lumbar spine, and the results are similar to those achieved in Sturesson et al' (1989) RSA analysis.

Surprisingly, Smidt et al (1995) showed, with a stereophotogrammetric analysis of skin markers in the reciprocal straddle position, a movement much greater than any of the other modern studies reviewed; 'The mean composite oblique–sagittal sacroiliac motion which occurred between the right and left straddle position was 9 degrees.' Of course, the greatest error of measurement in this technique is the calculation of the bony landmarks. However, the authors rejected data with a difference of more than 5 mm compared with the neutral standing position. The error of the method is not entirely clear.

ROENTGEN STEREOPHOTOGRAMMETRIC ANALYSIS

Selvik introduced RSA in Lund, Sweden, in 1972, and presented it further in his thesis 'A roentgen stereophotogrammetric method for the study of the kinematics of the skeletal system' (1974). RSA is a computerized system for the exact radiographic localization of landmarks in the human body.

Technique for sacroiliac motion analysis

Tantalum balls with a diameter of 0.8 mm are implanted into the pelvic bones, using an instrument with a cannula and a spring–piston–release mechanism–striker system that presses the ball into place. At least three, but usually between four and six, tantalum balls are placed geometrically well spread out in the 3-dimensional space.

In the X-ray room, two X-ray tubes are needed. Optimal requirements are two ceiling-suspended telescopic units with exposure synchronization. The X-ray films are placed in parallel in a calibration cage with a frame containing the tantalum balls. The relationship between the markers and the foci is established at the X-ray examination. This allows for free movements of the object. In the set-up used, it is possible to make horizontal and vertical exposures, and the object can move freely in front of the X-ray film as long as it is positioned at the cross-over point of the X-ray beams (Fig. 11.1).

The patients were examined in the following positions: (1) supine; (2) prone with hyperextension of the left leg; (3) prone with hyperextension of the right leg; (4) standing; and (5) sitting with straight knees.

Because of physical restrictions, some positions are impossible to examine. For example, one leg superimposed on the pelvis makes it impossible to identify the markers in the object and in the calibration frame on the X-ray films. Because of this, only a few observations concern sitting. The two-dimensional coordinates of the markers in the frame and on the X-ray films are registered on a digitalizing table with the aid of a television camera with a magnification factor of about 20 and a resolution of about 20 µm. The computations are then made with the use of fairly sophisticated mathematics, transforming the two-dimensional image coordinates into three-dimensional laboratory coordinate system (KINLAB, KINERR, X-RAY 90; RSA BioMedical Innovations AB, Umeå, Sweden).

In the study, the sacrum was defined as the fixed segment, and the movements were described as rotation around and translation along the axis, as illustrated in Fig. 11.2. The rotation around

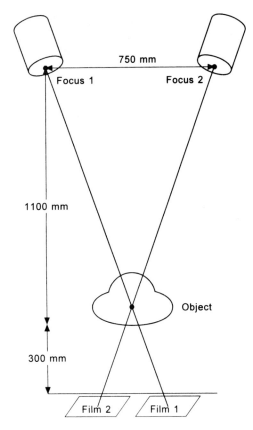

Fig. 11.1   The positions of X-ray tubes (focus 1 and 2), object, and X-ray films for the examination.

the helical axis was also analysed. The mean error for rotation and translation was 0.1–0.2° and 0.1 mm respectively.

Patient population

In the initial study (Sturesson et al 1989), 25 patients were included. The data now include 34 patients: 28 women (19–45 years of age) and 6 men (18–45 years old). The additional patients were included in other studies of the pelvis, but the basic movement analysis is the same. Twenty-one patients had unilateral and 13 bilateral sacroiliac (SI) pain. SI pain was diagnosed when the patients had positive results on two of three tests – the flexion–adduction test, the hyperextension test, and the sacral springing test (Lewit 1984) – and a pain distribution like that seen in posterior pelvic pain (Östgaard et al 1991).

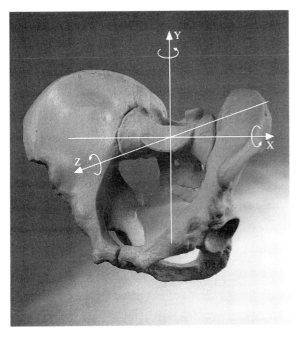

Fig. 11.2 The pelvis with the rotational axes.

Movement analysis

Supine to standing. The sacrum was shown to rotate forwards relative to the ilia (nutation) when standing up from a supine position. As shown in Table 11.1, the rotation was equal on both sides, and the mean rotation was 1.3° around the helical axis. Although the rotation was rather small, more than 90% of the movement occurred around the X-axis. The mean rotation around the sagittal (Z) axis and the rotation around the longitudinal (Y) axis are close to zero. The range

reflects in some cases a widening in the posterior part of the SIJ and in other cases a closing movement (Y-axis). The widening or closing pattern is also seen around the Z-axis but to a lesser degree. These movements around the Y- and Z-axes probably reflect the wide variation in the anatomy of the SIJ (Solonen 1957). The movements around the X-axis and the helical axis did not show statistical differences, so it can be said that the innominates move around the sacrum as a unit, or the sacrum moves symmetrically between the ilia.

Supine to sitting. Compared with the movement pattern from supine to standing, the movement from supine to sitting, both around the helical and the X-axis, shows an increase of about 25%. However, the most interesting observation is a small but constant inward movement of the iliac crests, noted as positive values around the Z-axis for the left side and negative values for the right (Table 11.2).

Standing to prone with hyperextension. The largest movement in the SIJ was found between the 'standing to prone with hyperextension' positions (Tables 11.3 and 11.4). In contrast to the other positions, the movement showed a significant difference between the provoked and the non-provoked side ($p < 0.0001$, paired t-test). Although the mean was close to zero, the range of movement around the Y-axis on the provoked side was also greater compared with that on the non-provoked side. The asymmetry in the SIJ probably enlarges the magnitude of the movement around the Y-axis at the end of the physio-

Table 11.1 Movements of the SIJs when changing from supine to standing position (degrees and mm)

Rotation around the:		n	Mean	Range
X-axis	Left	33	−1.2	−2.3 – 0
	Right	34	−1.2	−2.4 – 0.5
Y-axis	Left	30	0.0	−1.0 – 1.2
	Right	31	0.3	−0.2 – 0.9
Z-axis	Left	30	0.0	−0.4 – 0.5
	Right	31	0.0	−0.4 – 1.0
Helical axis	Left	29	1.3	0.2 – 2.3
	Right	30	1.3	0.5 – 2.5
Translation	Left	24	0.5	0.2 – 1.0
	Right	25	0.4	0.1 – 1.0

Table 11.2 Movements of the SIJs when changing from supine to sitting position with straight legs (degrees and mm)

Rotation around the:		n	Mean	Range
X-axis	Left	11	−1.4	−2.2 – 0.4
	Right	11	−1.4	−2.5 – 0.6
Y-axis	Left	11	0.1	0.6 – 1.1
	Right	11	0.4	−0.4 – 1.1
Z-axis	Left	11	0.5	0.2 – 0.8
	Right	11	−0.3	−0.7 – 0
Helical axis	Left	11	1.5	0.7 – 2.3
	Right	11	1.6	0.8 – 2.6
Translation	Left	11	0.5	0.1 – 1.2
	Right	11	0.5	0.4 – 0.8

Table 11.3 Movements of the SIJs when changing position from standing to prone with the left leg hyperextended (degrees and mm)

Rotation around the:		n	Mean	Range
X-axis	Left	24	2.0	0.8 – 3.3
	Right	25	1.7	0.4 – 3.1
Y-axis	Left	24	−0.2	−1.3 – 2.4
	Right	24	0.0	−0.9 – 1.2
Z-axis	Left	24	−0.1	−0.6 – 0.8
	Right	25	0.0	−0.5 – 0.5
Helical axis	Left	24	2.2	0.9 – 3.9
	Right	24	1.7	0.6 – 3.0
Translation	Left	16	0.7	0.3 – 1.6
	Right	17	0.5	0.2 – 1.2

Table 11.4 Movements of the SIJs when changing position from standing to prone with the right leg hyperextended (degrees and mm)

Rotation around the:		n	Mean	Range
X-axis	Left	23	1.6	0.6 – 3.1
	Right	24	2.1	0.8 – 3.6
Y-axis	Left	23	−0.5	−1.8 – 0.1
	Right	24	−0.2	−1.1 – 2.0
Z-axis	Left	23	0.0	−0.4 – 0.8
	Right	24	0.2	−0.4 – 0.8
Helical axis	Left	23	1.7	0.7 – 3.2
	Right	24	2.2	1.3 – 3.8
Translation	Left	16	0.6	0.3 – 1.6
	Right	18	0.7	0.3 – 1.6

Table 11.5 Movements of the SIJs around the X-axis and helical axis when changing from supine to standing position, split by gender (degrees)

Rotation around the:		n	Mean	Range
X-axis	Male	12	−0.7	−0.1 – 1.2
	Female	55	−1.3	0.0 – 2.4
Helical axis	Male	10	0.7	0.2 – 1.3
	Female	52	1.4	0.6 – 2.5

Table 11.6 Movements of the SIJs around the X-axis and helical axis when changing from supine to standing position in patient with unilateral respectively bilateral symptoms (degrees)

Rotation around the:		n	Mean	Range
X-axis	Unilateral	41	−1.0	0 – 2.0
	Bilateral	26	−1.4	−0.6 – 2.4
Helical axis	Unilateral	35	1.2	0.2 – 2.2
	Bilateral	26	1.5	0.7 – 2.5

symptoms. In 'supine to standing', the mean rotation was 1.4° around the X-axis and 1.5° around the helical axis in the group with bilateral symptoms, and 1.1° and 1.2° respectively in the group with unilateral symptoms (X-axis, $p = 0.0045$; helical axis, $p = 0.0238$; unpaired t-test) (Table 11.6).

Among the patients with unilateral symptoms, the mean mobility around both the X- and helical axis of the symptomatic joints was equal to the mobility of the asymptomatic joints. The standard deviations were about the same for symptomatic and asymptomatic joints.

logic movement, although the force is directed around the X-axis.

Men versus women. The mean mobility of the SIJs for men was about 40% smaller than the movement registered for women in moving from supine to standing (X-axis, $p = 0.0002$; helical axis, $p < 0.0001$; unpaired t-test) (Table 11.5). Between the positions 'standing' and 'prone with hyperextension' the mean difference between men and women was about 30%.

Age. With age, there was no decrease in total mobility. In fact, there was a statistically significant increase with age from supine to sitting, ($r = 0.7$, $n = 11$, $p < 0.05$) and standing to prone with hyperextension ($r = 0.6$ $n = 15$, $p < 0.01$, regression analysis).

Hypermobility. Interestingly, the movements in patients with bilateral symptoms ($n = 13$) were larger than those in the group with unilateral

DISCUSSION

The first implantation of tantalum markers in patients occurred in 1973. In 1990 it was calculated that 2000 patients had been investigated using about 20 000 tantalum balls. To date, about 40 000 tantalum balls have been implanted in 4000 patients, mostly in Sweden but also in the Netherlands and USA.

RSA has taken the role as the gold standard in determining mobility in orthopedic research concerning growth, small movements in joints and tendons, and micromotion of arthroplasties. The error of the method is so small that hardly any other technique can compete in terms of precision.

As all methods, it has its drawbacks; for example, the procedure is time-consuming. Furthermore, there is a need for technical skill in all the different steps, and for the support of an engineer with knowledge of kinematic analysis. Because of the radiation dose, RSA cannot be used on volunteers. The dose-equivalent of radiation in patients examined with 8–10 double exposures on the pelvic bones has been shown to vary between 2.3 and 7.2 mSv (Sturesson et al 1989). This is equal to the radiation dose of an ordinary plain X-ray of the lower back and pelvis.

As far as the SIJ is concerned, the identical movements of symptomatic and asymptomatic joints show that RSA cannot identify an SIJ dysfunction. However, we have shown that there are probably small differences in mobility between patients with unilateral and bilateral symptoms (Table 11.6). It might be that patients with unilateral symptoms and those with bilateral symptoms reflect groups with a different etiology. Good evidence is lacking, but it can be postulated that pain in patients with unilateral symptoms is primarily caused by trauma or reactive arthritis. In patients with bilateral symptoms, the cause could be overload, for example after pregnancy, especially among women with relatively larger SIJ mobility. The SIJs are probably comparable to other joints, and hypermobility is likely to involve a subgroup of individuals in the upper range of the normal distribution of mobility.

Kissling and Jacob (1995), using Kirschner wires in both ilia and sacrum, obtained similar results with stereophotogrammetry as were found with RSA. The main advantage of their technique is the lack of radiation. However, the procedures and analysing technique appear to be more complicated for the patient. Furthermore,

the sacral bone is rather thin in the central part and it is difficult to get a good grip for the Kirschner wires. They can be placed in the lateral part of sacrum but there they will be influenced by the large dorsal sacroiliac ligaments, thus affecting the accuracy.

Non-invasive techniques using different type of skin markers probably measure a complex motion, involving also the connective tissue and skin. In themselves, they can not reflect real SIJ motion, but if compared with data obtained with RSA or the Kirschner wire technique, they can be of value in showing, for example, reduced mobility.

CONCLUSIONS

1. RSA is a technique for measuring small SIJ movements with a high accuracy and specificity. The results probably reflect real SIJ movements. Another invasive technique using Kirschner wires shows a similar pattern of movement in the SIJ.
2. The RSA results show the following:
   a. The SIJ movements are very small.
   b. SIJ mobility in men is on average 30–40% less than that in women.
   c. Small differences occur between patients with unilateral and patients with bilateral pain.
   d. No significant differences occur in mobility between symptomatic and asymptomatic joints in patients with unilateral symptoms.
3. For clinical use, no technique measuring mobility can as yet be recommended because none can reveal an SIJ disorder. RSA and other mobility-measuring techniques can be recommended only for further research, for example to study healing after SIJ arthrodesis and the effect of external fixation.

REFERENCES

Colachis S C Jr, Worden R E, Brechtol C O, Strohm B R 1963 Movement of the sacroiliac joint in the adult male: a preliminary report. Archives of Physical Medicine and Rehabilitation 44: 490–498
Egund N, Olsson T H, Schmid H, Selvik G 1978 Movements in the sacroiliac joints demonstrated with roentgen stereophotogrammetry. Acta Radiologica Diagnostica 19: 833–846
Grieve E F M 1983 Mechanical dysfunction of the sacro-iliac joint. International Rehabilitation Medicine 5: 46–52

Kissling R O, Jacob H A C 1995 The mobility of the sacro-iliac joint in healthy subjects. In: Vleeming A, Mooney V, Dorman T, Snijders C J (eds) Second interdisciplinary world congress on low back pain. San Diego, CA, 9–11 November, pp 411–422
Lewit K 1984 Manuelle Medicin im Rahmen der Medizinischen Rehabilitation, 4th edn. Urban & Schwarzenberg, Munich
Miller J A A, Schultz A B, Andersson G B J 1987 Load-displacement behavior of sacro-iliac joints. Journal of Orthopedic Research 5: 92–101
Östgaard H C, Andersson G B J, Karlsson K 1191 Prevalence

of back pain in pregnancy. Spine 16: 548–552

Selvik G 1974 A roentgen stereophotogrammetric method for the study of the kinematics of the skeletal system. AV-centralen, Lund, Sweden. Reprinted 1989 Acta Orthopaedica Scandinavica 60: (supplement) 232

Smidt G L, McQuade K, Wei S-H, Barakatt E 1995 Sacroiliac kinematics for reciprocal straddle positions. Spine 20: 1047–1054

Solonen K 1957 The sacroiliac joint in the light of anatomical, roentgenological and clinical studies. Acta Orthopaedica Scandinavica (supplement 27)

Sturesson B, Selvik G, Udén A 1989 Movements of the sacroiliac joints. A roentgen stereophotogrammetric analysis. Spine 14: 162–165

Vleeming A, Van Wingerden J P, Dijkstra P F, Stoeckart R, Snijders C J, Stijnen T 1992 Mobility in the sacroiliac joints in the elderly: a kinematic and radiological study. Clinical Biomechanics 7: 170–176

Weisl H 1955 The movements of the sacro-iliac joint. Acta Anatomica 23: 80–91

12. The mobility of sacroiliac joints in healthy subjects

R. O. Kissling   H. A. C. Jacob

INTRODUCTION

The sacroiliac joint (SIJ) has very great significance in manipulative medicine, and the phenomenon of 'blocking' has been a concern of this branch of medicine for many years. As suggested by Vleeming et al (1990), disorders can occur in the joint when, in special circumstances, the rough surfaces of the joint, with their peaks and troughs, come to rest in a pathological relationship, with peak lying opposite peak and trough opposite trough.

Since no information was available on the extent of normal motion in the SIJ of healthy individuals, we set off to investigate the movement of these joints in vivo in a collective of 15 males and 9 females within the age group 20–50 years. At the same time, we conducted anatomic studies to explore the local nervous system and to trace the innervation of the joint proper, as well as that of its ligaments, as far as possible. This was found to be necessary in order to correlate hypermobility with the clinical manifestation of SIJ disorders.

A review of the literature on this subject known to us has revealed that the reported extent of motion observed in patients varies from about 15° (Pitkin & Pheasant 1936) to less than 3° (Egund et al 1978, Sturesson et al 1989). These investigations were, however, carried out on patients with SIJ disorders.

Recently, Vleeming et al (1992) have reported on the mobility of the SIJ in the elderly, but as observed in embalmed preparations. Therefore, since no data were available on the motion of the SIJ of healthy men and women, we felt urged to investigate this matter closely.

Also, apart from that of Solonen (1957), no significant work has so far appeared on the innervation of the SIJ. Solonen performed his study on nine cadavers. By macroscopic and dissecting microscopic observation, he found ventral innervation from nerve roots L3–S2 and from the superior gluteal nerve. In one instance, this author found the obturator nerve (L2–4) to be connected with the lumbosacral trunk via two communicating rami. In all cases studied, Solonen (1957) found innervation from S1 and S2 on the dorsal side of the joint, but he attributed less significance to this than to the ventral innervation.

Because of the lack of other studies, we were interested to know whether Solonen's work under the dissecting microscope could be confirmed and whether thick myelinated axons could be detected as evidence of specific, encapsulated proprioceptors.

MOTION STUDIES

Materials and methods

Fifteen men and 9 women between 20 and 50 years of age (mean age 34.0 years) volunteered to take part in this study. With one exception, all were healthy, had no pain affecting the vertebral column or pelvic girdle, did not show any external or static asymmetries, and had no clinical articular restriction in the SIJ. The 3 women between 30 and 40 years of age were mothers. The only exception, deliberately included for investigation, was subject No. 7 (35 years old), a former top-class track athlete who had suffered for many years from symptoms of disorder in the region of both SIJs.

The age distribution (Fig. 12.1) shows 3 female subjects per decade between 20 and 50 years,

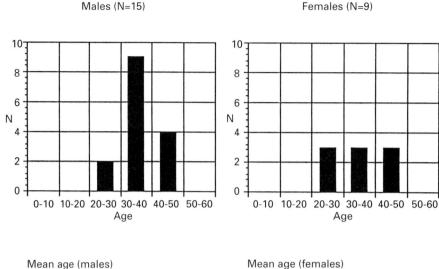

Mean age (males)
20-30 yrs.: 26.0 (2 subjects)
30-40 yrs.: 33.9 (9 subjects)
40-50 yrs.: 44.3 (4 subjects)

Mean age (females)
20-30 yrs.: 23.0 (3 subjects)
30-40 yrs.: 34.0 (3 subjects)
40-50 yrs.: 43.3 (3 subjects)

Fig. 12.1   Distribution of subjects according to age groups.

whereas for the men, subjects in the 30–40 years age group predominate.

Profession showed a predominance of mixed professional occupations, which results from the fact that the male and female subjects were mostly recruited in hospitals (physicians, nurses, and physiotherapists).

In order to observe the relative movement between ilia and sacrum, marker triads were rigidly attached to these bones by means of Kirschner wires (Fig. 12.2). The following were implanted:

- a Kirschner wire, 3 mm in diameter, into each posterior superior iliac spine
- three Kirschner wires, each 1.6 mm in diameter, into the crista sacralis at S2, forming a tripod.

A marker-cross with marker beads of 5 mm diameter was attached by means of clips to each of the 3 mm thick Kirschner wires and to the tripod. The implantations were carried out transcutaneously under local anesthesia.

Shortly after the Kirschner wires were surgically implanted and the marker triads fixed firmly to them, the test subject was asked to stand erect

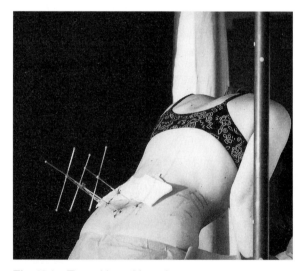

Fig. 12.2   Test subject with markers.

between two stationary, reference poles. Stereophotographs were taken in this position.

Following this initial situation, and as practiced by Egund et al (1978), the subject was requested to adopt the following postures: maximum possible anteflexion; maximum possible retroflexion; one-legged stance, left; and one-legged stance, right.

One-legged stance was performed with flexion in the unloaded hip of about 60°. All subjects received antibiotic prophylaxis with oral cefadroxil 1000 mg on the day of the investigation and 1000 mg the next day. No serious side-effects or complications occurred. An enquiry 3 months after the investigation showed that no symptoms or impairment of function had occurred.

The manner in which the measurements were carried out and the mathematical methods chosen to determine the spatial motion of the iliac marker triads with respect to that fixed to the sacrum have been presented in detail elsewhere (Jacob & Kissling 1995). However, to give the interested reader an understanding of the procedure adopted without turning to the original articles, a brief description will be given.

Two reflex cameras with lenses of 200 mm focal length were used to capture the position of the markers in space. The cameras were mounted on tripods about 5.5 m apart and were simultaneously triggered by a pneumatic actuator by a remotely controlled switch. The spatial coordinates of the cameras were determined by means of a calibration device that specified the origin of the Cartesian coordinate system and the direction of the principal planes (Fig. 12.3). Also in the view of each camera were two stationary vertical poles between which the subject was requested to stand. Each pole had two spots of 5 mm, so placed that all four spots were visible at all times. These four spots, which appeared on every color slide taken, facilitated determination of the picture coordinates (i.e. two-dimensional coordinates) of each marker point on each picture. Subsequently, the two pairs of two-dimensional coordinates were used, together with the known spatial positions of the two cameras, to find the position of each marker point in space.

The triad of marker points (centers of the 5 mm diameter beads) rigidly attached to each bone, being non-colinear in their arrangement, allow a local coordinate system to be attributed to the bone. Thus, it is possible to observe the relative movement of each local system with respect to another.

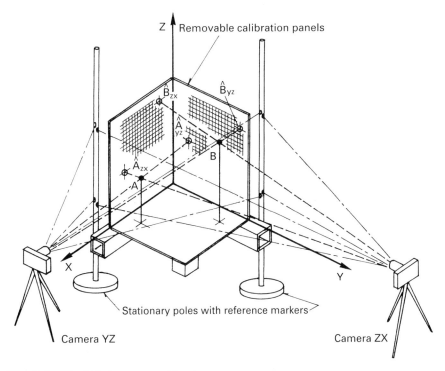

Fig. 12.3 The 3-D photogrammetric set-up.

The general movement can always be described as a combination of rotation and translation. This combination leads to the concept of the helical axis that was probably first described by Panjabi and White (1971) in biomechanics. Having determined the position and direction of the helical axis and the degree of rotation and translation about this axis in one of the local systems, it then becomes necessary to present these data in relation to anatomic landmarks. To do this, the spatial positions of the posterior and superior iliac spines on both sides, as well as the upper margin of the pubic symphysis were determined by palpation using special 'pointers' (Jacob & Kissling 1995).

Results

Table 12.1 shows the average rotation and translation values with the range of variations for the SIJ of the men aged between 20 and 50 years

($n = 14$). Subject No. 7, the only patient with a recurrent SIJ problem, described as 'blockages', will be considered separately (Table 12.2). Table 12.3 shows the average rotation and translation with the range of variation for the SIJ of the women aged between 20 and 50 years ($n = 7$).

Two female subjects (aged 22 and 39 years) had to be excluded from the analysis because their implants moved during measurements.

A large individual variability was found but, taken as a whole, the movement axes were similarly aligned and the overall pattern was comparable. Figure 12.4 is an example of the helical axes of both SIJs represented three-dimensionally. To be able to compare the results between the test subjects and also with those reported in literature, the movement about the helical axis has been expressed by three components of rotation and translation, in the sagittal, frontal, and horizontal planes (Jacob & Kissling 1995). Table 12.4 shows the results in the form

Table 12.1 Average rotation and translation, with range of movements, in the SIJs of males aged 20–50 years ($n = 14$)

	Rotation (°)			Translation (mm)		
	Average	Standard deviation	Range	Average	Standard deviation	Max. value
Anteflexion of the lumbar spine	1.66	0.78	0.4–3.7	1.03	0.84	3.3
Retroflexion of the lumbar spine	1.25	0.59	0.4–2.5	0.60	0.29	1.2
One-legged stance left	1.36	0.69	0.4–3.1	0.59	0.39	1.5
One-legged stance right	1.31	0.73	0.5–3.4	0.65	0.41	1.7

Table 12.2 Average rotation and translation, with range of movements, in the SIJs of females aged 20–50 years ($n = 7$)

	Rotation (°)			Translation (mm)		
	Average	Standard deviation	Range	Average	Standard deviation	Max. value
Anteflexion of the lumbar spine	1.78	1.04	0.5–4.3	0.75	0.54	2.00
Retroflexion of the lumbar spine	1.54	1.00	0.2–3.1	0.73	0.54	1.40
One-legged stance left	1.71	1.12	0.5–3.7	1.56	0.86	3.30
One-legged stance right	1.69	1.39	0.3–5.0	1.11	0.97	3.89

Table 12.3   Rotation and translation of subject No. 7 with hypermobility of his SIJs

	Rotation (°)		Translation (mm)	
	Right SIJ	Left SIJ	Right SIJ	Left SIJ
Anteflexion of the lumbar spine	1.8	1.7	1.36	0.22
Retroflexion of the lumbar spine	6.4	5.6	2.52	0.61
One-legged stance left	8.2	7.7	0.22	0.22
One-legged stance right	8.7	8.7	0.14	0.10

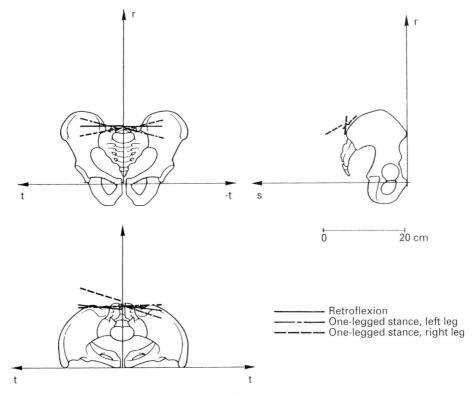

Fig. 12.4   Example of 3-D motion axes. Subject W. Ch., aged 35 years.

of mean values and standard deviations for the collective of the 21 healthy volunteers evaluated.

NEUROANATOMIC STUDIES

Adult SIJ

For macroscopic examination, cadavers fixed with formalin or Tegodor (Goldschmidt Ltd, Zurich, Switzerland) were used. These were intended for dissection courses at the Institute of Anatomy, University of Zurich, Switzerland. Four male and 4 female pelves were sagittally sectioned. Five male and 2 female bodies were used for dissection of the ventral side. The dorsal part of the joint was dissected in 4 specimens (2 male and 2 female). Dissection was performed with the aid of a Zeiss surgical microscope providing up to × 40 magnification.

Table 12.4 Results of analysis of motion (rotation and translation components in the sagittal, frontal, and horizontal planes) for the 21 men and women

Case*	Variable†	Mean	Standard deviation	Minimum	Maximum
1	φ	1.7°	0.86	0.4	4.3
	α	0.83°	0.81	0	3.6
	β	0.59°	0.53	0	1.7
	γ	1.11°	0.78	0.1	3.8
	Tr	0.45 mm	0.51	0	2.0
	Ts	0.40 mm	0.45	0	2.4
	Tt	0.71 mm	0.75	0	3.3
2	φ	1.34°	0.74	0.2	3.1
	α	0.73°	0.60	0	2.3
	β	0.44°	0.46	0	2.0
	γ	0.91°	0.61	0	2.9
	Tr	0.36 mm	0.29	0	1.2
	Ts	0.27 mm	0.31	0	1.4
	Tt	0.45 mm	0.39	0	1.4
3	φ	1.45°	0.88	0.3	5.0
	α	0.77°	0.68	0	3.1
	β	0.50°	0.39	0	1.7
	γ	0.97°	0.82	0.1	4.4
	Tr	0.45 mm	0.56	0	3.3
	Ts	0.34 mm	0.46	0	3.8
	Tt	0.62 mm	0.72	0	4.1

*Case 1, from standing erect on both feet to a maximum of anteflexion; case 2, from standing erect on both feet to a maximum of retroflexion; case 3, from standing erect on both feet to one-legged stance (both SIJs for each foot).

†φ, total rotation; α, rotation about a vertical axis; β, rotation about a horizontal axis lying in the sagittal plane; γ, rotation about a horizontal axis lying in the frontal plane; Tr, absolute translation along a vertical axis; Ts, absolute translation along a horizontal axis in the sagittal plane; Tt, absolute translation along a horizontal axis in the frontal plane.

Histology. To check that all strands classed as nerve fibers during dissection had been correctly identified, all 'nervoid' structures were examined histologically. They were further fixed in 2.5% glutaraldehyde in 0.1 M phosphate buffer (pH 7.4), treated with 1% OsO_4 solution and embedded in Epon. Semi-thin sections of 1–2 μm were stained with toluidine and examined under the light microscope.

Fetal SIJ

A 14- and a 16-week-old fetus were available, having been obtained for examination after therapeutic abortion. The fetal pelves were fixed in 4% phosphate-buffered formalin and decalcified in phosphate-buffered 4% EDTA solution. After cryoprotection in 18% sucrose solution, frozen sections 18–20 μm in thickness were prepared.

A series of sections was obtained for immunocytochemical detection of neurofilaments, and an alternating series was obtained for H&E counterstaining. Nerve fibers were detected immunocytochemically with monoclonal anti-neurofilament antibodies and FITC-labeled secondary antibodies.

Results

Adult SIJ

Dorsal aspect. After emerging from the posterior sacral foramina, the dorsal rami of spinal nerves S1–4 lie in the loose connective tissue that covers the dorsal ligaments of the SIJ. The trunks of the dorsal rami are connected to each other by long anastomoses. Fine branches run to the dorsal ligaments (interosseous sacroiliac [SI] ligaments, and short and long dorsal SI ligaments). Branches from S3 and S4 also run to the sacrotuberous and sacrospinal ligaments. The dorsal rami run further laterally under the superficial and deep layers of the long dorsal SI ligament, pierce the sacral origin of the gluteus maximus muscle, giving off fine branches, and continue further as the nervi clunium medii to the skin.

Ventral aspect. Even with the most careful microscopic dissection, nerve branches from the ventral nerve roots to the SIJ could not be found in any of the preparations. In many cases, it seemed as if branches ran from the sacral plexus to the ventral SIJ ligaments. However, closer inspection always revealed them to be vessels, mostly branches from the internal iliac artery, which passed through the sacral plexus and penetrated into the underlying ligaments.

Histology. Histological examination of the dissected structures confirmed the presence of fine nerve fibers in many cases. Apart from numerous unmyelinated and thin myelinated axons, there were also numerous myelinated fibers with diameters of about 6–8 μm (Grob et al 1995).

Fetal SIJ

In the 16-week-old fetus, which already had a formed joint cleft, we found neurofilament-positive nerve fibers in significant numbers only in the dorsal mesenchyma of the joint bed. Only two questionable neurofilament-positive axons could be made out in the ventral ligament bed, the source of which could not be reliably determined (possibly sacral plexus).

In the 14-week-old fetus, neurofilament-positive fibers were also found only dorsally in the immediate vicinity of the joint cleft.

DISCUSSION

This procedure (with a surgical microscope) and the histological and immunocytochemical examination of eight pelves shows that the innervation of the SIJ and its ligaments is derived exclusively from dorsal branches of the sacral spinal nerves.

On the basis of the findings of this work, it must be assumed that if there is any innervation of the ventral ligaments of the SIJ, this must also derive from dorsal spinal nerve branches that reach the joint from the dorsal side. This basically agrees with the embryogenetic features in that the vertebral joints are also innervated from the dorsal

roots and the sacrum can be phylogenetically and ontogenetically considered as five fused vertebrae.

The ligaments located immediately dorsal to the joint and probably the joint capsule itself are innervated by branches from S1 and S2, whereas especially the sacrotuberous ligament is innervated by S2–4.

All dorsal nerve trunks pass between the layers of the long SI ligament, pierce the origin of the gluteus maximus muscle, and reach the skin as the nervi clunium medii (Fig. 12.5).

The numerous thick myelinated axons in the nerve branches to the SIJ ligaments indicate the presence of special encapsulated mechanoreceptors and nociceptors (Halata & Strasmann 1990).

The small intra-articular alterations in this joint can lead to the transmission of referred pain signals through the dorsal S1 (and S2) branches and the nervi clunium medii to the robust dorsal SI ligaments and especially the origin of the gluteus maximus muscle, which would explain the zones of irritation considered in manipulative therapy for disorders of the SIJ.

It is generally recognized that the normal mobility in the SIJ must be very slight. As mentioned above, direct comparison with the method and the measurements of Egund et al (1978) and Sturesson et al (1989) is not possible. The results they obtained with patients were, however, similar to ours (Table 12.4 above).

No statistically significant differences in mobility for the four measured changes in position could be found. The large interindividual range of variation of the measurements must be pointed out. The tendency to somewhat larger rotation in the female subjects, together with slightly greater translations, might indicate greater movement within the pelvic girdle in women than in men. A reduction in the mobility of the SIJ with age in both sexes could not be confirmed. This is in agreement (up to the upper age limit of the subjects investigated here at least) with the data of Vleeming et al (1990) and Sturesson et al (1989).

The three female subjects aged between 30 and 40 years were all mothers and showed no greater mobility of the SIJ in comparison with those of the two other age categories (who had not given birth) or the values for men.

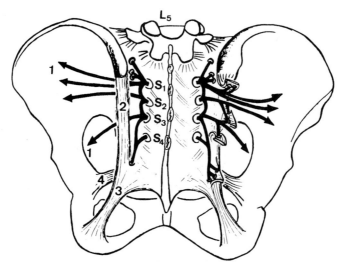

Fig. 12.5 Diagram of the innervation of the human SIJ and its ligaments. Left: View of intact long dorsal SI ligament (2). Right: Superficial layer of the long dorsal SI ligament lifted away, but the thickness of the revealed nerves is not shown to scale. 1, nervi clunium medii; 3, sacrotuberous ligament; 4, sacrospinal ligament.

On the basis of these results, hypomobility, as low as 0.3° of rotation, obviously did not give rise to problems in the group of subjects between 20 and 50 years of age: they never suffered from clinical symptoms of SIJ disorder.

Subject No. 7 on the other hand, the only *patient* investigated, had suffered for years from recurrent, bilateral SIJ hypomobility. The measurements obtained in a symptom-free interval are shown in Table 12.3 above. The values show distinctly greater rotations than in all the other male and female subjects, with the exception of those in anteflexion of the lumbar spine. The translation movement during ante- and retroflexion of the lumbar spine is also greater than the male average, but lower when standing on one leg (either left or right). However, these lower translation values are also associated with the greatest rotation values, with no significant difference between sides. This is therefore probably a case of rotatory hyper- mobility during imitation of walking and move- ment of the trunk. Based on this one case in which SIJ problems were known occasionally to develop, we tentatively hypothesize that hyper- mobility (greater than 6° of rotation) in the

asymptomatic phase might be a characteristic of such patients.

CONCLUSIONS

1. The innervation of the SIJ and its ligaments is derived exclusively from the dorsal branches of the sacral spinal nerves.

2. All dorsal nerve trunks pass between the layers of the sacrotuberal ligament and, after piercing the origin of the gluteus maximus muscle, reach the skin as the nervi clunium medii.

3. In healthy individuals between 20 and 50 years of age with no record of SI disorders, the average total rotational motion in the SIJ between standing erect on both feet and one- legged stance is about 2° (range 0.4–4.3°).

4. No significant differences are observed with regard to sex, age or parturition.

5. Based on one case in which definite prob- lems with the SIJ were occasionally encountered, we tentatively hypothesize that hypermobility (greater than 6% rotation) in the asymptomatic phase might be a characteristic of such patients. The numerous thick myelinated axons in the nerve branches to the SIJ ligaments indicate the

presence of special encapsulated mechanoreceptors and nociceptors, as shown by Halata and Strasmann (1990). This, and the relation of these

nerves to the nervi clunium medii, probably explains the symptoms of muscle pain in such patients.

REFERENCES

Egund N, Olson T H, Schmid H, Selvik G 1978 Movements in the sacroiliac joints demonstrated with roentgen stereophotogrammetry. Acta Radiologica Diagnostica 19(5): 833–846

Grob K R, Neuhuber W L, Kissling R 1995 Die Innervation des Sacroiliacalgelenkes beim Menschen. Zeitschrift für Rheumatologie 54: 117–122

Halata Z, Strasmann T 1990 The ultrastructure of mechanoreceptors in the musculoskeletal system of mammals. In: Zenker W, Neuhuber W L (eds) The primary afferent neuron. Plenum Press, New York, pp 51–65

Jacob H A C, Kissling R O 1995 The mobility of the sacroiliac joints in healthy volunteers between 20 and 50 years of age. Clinical Biomechanics 10(7): 352–361

Panjabi M M, White A A 1971 A mathematical approach for 3-D analysis of the mechanics of the spine. Journal of Biomechanics 4: 203–211

Pitkin H C, Pheasant H C 1936 Sacarthrogenic telalgia. Journal of Bone and Joint Surgery (US) 18: 365–374

Solonen K A 1957 The sacroiliac joint in the light of anatomical roentgenological and clinical studies. Acta Orthopedica Scandinavia (supplement)28: 1–127

Sturesson B, Selvik G A, Udén U 1989 Movements of the sacroiliac joints. Spine 14(2): 162–165

Vleeming A, Volkers A C W, Snijders C J, Stoeckart R 1990 Relation between form and function in the sacroiliac joint. 2: Biomechanical aspects. Spine 15: 133–135

Vleeming A, Van Wingerden J P, Dijkstra P F, Stoeckart R, Snijders C J, Stijnen T 1992 Mobility of the sacroiliac joints in the elderly. Clinical Biomechanics 7: 170–176

13. Interinnominate range of motion

G. L. Smidt

INTRODUCTION

In the erect position, superincumbent body weight is transmitted and controlled onto the sacrum by the wedge-shaped presacral disc, facet joints, and surrounding ligamentous structures and muscles (Schmorl & Junghanns 1971). The weight is further distributed and transmitted to the pelvis via the two crescent-shaped sacroiliac joints (SIJs). With the convexity directed anterior and slightly inferior, the pair of SIJs consists of a small synovial cavity with surrounding ligaments and three sets of accessory ligaments (sacrotuberous, sacrospinous, and iliolumbar). The joint surface is fibrocartilage on the iliac side and hyaline cartilage on the sacral side (Esses & Botsford 1991). Inflammatory (Hollingsworth et al 1983, Weisz & Green 1986), degenerative joint (Firoozmia et al 1984, Weisz & Green 1986), and inflammatory conditions (Hooge & Li 1981, Malarvista et al 1965) represent clinical abnormalities reported at the SIJ.

Although individual SIJs may vary somewhat in their biomechanics, Pitkin & Pheasant (1936) hypothesized that two general types of motion occur between the innominate bones and the sacrum. One type involves the sacrum moving between the two 'fixed' (like-positioned) innominate bones. The sacrum flexes (or anteriorly rotates) when the sacral promontory moves anteriorly and inferiorly. Posterior and superior movement of the sacral promontory occurs with sacral extension (posterior rotation). In pure spinal flexion and extension, the sacrum will flex and extend respectively. The axis of rotation for this type of movement, through the subject of varied opinion, may be in the region of the SIJ (Kapanji 1974, Mitchell et al 1979, Pitkin & Pheasant 1936, Porterfield & DeRosa 1991, Weisl 1955). The other postulated type of intrapelvic movement occurs when the innominate bones move in opposite directions relative to the sacrum (Pitkin & Pheasant 1936). This occurs in most activities except pure spinal flexion and extension.

Several attempts to quantify sacroiliac (SI) motion have been made using a variety of methods in both in vivo and in vitro studies. The majority of these studies report an average translation of about 3 mm and an average angular displacement of less than $4°$ (Egund et al 1978, Miller et al 1987, Reynolds 1980, Shafer 1987, Scholten et al 1989, Sturesson et al 1989). Others have reported average rotation values in the vicinity of $9°$ and as high as $19°$ (Lavignolle et al 1982, Pitkin & Pheasant 1936). If the motion at the SIJs, is negligible or non-existent, it stands to reason that these joints may not be a direct or indirect source of low back or posterior pelvic pain. If, however, considerable motion is available, the opposite seems true. The issues of interinnominate asymmetry (Smidt et al 1995) and joint flexibility exercises (Turoff 1991) would appear especially clinically relevant if a significant SI range of motion is present. Previous studies have reported motion for body position which in the main did not passively stretch the SIJ to the extreme, thus precluding elucidation of the full joint range of motion.

PURPOSE

It is the purpose of this chapter to report on efforts to determine the interinnominate range of motion utilizing several extreme passive body positions.

METHODS

Two studies were performed: (1) men and women (*n* = 32) in a constrained straddle position; and (2) normal young men and women, normals and collegiate gymnasts (*n* = 34) matched for age, sex, and weight. The Metrecom Skeletal Analysis System (Metrecom, Faro Technologies Inc, Lake Mary, FL, USA) was used to determine the coordinates of the anterior and posterior superior spines bilaterally. These coordinates were used to calculate unit vectors from which the measures of interinnominate range of motion were determined. These measures were acquired for two different planes and reported as oblique sagittal and oblique transverse angles. The details of the method can be found elsewhere (Barakatt et al 1996, Smidt et al 1995).

Subjects were placed in extreme static reciprocal hip positions bilaterally. The positions were the straddle position with pelvic belt, unilateral ischial elevation, unilateral leg elevation and the half-kneel stretch. The test–retest accuracy of the measures was 2.2° for the oblique sagittal measures and 1.9° for the oblique transverse. The average intraclass correlations, which reflect good reliability, were 0.88 for the oblique sagittal and 0.95 for the oblique transverse.

RESULTS

The descriptive data for the oblique sagittal range of motion is shown in Fig. 13.1. The least motion was found for the reciprocal straddle positions, so it seems that the posterior pelvic belt

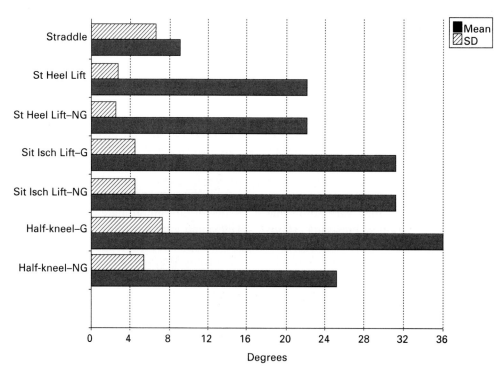

Fig. 13.1 Oblique sagittal interinnominate motion. Straddle = standing maximum reciprocal hip flexion and extension with knees extended. Pelvic belt across sacrum to minimize transverse rotation. St Heel Lift–unilateral heel lift in standing for gymnasts. St Heel Lift–NG = unilateral heel lift in standing for non-gymnasts. Sit Isch Lift–G = unilateral ischial lift in sitting for gymnasts. Sit Isch Lift–NG = unilateral ischial lift in sitting for non-gymnasts. Half-kneel–G = maximal reciprocal hip flexion and extension in the kneeling position for gymnasts. Half-kneel–NG = maximal reciprocal hip flexion and extension in the kneeling position for non-gymnasts.

significantly constrains interinnominate motion. The interinnominate motion for the other positions was greater than 20°, with the gymnasts, at 36°, having the most. The two intervening SIJs must necessarily accommodate this interinnominate motion. So for the reciprocal body positions, each SIJ, if equal in all way biologically and mechanically, would probably accommodate half of the measures for the oblique sagittal measures. For example, in the case of the gymnasts, there would be a range of motion of 18° at each SIJ.

While in the right leg elevated posture, the right ischium elevated posture, and the left half-kneel posture, the right innominate bone was more posteriorly rotated relative to the left when compared with standing in all subjects. Conversely, the right innominate bone was more anteriorly rotated relative to the left when compared with standing while in the left leg elevated, left ischium elevated, and right half-kneel postures in all subjects.

Oblique transverse interinnominate motion was also evident. The maximum average measures of

7° were obtained for the half-kneel and ischial elevated position in the gymnasts (Fig. 13.2). For the majority of the positions, the transverse plane motion was in the direction of external rotation.

If the half-kneel postures were not considered, there was no significant difference between gymnasts and non-gymnasts for the oblique sagittal inter-innominate (OSI) motion. This, combined with the fact that gymnasts have significantly greater stride angles (hip angles formed between the left and right thighs in extreme reciprocal stride position) than do non-gymnasts, suggests that gymnasts have great mobility across the hip joints and possibly the lumbar spine, but not at the SIJ. A significantly greater stride angle in gymnasts may be due to their frequent passive exercise regimens.

The stand to left ischium elevated OSI composite motion was found to be larger than the OSI composite motions of stand to right ischium elevated, stand to left leg elevated, and stand to right leg elevated postures. These results suggest

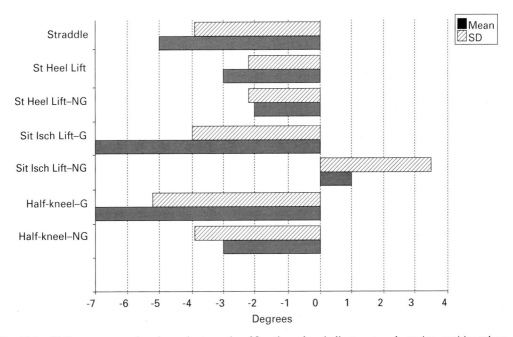

Fig. 13.2 Oblique transverse interinnominate motion. Negative values indicate external rotation, positive values internal rotation. For key see Fig. 13.1.

that standing with one leg on a 4 cm block does not maximize OSI composite motions, whereas sitting with one ischium on a 4 cm block does. If OSI composite motions were not maximized with the reciprocal modified standing posture, symmetrical motion would be observed, since similar forces are placed on each side of the pelvis to elicit the motion.

Symmetry of OSI composite motions of stand to left leg elevated posture combination versus stand to right leg elevated posture combination may give some support to clinicians who evaluate SI movement using the Gillet (kinetic) test. The Gillet test is intended to assess SIJ motion by tracking the posterior superior iliac spine (PSIS) with respect to the second sacral tubercle landmarks during standing hip flexion. The mean OSI composite motion of stand to left leg elevated was −11.2°, and the mean OSI composite motion of stand to right leg elevated was 11.0°. This finding suggests that one may see symmetrical reciprocal OSI composite motions in individuals without low back pain.

DISCUSSION

The two studies in this chapter appear to be the first attempts to use extreme passive hip positions indirectly to elucidate SI range of motion in the form of interinnominate composite motion. Relative to the oblique sagittal interinnominate motion:

1. The magnitude of the SI range of motion was:
    a. large and variable among subjects
    b. diminished with external pelvic constraint
    c. similar for men and women
    d. similar for gymnasts and non-gymnasts, although the largest average range of motion of 36° was found for the gymnasts.
2. A significant SI range of motion was present even for unilateral heel and ischial left positions.
3. For the reciprocal lower extremity positions, the angular displacement direction of the innominates and thighs tended to be in the same direction unilaterally.

Relative to the oblique transverse interinnominate motion, the largest motion (7°) was found for the half-kneel stretch and ischial left positions. Also, the direction of motion for the positions tested was predominately towards external rotation.

The results clearly show that normal young subjects possess a significant amount of inter-innominate range of motion. As such, it seems reasonable to expect that the SIJs can be a primary source of pain. Furthermore, this significant motion has obvious implications for potential strain on all biological structures that traverse the SIJ and structures that are connected to the pelvis and lumbar spine directly or indirectly. The significant resultant sacral motion also obviously impacts on the lumbosacral junction and its superincumbent segments and structures.

Since a significant interinnominate range of motion has now been established in normal subjects, the author suggests that the SIJs be viewed clinically in a generic sense like any other synovial joint. As with other joints, care should be taken to differentiate between passive range of motion, passive motion, active motion, resisted motion, and whether tests or treatments are carried out under loaded or unloaded conditions. Our understanding and hopefully treatment effectiveness should be enhanced by a mindset for the sacro-iliac joints which is akin to other joints of clinical concern.

CONCLUSIONS

1. Placing normal young subjects in extreme reciprocal hip positions has revealed that large amounts of SI motion are present at the SIJs.
2. The majority of this motion seems to occur in an oblique sagittal plane, but some motion is also present in the transverse plane.
3. The SI motion for gymnasts was slightly greater than that for non-gymnasts.

REFERENCES

Barakatt E, Smidt G L, Dawson J D, Wei S H, Heiss D C 1996 Interinnominate motion and symmetry: comparison between gymnasts and non-gymnasts, Journal of Orthopedic and Sports Physical Therapy 23(5): 309–319

Egund N, Olsson T H, Schmid H, Selvik G 1978 Movements in the sacroiliac joints demonstrated with Roentgen stereophotogrammetry. Acta Radiologica 19: 833–846

Esses S I, Botsford D J 1991 Surgical anatomy and operative approaches to the spine. In: Frymoyer J W (ed.) The adult spine. Raven Press, New York, pp 2095–2106

Firoozmia H, Golimbu C, Rafii M, Kricheff I, Marshall C, Beranbaum E R 1984 Computed tomography of sacroiliac joints: comparison with complex-motion tomography. Journal of Computer Assisted Tomography 8: 31–39

Hollingsworth P N, Owen E T, Dawkins R L 1983 Correlation of HLA B27 with radiographic abnormalities of the sacroiliac joints and with other stigmata of ankylosing spondylitis. Clinical Rheumatology 9: 307–322

Hooge W A, Li D 1981 CT of sacro-iliac joints in secondary hyperparathyroidism. Canadian Association Radiology 32: 42–44

Kapanji I 1974 The physiology of the joints, vol. 3, The trunk and the vertebral column, 2nd edn. Churchill Livingstone, Edinburgh

Lavignolle B, Vital J M, Senegas J et al 1982 An approach to the functional anatomy of the sacroiliac joints in vivo. Clinical Anatomy 5: 169–176

Malarvista S E, Seegmiller J E, Hathaway B E, Sokoloff L 1965 Sacroiliac gait. Journal of the American Medical Association 194: 954–956

Miller J A A, Schultz A B, Andersson G B J 1987 Load displacement behaviors of sacroiliac joints. Journal of Orthopedic Research 5: 92–101

Mitchell F Jr, Moran P, Pruzzo N 1979 An evaluation and treatment manual of osteopathic muscle energy procedures, 1st edn. Mitchell, Moran & Pruzzo, Valley Park, MO

Pitkin H, Pheasant H 1936 Sacrothrogenetic telagia. II: a study of sacral mobility. Journal of Bone and Joint Surgery (US) 18(2): 365–374

Porterfield J, De Rosa C 1991 Mechanical low back pain. WB Saunders, Philadelphia

Reynolds H H 1980 Three dimensional kinematics in the pelvic girdle. Journal of the American Osteopathic Association 80: 277–280

Schmorl G, Junghanns H 1971 The human spine in health and disease, 2nd edn. Translated by E F Besermann. Grune & Stratton, New York

Scholten P J M, Schultz A B, Luchico C W, Miller J A A 1989 Motions and loads within the human pelvis: a biomechanical model study. Journal of Orthopedic Research 6: 840–850

Shafer R C (ed.) 1987 The lumbar spine and pelvic clinical biomechanics, 2nd edn. Williams & Wilkins, Baltimore

Smidt G S, McQuade K, Wei S H, Barakatt E 1995 Sacroiliac kinematics for reciprocal stride positions. Spine 20(9): 1047–1054

Sturesson B, Selvik G, Udén A 1989 Movements of the sacroiliac joints: a roentgen stereophotogrammetry analysis. Spine 14: 162–165

Turoff F 1991 Artistic gymnastics: a comprehensive guide to performing and teaching skills for beginners and advanced beginners. William C. Brown, Dubuque, IA

Weisl H 1955 The movements of the sacroiliac joint. Acta Anatomica 23: 80–91

Weisz G M, Green L 1986 Progressive sacro-iliac obliteration in Forestier disease. International Orthopedic 10: 47–51

The lumbopelvic rhythm

14. The combined function of spine, pelvis, and legs when lifting with a straight back

M. A. Adams   P. Dolan

INTRODUCTION

The fact that so many people injure their backs while lifting weights has created a widespread concern to determine the 'best' way to lift. Unfortunately, many biomechanical analyses concentrate on only one aspect of the problem, such as the compressive or shear force acting on the lumbar spine (Potvin et al 1991a, 1991b), the activity of the back muscles (Dolan et al 1994a) or leg muscles (Schipplein et al 1990), or spinal shrinkage (van Dieen et al 1994). Lifting is done by the whole body, and any recommendations on how to lift must not disregard any one part in favor of the others.

So many factors need to be taken into account that the problem of how best to lift appears very complicated. One solution is to construct elaborate mathematical models to cope with all of the complexity and, in effect, to reinvent the technique of lifting. A simpler and more humble approach is to assess the validity of 'common-sense' advice that has stood the test of time. One such piece of advice, which has been in widespread use for a long time, is to 'lift with a straight back', and photographic evidence shows that many experienced weightlifters do exactly this (see, for example, McGill & Norman 1988). In this chapter, we examine the implications of 'keeping a straight back' for all of the major structures involved in lifting, including the lumbar spine, the sacroiliac joints (SIJs) and the back and leg muscles. These structures are all linked by the lumbodorsal fascia, and we examine the evidence that it coordinates the function of the other structures during lifting.

What does a 'straight back' actually mean? Not 'the shape of the back during erect standing' because standing actually *increases* the spine's curves, rather than reduces them (Adams et al 1988). A straight back involves considerable lumbar flexion, and some thoracic extension, in order to flatten the curves naturally present in an unloaded cadaver spine (Adams & Dolan 1991, Dolan et al 1994a, 1994b). As far as the lumbar spine is concerned, it is useful to distinguish between 'straight back' (or 'flat back') postures, which flex (flatten) the lumbar lordosis, and 'lordotic' (or 'erect') postures, which preserve or exaggerate the lumbar lordosis (Fig. 14.1).

Lumbar curvature, as defined in Fig. 14.1, affects the mechanics of lifting in several ways. First, it determines the relative orientation of adjacent lumbar vertebral bodies and thereby affects the distribution of stress acting in the intervertebral discs. Second, it influences the distribution of loading between the discs, the apophyseal (facet) joints, and the ligaments of the neural arch. Third, lumbar curvature affects the action of the back muscles by changing their length and, to a lesser extent, their line of action. Fourth, it alters the tension in the lumbodorsal fascia, thereby affecting all of the structures involved in lifting, including some which are remote from the lumbar spine.

These effects will be considered in more detail below, and the final discussion will then summarize the benefits of 'keeping a straight back' during lifting. First of all, however, we will consider some basic mechanical concepts related to lifting.

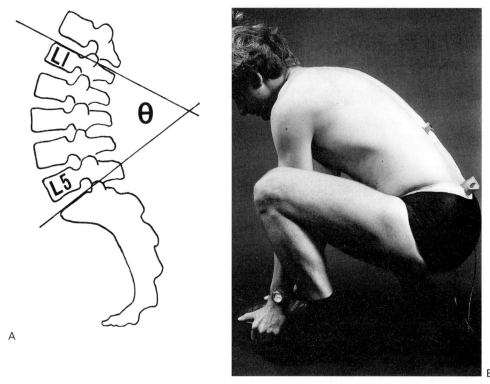

Fig. 14.1   (A) The curvature of a cadaver lumbar spine can be designated by the angle (θ) as defined in the figure. This curvature is increased in 'lordotic' postures such as standing erect, and reduced in 'straight back' (flexed) postures. (B) The lumbar and lower thoracic spine are approximately straight when lifting a weight from the ground.

MECHANICS OF LIFTING

Moment arm analysis

During lifting movements, the upper body pivots about centers of rotation which lie in the nucleus pulposus of each intervertebral disc (Pearcy & Bogduk 1988). Confirmation of this comes from the simple observation that lumbar flexion increases the height of the posterior annulus and decreases the height of the anterior annulus (Adams & Hutton 1982). Tensile forces in structures lying posterior to each pivot must generate an extensor moment (a moment is a force multiplied by a distance), which opposes the flexor moment due to the weight of the upper body and the object being lifted. During a very slow or static lift, when inertial forces can be discounted, the extensor and flexor moments must balance, as shown in Fig. 14.2. During rapid movements, much higher extensor moments may be required

to accelerate the upper body into the upright position (Dolan et al 1994a).

Compressive penalty

The required extensor moment may be generated by tension in many structures, including the posterior annulus fibrosus, the ligaments of the neural arch, the erector spinae muscles, and the lumbodorsal fascia. Since the extensor moment generated by each structure is equal to the tensile force acting in it multiplied by the lever arm between that structure and the center of rotation in the disc, it is apparent that some structures are better placed than others to assist in lifting: those which lie furthest from the pivot can generate a high extensor moment with only a small tensile force. This is advantageous, because these tensile forces all act to pull the vertebrae closer together and thus compress the intervertebral disc. In

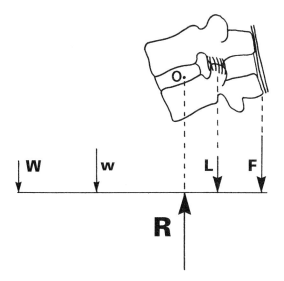

Fig. 14.2   During lifting, the spine pivots about a center of rotation (O) near the middle of each intervertebral disc. The forward bending moment arising from the weight lifted (W) and from upper body weight (w) must be balanced by the extensor moment generated by tensile structures lying posterior to O. Only two of these are shown: the lumbodorsal fascia (F) and the ligaments of the apophyseal joints (L). The ligaments act on a shorter lever arm than the fascia, so must exert a higher compressive 'penalty' on the disc. The lumbar back muscles lie between L and F.

general, the greater the lever arm, the greater the extensor moment for the same compressive 'penalty' on the disc (Fig. 14.2).

Strain energy

Tension in elastic tissues such as ligaments and fascia can reduce the metabolic cost of lifting, because 'strain energy' stored during forward bending can be recovered later when straightening up. The strain energy stored in each tissue is equal to the area under its force–deformation curve, so is approximately proportional to the maximum stretching of the structure multiplied by the maximum tension acting in it.

LUMBAR CURVATURE AND THE DISTRIBUTION OF STRESS WITHIN LUMBAR INTERVERTEBRAL DISCS

The height of intervertebral discs (6–12 mm) is small compared with their anteroposterior diameter

(30–45 mm), so small angulations of adjacent vertebral bodies in the sagittal plane greatly deform the annulus fibrosus in the vertical direction; for example, a flexion angle of 10–12° can stretch the posterior annulus by 50% or more and compress the anterior annulus by approximately 30% (Adams & Hutton 1982). It is not surprising, therefore, that experiments on cadaveric lumbar motion segments have shown that lumbar curvature has a profound effect on stress distributions within the disc. For example, lordotic postures create concentrations of vertical compressive stress within the posterior annulus (Adams et al 1994b, McNally & Adams 1992) (Fig. 14.3), particularly following sustained 'creep' loading (Adams et al 1996), or following damage to an adjacent vertebra (Adams et al 1993). Repetitive loading in a lordotic posture can cause 'hairpin bend' deformations of lamellae within the posterior annulus, leading to posterior bulging of the disc (Adams et al 1988) (Fig. 14.3B). Moderate flexion of lumbar motion segments brings the endplates approximately parallel and equalizes compressive stress across the whole disc (Adams et al 1993, 1994a) (Fig. 14.3A). Flexion right up to the elastic limit of the intervertebral ligaments can generate peaks of compressive stress in the anterior annulus (Adams et al 1994b) and high tensile stresses in the posterior annulus (Adams et al 1994a). Flexion just beyond this limit stretches and thins the posterior annulus to such an extent that the disc can prolapse posteriorly if it is simultaneously subjected to a high compressive force (Adams & Hutton 1982, 1985).

The posterior annulus fibrosus resists anterior bending rather like a ligament would (Adams et al 1994a), but its proximity to the center of rotation means that it generates only a small extensor moment and applies a very high compressive penalty to the rest of the disc. When stretched vertically, the posterior annulus fails at a stress of 9 MPa and a strain of 34% respectively (Green et al 1993). The small resting length of the posterior annulus means that total stretch at failure is less than 3 mm, so there is little potential for energy storage. Even this potential will not normally be realized, because the intervertebral ligaments prevent the posterior annulus from

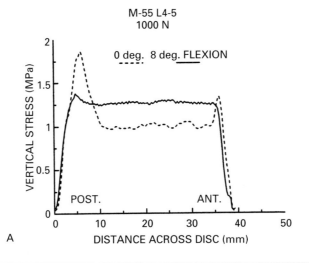

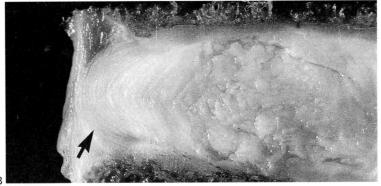

Fig. 14.3 (A) The distribution of vertical compressive stress across the midsagittal diameter of a typical L4–5 intervertebral disc loaded with a compressive force of 1000 N. (male, 55 years old, posterior on left). Lordotic postures ('0 deg.') are characterized by a stress peak in the posterior annulus. Moderate flexion removes this peak but increases slightly the pressure in the nucleus pulposus. (B) A disc of similar age cut through in the midsagittal plane after sustained loading in simulated lordotic posture. (The anterior annulus is missing from this close-up.) Note the bulging of the lamellae in the posterior annulus (arrowed).

being stretched to its elastic limit (Adams et al 1994a). Ligament protection is valuable because the posterior annulus is frequently a source of severe low back pain (Kuslich et al 1991). In any case, the discs are not well suited to store energy because they are avascular and therefore unable to dissipate that proportion of the stored energy which is lost as heat (hysteresis energy). Thermal damage to collagen and to cells may well be a problem in large, poorly vascularized skeletal tissues (Wilson & Goodship 1994).

LUMBAR CURVATURE AND THE DISTRIBUTION OF LOAD BETWEEN DISCS, LIGAMENTS, AND FACETS

Lordotic postures generate high contact stresses in the lower margins of the apophyseal joints and can cause extra-articular impingement of the inferior articular processes on the lamina below, especially following sustained loading (Dunlop et al 1984). This slightly reduces the compressive stresses within the disc, especially in the nucleus

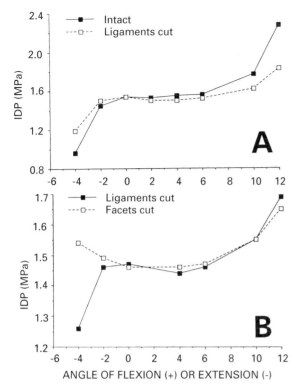

Fig. 14.4 Intradiscal pressure (IDP) measured in a cadaveric motion segment varies with the angle of flexion or extension, even though the applied compressive force is constant (2 kN). (A) Cutting the ligaments of the neural arch reduces IDP in flexion by removing ligament prestress. (B) Removing the bony surfaces of the apophyseal (facet) joints increases IDP in extension because the facets no longer resist part of the compressive force. (Adapted from Adams et al 1994b.)

pulposus (Adams et al 1994b). Only a few degrees of flexion are required to relieve the apophyseal joints of all axial loading (Adams & Hutton 1980). *Full* flexion, however, generates high tensile forces in the ligaments of the neural arch (Adams et al 1980), and ligament tension increases the pressure in the center of the disc. Figure 14.4 shows how redistributions of load between discs, apophyseal joints, and ligaments, arising from changes in lumbar curvature, can result in large variations in intradiscal pressure, even though the compressive force acting on the spine remains constant.

Most intervertebral ligaments act on shorter lever arms than the back muscles, so the maximum extensor moment that they generate when the motion segment is fully flexed (approximately 35 Nm; Adams et al 1980) is associated with a

high compressive penalty on the discs. When a cadaveric 'motion segment' is flexed right up to its elastic limit, the combined tension in all of the intervertebral ligaments ranges from approximately 300 N to 3000 N, depending on specimen size and age (Adams et al 1980). However, the shortness of these ligaments means that they are stretched by only 2–8 mm at the elastic limit (Adams et al 1980), and the protective action of the back muscles ensures that this limit is not normally reached in life (Adams & Hutton 1986a). Therefore, the intervertebral ligaments are not important energy stores during lifting. Their main function may be to protect the disc from excessive bending rather than to assist the back muscles during lifting.

The compressive strength of motion segments positioned in moderate flexion can be particularly high (Hutton & Adams 1982), whereas more substantial flexion, to approximately 75% of the full range allowed by the intervertebral ligaments, causes motion segment strength to be similar to that found in lordosis (Adams et al 1994b). Evidently, the beneficial effect of an even stress *distribution* in the disc in flexion is partially offset by a slight overall increase in *magnitude*. Fully flexed or hyperflexed specimens are probably weaker (Adams & Hutton 1982, Granhed et al 1989) presumably because of the extra forces exerted on the disc by the stretched ligaments (Fig. 14.4A), and because the posterior annulus is stretched and thinned (Adams & Hutton 1982, 1986b).

Evidence in this and the previous section indicates that the lumbar spine is best able to distribute high compressive loading when positioned in the moderately flexed ('flat back') posture. Lordotic postures generate stress concentrations in the posterior annulus and apophyseal joints, whereas full flexion increases the risk of injury to the discs, ligaments, and vertebral bodies.

LUMBAR CURVATURE AND THE ACTION OF THE BACK MUSCLES

Muscles contain collagenous tissues that are capable of resisting externally applied tensile forces. The perimysium, epimysium, and endomysium form a strong 'honeycomb' structure that can transmit high tensile forces from one tendon to another without assistance from the muscle cells (Pursloe 1989). Fibers within these sheets generally run at an oblique angle to the muscle axis, and this angle diminishes when the muscle is stretched (Pursloe 1989). Post mortem rectus abdominis muscle can withstand tensile stresses of approximately 14 N/cm^2 once rigor mortis subsides (Katake 1961), so the average cross-sectional area of the lumbar extensor muscles (40 cm^2; McGill et al 1988) suggests that they, and their tendons, can withstand tensile forces of up to 560 N while remaining electrically inactive. This may be an underestimate, because different muscles have different proportions of collagenous fibers within them, and the back muscles might be expected to have a particularly high collagen content and hence passive strength.

A recent claim that lumbar flexion decreases the lever arms of the back muscles (Tveit et al 1994) may be explained by the erector spinae being squashed when the subjects tried to adopt a flexed posture inside the confines of a magnetic resonance imaging scanner! Certainly, this finding receives little support from a more comprehensive study performed on subjects in more natural postures (Bogduk et al 1992, MacIntosh et al 1993). Flexion reverses the forward shear force that the back muscles normally exert on the L5 vertebra (MacIntosh et al 1993).

The center of the lumbar back extensor muscles lies approximately 5.9 cm posterior to the center of the discs (McGill et al 1988), so the passive tissues within them are better able to generate extensor moments than are the intervertebral ligaments. Muscles of the thoracic spine are better positioned to generate extensor moments (active and passive) because they are connected to the sacrum by a long tendon lying approximately 8.5 cm posterior to the center of the lumbar discs (McGill et al 1988). In full flexion, collagen fiber reorientation allows the back muscles to be stretched by 15–59% (MacIntosh et al 1993). Note, however, that this stretching is measured relative to the upright standing position, in which the lumbar spine is extended (Adams et al 1988) and the muscles correspondingly shortened relative to their resting position. The passive strength of the back muscles and tendons,

combined with their great length and ability to be stretched, means that their energy storage capacity is high.

LUMBAR CURVATURE AND TENSION IN THE LUMBODORSAL FASCIA

The lumbodorsal fascia consists of several broad collagenous sheets, the strongest and most posterior of which overlies the erector spinae muscles (Vleeming et al 1995). Its precise mechanical function is disputed, but its strength is undeniable. Experiments on small tissue samples indicate that the posterior layer alone can resist 335 N in the caudocephalad direction (Tesh et al 1987). This probably underestimates its strength in situ, because the act of cutting out a small sample of tissue disrupts the collagen network and reduces tissue strength; experiments on small samples of annulus fibrosus suggest that they have only 44% of the strength they would have in an intact disc (Adams & Green 1993). In effect, collagen fibers behave like the chopped fibers in fiberglass, in that their ability to reinforce the surrounding matrix is proportional to their length. If these results can be applied to the lumbodorsal fascia, the posterior layer alone could resist a longitudinal force of 760 N. This figure does not include those fibers of the supraspinous ligament which span more than one spinous process. Much of the supraspinous ligament passes from the upper lumbar spine to the sacrum, with only loose attachments to the lower lumbar spinous processes, and it is barely distinguishable from the midline thickening of the lumbodorsal fascia. The 'untethered' portion may explain the apparent difference in strength of the 'supraspinous ligament' in motion segments from the lower and upper lumbar levels. This difference is approximately 450 N in old cadavers (Myklebust et al 1988), suggesting that the untethered portion of the supraspinous ligament may be at least this strong. In young individuals, it may be even stronger. Its mechanical role will be similar to that of the fascia, and their combined strength may exceed 1 kN.

The lumbodorsal fascia can generate large extensor moments with the lowest compressive penalty because it lies approximately 9 cm posterior to the center of the intervertebral discs (Tracy et al 1989). The maximum stretching of the lumbodorsal fascia in full flexion may be approximately 30%, or 15 cm. If the fascia and supraspinous ligament do indeed have a combined strength of over 1 kN, as suggested above, they have the potential to store large amounts of strain energy. The precise relationship between lumbar curvature and tension in the lumbodorsal fascia is considered in the section 'Lumbar curvature during lifting' below.

LUMBAR CURVATURE AND FUNCTION OF THE SIJs

A flat back stretches the lumbodorsal fascia. Tension in the fascia then stabilizes the SIJ by pressing the opposing undulating surfaces closely together and increasing their resistance to shearing movements (Snijders et al 1995). This 'force closure' (Vleeming et al 1995) of the SIJs is treated in detail in other chapters of this book.

LUMBAR CURVATURE DURING LIFTING

The previous sections have described the mechanical benefits of lifting with a flat back. Elite weightlifters evidently take full advantage of these mechanisms because they have been shown by videofluoroscopic analysis to flex their lumbar spine by a moderate amount during extreme lifting (Cholewicki & McGill 1992). It is pertinent now to consider whether or not average people also lift with a straight back in the manner shown by the experts and the subject in Fig. 14.1. This is a confused topic because several authors have claimed that subjects 'maintained a normal lordosis' during lifting, even though accompanying photographs show that this is plainly not the case.

Objective dynamic measurements of lumbar curvature can be made in vivo using small goniometers attached to the skin surface overlying the L1 and S1 spinous processes. Such skin surface measurements can correlate well with the angular movements of the underlying vertebrae (Adams et al 1986), and they show that people have a natural tendency to flex their lumbar spine during daily activities (Dolan et al 1988),

especially when lifting objects from the floor (Adams & Dolan 1991, Dolan et al 1994a, 1994b). Lifting a 10 kg weight with the knees bent normally requires that the lumbar spine be flexed by 80–85% of its in vivo range between erect standing (0%) and full flexion (100%). Even when trained subjects tried their best to lift weights with a full lordosis, they averaged 57% lumbar flexion (Dolan et al 1994b). Lifting 10 kg from the floor with the knees straight usually requires 90–95% of lumbar flexion (Dolan et al 1994a, 1994b).

Comparisons between the ranges of movement observed in cadaveric spines and living people suggest that people do not flex right up to the elastic limit of their osteoligamentous lumbar spine, and that '100% flexion' in vivo means that lumbar motion segments are flexed approximately 70% of the way to their elastic limit (Adams & Dolan 1991). Further comparisons with the bending stiffness properties of lumbar motion segments indicates that '80% flexion' in vivo generates a bending moment on the osteoligamentous lumbar spine of only 8 Nm, which is approximately 14% of that required to cause the slightest detectable damage to a motion segment (Adams & Dolan 1991). For '100% flexion' in vivo, the equivalent bending moment is 21 Nm, which is 35% of that required to cause damage. Fatigue damage may possibly accumulate at 35% of the failure load, so it can be assumed that, for a living person, '80% flexion' is safe and 'moderate', whereas 100% may not be.

The question now is, can flexing the lumbar spine to 80% of its full range in vivo generate substantial antiflexion forces in the passive tissues posterior to the spine? In an attempt to answer this question, we developed a technique for estimating the size of the antiflexion moment generated by passive (i.e. electrically silent) tissues in living people (Dolan et al 1994b). Healthy subjects adopted a stooped posture and pulled up with increasing force on a load cell attached to the ground (Fig. 14.5, upper part). The lever arms shown in Fig. 14.5 were measured, and the total antiflexion (extensor) moment was calculated from the load cell data and from the position of the upper body. Extensor moment was plotted against electromyographic (EMG)

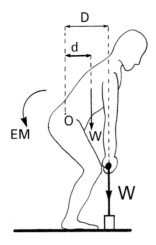

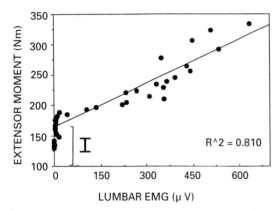

Fig. 14.5 (Upper) Subjects pulled up with increasing force on a load cell attached to the floor. The total extensor moment generated by active and passive tissues (EM) was calculated from the load cell force W, upper body weight w, and the lever arms D and d. (Lower) When extensor moment was plotted against the EMG activity of the back muscles, there was an intercept 'I' which denotes a 'passive' extensor moment unrelated to back muscle activity. (Adapted from Dolan et al 1994b.)

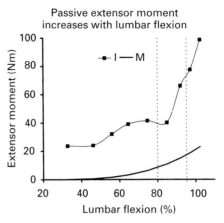

Fig. 14.6 The upper curve shows that the total 'passive' extensor moment *I* increases with lumbar flexion, where 100% flexion refers to the toe-touching posture in life (data from Dolan et al 1994b). During lifting, peak lumbar flexion is usually in the range shown by the dotted lines; in this range, only a small proportion of *I* is attributable to the intervertebral discs and ligaments. This component of *I* is denoted *M*. (Data from Adams & Dolan 1991.)

activity in the erector spinae muscles, recorded using skin surface electrodes at the levels of T10 and L3. The relationship between extensor moment and EMG activity was linear, with an intercept on the extensor moment axis (Fig. 14.5, lower part). This intercept, *I*, was a measure of the total extensor moment produced by the subject when the back muscles first began to contract; it is a direct measure of the extensor moment associated with passive tissues of the trunk. Each subject repeated his or her isometric pulls on the load cell while positioned in varying amounts of

lumbar flexion, and the dependence of *I* on lumbar flexion is shown in Fig. 14.6. *I* rises rapidly to 100 Nm as the limit of lumbar flexion is approached, and does not fall below 20 Nm even when the back is upright. Clearly, at least 20 Nm of *I* is not attributable to stretched tissues posterior to the center of rotation, but the remaining 80 Nm probably is. Note that *I includes* the passive resistance of tissues present in a motion segment; this component is shown separately in Fig. 14.6 as *M*. Figure 14.6 answers the question posed above: lumbar flexion to 80% can indeed generate a considerable extensor moment in passive tissues. Very little of this is attributable to the posterior annulus or intervertebral ligaments, which impose high compressive penalties on the discs, and most of it probably comes from the lumbodorsal fascia.

DISCUSSION

The evidence presented above indicates that the lumbar spine is best able to resist high compressive forces when flexed by approximately 80% of the range between erect standing and full flexion. This is sufficient for the passive tissues posterior to the spine to generate substantial extensor moments. The tissues most involved act far from the center of rotation and thus exert a small compressive penalty on the discs. They are also capable of storing a large amount of strain energy and so reduce the metabolic cost of lifting. Tension in the lumbodorsal fascia also helps to stabilize the SIJ.

The mechanisms by which passive tissues are put under tension are debatable. In a stooped posture, gravity alone will force the upper body forwards into more flexion, but it seems likely that there is more to it than this. The lower part of Fig. 14.5 shows that the passive antiflexion moment can increase during an isometric pull, even though the erector spinae remain electrically silent and the lumbar flexion angle is constant. The activity of muscles remote from our electrodes might be responsible for this. Skin surface electrodes have a large pick-up area, and additional experiments have demonstrated electrical silence in all of the muscles close to the lumbar and thoracic spine in flexed postures (Dolan et al 1994b, Floyd & Silver 1955). This suggests that the 'passive' extensor moment may be generated, or increased, in the lumbar region by remote muscles such as the abdominals and gluteals.

In theory, at least, the sideways pull of the abdominal muscles could generate a longitudinal tension in the lumbodorsal fascia (Gracovetsky et al 1981). This mechanism requires that the junction between muscle and fascia is strong, and recent dissections in our own laboratory (Waldron 1995, unpublished results) have confirmed that this is the case. The latissimus dorsi could also pull strongly on the lumbodorsal fascia, but our recent EMG studies (Dolan et al 1994b) and a mathematical model (McGill & Norman 1988) suggest that they do not, at least during normal lifting movements where the weight does not have to be pulled towards the body. Perhaps the best candidate for the role of tensioning the lumbodorsal fascia is the gluteal muscle group. These powerful muscles extend the hip joint, but gluteus maximus also attaches strongly to the inferior margins of the lumbodorsal fascia and may well be able to tension it when it is already stretched in a flat back posture (Vleeming et al 1995). The abdominal muscles may then serve mainly to prevent lateral contraction of the fascia

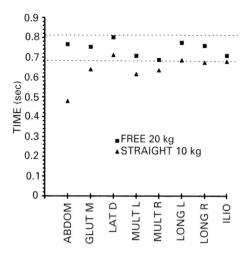

Fig. 14.7 Subjects lifted weights from the ground using either a freestyle ('free') or straight–legged technique, while the EMG signal was recorded from various muscle groups, including the external obliques (ABDOM), gluteus maximus (GLUT M) and latissimus dorsi (LAT D). The Y axis shows the time of the peak EMG signal relative to the time when the weight left the ground, after correction for electromechanical delay (mean values, $n = 15$). Note that the peaks for the first three muscle groups lie within 0.05 s of each other during the freestyle lift. (Waldron et al, 1996, unpublished results.)

and help to stabilize the lumbar spine in the frontal plane (Tesh et al 1987). Preliminary EMG studies in our laboratory support this concept of concerted action by the abdominals, gluteals, and latissimus dorsi to increase or maintain tension in the lumbodorsal fascia during lifting (Fig. 14.7). The degree of synchrony shown in Fig. 14.7 suggests that a stretched lumbodorsal fascia may have a proprioceptive function that allows it to coordinate the activity of the major muscle groups attached to it.

A flat back may have other advantages. It influences the transportation of metabolites to the chondrocytes within the avascular intervertebral discs by increasing the surface area of the posterior annulus and shortening the diffusion path length between the disc periphery and cells in the inner posterior annulus (Adams & Hutton 1986b). This is the region of the disc with the most precarious nutrient supply (Maroudas et al 1975). Flexed postures also increase the fluid exchange within the nucleus pulposus (Adams & Hutton 1983) and thereby increase the movement of large molecular weight solutes to and from the chondrocytes.

The traditional advocacy of lordotic postures appears to be based upon the finding that they reduce intradiscal pressure (Andersson et al 1974). We now know that this occurs because compressive force is transferred onto the posterior annulus and apophyseal joints, which are both innervated, without any compensatory increase in the spine's compressive strength (see above). Lordosis has also been advocated because it helps the back muscles to limit the anterior shear force acting on the lower lumbar vertebrae to 250 N (MacIntosh et al 1993, Potvin et al 1991b). However, the neural arch can resist shear forces of approximately 2 kN (Cyron et al 1976), so this may not be of much consequence. The 'arch' theory of the spine proposes some benefits from a lumbar lordosis (Aspden 1989), but this theory ignores differences in the mechanical properties of different spinal tissues and contains a substantial error (Adams 1989).

Although it appears advantageous to flatten the lumbar spine during lifting, it is undoubtedly important to avoid full flexion or hyperflexion because of the attendant risk of disc prolapse (Adams & Hutton 1982, 1985). Bending the knees and *attempting* to maintain a lordosis results in the lumbar spine being flexed by approximately 60–80% of its full range, which is just about right. Therefore the traditional advice to 'keep your back straight' or even 'preserve the hollow in your back' is probably good advice, even though it does not produce quite the effect that was intended. However, it is necessary to distinguish between what people actually *do* and what they are *trying* to do if the mechanics of lifting are to be understood.

CONCLUSIONS

1. Lifting is best done with the lumbar spine flexed by approximately 80% of its full range between erect standing and touching the toes. The lumbar lordosis is then flattened.

2. This 'flat back' posture evens up the distribution of compressive stress within the intervertebral discs and unloads the apophyseal joints, but does not reduce the spine's compressive strength.

3. A flat back posture maximizes back muscle strength and allows stretched passive tissues posterior to the spine to assist the muscles in two ways: by generating an extensor moment, without a high compressive penalty, and by storing elastic strain energy, thereby reducing the metabolic cost of lifting.

4. Tension in these passive tissues helps to stabilize the SIJ.

5. Muscles such as the gluteals and abdominals are probably able to increase the passive tissue contribution to lifting by pulling on the lumbodorsal fascia, and tension in the lumbodorsal fascia may help to synchronize the action of these large muscle groups during lifting.

REFERENCES

Adams M A 1989 Letter to the Editor. Spine 14: 1272

Adams M A, Dolan P 1991 A technique for quantifying bending moment acting on the lumbar spine in-vivo. Journal of Biomechanics 24: 117–126

Adams M A, Green T P 1993 Tensile properties of the annulus fibrosus. Part I: The contribution of fibre–matrix interactions to tensile stiffness and strength. European Spine Journal 2: 203–208

Adams M A, Hutton W C 1980 The effect of posture on the role of the apophyseal joints in resisting intervertebral compressive force. Journal of Bone and Joint Surgery (UK) 62: 358–362

Adams M A, Hutton W C 1982 Prolapsed intervertebral disc. A hyperflexion injury. Spine 7: 184–191

Adams M A, Hutton W C 1983 The effect of posture on the fluid content of lumbar intervertebral discs. Spine 8: 665–671

Adams M A, Hutton W C 1985 Gradual disc prolapse. Spine 10: 524–531

Adams M A, Hutton W C 1986a Has the lumbar spine a margin of safety in forward bending? Clinical Biomechanics 1: 3–6

Adams M A, Hutton W C 1986b The effect of posture on diffusion into lumbar intervertebral discs. Journal of Anatomy 147: 121–134

Adams M A, Hutton W C, Stott J R R 1980 The resistance to flexion of the lumbar intervertebral joint. Spine 5: 245–253

Adams M A, Dolan P, Marx C, Hutton W C 1986 An electronic inclinometer technique for measuring lumbar curvature. Clinical Biomechanics 1: 30–34

Adams M A, Dolan P, Hutton W C 1988 The lumbar spine in backward bending. Spine 13(9): 1019–1026

Adams M A, McNally D S, Wagstaff J, Goodship A E 1993 Abnormal stress concentrations in lumbar intervertebral discs following damage to the vertebral body: a cause of disc failure. European Spine Society (Acromed) Award paper. European Spine Journal 1: 214–221

Adams M A, Green T P, Dolan P 1994a The strength in anterior bending of lumbar intervertebral discs. Spine 19(19): 2197–2203

Adams M A, McNally D S, Chinn H, Dolan P 1994b Posture and the compressive strength of the lumbar spine. International Society of Biomechanics Award Paper. Clinical Biomechanics 9: 5–14

Adams M A, McMillan D W, Green T P, Dolan P 1996 Sustained loading generates stress concentration in lumbar intervertebral discs. Spine 21: 434–438

Andersson G B J, Ortengren R, Nachemson A, Elfstrom G 1974 Lumbar disc pressure and myoelectric back muscle activity during sitting. Part I: Studies on an experimental chair. Scandinavian Journal of Rehabilitation Medicine 6: 104–114

Aspden R M 1989 The spine as an arch: a new mathematical model. Spine 14: 266–274

Bogduk N, Macintosh J E, Pearcy M J 1992 A universal model of the lumbar back muscles in the upright position. Spine 17(8): 897–913

Cholewicki J, McGill S M 1992 Lumbar posterior ligament involvement during extremely heavy lifts estimated from fluoroscopic measurements. Journal of Biomechanics 25(1): 17–28

Cyron B M, Hutton W C, Troup J D G 1976 Spondylolytic fractures. Journal of Bone and Joint Surgery (UK) 58: 462–466

Dolan P, Adams M A, Hutton W C 1988 Commonly adopted postures and their effect on the lumbar spine. Spine 13: 197–201

Dolan P, Earley M, Adams M A 1994a Bending and compressive stresses acting on the lumbar spine during lifting activities. Journal of Biomechanics 27: 1237–1248

Dolan P, Mannion A F, Adams M A 1994b Passive tissues help the back muscles to generate extensor moments during lifting. Journal of Biomechanics 27: 1077–1085

Dunlop R B, Adams M A, Hutton W C 1984 Disc space narrowing and the lumbar facet joints. Journal of Bone and Joint Surgery (UK) 66: 706–710

Floyd W F, Silver P H S 1955 The function of the erectores spinae muscles in certain movements and postures in man. Journal of Physiology 129: 184–203

Gracovetsky S, Farfan H F, Lamy C 1981 The mechanism of the lumbar spine. Spine 6: 249–262

Granhed H, Jonson R, Hansson T 1989 Mineral content and strength of lumbar vertebrae: a cadaver study. Acta Orthopaedica Scandinavica 60(1): 105–109

Green T P, Adams M A, Dolan P 1993 Tensile properties of the annulus fibrosus. II: Ultimate tensile strength and fatigue life. European Spine Journal 2: 209–214

Hutton W C, Adams M A 1982 Can the lumbar spine be crushed in heavy lifting? Spine 7: 309–313

Katake K 1961 Studies on the strength of human skeletal muscles. J Kyoto Pref Med Univ 69: 463–483

Kuslich S D, Ulstrom C L, Michael C J 1991 The tissue origin of low back pain and sciatica. Orthopaedic Clinics of North America 22(2): 181–187

MacIntosh J E, Bogduk N, Pearcy M J 1993 The effects of

flexion on the geometry and actions of the lumbar erector spinae. Spine 18: 884–893

McGill S M, Norman R W 1988 Potential of lumbodorsal fascia forces to generate back extension moments during squat lifts. Journal of Biomedical Engineering 10: 312–318

McGill S M, Patt N, Norman R W 1988 Measurement of the trunk musculature of active males using CT scan radiography: implications for force and moment generating capacity about the L4/L5 joint. Journal of Biomechanics 21(4): 329–341

McNally D S, Adams M A 1992 Internal intervertebral disc mechanics as revealed by stress profilometry. Spine 17(1): 66–73

Maroudas A, Stockwell R A, Nachemson A, Urban J 1975 Factors involved in the nutrition of the human lumbar intervertebral disc: cellularity and diffusion of glucose in vitro. Journal of Anatomy 120: 113–130

Myklebust J B, Pintar F, Yoganandan N, et al 1988 Tensile strength of spinal ligaments. Spine 13: 526–531

Pearcy M J, Bogduk N 1988 Instantaneous axes of rotation of the lumbar intervertebral joints. Spine 13(9): 1033–1041

Potvin J R, McGill S M, Norman R W 1991a Trunk muscle and lumbar ligament contributions to dynamic lifts with varying degrees of trunk flexion. Spine 16(9): 1099–1108

Potvin J R, Norman R W, McGill S M 1991b Reduction in anterior shear forces on the L4/L5 disc by the lumbar musculature. Clinical Biomechanics 6: 88–96

Pursloe P P 1989 Strain–induced reorientation of an intramuscular connective tissue network: implications for passive muscle elasticity. Journal of Biomechanics 22: 21–31

Schipplein O D, Trajimow J H, Andersson G B J, Andriacchi T P 1990 Relationship between moments at the L5–S1 level, hip and knee joint when lifting. Journal of Biomechanics 23(9): 907–912

Snijders C J, Vleeming A, Stoeckart R, Kleinrensink G J, Mens J M A 1995 Biomechanics of sacroiliac joint stability: validation experiments on the concept of self–locking. In: Vleeming A, Mooney V, Dorman T, Snijders C J (eds) Second interdisciplinary world congress on low back pain. San Diego, CA, 9–11 November, pp 75–92

Tesh K M, Shaw Dunn J, Evans J H 1987 The abdominal muscles and vertebral stability. Spine 12: 501–508

Tracy M F, Gibson M J, Szypryt E P, Rutherford A, Corlett E N 1989 The geometry of the muscles of the lumbar spine determined by magnetic resonance imaging. Spine 14: 186–193

Tveit P, Daggfeldt K, Hetland S, Thorstensson A 1994 Erector spinae lever arm length variations with changes in spinal curvature. Spine 19(2): 199–204

van Dieen J H, Creemers M, Draisma I, Toussaint H M 1994 Repetitive lifting and spinal shrinkage, effects of age and lifting technique. Clinical Biomechanics 9: 367–374

Vleeming A, Pool-Goudzwaard A L, Stoeckart R, van Wingerden J-P, Snijders C J 1995 The posterior layer of the thoracolumbar fascia. Its function in load transfer from spine to legs. Spine 20: 753–758

Wilson A M, Goodship A E 1994 Exercise–induced hyperthermia as a possible mechanism for tendon degeneration. Journal of Biomechanics 27: 899–905

15. The role of the hamstrings in pelvic and spinal function

*J.-P. van Wingerden   A. Vleeming   G.-J. Kleinrensink
R. Stoeckart*

INTRODUCTION

Normal daily functions, such as standing, walking and bending forward, can only be efficiently performed with a stable pelvis. In this respect, extrinsic and intrinsic pelvic stability have to be distinguished. Extrinsic pelvic stability refers to the stability of the pelvis as a whole relative to the legs moving in the hip joints, whereas intrinsic stability refers to the stability of the sacroiliac joints (SIJs) and the public symphysis.

Since the hamstrings attach to the ischial tuberosities, they play an important role in extrinsic pelvic stability. However, the role of the hamstrings with respect to the intrinsic pelvic stability is less obvious. This also holds for the hamstring influence on the coupled motion of the lumbar spine and pelvis during forward bending, the *lumbopelvic rhythm*. In this chapter, the function of the hamstrings with respect to both intrinsic and extrinsic pelvic stability, and their effect on the lumbopelvic rhythm, will be discussed. Of course, questions related to the role of the hamstrings are not merely of academic interest since 'short' hamstrings are often found in low back pain patients (Gajdosik et al 1990, Göeken 1988).

INTRINSIC PELVIS STABILITY

From the perspective of standard anatomical textbooks, the role of the hamstrings in intrinsic pelvic stability is limited. Although the ischial tuberosity is referred to as the site of attachment of both the hamstrings and the sacrotuberous ligament, these structures are viewed as being separate structures. From this viewpoint, the sacrotuberous ligament is mainly seen as a 'passive' structure.

However, in the region of the ischial tuberosity, a distinct difference was found between the lateral and medial parts of the sacrotuberous ligament. The lateral part of the hamstrings, the long head of the biceps femoris, frequently attaches to the sacrotuberous ligament via a firm tendon (Vleeming et al 1989a, 1989b). Force of the biceps femoris can apparently be transferred to the sacrotuberous ligament. In 6 out of 10 dissections, hardly any connection was found between the ischial tuberosity and the combination of the biceps femoris and the lateral part of the sacrotuberous ligament (van Wingerden et al 1993). Here a sliding mechanism, the ischial bursa, was found between the tendon ligament and the ischial tuberosity. In the other preparations, the biceps femoris tendon and lateral part of the sacrotuberous ligament were fixed to the ischial tuberosity. In all preparations, the medial part of the sacrotuberous ligament was connected to the ischial tuberosity as usually described.

In a biomechanical study, it was shown that a distally directed tension applied to the biceps femoris tendon was transferred to the sacrotuberous ligament in *all* preparations. This was surprising but can be explained by the occurrence of superficial fibers passing between the biceps femoris tendon and the sacrotuberous ligament, even in preparations where the biceps femoris tendon is fixed to the tuberosity (van Wingerden et al 1993).

Obviously, force from the biceps femoris muscle can lead to increased tension of the sacrotuberous ligament in various ways. Since increased tension of the sacrotuberous ligament diminishes the range of SIJ motion, the biceps femoris can play a role in stabilization of the SIJ (Vleeming et al 1989).

Because of this relationship, the phenomenon of 'short' hamstrings needs particular attention. Generally speaking, 'short' hamstrings are considered to be a pathologic side-effect of low back pain (Gajdosik et al 1990, 1992, Göeken 1988). However, 'short' hamstrings due to increased hamstring tension in patients with pelvic instability might well be a beneficial compensatory mechanism.

EXTRINSIC PELVIC STABILITY

Coupled motion of pelvis and lumbar spine in seated subjects

Several studies have shown that the movements of the spine and pelvis are coupled (Adams et al 1986, Gajdosik et al 1992, Gracovetsky et al 1990, Sihvonen et al 1991, Stokes & Abery 1980, Toppenberg & Bullock 1986). Cailliet (1968) describes a lumbopelvic rhythm similar to the scapulothoracic rhythm. Recently, Paquet et al (1994) demonstrated differences in the lumbar–pelvic rhythm between low back pain patients and healthy subjects.

Because of the role of the hamstrings in extrinsic pelvic stabilization, it seems obvious that the relatively high hamstring tension often found in low back pain patients affects the lumbopelvic rhythm (Snijders et al 1993, Vleeming et al 1989a, 1989b). However, the relationship between hamstring tension and the coupled motion of the pelvis and lumbar spine is unclear (Mellin 1988). Therefore, the effect of passive hamstring stiffness on lumbar spine and pelvic motion during forward bending was assessed in healthy seated subjects. Increased hamstring stiffness was simulated by extending the knee (from 45° to 15° flexion). This caused a statistically significant increase in the contribution of the lumbar spine to forward bending (van Wingerden et al 1995).

Coupled motion of pelvis and lumbar spine in standing subjects

The effect of passive hamstring stiffness on the lumbopelvic rhythm concerned healthy subjects in a seated posture. Whether this effect also occurred when bending from a standing position had not been demonstrated. We therefore analysed the lumbopelvic rhythm during forward bending from a standing position in both healthy subjects ($n = 46$) and low back pain patients ($n = 31$).

Healthy subjects

In the healthy subjects (13 males and 33 females, average age 21.4 ± 2.4 years), a specific lumbar–pelvic rhythm was found during forward bending from a standing position. Three phases could be distinguished:

1. In the first phase, forward bending is mainly caused by the lumbar spine ($65 \pm 8\%$).
2. The second phase is characterized by a smooth transition.
3. The third phase is characterized by a very limited contribution of the lumbar spine ($28 \pm 12\%$); forward bending mainly occurs in the hip joints.

This observation of a specific relation between pelvic and lumbar motion confirms a recent study of Nelson et al (1995).

Low back pain patients

In chronic low back pain patients (13 males and 18 females, average age 41.7 ± 9.7 years), the lumbopelvic rhythm was significantly different from that of healthy subjects. The patients tend to keep the lumbar spine lordosed ('hollow') during the first phase, which results in a somewhat smaller contribution of the lumbar spine ($55 \pm 16\%$). In the third phase, the contribution of the lumbar spine to flexion of the patients ($37 \pm 16\%$) is larger than that of the healthy subjects.

Because of the age difference, the resulting differences between patients and healthy subjects must be interpreted with caution. Nevertheless, several questions arise, one being whether these findings can be related to the 'short' hamstring phenomenon, as found in low back pain patients (Gajdosik et al 1990, 1992).

In low back pain patients, bending forward is often painful because the load on the spine increases during this motion (see Chapter 14 in this volume). Whether motion takes place in the lumbar spine or in the hip joints (pelvis tilting forward), the motion is painful and must be limited. Increased hamstring tension prevents the pelvis from tilting forward, which diminishes the forward-bent position of the spine, consequently reducing spinal load (see Chapter 14). In this respect, an increase of hamstring tension might well be part of a defensive arthrokinematic reflex mechanism of the body to diminish spinal load. Whatever mechanism causes increase of the hamstring tension, it can be assumed that the capacity of the spine to handle loads will be negatively affected (Adams & Dolan 1995, Dolan et al 1994, Gracovetsky et al 1989, Macintosh et al 1987).

Low back pain patients are known to persist in deviated motion patterns even after the actual lesion has resolved (see Chapter 36 in this volume). In these cases, the spine will not resume its normal capacity (see Chapter 14). In these cases,

training of a 'natural' lumbopelvic rhythm might be an essential part of low back pain therapy.

CONCLUSIONS

1. There is a functional–anatomic connection between the biceps femoris muscle and the sacrotuberous ligament.

2. The biceps femoris, usually classified as a leg muscle, also plays a role in the intrinsic (i.e. stability of the SIJ) and extrinsic stability of the pelvis.

3. When healthy subjects bend forward, a specific coupled motion exists between the pelvis and the lumbar spine: the lumbopelvic rhythm.

4. In low back pain patients, this lumbopelvic rhythm seems to differ from that of the healthy subjects, although the influence of age on the lumbopelvic rhythm has not yet been established.

5. 'Normalizing' the lumbopelvic rhythm might be beneficial in low back pain patients.

REFERENCES

Adams M, Dolan P 1995 Posture and spinal mechanisms during lifting. In: Vleeming A, Mooney V, Dorman T, Snijders C J (eds) Second interdisciplinary world congress on low back pain. San Diego, CA, 9–11 November, pp 19–20

Adams M A, Dolan P, Marx C, Hutton W C 1986 An electronic inclinometer for measuring lumbar curvature. Clinical Biomechanics 1: 130–134

Cailliet R 1968 Low back pain syndrome, 2nd edn. FA Davis, Philadelphia

Dolan P, Mannion A F, Adams M A 1994 Passive tissues help the back muscles to generate extensor moments during lifting. Journal of Biomechanics 27(8): 1077–1085

Gajdosik R L, Giuliani C A, Bohannon R W 1990 Passive compliance and length of the hamstring muscles of healthy men and women. Clinical Biomechanics 5: 23–29

Gajdosik R L, Hatcher C K, Whitsell S 1992 Influence of short hamstring muscles on the pelvis and lumbar spine in standing and during the toe-touch test. Clinical Biomechanics 7: 38–42

Göeken L N H 1988 Straight-leg raising in 'short hamstrings'. Dissertation, RU Groningen, The Netherlands

Gracovetsky S, Kary M, Pitchen I, Levy S, Ben Said R 1989 The importance of pelvic tilt in reducing compressive stress in the spine during flexion–extension exercises. Spine 14: 412–416

Gracovetsky S, Kary M, Levy S, Ben Said R, Pitchen I, Helie J 1990 Analysis of spinal and muscular activity during flexion/extension and free lifts. Spine 15: 1333–1339

Macintosh J E, Bogduk N, Gracovetsky S 1987 The biomechanics of the thoracolumbar fascia. Clinical Biomechanics 2: 78–83

Mellin G 1988 Correlations of hip mobility with degree of back pain and lumbar spinal mobility in chronic low-back pain patients. Spine 13: 668–670

Nelson J M, Walmsley R P, Stevenson J M 1995 Relative lumbar and pelvic motion during loaded spinal flexion/extension. Spine 20(3): 199–204

Paquet N, Malouin F, Richards C L 1994 Hip–spine movement interaction and muscle activation patterns during sagittal movement in low back pain patients. Spine 19(5): 596–603

Sihvonen T, Partanen J, Häninnen O, Soimakallio S 1991 Electric behaviour of low back muscles during lumbar pelvic rhythm in low back pain patients and healthy controls. Archives of Physical Medicine and Rehabilitation 72: 1080–1087

Snijders C J, Vleeming A, Stoeckart R 1993 Transfer of lumbosacral load to iliac bones and legs, parts 1 and 2. Clinical Biomechanics 8: 285–294

Stokes I A, Abery J M 1980 Influence of the hamstring muscles on lumbar spine curvature in sitting. Spine 5(6): 525–528

Toppenberg R, Bullock M 1986 The interrelation of spinal curves, pelvic tilt and muscle length in the adolescent female. Australian Journal of Physiotherapy 32: 6–12

van Wingerden J P, Vleeming A, Snijders C J, Stoeckart R 1993 A functional–anatomical approach to the spine–pelvis mechanism: interaction between the biceps femoris muscle and the sacrotuberous ligament. European Spine Journal 2: 140–144

van Wingerden J P, Vleeming A, Stam H J, Stoeckart R 1995 Interaction of spine and legs: influence of hamstring tension on lumbo-pelvic rhythm. In: Vleeming A, Mooney V, Dorman T, Snijders C J (eds) Second interdisciplinary world congress on low back pain. San Diego, CA, 9–11 November, pp 111–121

Vleeming A, Stoeckart R, Snijders C J 1989a The sacrotuberous ligament: a conceptual approach to its

dynamic role in stabilizing the sacroiliac joint. Clinical Biomechanics 4: 201–203
Vleeming A, van Wingerden J P, Snijders C J, Stoeckart R, Stijnen T 1989b Load application to the sacrotuberous ligament: influences on sacroiliac joint mechanics. Clinical Biomechanics 4: 204–209
Vleeming A, Pool-Goudzwaard A L, Stoeckart R, van Wingerden J P, Snijders C J 1995 The posterior layer of the thoracolumbar fascia: its function in load transfer from spine to legs. Spine 20(7): 753–758

Evolution and gait

16. Evolutionary aspects of the human lumbosacral spine and their bearing on the function of the lumbar intervertebral and sacroiliac joints

C. O. Lovejoy   B. Latimer

INTRODUCTION

Normal spine function is central to an understanding of both its pathological states and their mechanical effects. Our knowledge of that function therefore has an important bearing on clinical practice. This paper approaches the question of modern human lumbar spine and sacroiliac (SI) function from the point of view of comparative anatomy, especially that of higher primates, and an examination of the evolutionary history of our species. It documents relatively recent and dramatic anatomic changes in the human vertebral column and pelvic girdle, which carry implications for normal anatomic function of the lumbar spine and sacroiliac joint (SIJ). Before turning directly to the natural history of these structures, however, it may prove useful first to discuss some relevant aspects of the manner in which human locomotion has been traditionally analysed.

Human gait has been studied intensively for several decades. Most of the data that have been gathered, however, have been obtained from observations of quiet walking on level, even substrata. While such data are valuable for the solution of many clinical problems (for example the design of prostheses), they are nevertheless likely, if relied on principally or exclusively, to give an incomplete understanding of the roles of various elements of our musculoskeletal system during upright locomotion. The earlier species from which we have evolved (and from whom we have inherited our musculoskeletal system; see below) would have used bipedal progression under much more demanding conditions than we do. In as much as the energy levels of limb segments and the stress borne by their joints are much greater during

running than during walking, running has almost certainly served as the primary agency of natural selection. In fact, the avoidance of debilitating injury under such demanding conditions has probably been *the* primary design criterion of our evolving lower limb; yet the chances of suffering such injury during quiet walking on an invariant, level substratum are virtually nil.

We do not wish to imply that the kinematic, electromyographic (EMG), and force platform data that have been gathered for human walking should be ignored. Indeed, they are, without question, a valuable source of information about the manner in which our anatomic structures coordinate during locomotion, and much of what has been learned about walking can generally be extended to running. However, care must be taken in interpreting what constitute primary adaptations to upright locomotion when such an interpretation is solely reliant on data gathered from walking. An obvious case in point is the frequent citation of 'Duchenne's observation' that complete paralysis of the gluteus maximus in no way disturbs relaxed walking (Basmajian & de Luca 1985). The gluteus maximus has long been viewed as a pivotal adaptation to upright locomotion in humans: it almost certainly plays a central role in human walking and/or running (Basmajian & de Luca 1985).

A primary intent of most laboratory studies of human gait has been to establish kinetic and kinematic standards for comparison with the pathological and/or reconstructed gait patterns of patients. Such data are clearly ideal for this particular purpose. At the same time, however, the 'normal' gait of an individual is an acquired rhythmic movement that minimizes energy consumption and muscular effort. That such a minimization of effort should be achieved by each individual is hardly surprising and should not be assumed to imply that the human musculoskeletal frame has been 'optimally designed' by natural selection to achieve an absolute minimization of effort – individuals will naturally acquire those habitual movement patterns which minimize fatigue during walking. Indeed, it is now clear that human bipedality is no more or less energy-costly than most other forms of mammalian locomotion (Alexander 1991, Taylor & Rowntree 1973), and that energy consumption has, in general, not been a particularly important design criterion in mammalian limbs (Taylor et al 1974).

Two approaches can be applied to human locomotion. First, we can analyse our musculoskeletal system with respect to the probable role of each structural change in the emergence of bipedality from a non-bipedal ancestor. This can be called the *adaptive* or *natural selective* method. A second approach is to define kinetic and kinematic standards of quiet normal walking in average healthy individuals, which can then be used as comparative normal standards. This might be called the *clinical* method. It is important to distinguish between these two types of analysis because the questions which each can answer are quite different. As an example, let us suppose that *clinical* normalcy of gait can regularly be achieved by the elimination of motion at some particular joint. Arthrodesis may therefore be fully indicated as an effective solution

to this clinical problem. This should have little or no bearing, however, on our interpretation of the *original adaptive value* of motion at the joint, nor on our attempts to understand its primary functional role in general human locomotion. The modification of a structure that has no apparent negative effects on quiet level walking should not be used to judge the evolutionary significance of the structure. Therefore, the analyses and discussions presented here will be primarily at the adaptive rather than the clinical level of analysis.

COMPARATIVE ANATOMY OF THE HUMAN LUMBOSACRAL SPINE

While the primary role of any terrestrial animal's limb is the production of the substrate–reaction forces necessary for propulsion, the limb's capacity to insulate itself from the high and therefore potentially destructive loads imposed by locomotion is also of vital importance. Indeed, the protection of soft tissue structures in the limb, and especially its non-renewable cartilaginous joint surfaces, is likely to have been a pivotal design criterion for mammalian limbs (Currey 1984).

A common mammal is shown in Fig. 16.1 during active locomotion. The musculoskeletal advantages of quadrupedality are not limited merely to the more favorable distribution of body mass over four as opposed to two limbs. Although ground reaction imposes substantial compressive and bending loads

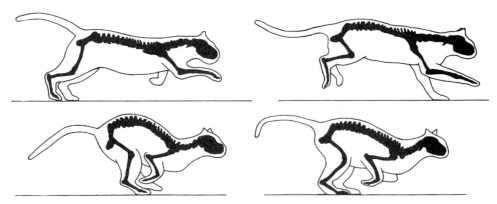

Fig. 16.1 Four positions of the fore- and hindlimbs in the locomotor cycle of the domestic cat. The position of the scapulohumeral joint at forefoot contact permits the triceps and serratus magnus to contract eccentrically, thereby mollifying the effects of forelimb–substratum contact. In bipeds, such energy dissipation must be borne exclusively by the hindlimb, which is normally to near-to-full extension. This makes potential energy-absorbing mechanisms, such as eccentric contraction of the gluteus maximus and the erector spinae, exceptionally important adaptations in humans and their ancestors.

on the animal's forelimb, numerous mechanisms capable of dissipating these loads are available (Biewener 1983).

Eccentric contraction of the triceps muscle during the support phase of gait is an excellent example. It is ideally disposed to mollify the potentially damaging effects of body mass inertia because it has a high cross-sectional area, its contraction can be phased over a significant time period of forefoot contact with the substrate, and its relatively short moment arm requires only a minimal vertical translation of body mass to accomplish this task. Because the forelimb's attachment to the thorax is almost exclusively by muscle, the shoulder joint is also favorably disposed to energy dissipation. The attachment of serratus magnus, for example, is ideally suited to eccentrically resist translation of the vertebral border of the scapula as the latter is thrust across the thoracic wall by the anteroposteriorly oriented humeral head during forelimb–ground contact. In general, the forelimb skeleton of cursorial mammals is an excellent energy absorber.

Old World monkeys (cercopithecoids) are arboreal quadrupedal primates that retain the primary advantages of these important functional features of the forelimb, including posteriorly directed humeral heads and short vertebral scapular borders with prominent serratus magnus muscles (Hartman & Straus 1933). In fact, simultaneous EMG and force platform analysis of their quadrupedal walking indicates that their forelimbs play an even more prominent role than in other mammals. 'The forelimbs of non-human primates work to a relatively greater degree [than other quadrupedal mammals] to steer and brake, while the hindlimbs support and accelerate … This differentiation between the forelimb and the hindlimbs, specifically the greater degree of body support by the hindlimbs, must have been crucial in the pre-adaptation of our ancestors to bipedalism' (Kimura 1985). Old World monkeys also exhibit long flexible lumbar spines (an average of seven vertebrae; Schultz 1968), which play an important role in leaping, running, and arboreal clambering.

Both the forelimbs and hindlimbs of our closest living relatives, the African great apes, have been greatly modified and have not retained these more generalized adaptations of Old World monkeys. The chimpanzee and gorilla are best characterized as terrestrial quadrupeds that have retained unique climbing adaptations as a central part of their feeding strategy (Teleki 1981). While the arboreal activities of gorillas are restricted by their great body mass, chimpanzees are more agile and are regular arboreal feeders (Teleki 1981). Their forelimbs have a number of specialized adaptations that have enhanced mobility and scapulohumeral rhythm during abduction. These include a craniocaudally expanded vertebral scapular border, a more mediolaterally oriented humeral head, an anteroposteriorly compressed thoracic cage, such that the scapular glenoid faces more laterally instead of anteriorly as in Old World monkeys (Ashton & Oxnard 1964, Keith 1923), and an intra-articular meniscus that isolates the ulna from the wrist joint and enhances pronation and supination (Lewis 1974). All of these adaptations are shared with humans.

While the chimpanzee pelvis (Fig. 16.2) retains the general overall form of that of Old World monkeys (and therefore differs dramatically from our own), it also bears unique specializations not seen in monkeys. It exhibits a very narrow sacrum with a craniocaudally elongated auricular surface. Its iliac blades are elongated cranially, and its lumbar column has been reduced to only three or four vertebrae (the ape thoracic column contains 13 vertebrae and ribs). The lower two lumbar vertebrae are completely immobilized by strong ligamentous investment with the cranially elongated iliac blades. In concert, these features have resulted in an unusually rigid lower thorax, with the iliac crest and most inferior rib separated only by a distance equal to an average intercostal space. The rigidity of the chimpanzee lower thorax serves as a base of support for the quadrumanual climbing and clambering of a large-bodied arboreal feeder with four highly mobile limbs (Cartmill & Milton 1977). In addition, such rigidity (as maintained by, *inter alia*, the internal and external obliques, the transversus, and the transversus fascia) may serve to protect their lower back from excessive spinal flexion, extension, and rotation. Chimpanzees are among the most large-bodied of all arboreal mammals (Nowak 1991) and have powerful and massive hindlimbs. They engage in acrobatic

A

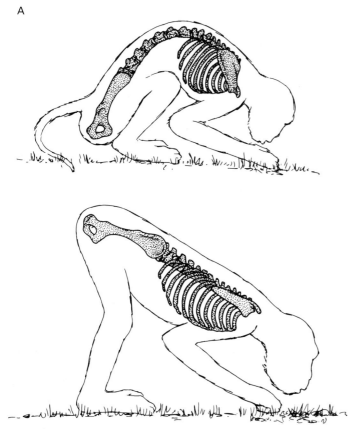

B

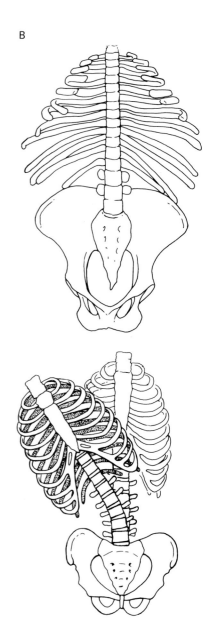

Fig. 16.2   (A.) Lateral views of the spine and pelvis of an adult Old World monkey (top) and chimpanzee (bottom). A flexible lumbar spine is retained in the monkey as part of its locomotor complex, but virtually all flexibility has been eliminated from the lumbar column of the chimpanzee by reduction in lumbar number and a cranial expansion of the iliac blades above the SIJ so as to 'capture' the lower two lumbar vertebrae. This is made specially apparent from the frontal views in (B) of an adult gorilla (top) and human (bottom). Note that lateral as well as anteroposterior flexibility characterizes the human lumbar spine while almost complete rigidity is maintained in the gorilla by its short lumbar column and cranially extended iliac blades.

climbing, leaping, and suspension. Without the strong attachment between their pelvic frame and thorax, their lumbar region could be subjected to extremely high inertial forces, tending to excessively flex, extend, and rotate it. These forces are well contained by the approximation of their iliac crest and thorax, which is in turn accomplished by both a superiorward extension of the iliac blade and a reduction in the number of lumbar vertebrae.

The so-called 'lesser apes', the Gibbons and Siamangs, which are even more acrobatic arborealists, appear to have avoided similar problems by a combination of moderate spinal reduction (an average of five lumbar vertebrae) and a strong limitation on total body mass (less than 13 kg). These differences between the human frame and those of other primates provide an appropriate context within which to discuss the emergence of bipedality.

Some special requirements of human bipedality

Human locomotion imposes tasks upon our hind-limb that are normally performed by both fore-*and* hindlimbs in quadrupedal mammals. From heel strike to foot flat, the net horizontal ground reaction acting on the human lower limb skeleton is posteriorly directed, and during fast walking and running, transarticular forces in the lower limb may approach several multiples of body weight. The human leg must therefore be both an impulse producer and an effective energy absorber.

This task is made very difficult by our ortho-grade posture. At heel strike, the supporting limb is maintained in an almost completely extended condition. Excessive flexion of the knee (which could serve to dissipate some of its kinetic energy by allowing eccentric contraction of the quadriceps) would result in large vertical oscillations of the trunk's center of mass, which would lead to rapid fatigue of the muscle. During quiet walking on a level substratum, however, there *is* sufficient knee flexion (approximately 15°) and eccentric con-traction of the quadriceps to achieve the necessary levels of force dissipation. The knee serves largely as an energy-*absorbing* device during *level walking*, and thus contributes little to propulsion at low speeds (Meglan & Todd 1994).

During active running, changes in direction, or the negotiation of significant grades, however, the energy absorption function of our lower limb is compromised by the requirement that it must remain near full extension. For example, during running and sprinting, a torque is generated about the supporting hip at foot–substratum contact, which tends to rotate the trunk forward. This will occur with each heel strike unless the postero-superiorly directed ground reaction (translated to the hip joint by the lower limb) and the antero-inferiorly directed momentum of the head, arms, and trunk are colinear, which is virtually never the case in normal running. This torque would induce significant trunk flexion at the initiation of each stance phase were it not for the synchronized actions of gluteus maximus and the epaxial mus-culature, especially the erector spinae (see DonTigny 1990, and Greenman 1990, for dis-cussions of the eccentric actions of these muscles

during level walking). Contraction of the gluteus maximus can therefore aid in the dissipation of ground reaction forces acting at the hip, and the epaxial muscles can play a similar role with respect to the lumbar spine. That is, the trunk is not only stabilized and prevented from anteriorward ro-tation, but some of the otherwise potentially de-structive transarticular forces of the lower limb and spine are also dissipated by their eccentric con-traction. Without this energy-absorbing mechanism, active bipedality could result in excessive loads on the lower limb skeleton.

The critical role of the gluteus maximus and epaxial muscles in human evolution can be demon-strated further by comparison of our lumbosacral anatomy with that of the primates reviewed above. While the detailed structure of the gluteus maximus (or gluteus superficialis) differs significantly in apes and Old World monkeys, it remains a relatively small abductor/extensor of the hip in all non-human primates (see the discussion in Robinson 1972). Only in humans has it become the single largest muscle in the body (judged on the basis of cross-sectional area). In humans, it is positioned eccentrically to resist medial rotation of the ipsi-lateral hip imposed by foot–substratum contact. Likewise, only humans possess a posteriorly con-cave lumbar lordosis (which is reduced by the anteroinferiorly directed inertial trunk vector at heel strike). This potential motion allows the erector spinae also to contract eccentrically, and their capacity to do so has been further amplified by a ventral invagination of the entire vertebral column (into the thorax) and a more dorsal positioning of our costal angles. This relocation of the spine has enhanced the potential eccentric capacity of the erector spinae, just as a dorsal extension of the retroauricular mass of the ilium has increased the moment arm and eccentric capacity of the gluteus maximus. These human adaptations are unique among primates.

Of particular interest to the present discussion, therefore, is the SIJ of non-human primates. Two sources of evidence are available which indicate that it is essentially a non-mobile joint in all of the taxa discussed above. First, its surface topo-graphy, which will be reviewed more closely below, is highly reticulated and complex, making relative motion between the sacrum and ilium difficult, given its extensive capsule. Second, the pubic symphysis of many primates is regularly fused, thus obviating any mobility at the SIJ (Lovejoy et al 1996).

Evidence from the recent human fossil record

Chimpanzees and humans are very closely related, and share a common ancestor that dates back only about 6–9 MYBP (million years before present). DNA hybridization indicates nucleotide base pair sequence identity of greater than 98.5% (Kohne et al 1972). Because there is, to date, virtually no fossil record for apes, we have no direct knowledge of the skeletal structure of the last common ancestor of chimpanzees and humans. The locomotor pattern of that ancestor is unknown and controversial, with opinions ranging from one of knuckle-walking (Washburn 1960) to a more generalized arboreal-suspensory (Tuttle 1967) or even quadrupedal pattern (Straus 1949). Although an unresolved and interesting problem, it does not obstruct the heuristic value of an anatomical comparison of the lower limb of apes and humans, and what is known of the emergence of the latter from the fossil record.

It should also be noted that, in addition to the very close genetic similarity with the great apes, the overall anatomic structure that they share with humans also makes it highly probable that humans and chimpanzees evolved from a common ancestor that already possessed most hominoid specializations of the thorax, abdomen, mediastinum, and upper limb (Keith 1923). It is therefore very possible that the human lower limb evolved from one similar to that which characterizes modern anthropoid apes (but see below).

At present, the earliest and best evidence for the emergence of the modern human lower limb skeleton is provided by fossils recovered from the site of Hadar, Ethiopia (Johanson et al 1982). The best known of these fossils is AL-288-1, commonly known as 'Lucy' and assigned to the species *Australopithecus afarensis*. This partial skeleton includes the oldest known (*c.* 3.1 MYBP; Walter & Aronson 1993), hominid pelvis and spine (Johanson et al 1982, Lovejoy 1979). Several presacral vertebrae were preserved along with a complete

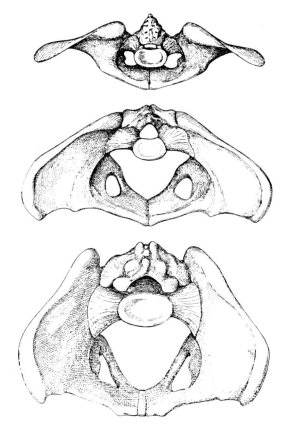

Fig. 16.3 Top views of the pelvis of a chimpanzee (top), AL-288-1 (middle), and modern human female (bottom), with each in the approximate anatomic position for bipedal walking and standing. Note the great expansion of the iliac blades in order to provide a lateral position for the gluteus minimus and gluteus medius during the single support phase of walking in the australopithecine and human. Note the much more cylindrical birth canal in the latter. (After Lovejoy 1988.)

sacrum and left innominate. The innominate had suffered extensive breakage and required considerable restoration (Lovejoy 1979). A right innominate was sculpted by mirror imaging. This provides a complete pelvic girdle of this early hominid (Figs 16.3 and 16.4).

The AL-288-1 pelvis differs dramatically from that of a chimpanzee, the primary adaptations to bipedality already being present. It also differs substantially, however, from that of a modern human pelvis, and these differences have a strong bearing on its evolutionary pattern of emergence from a more quadrupedal type of pelvis (whether like that of the modern chimpanzee or a more generalized form).

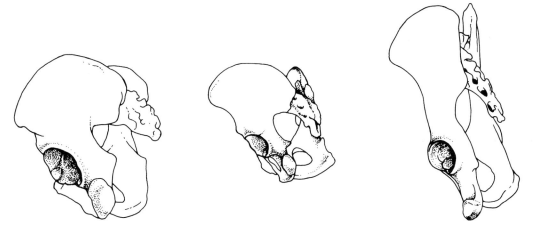

Fig. 16.4   Three-quarter lateral views of an adult human (left), AL-288-1 (middle), and chimpanzee (right), again approximating their anatomic positions during bipedal standing and walking. Note the complete reorganization of the two hominid pelvises and their distinct structural changes from that of the chimpanzee, including a reorientation of acetabular position, reduction and retroflexion of the ischial ramus, broadening of the sacrum, formation of a true greater sciatic notch, and dramatic superoinferior shortening of the entire os coxa, especially the iliac blades.

In superior view (Fig. 16.3), it is obvious that the pelvis of AL-288-1 is remarkably platypelloid, with a Caldwell–Malloy index (i.e. the anteroposterior length of the pelvic midplane divided by its mediolateral breadth) very close to 50, well below anything seen in modern humans. It is probable that this transversely elliptical form was the result of structural limitations imposed on the transformation of a quadrupedal pelvis into one well adapted to bipedality (Tague & Lovejoy 1986). The iliac blades of the chimpanzee lie almost directly in the coronal plane. In order for the gluteus medius and minimus to function adequately as abductors and prevent pelvic tilt during single support phase, their origin must be made to lie substantially closer to the parasaggital plane. However, given the narrowness of the chimpanzee sacrum, a simple rotation of the chimpanzee ilia at their SIJ would have eliminated virtually all of the space of the false pelvis that normally accommodates the viscera (see Tague & Lovejoy 1986). It is clear from the pelvis of AL-288-1 that an anatomic compromise was employed.

First, there was a dramatic increase in the width of the sacrum, a change that accommodated what would otherwise have been a severely compromised false pelvis. In addition, there was a marked anteroposterior expansion in the length of the iliac crest, as well as the introduction of a substantial anteriorly directed bend in the ilium at a point sufficiently lateral to the SIJ to preserve a large abdominal space (Fig. 16.3). These latter changes repositioned the abductors into the parasaggital plane and provided them with a long lever arm with which to control pelvic tilt during single support phase. In combination with sacral widening, modifications in hip musculoskeletal mechanics permitted habitual bipedality while still retaining an ample visceral volume of the false pelvis.

ADAPTATIONS OF THE HUMAN SIJ TO BIPEDALITY

These alterations of the early hominid pelvis placed the anterior gluteals in a position from which to control pelvic tilt during the single support phase of bipedality. These same changes, however, also resulted in a dramatic *increase* in the load arm of body weight during single support. The combination of the corresponding increase in the required contraction of gluteus medius and minimus and the support of all the body mass by only one hind limb imposed substantially higher shear on the supporting SIJ. One simple and direct response has been an enlargement of its surface area. Fig. 16.5 shows the average area of the iliac auricular

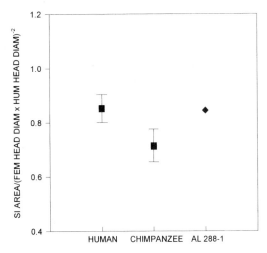

Fig. 16.5   Area of the SIJ divided by the square root of the product of the diameters of the humeral and femoral heads (as general indicators of body size) for 30 humans, 30 chimpanzees, and AL-288-1. The latter lies near the human mean value. Means and standard deviations are indicated.

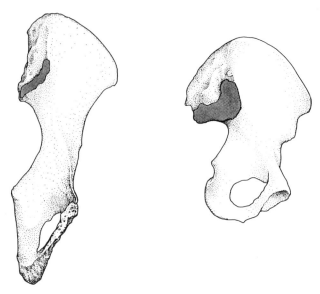

Fig. 16.6   General form of the auricular surface in an adult chimpanzee (left) and human (right). Note the elongated form of the surface in the chimpanzee and its larger and more ovoid and compact condition in the human. In chimpanzees, the surface is often subdivided into two or more separate segments, giving it an archipelago-like appearance. See text for further discussion.

surface relative to the geometric average of humeral and femoral head diameters of chimpanzees and humans (the square root of their product), the latter serving as a simple index of body mass. Both the AL-288-1 and modern human SIJs show distinctive enlargement of surface area.

The SIJ has also undergone a marked change in shape. As can be seen in the comparisons provided in Fig. 16.6, this articulation in hominids has become more compact, in addition to incorporating (as noted earlier) significantly more area. Of particular importance is its obvious change in form. Rather than the elongate, archipelago-like disposition seen in the chimpanzee, the hominid SIJ is a much more concentrated structure. This has had the important effect of permitting moderate sacral nutation and counternutation during locomotion, a phenomenon almost certainly absent in the chimpanzee because of its reticulated SIJ complex.

The craniocaudal elongation of the SIJ in the chimpanzee greatly restricts any significant capsular elongation. Any relative rotation between the ilium and sacrum will cause the fibers at the superior and inferior extremities of its SIJ to reach their elastic limits well before those nearer its midsection have been distended. Because of the greatly reduced craniocaudal height and

more ovoid form of the joint surface in modern humans, the same degree of SI angular displacement during nutation results in a more uniform resistance by a much greater mass of ligamentous tissue (especially those fibers attached along the iliac tuberosity).

If stretching of a periarticular ligamentous environment is viewed at least in part as a potentially important energy dissipation device, the human SIJ is a much more favorably designed structure. This can be demonstrated by using a simple index commonly employed in engineering, which is the ratio between the perimeter of a bearing surface and the square root of its area. Figure 16.7 provides the results of such a comparison for 30 chimpanzees and 30 humans. In short, the human SIJ has much less inherent rigidity than that of a chimpanzee, and its motion is therefore much more favorably disposed to serve as a potential locus of kinetic energy dissipation during sacral nutation. This carries clinical implications: even the retention of slight motion in the SIJ may serve to protect the remainder of the spine from suffering excessive loads.

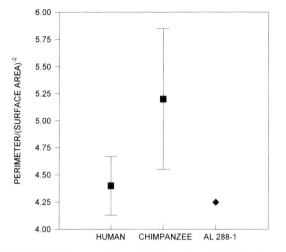

Fig. 16.7 Perimeter of the auricular surface divided by its area for 30 humans, 30 chimpanzees, and AL-288-1. Means and standard deviations are provided.

There are two possible ways to view these changes in the human SIJ. First, the change in shape in the joint (in particular its more ovoid form) may simply be an epiphenomenon of the dramatic superoinferior iliac shortening that occurred in early hominids. Alternatively, it may have resulted from natural selection to enhance mobility in the joint. In addition to allowing the capsule and surrounding musculature eccentrically to dissipate kinetic energy during the single support phase, such mobility is also an important element of parturition in both humans and our bipedal ancestors (Tague & Lovejoy 1986). It is thus not possible to state that mobility of the SIJ is a *direct* adaptation to bipedal progression *per se*; it may be more a consequence of the requirements of parturition, a functional consequence of other evolutionary changes in the pelvis, or a combination of these plus the eccentric protective role that it permits. It does seem clear, however, that whatever its initial cause, it has become an important energy-absorptive link in the human kinematic chain, especially when viewed in light of the concurrent changes that took place in the lumbar spine.

Adaptations of the lumbar spine

One of the most fundamental adaptations of the human frame to bipedality is its lumbar lordosis and the accompanying angulation of the sacrum within the body of the pelvis. In bipedal locomotion, the center of mass of the trunk must consistently lie near a vertical axis through the feet when the trunk is held vertically erect. If the knee and hip joints lie near this axis, only minimal muscular effort is required to maintain their full extension. In order to attain such a favorable position for the hip and knee joints, a lumbar lordosis has emerged which displaces the trunk's center of mass more anteriorly. This lordosis causes the human sacrum to tilt ventrally, which in turn approximates both the SIJ and the hip joint along a vertical axis through the feet in the erect stance, minimizing the necessary magnitudes of any extension moments at these joints. As a consequence, the superior plane of the first sacral vertebra is tilted ventrally and the lumbar column is correspondingly lordosed.

As was pointed out earlier, the lower spine and pelvic ring of anthropoid apes comprise an unusually rigid structure, the paramount feature being a reduction in the number of lumbar vertebrae to an average of four (Schultz 1968). This has the effect of spatially approximating the last (13th) rib to the iliac crest and greatly limiting any lateral mobility of the torso. Furthermore, because of the conformation of the facets and orientation of the ape lumbar spinous processes (see below), the lower spine is essentially incapable of achieving any significant lordosis.

In view of the chimpanzee condition, the extensive bipedal adaptations of the pelvis in AL-288-1 should also have been accompanied by substantial changes in lumbar morphology. One such alteration is directly related to lumbar lordosis and is easily understood in the context of modern humans. When seen in dorsal view (Fig. 16.8), the human lumbar column is unique among extant mammals in showing a progressive increase in the transverse distances between the left and right vertebral articular facets. This results in a caudally directed pyramidal configuration (Latimer & Ward 1993), and differs dramatically from the ape condition, wherein the lumbar facet distances are either parallel or spatially convergent as they approach the sacrum. The human lumbar lordosis can develop only if the lumbar facets have the pyramidal configuration enabling superoinferiorly contiguous

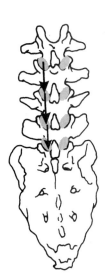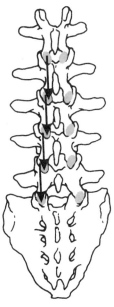

Fig. 16.8 Dorsal view of the lumbar vertebral column and sacrum of a chimpanzee (left) and modern human (right). Note the great breadth of the human sacrum and the progressive increase in mediolateral separation of the articular facets in the human lumbar column. In chimpanzees, these distances often become reduced with increasingly more caudal position of the lumbar vertebrae. The arrows indicate the pathway of potential imbrication. See text for further discussion.

Table 16.1 Interfacet distances of lumbosacral vertebrae of hominoids

Vertebral level	Humans with five lumbars		Humans with six lumbars		Chimpanzees		AL-288-1
	Mean	SD	Mean	SD	Mean	SD	
Six	27.5	3.5	28.4	2.8	20.9	1.8	
Five	26.9	3.0	29.4	2.8	22.8	2.7	
Four	27.4	2.1	31.5	2.4	25.0	2.3	
Three	29.6	2.5	33.0	2.8	27.3	2.6	22.9
Two	32.5	3.9	35.0	2.0	27.0	2.5	
One	37.4	3.5	39.2	2.9	25.9	2.6	
Sacrum	43.8	2.7	41.4	5.1	23.7	2.7	28.9*

*This must be considered a minimum value because of some crushing of the specimen.

facets to imbricate, thereby avoiding direct contact with intervening structures such as the laminae or the pars interarticularis. Inadequate spatial separation between contiguous superior and inferior lumbar facets can result in these structures pinching the intervening laminar region, a pressure that potentially contributes to the developmental sequelae of the uniquely human vertebral condition of spondylolysis (Latimer & Ward 1993).

Although apes and humans show equivalent patterns of interfacet distances in their thoracic columns, they diverge markedly in their lumbar columns (Fig. 16.8; Table 16.1). In the absence of the pyramidal facet configuration, the ape lumbar spine is anatomically incapable of achieving a human-like lordosis. This is further demonstrated in the lack of dorsally directed vertebral wedging and the caudally directed spinous processes of the ape lumbars, both features that further mitigate against their achieving any significant lordosis.

Although the AL-288-1 lumbar spine is represented by only one complete vertebra (probably L3), when this specimen is compared to its associated *sacrum* it is clear that the interfacet distances differ dramatically in a manner comparable to those seen in modern humans. This demonstrates that by roughly 3.1 million years ago, the anatomic adjustments for lumbar lordosis had already taken place, and it is likely that they are ancient, primary adaptations to bipedality.

In addition to AL-288-1, there are now two other early hominid specimens with nearly complete lumbar columns, adding to our ability further to track the early evolution of the human lumbar spine. One of these is from the South African cave site of Sterkfontein (STS 14; Robinson 1972), and the other is from the site of Nariokotome on the west side of Lake Turkana, Kenya (WT 15000; Walker & Leakey 1993). The South African specimen represents the species *Australopithecus africanus* (a probable lineal descendant of *A. afarensis* of *c.* 2.5 MYBP) and the Kenyan specimen, *Homo erectus* (*c.* 1.5 MYBP; Walker & Leakey 1993).

In each of these individuals, the number of lumbar vertebrae is six (Latimer & Ward 1993, Robinson 1972) rather than five. It is therefore probable that the modal number of lumbar vertebrae in our immediate ancestors was six, rather than five, which characterizes over 95% of modern humans (Schultz 1968).

This raises an interesting potential evolutionary paradox, since the modern African apes exhibit a modal condition of only four lumbar and 13 thoracic vertebrae, while the lesser apes (the Gibbons and Siamangs) retain the more primitive mode of five lumbar (and 13 thoracic) vertebrae.

There are thus two possible routes for the emergence of our lumbar column. First, these early bipeds may have experienced a reversal of the evolutionary trend of lumbar reduction and 're-evolved' an elongated lower back from one like that of modern pongids. Modern apes have at least one more segment in their sacra than do humans (as well as one extra thoracic segment) (Schultz 1968), and such reversal of a meristic structure would therefore have not been evolutionarily difficult.

A second possibility is that the common ancestor of the African apes and humans retained the less specialized condition of lower back reduction and exhibited a more mobile back structure, like Gibbons. This is an interesting evolutionary problem, but it involves complex phylogenetic issues which need not concern us further here.

In either of the two scenarios just cited, the modern human condition of five lumbar elements represents a refinement of a simpler and earlier means of achieving lordosis by means of a modal number of six rather than five lumbar elements in our early bipedal ancestors. Based on WT 15000, this transition must have occurred some time after early *H. erectus*. In any case, it is clear that increased lumbar mobility played a prominent role in the emergence of hominid bipedality.

One additional adaptive feature of the modern human lumbar spine can now also be appreciated as a functional correlate of changes related directly to bipedality. At heel strike, there regularly occurs in human walking a spinal rotation and translation, normally resisted by the erector spinae contra-lateral to the limb entering the stance phase (see above). If not controlled, such spinal rotation has a significant potential for injury by causing excessive torsional stresses on the annular fibroses. Their ability to passively resist such rotation has been markedly augmented in modern humans by a substantial increase in the diameters of the vertebral bodies. This increase in diameter has correspondingly increased the magnitude of the resisting torque generated by passive elongation of the fibers of each vertebra's annulus fibrosis. That this is probably the case receives strong support from the progressive distal increase in centrum diameter within the human lumbar spine. Unlike in humans, the dimensions of the lumbar bodies of apes do not change substantially with increasingly more distal position in the column, but, as noted above, their column is deeply invaginated into the space between the upper ilia and is closely approximated by the thirteenth rib. Their columns are thus quite rigid. The progressive enlargement in humans probably represents, therefore, a simple adaptive mechanism that provides the annular fibroses of the lower lumbar vertebrae with a greatly enhanced ability passively to resist the torsional stresses imposed by supporting a large trunk on a lumbar column that lacks the structural rigidity of apes' lumbar columns.

The diameters of the vertebrae in the hominid fossil spines, although relatively larger than those of apes, appear to be slightly smaller, on average, that those of modern humans. Larger inter-vertebral discs and the advantage afforded to their annular fibroses (the polar moment of inertia, J, varies with the fourth power of the radius) may have coincided with the reduction to five lumbar elements as part of a two-step evolutionary process.

The first of these two steps was most probably the change to 12 thoracic and six lumbar vertebrae and a slight-to-moderate expansion in vertebral surface areas. These changes in early hominids were probably related to the mechanical requirements of bipedality, specifically the necessity to enhance spinal mobility and to create a sufficient lordosis to allow locomotion without excessive flexion of the hip and knee during upright walking.

The second phase of vertebral evolution, that of the reduction to five lumbar vertebrae and an enlargement of vertebral areal dimensions, appears to have taken place sometime after 1.5 MYBP. These latter two changes probably occurred together, given that the reduction of one lumbar element would also result in greater relative rotation of the remaining vertebrae and discs (the expansion of the vertebral centrum greatly enhancing the intervertebral disc's ability to resist torsional stresses; see above). In addition, the greater longevity of hominids may also have played a role in the expansion of the spine's areal dimensions because any significant increase in longevity would subject the spine to a greater number of loading cycles.

CONCLUSIONS

1. The comparative anatomy and evolutionary history of the human lumbar spine and pelvis suggest that both have undergone relatively recent major reorganization and alteration of function.

2. Anatomical specializations of the human lumbar spine and SIJ represent critically important adaptations to the kinetic effects of bipedality. Especially important are those changes which permit lumbar lordosis and sacral nutation/counternutation, because each of these appears to be an important mechanism of energy dissipation, especially during very active locomotion. Neither of these movements is permitted by the anatomic structure of our nearest relatives, the great apes. Each therefore is very clearly an important and relatively recent adaptation to upright locomotion.

3. These changes have required modifications of the size and structure of the lumbar vertebrae and SIJ. The interfacet distances of the lumbar vertebrae of hominids progressively increase distally, so as to allow their imbrication during flexion/extension of the lumbar spine. The SIJ has become ovoid and compact so as to allow nutation/counternutation. These anatomic features differ markedly from those in other primates.

4. The evolution of the hominid lumbosacral spine appears to have taken place in two distinct phases. The first of these was the appearance of a long lumbar column (an average of 6 lumbar vertebrae), accompanied by a progressive increase in the interfacet distance of each more distal vertebral arch. These adaptations permitted lumbar lordosis and obviated the need for flexion of the hip and knee during bipedal gait. In the second phase, the lumbar column became somewhat more compact, with the average number of lumbar vertebrae becoming five, rather than six, and with the introduction of a progressive increase in the diameter of each more distal lumbar body, so as to better resist the torsional forces acting on the annular fibroses imposed during active bipedal gait.

REFERENCES

Alexander R M 1991 Characteristics and advantages of human bipedalism. In: Raynor J M V, Wootton R J (eds) Biomechanics in evolution. Cambridge University Press, Cambridge, pp 255–266

Ashton A E, Oxnard C E 1964 Functional adaptations of the primate shoulder girdle. Proceedings of the Zoological Society of London 142: 49–66

Basmajian J V, de Luca C J 1985 Muscles alive: their functions revealed by electromyography, 5th edn. Williams & Wilkins, Baltimore

Biewener A A 1983 Allometry of quadrupedal locomotion: the scaling of duty factor, bone curvature and limb orientation to body size. Journal of Experimental Biology 105: 147–171

Cartmill M, Milton K 1977 The lorisiform wrist joint and the evolution of 'brachiating' adaptations in the Hominoidea. American Journal of Physical Anthropology 47: 249–272

Currey J 1984 The mechanical adaptations of bones. Princeton University Press, Princeton, NJ

DonTigny R L 1990 Anterior dysfunction of the sacroiliac joint as a major factor in the etiology of idiopathic low back pain syndrome. Physical Therapy 70: 44–56

Greenman P E 1990 Clinical aspects of sacroiliac function in walking. Journal of Manual Medicine 6: 354–359

Hartman C G, Straus W L Jr 1933 The anatomy of the Rhesus monkey. Williams & Wilkins, Baltimore

Johanson D C, Lovejoy C O, Kimbel W H et al 1982 Morphology of the Pliocene partial hominid skeleton (A.L. 288–1) from the Hadar Formation, Ethiopia. American Journal of Physical Anthropology 57: 403–452

Keith A 1923 Man's posture: its evolution and disorders. British Medical Journal 1: 451–454, 499–502, 545–548, 587–590

Kimura T 1985 Bipedal and quadrupedal walking of primates: comparative dynamics. In: Kondo S (ed.) Primate morphophysiology, locomotor analyses and human bipedalism. University of Tokyo Press, Tokyo

Kohne D E, Chiscon J A, Hoyer B 1972 Evolution of primate DNA sequences. Journal of Human Evolution 1: 627–644

Latimer B M, Ward C V 1993 The thoracic and lumbar vertebrae. In: Walker A, Leakey R (eds) The Nariokotome *Homo erectus* skeleton. Harvard, Cambridge, MA

Lewis O J 1974 The wrist articulations of the anthropoidea. In: Jenkins F A Jr (ed.) Primate locomotion. Academic Press, New York, pp 143–170

Lovejoy C O 1979 A reconstruction of the pelvis of A.L.-288-1 (Hadar Formation, Ethiopia). American Journal of Physical Anthropology 50: 413

Lovejoy C O 1988 Evolution of human walking. Scientific American 259: 118–125

Lovejoy C O, Meindl R S, Tague R G, Latimer B M 1996 The senescent biology of the hominoid pelvis: its bearing on the pubic symphysis and auricular surface as age-at-death indicators in the human skeleton. Rivisita de Anthropologia 73:

Meglan D, Todd F 1994 Kinetics of human locomotion. In: Rose J, Gamble J G (eds) Human walking, 2nd edn. Williams & Wilkins, Baltimore

Nowak R M 1991 Walker's mammals of the world, vols I and II, 5th edn. Johns Hopkins University Press, Baltimore

Robinson J T 1972 Early hominid posture and locomotion. University of Chicago Press, Chicago

Schultz A H 1968 The recent hominoid primates. In: Washburn S L, Jay P C (eds) Perspectives on human evolution, 1. Holt, Rinehart & Winston, New York, pp 122–195

Straus W L Jr 1949 The riddle of man's ancestry. Quarterly Review of Biology 24: 200–223

Tague R G, Lovejoy C O 1986 The obstetric pelvis of Al-288-1 (Lucy). Journal of Human Evolution 15: 237–255

Taylor C R, Rowntree V J 1973 Running on two or on four legs: which consumes more energy? Science 179: 186–187

Taylor C R, Shkolnik A, Dmi'el R, Baharav D, Borut A 1974 Running in cheetahs, gazelles, and goats: energy cost and limb configuration. American Journal of Physiology 227: 848–850

Teleki G 1981 The omnivorous diet and eclectic feeding habits of chimpanzees in Gombe National Park, Tanzania. In: Harding R S O, Teleki G (eds) Omnivorous primates: gathering and hunting in human evolution. Columbia University Press, New York, pp 303–343

Tuttle R H 1967 Knuckle-walking and the evolution of hominoid hands. American Journal of Physical Anthropology 26: 171–206

Walker A, Leakey R E (eds.) 1993 The Nariokotome *Homo erectus* skeleton. Harvard University Press, Cambridge, MA

Walter R C, Aronson J L 1993 Age and source of the Sidi Hakoma Tuff, Hadar Formation, Ethiopia. Journal of Human Evolution 25: 229–240

Washburn S L 1960 Tools and human evolution. Scientific American 203: 63–75

17. Elasticity in human and animal backs

R. McNeill Alexander

INTRODUCTION

This chapter will show how elastic structures aid our movements. A runner bounces along, using the principle of a bouncing ball. A well-executed jump makes use of the recoil of elastic structures, and elastic structures cushion the impacts of our feet on the ground. We have to consider all the structures involved, but we will focus particularly on the back, asking how much its elasticity can contribute to movement.

RUNNING

Legs and feet

While a foot is on the ground, in walking or running, the force it exerts on the ground remains more or less in line with the legs. Consequently, the body is decelerated and then accelerated – it loses and then regains kinetic energy. If the deceleration depended on muscles functioning as brakes (doing negative work), the kinetic energy involved would be lost as heat and would have to be replaced by (positive) muscular work, at large metabolic cost.

The metabolic cost of locomotion is reduced by two distinct mechanisms (Cavagna et al 1977). In walking, the body's potential energy rises as the kinetic energy falls, and vice versa: energy is conserved by the principle of the pendulum, by moving it back and forth between the kinetic and potential forms. In running, however, the potential energy changes are in phase with the kinetic energy changes and the pendulum principle cannot operate. Instead, energy is saved in running by the principle of the bouncing ball – elastic strain energy rises as kinetic and potential energy

fall, and vice versa – so that energy is again conserved.

Tendons (especially the Achilles tendon) are the most important of the springs that save energy in running (Alexander & Bennet-Clark 1977). Tendon is an excellent elastic material, returning in its elastic recoil 93% of the work done to stretch it (Ker 1981). Its energy-saving role is supplemented by the arch of the foot, which is also a reasonably good spring (Ker et al 1987).

A 70 kg man running at a good marathon speed loses and regains about 100 J of (kinetic plus potential) energy at each footfall. Of this, about 35 J is converted to strain energy in the Achilles tendon and 17 J to strain energy in the arch of the foot (Ker et al 1987). Thus the work required of the muscles is roughly halved. A further saving of 6–8 J may be made by elastic storage in the soles of running shoes (Alexander & Bennett 1989).

The sacroiliac joint

The sacroiliac joint (SIJ) can move only a little, but Dorman (1992) has suggested that its elasticity may be important. We will assess its likely significance in running, using the very limited data that are available.

Miller et al (1987) have investigated the elastic properties of the SIJ. We can use their data to assess the joint's possible role, but first we must estimate the loads that act on it. The peak force on the foot of a 70 kg man, running at marathon speed, is about 1900 N acting vertically (Ker et al 1987). The force transmitted across the SIJ is presumably less, because the weight and inertia of the support leg do not contribute to it; we can estimate it as 1500 N. It can be calculated from the measurements of Miller et al (1987), of SIJ displacement under vertical load, that a 1500 N force would cause a displacement of up to 5 mm, storing no more than 4 J of strain energy. This is small compared with the estimates of 35 J and 17 J for strain energy in the Achilles tendon and the arch of the foot.

Our roughly estimated force of 1500 N can be expected to act through (or at least near) the center of mass of the upper body, roughly 5 cm in front of the SIJs. The moment about a transverse axis through the SIJs can thus be estimated as 75 N m. Excluding one aberrant specimen, Miller et al (1987) found that moments of this size caused a 1–2° rotation of the SIJ, storing (we can calculate) around 1 J of strain energy. This would be a negligible contribution to energy-saving in running. Even the small contributions calculated in this section are over-estimates because we have ignored the effects of the contralateral joint and of the ligaments, which would have further restricted movement.

Our estimates are very rough but seem sufficient to show that the SIJ is not an important energy-saving spring. They might have to be modified if account could be taken of the unknown forces in muscles such as the parts of the longissimus that insert on the pelvis and the oblique abdominal muscles, which cross the SIJ, but it seems most unlikely that this would change the conclusion.

The longissimus aponeurosis

Alexander et al (1985) showed how the aponeurosis of the longissimus muscle (close under the skin of the back) may serve as an energy-saving spring when quadrupedal mammals gallop. At the stage of the stride when the back is most bent, the fore legs have been swinging backwards and are about to swing forwards, and the hind legs have been swinging forwards and are about to swing back; all four legs lose and regain kinetic energy. The suggestion was that much of the energy was stored as strain energy in the aponeurosis, and returned by elastic recoil. Mechanical tests on strips cut from the aponeurosis of deer showed that it had good elastic properties and could function as proposed.

The aponeurosis cannot store useful quantities of strain energy in human running, in which the back is kept fairly straight and longissimus forces seem unlikely to be great.

The vertebral column

When large bending moments act on the back, tension in the longissimus muscle imposes axial compressive loads on the lumbar vertebrae. Alexander et al (1985) performed compressive tests on segments of the vertebral column of deer and showed that approximately equal quantities of strain energy are stored in the intervertebral discs and in the vertebral centra. However, for any given force in the longissimus muscle, only about one-third as much strain energy would be stored in the lumbar vertebral column, as in the aponeurosis.

Because of our vertical posture, the human vertebral column would be loaded in compression during the stance phase of running, even if there were no tension in the longissimus or other trunk muscles. Smeathers & Joanes' (1988) compressive tests enable us to estimate that a 1000 N load on the lumbar spine would compress it by 2 mm and store 1 J of strain energy. This is negligible as a contribution to elastic energy-saving in running. A load of 1000 N, or about half the peak ground force, has been used for this calculation, because about half the body mass is above the lumbar region.

So far we have considered the vertebral column only as a compression spring. Gál (1992) considered it as a flexion spring, measuring the flexural stiffness of the lumbar vertebral column of a tiger and other mammals, and considering its possible energy-saving role in galloping. She showed that the strain energy associated with flexion was too small to be important. The vertebral column does not recoil strongly enough, when bent and released, to make a useful contribution.

We have to conclude that the energy-saving springs that are important for running are in the legs and feet. Structures in the back – the SIJ, the aponeurosis, and the vertebral column itself – can contribute only in a trivial way to this energy-saving role.

JUMPING

A running jump is, essentially, a very big stride, and the principles that have been explained for running apply. This section is about standing jumps, in which we jump from a stationary position.

The most obvious technique of jumping starts from a squatting position, with the knees strongly bent. By forcefully extending the joints of our legs, we throw ourselves into the air. However, athletes prefer to make a countermovement, bending the knees immediately before extending them. Starting from a standing position with the legs straight, the knees are allowed to bend and the trunk falls, losing potential energy and gaining kinetic energy. The fall is halted by the extensor muscles, developing forces that store elastic strain energy in their tendons and in the ligaments of the arch of the foot. Then the muscles shorten and the tendons and ligaments recoil, throwing the body into the air. Thus much of the potential energy lost in the initial countermovement is stored as elastic strain energy and made available to help the jump (see Alexander 1995, where further complications are considered). Tests on volleyball players showed that they could jump on average 6 cm higher with a countermovement, than in a simple squat jump.

The extensor muscles of the back make a useful contribution to jumping: the work done as they contract, straightening the back, is added to the work done by the leg muscles, increasing the kinetic energy with which the body leaves the ground. But calculations like the ones we made for running would show that the elastic properties of the vertebral column and SIJs can contribute relatively little to the recoil that makes a countermovement effective. It is possible that the longissimus aponeurosis may make a significant contribution, but I have no information on its properties in humans. In any case, its contribution cannot be very large, because the part of the potential energy lost in the countermovement that is due to the bending of the back is quite

small. As in running, the important springs are the ones in the legs and feet.

WALKING

Energy economy in walking depends on the principle of the pendulum rather than of the bouncing ball (see above), so energy cannot be saved in the same manner as in running. Alexander (1986) suggested another possibility. It had been observed that African women walking with loads on their heads used remarkably little more energy than when they were not loaded. I suggested that if the back were a sufficiently compliant spring the vertical movements of the load, in the course of each step, might be much less than those of the body's center of gravity. Hence, carrying a load of x% of body mass might add less than x% to the energy cost of walking. I argued that the back was not in fact sufficiently compliant, but the suggestion was in any case misconceived; although the compliance might reduce the potential energy fluctuations of the load, it would increase elastic strain energy fluctuations correspondingly, and the work required of the leg muscles would be unchanged.

FOOT IMPACTS

A different function from the ones described so far is served by the properties of structures that cushion the impact of the foot on the ground: the heel of a running shoe, and the fatty pad under the calcaneus of the foot itself (Aerts et al 1995). Cushioning is needed because the foot is still moving when it hits the ground, so very large forces would act if it were brought to rest instantaneously. Even though cushioning is present, force plate records show substantial vertical force peaks at the impact, commonly 1500–2000 N in the first 20 ms of ground contact in running.

The sole of the foot comes completely to rest in the impact but higher parts of the leg do not. Nevertheless, we can think of an 'effective mass', which, if the whole of it were brought completely to rest, would produce the same force peak. Ker et al (1989) showed how the size of the force peak at impact, and the vertical velocity with which the foot hit the ground (measured from films; about

0.7 m/s), could be used to calculate the effective mass for running. They obtained a value of 3.6 kg, equivalent to a foot amputated a few centimetres below the knee.

This calculation tells us that very little of the impact force can be transmitted to the trunk, so the back cannot be very important in cushioning ground impacts. Nevertheless, a small shock wave is transmitted up the back and can be recorded in the head by means of an accelerometer held between the teeth. Alexander (1988) showed that the speed with which the shock wave travels is consistent with its being propagated up the vertebral column.

In walking (unsurprisingly), impact forces are much smaller.

CONCLUSIONS

1. The energy-saving springs that are important in running are in the legs and feet; structures in the back have only a minor role.

2. The elastic structures utilized in standing jumps are predominantly in the legs and feet, rather than the back.

3. A suggestion that the elastic compliance of the back saves energy, when loads are carried on the head, was misconceived.

4. Foot impacts in running are cushioned predominantly by the heel of the shoe and the fatty pad under the calcaneus.

REFERENCES

Aerts P, Ker R F, De Clerq D, Ilsley D W, Alexander R McN 1995 The mechanical properties of the human heel pad: a paradox resolved. Journal of Biomechanics 28: 1299–1308

Alexander R McN 1986 Making headway in Africa. Nature 319: 623–624

Alexander R McN 1988 Elastic mechanisms in animal movement. Cambridge University Press, Cambridge

Alexander R McN 1995 Leg design and jumping technique for humans, other vertebrates and insects. Philosophical Transactions of the Royal Society B 347: 235–248

Alexander R McN, Bennet-Clark H C 1977 Storage of elastic strain energy in muscle and other tissues. Nature 265: 114–117

Alexander R McN, Bennett M B 1989 How elastic is a running shoe? New Scientist 123(1673): 45–46

Alexander R McN, Dimery N J, Ker R F 1985 Elastic structures in the back and their role in galloping in some mammals. Journal of Zoology (A) 207: 467–482

Cavagna G A, Heglund N C, Taylor C R 1977 Mechanical work in terrestrial locomotion: two basic mechanisms for minimizing energy expenditure. American Journal of Physiology 233: R243–R261

Dorman T 1992 Storage and release of elastic energy in the pelvis: dysfunction, diagnosis and treatment. Journal of Orthopaedic Medicine 14: 54–62

Gál J M 1992 Spinal flexion and locomotor energetics in kangaroo, monkey, and tiger. Canadian Journal of Zoology 70: 2444–2451

Ker R F 1981 Dynamic tensile properties of the plantaris tendon of sheep. Journal of Experimental Biology 93: 283–302

Ker R F, Bennett M B, Bibby S R, Kester R C, Alexander R McN 1987 The spring in the arch of the human foot. Nature 325: 147–149

Ker R F, Bennett M B, Alexander R McN, Kester R C 1989 Foot strike and the properties of the human heel pad. Proceedings of the Institution of Mechanical Engineers 203: 191–196

Miller J A A, Schultz A B, Andersson G B J 1987 Load-displacement behaviour of sacroiliac joints. Journal of Orthopaedic Research 5: 92–101

Smeathers J E, Joanes D N 1988 Dynamic compression properties of human intervertebral joints: a comparison between fresh and thawed specimens. Journal of Biomechanics 21: 425–433

18. Instability of the sacroiliac joint and the consequences for gait

D. Lee

INTRODUCTION

Instability occurs when the functional integrity of a system that provides stability is lost. In the pelvic girdle, two systems contribute to stability: the osteoarticularligamentous and the myofascial. Together they provide a self-locking mechanism. The osteoarticularligamentous system provides form closure, and the myofascial system provides force closure (Snijders et al 1993, Vleeming et al 1990a) (see Chapters 3 and 6 in this volume).

Loss of the ligamentous support (form closure) will lead to instability of the sacroiliac joint (SIJ). Form closure can be evaluated clinically with specific stability tests that evaluate the ability of the SIJ to resist vertical and horizontal translation forces (shear) that are applied passively to the non-weight-bearing joint. These tests are described in detail elsewhere (see Chapter 37 in this volume). Loss of muscle strength and control (force closure) will lead to myofascial instability through the pelvic girdle. Force closure can be evaluated clinically with specific muscle tests (see Chapter 37).

During gait, the integrated function of the trunk and lower extremity muscles assist in load transference during the weight-bearing phase by increasing intra-articular compression (see Chapter 3 in this volume). Weakness, or non-synergistic recruitment of these muscle groups, reduces the force closure mechanism through the SIJ and leads to myofascial instability. The patient then adopts compensatory movement strategies to accommodate the weakness. These strategies can be observed during gait. Over time, they can lead to decompensation of the lower back, hip, and knee.

NORMAL GAIT

During the swing phase of the right leg, the right innominate bone rotates posteriorly relative to the sacrum (unilateral right sacral nutation or flexion) (Greenman 1992, Vleeming et al 1995a). This motion increases the tension of the sacrotuberous and interosseus ligament and prepares the joint for heel strike (Fig. 18.1). The increase in tension contributes to the force closure mechanism, augments the form closure mechanism, and therefore increases stability. Inman et al (1981) have shown that the hamstrings become active just

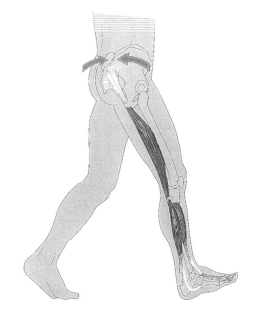

Fig. 18.1 At heel strike, the biceps femoris contracts and increases tension in the sacrotuberus ligament (Vleeming et al 1995a). This mechanism facilitates force closure of the SIJ. (Redrawn from Vleeming et al 1995a.)

before heel strike. Contraction of the biceps femoris increases the tension in the sacro-tuberous ligament, further contributing to the force closure mechanism.

During the single-leg stance phase of the right leg, the right innominate begins to rotate anteriorly relative to the sacrum (unilateral right sacral counternutation or extension). This motion is resisted by the long dorsal sacroiliac (SI) ligament (Vleeming et al 1995b). The hamstrings relax and the gluteus maximus becomes more active (Inman et al 1981) (Fig. 18.2). This occurs in conjunction with a counter-rotation of the trunk. The contralateral latissimus dorsi can be felt to fire during this motion. Together, these two muscles tense the thoracodorsal fascia and facilitate the force closure mechanism through the SIJ. The superincumbent body weight is thereby transferred to the lower extremity through a system that is stabilized through ligamentous and myofascial tension. From heel strike through midstance, the ipsilateral gluteus medius, minimus, and tensor fascia latae, and contralateral adductors are active to stabilize the pelvic girdle on the femoral head.

Muscle activity is much less in all groups during the double support phase since both legs receive the body weight.

In optimal gait, the center of gravity travels along a smooth sinusoidal curve both vertically and laterally. The displacement in both planes should be no more than 5 cm (Inman et al 1981).

UNSTABLE GAIT

The displacement of the center of gravity is exaggerated when the SIJ is unstable (insufficient in either form or force closure). The patient attempts to compensate for the lack of stability by reducing the shear forces through the SIJ. In a fully compensated gait, the patient transfers his or her weight laterally over the involved limb (compensated Trendelenburg sign), thus reducing the vertical shear forces through the joint (Fig. 18.3).

In a non-compensated gait pattern, the patient tends to demonstrate a true Trendelenburg sign. The pelvic girdle adducts excessively (on the weight-bearing leg) (Fig. 18.4). The femur abducts relative to the foot, thus bringing the center of

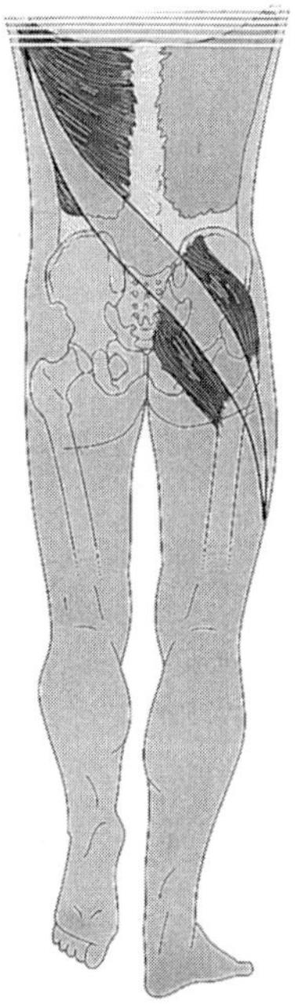

Fig. 18.2 Through midstance, the gluteus maximus contracts and facilitates the transmission of force through the thoracodorsal fascia.

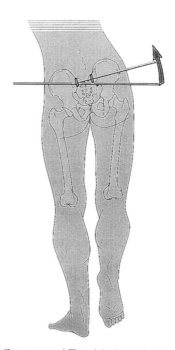

Fig. 18.3 Compensated Trendelenburg sign.

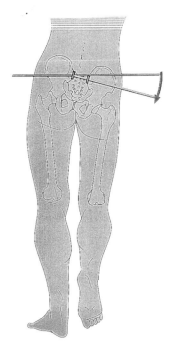

Fig. 18.4   Non-compensated Trendelenburg sign.

gravity closer to the SIJ, which reduces the vertical shear force. This gait pattern is also seen when the SIJ is stable and the gluteus medius weak or poorly recruited.

Clinically, the gluteus maximus appears to become inhibited whenever the SIJ is irritated or in dysfunction. The consequences to gait can be catastrophic when the gluteus maximus is weak. The stride length shortens and the hamstrings are overused to compensate for the loss of hip extensor power. The hamstrings are not ideally situated to provide a force closure mechanism and, in time, the SIJ can become hypermobile. This is often seen in athletes with repetitive hamstring strains. The hamstrings remain overused and vulnerable to intramuscular tears.

CONCLUSIONS

1. Instability of the pelvic girdle can become an extremely debilitating condition.
2. Instability of the pelvic girdle is reflected in the gait pattern.
3. Early identification can prevent the excessive loss of muscle power and the subsequent breakdown of the force closure mechanism.

REFERENCES

Greenman P E 1992 Clinical aspects of sacroiliac function in walking. In: Vleeming A, Mooney V, Snijders C J, Dorman T (eds) First interdisciplinary world congress on low back pain and its relation to the sacroiliac joint. San Diego, CA, 5–6 November, pp 353–359

Inman V T, Ralston H J, Todd F 1981 Human walking. Williams & Wilkins, Baltimore

Snijders C J, Vleeming A, Stoeckart R 1993 Transfer of lumbosacral load to iliac bones and legs. Part 1: Biomechanics of self-bracing of the sacroiliac joints and its significance for treatment and exercise. Clinical Biomechanics 8: 285–294

Vleeming A, Snijders C J, Stoeckart R, Mens J M A 1955a A new light on low back pain. In: Vleeming A, Mooney V, Dorman T, Snijders C J (eds) Second interdisciplinary world congress on low back pain. San Diego, CA, 9–11 November, pp 149–168

Vleeming A, Pool-Goudzwaard A L, Hammudoghlu D, Stoeckart R, Snijders C J, Mens J M A 1995b The function of the long dorsal sacroiliac ligament: its implication for understanding low back pain. In: Vleeming A, Mooney V, Dorman T, Snijders C J (eds) Second interdisciplinary world congress on low back pain. San Diego, CA, 9–11 November, pp 123–137

19. Clinical aspects of the sacroiliac joint in walking

P. E. Greenman

INTRODUCTION

Walking as an exercise for enhanced physical fitness has many positive attributes (Rippe et al 1986). If pursued at a rapid pace, the aerobic conditioning capacity is almost as great as in jogging and running, but with less risk of injury and progressive degenerative joint disease of the lower extremities. In addition to cardiovascular conditioning, walking provides biomechanical exercise for the total musculoskeletal system, including the upper and lower extremities and the trunk and pelvis. To be biomechanically efficient, the gait should be cross-patterned, with alternating arm swing and leg movement, and as symmetrical as possible. Walking has many advantages. It can be done in many places by anyone with appropriate shock-absorbing shoes and the available time. The American Medical Association's council on scientific affairs has stated, 'walking is a most convenient and adaptable form of exercise' (Dan 1988). In the presence of lower back and lower extremity pain, walking is frequently an activity that contributes to the patient's pain and disability. In those patients, it is an appropriate therapeutic goal to establish the maximal biomechanical capacity for symmetrical gait within the musculoskeletal system.

Lower back pain with or without lower extremity radiation is a frequent patient presentation to the health-care delivery system. It constitutes 25% of worker's compensation claims but consumes 80% of worker's compensation costs. It presents a major diagnostic challenge to health-care practitioners. Between 60 and 80% of cases defy specific diagnosis and are classified as idiopathic (Kirkaldy-Willis & Hill 1979).

The role of the sacroiliac joint (SIJ) in lower back and lower extremity pain has recently gained more attention and understanding. The anatomy, radiology and other imaging studies, and the pathology of the joint have been extensively reviewed by Bellamy et al (1983). This excellent review does not deal with the dysfunctional biomechanics of the sacroiliac (SI) mechanism viewed by many practitioners as being highly significant in back pain patients. These authors do, however, note that a discrepancy in leg length of 1.0 cm or more causes torsion to occur in the pelvic girdle, resulting in changes in the sacrum and pubis that frequently result in SI pain. It is further pointed out that the most reliable clinical sign of instability of the SIJ is disruption at the symphysis pubis, resulting in increased mobility when alternately weight-bearing on either leg.

The SIJ was eloquently reviewed from the perspective of the anatomy, biomechanics, and structural diagnosis by Beal (1982). This excellent review concluded that the motion at the SIJ was highly variable and of small quantity, and that there were marked variations in the anatomy of the joint surface. Beal also concluded that structural diagnosis of SIJ dysfunction required high-level skill in testing joint motion, analysing tissue texture, and assessing asymmetry of pelvic landmarks. Great care must be used in this process to differentiate accurately between normal and abnormal mobility.

ANATOMY

The anatomy of the lower back and pelvis has been covered in previous chapters and has been eloquently reviewed by Alderink (1991). There

235

are certain features of the anatomy that relate to the biomechanics of gait which need to be highlighted.

Conceptually, the junction of the lower extremity and the trunk can be viewed as being at the two SIJs with the two innominates functioning as lower extremity bones. Gracovetsky (see Chapter 20) has demonstrated that an individual with no lower extremities can perform a classic cross-pattern walking cycle with the ground contact being the two ischial tuberosities. The SIJs have two major components: a ventrally placed synovial joint and an extensive dorsal ligamentous component. The articular surfaces of the SIJ have extensive elevations and depressions (Vleeming et al 1990a, Weisl 1954), with a central depression on the sacral side. The sacral concavity and iliac convexity, and other elevations and depressions, increasingly develop over time (Bowen & Cassidy 1981). The contour of the joint begins to develop its uneven articular surfaces during the second and third decades. Well into the seventh decade, there is continued movement, but the interdigitating groves of the joint are better developed. It is interesting to note that the age of the greatest incidence of disabling back pain, the third and fourth decades, is a time at which the joint is well formed and quite mobile, yet is frequently dysfunctional. In childhood and early adolescence, the joint is not well formed, glides quite easily and is apparently not frequently involved in restricted dysfunction. In one's fifties, the joint begins to have less flexibility, and increased interdigitation of the opposing joint surfaces results in reduced mobility. Disabling mechanical back pain is less common in this age. The SIJs have the capacity for rotation and translation determined in large measure by the joint shape and ligamentous attachments. The axis of rotation varies considerably between individuals, and the combined rotation and translation that occur contributes to ligamentous tension which would absorb energy, and result in the concept that the SIJs function as shock-absorbing structures (Wilder et al 1980).

The ligamentous portion of the SIJ is extensive and has several significant relationships. The anterior SI ligament is quite thin and can basically be viewed as the anterior extension of the capsule of the synovial portion of the joint. The iliolumbar ligaments from the transverse processes of L4 and L5 not only attach to the iliac crest, but also have extensions that blend caudally with the anterior SI ligaments. The posterior SI ligaments are extensive and multilayered. The deepest component is extremely short and horizontally oriented. As the layers become more superficial, they result in the vertical portion of the posterior SI ligament, which blends into the sacrotuberous ligament ultimately becoming continuous with the hamstring fascia of the posterior thigh. The SIJ and its ligamentous components are extensively innervated from the lower lumbar and upper sacral roots.

There are no muscle prime movers for motion of the SIJ. The bony pelvic ring responds to mass action of muscles from the trunk above and the lower extremities below. The piriformis muscle is as close to a prime mover as exists. It takes origin from the anterior surface of S2, 3, and 4, and traverses the sciatic notch to insert into the greater trochanter of the femur. Its primary action is external rotation and abduction of the femur. There is some question of the possibility of the muscle functioning as an internal rotator if the hip joint is flexed beyond 90°. The piriformis is a muscle that becomes easily facilitated, resulting in shortness and tightness. Asymmetric length and tone of the piriformis is a frequent clinical finding in the presence of SI dysfunction.

The abdominal musculature attaches to the iliac crest and inguinal ligament, with the rectus abdominis muscle attaching directly to the pubis. The adductor group of the medial thigh attaches to the inferior ramus of the pubis. Muscle imbalance between the abdominals above, particularly the rectus abdominis, and the adductors below appears to contribute to the persistence of dysfunction at the symphysis pubis.

The psoas major muscle links the thoracolumbar junction and lumbar vertebra with the hip joint while passing over the anterior aspect of the SIJ. The quadratus lumborum links the twelfth rib with the lumbar vertebra and the iliac crest. These two trunk muscles can be viewed as lower extremity muscles in that they influence function of the innominate bones as well as the femur through the hip joint. Imbalance of right and left can significantly influence the participation of the innominate bone in the walking cycle.

Lower extremity muscles that influence pelvic function in addition to the adductors are the gluteals, hamstrings, and quadriceps groups. The rectus femoris muscle of the anterior thigh is a two-joint muscle, attaching proximally to the anterior inferior iliac spine of the innominate and distally to the tibia; when dysfunctional, this muscle becomes facilitated, short, and tight. The other three components of the quadriceps group are one-joint muscles, which, when dysfunctional, become inhibited. Shortness and tightness of the rectus femoris is frequently associated with tightness of the psoas muscle and can restrict the anterior capsule of the hip joint. The gluteus minimus and medius are hip abductors and weak internal rotators. The gluteus maximus is primarily a hip extensor. The glutei when dysfunctional become inhibited and result in weakness. A major problem in the gait results from tightness of the psoas and rectus femoris anteriorly and weakness of the glutei posteriorly. The hamstring group links the ischial tuberosity of the innominate with the lower extremity. The biceps femoris attaches distally to the head of the fibula and responds to altered functional capacity of the lower portion of the lower extremity, particularly ankle mechanics. The proximal tibiofibular articulation becomes dysfunctional in the presence of biomechanical fault of the foot and ankle. Good foot, ankle, and knee mechanics are all essential components of normal gait. It can be seen that there is an extensive and continuous linkage of myofascial elements from the foot through the thoracolumbar junction that can influence SI motion, both normal and dysfunctional.

Other muscles that relate to the osseous pelvis are those in the pelvic and urogenital diaphragms. While they appear to have little function in the mechanics of pelvic girdle mobility, they respond to alteration in pelvic girdle function with imbalance and contribute to symptoms relative to the lower urinary, genital, and rectal viscera. Urgency, frequency, dysuria, and dyspareunia are frequently associated with dysfunction at the symphysis pubis.

BIOMECHANICS

The motions within the pelvic girdle can be viewed from the perspective of the symphysis pubis, one innominate in relation to one side of the sacrum, and the sacrum between the two innominates. Each motion contributes a small component to overall pelvic mobility during gait.

Movement at the symphysis pubis consists of two components. There is a superior-to-inferior translatory movement that occurs during one-legged standing (Chamberlain 1930). Normally, the right and left pubic bone is found in the same relationship to the horizontal plane. On prolonged one-legged standing, the ipsilateral pube moves cephalward. This should return to normal on standing on the opposite leg or on prolonged two-legged standing. Habitual one-legged standing results in muscle imbalance between the abdominals above and the adductors below, restricting the pubic bone in aberrant relationship with its fellow. This dysfunctional relationship interferes with the other major motion available at the symphysis pubis.

The symphysis serves as the axis of rotation for the alternating anterior and posterior rotation of the right and left innominate bones (Pitkin & Pheasant 1936). These authors used an inclinometer method for evaluating motion within the pelvis and described the alternating anterior and posterior rotation of the innominates. They felt that the sacrum responded with bilateral bending and rotation as coupled movements in response to ilial movement. The introduction of Kirschner wires into both innominates was used to assess the relative mobility of one innominate to the other (Colachis et al 1963). Nine test positions were used, and the relative movement was measured. These authors concluded that there were angular and parallel movements in addition to rotation, and that mobility was not about a fixed mechanical axis. The greatest movement demonstrated was in forward bending while standing. Studies of fresh cadavers monitoring load displacement behavior showed differences in the axis of rotation from one specimen to another (Miller et al 1987). Torsion was the cause of the greatest number of single joints to fail. There was a difference when one or both ilia were fixed:

when both ilia were fixed motion was small; with only one ilium fixed, mobility was greater and appeared to simulate behavior during a one-legged stance in vivo. The methodology did not allow for measurement of all coupled movements.

Lavignolle et al (1983) used radiographic photogrammetric methodology in cadavers and in vivo, measuring the right and left innominate bones in relation to the sacrum and to each other. The sacrum was fixed to reduce the influence of mobility at the lumbar spine and lumbosacral junction. The exact axes of rotation varied between subjects but were found to be in a relatively constant area and basically in the oblique direction. These authors refuted older studies that described motion in an antero-posterior axis. The amplitude of movement varied by subject but rotation averaged 10–12°, with translation of up to 6 mm in young adults.

One of the earliest studies assessing sacral motion in relation to the innominate was performed by Strachan et al (1938), who studied sacral movement induced by movement through the lumbar spine with one innominate being fixed. They demonstrated coupled side-bending and rotation to opposite sides in most specimens. The coupling seemed to vary depending upon how the motion was introduced through the lumbar spine and may have been biased by the unilateral preparation. Subsequent studies have usually identified that coupling of side-bending and rotation is to opposite sides. A report by Stevens (1992) eloquently described side-bending and axial rotation of the sacrum. Utilizing a goniometric measurement technique in both the standing and seated positions, he demonstrated coupled behavior of side-bending and rotation to opposite sides in neutral and extended posture. In the forward-bent posture, sacral side-bending and rotation occurred in the same direction. He further demonstrated coupled side-bending and rotation to the opposite side in the upper lumbar segments, and side-bending and rotation to the same side at the lumbosacral junction. Asymmetric movement was identified in symptomatic patients. The restriction was reversible by manual treatment, resulting in restored normal range of motion.

The contour of the SIJ with ridges and depressions has high friction coefficients and influences the amount of mobility available (Vleeming et al 1990b). Dorman (1994) postulated that, during gait, the SIJ has a clutch function, with bracing on the stance side resulting in close-packing of the joint and allowing loose-packing of the contralateral SIJ for mobility through the swing phase. The SI ligaments were viewed as essential components in this process, and compromise of the ligamentous structures might lead to symptoms, including pain and occasional falls. Vleeming et al (1995) described both form and force closure of the SI mechanism, providing a self-locking mechanism for stability and mobility. Form closure depends on the shape of the SIJs, their contours, and the associated friction. Ligamentous tension and muscle behavior are essential for stability of the SI mechanism. These authors link the behavior of myofascial elements of the trunk with those of the lower extremity as part of normal SI integrated function. Gracovetsky (1995) links motion of the pelvis and spine during gait with functions of lower extremity and trunk muscles in transferring energy to activate the 'spinal engine'.

These studies, and many others, have demonstrated the difficulty of identifying all the motions available within the pelvic girdle complex. Suffice it to say, one can conclude that there is normal anterior and posterior rotation of the two innominates associated with an axis through the symphysis pubis. In addition to this motion of one innominate with the contralateral one, there is also a repeating anterior and posterior rotational movement available of one innominate on one side of the sacrum. This has some axis posterior in the pelvis. The sacrum has a primary motion of nutation and counternutation, with some accompanying translation around a variable transverse axis. Since asymmetry between the right and left SIJs is the rule rather than the exception, asymmetry of this nutation and counternutation movement can be expected. The sacrum also has the capacity of side-bending and rotating between the two innominates. This coupled motion appears to be primarily to opposite sides. The coupling of lumbar side-bending and rotation with sacral side-bending and rotation is less clear. This is the result of the lumbar spine having the capability of side-bending and rotation to opposite sides in the upper levels, and side-bending and rotation to the same side at L5. All of these motions, resulting from multiple muscle activities, are essential for symmetrical gait.

GAIT

Most descriptions of gait focus upon the lower extremity up to the junction of the femur with the acetabulum of the innominate bone, with resultant overall rotation of the pelvis (Inman et al 1981). The function of the lower limb through gait is highly complex at a number of joints: the foot, ankle, knee, and hip (Dillingham et al 1992). The individual given credit for the development of the muscle energy system of manual medicine, Fred L. Mitchell, in his classic article 'Structural pelvic function' (1965), provided a description of SI movement during the walking cycle. Much of the confusion in gait analysis occurs because of differing descriptions of which bone is moving in what direction in relationship to another, either from above downward or below upward, and whether it is the first step or one that is continuous in the cycle. It has been shown that the whole pelvis will rotate in three-dimensional space with one leg at heel strike and the other at toe-off (Schmidt et al 1995). Schmidt et al's study concluded that there was substantial angular movement at the SIJs but it did not describe the function of the sacrum during the change from right to left straddled positions.

Lee (1989) eloquently describes the kinetics and kinematics of the sacrum, lumbar spine, innominates, and hip joints. Her description of the gait is congruent with Mitchell's, with the exception of the related side-bending and rotational behavior of the lumbar spine on the sacrum. Mitchell described the lumbar spine as having coupled side-bending and rotation to opposite sides as far down as the lumbosacral junction. He viewed that the sacrum would always rotate and side-bend to the opposite side of the lumbar spine. Lee's description is slightly different. She describes the L5 segment as side-bending and rotating to the same side, in agreement with research available since the time of Mitchell. She

describes the transition between lumbar and sacral rotation as occurring perhaps at the L4 level rather than at the L5/S1 level. Both authors agree on neutral side-bending and rotation coupling to opposite sides in the upper lumbar segments, and that the sacrum side-bends and rotates to opposite sides on a hypothetical oblique axis.

The following describes gait from the perspective of the sequences occurring once gait has been established, rather than of the first step. The description is limited to the combined activities of the right and left innominates, the sacrum, and the lumbar spine. The two innominate bones alternately rotate forward and backward synchronously, and the entire pelvis rotates from right to left around a vertical axis, with the shoulder girdle rotating in the opposite direction during classic cross-patterned gait. As the innominates rotate anteriorly and posteriorly, there is a changing center of gravity of the trunk over the hip joints. This anterior–posterior rotation of the innominates occurs around an anterior axis at the symphysis pubis and a posterior axis on each side for each SIJ, described as iliosacral motion. The sacrum appears to move alternately in a 'wobbling' fashion, with side-bending and rotation coupled to opposite sides and following the induced pelvic rotation. The lumbar spine will side-bend and rotate to opposite sides in an alternating fashion.

At the time of right heel strike and left toe-off, the right innominate is rotated posteriorly and the left innominate anteriorly to the maximum (Fig. 19.1). The sacrum is level and the lumbar spine straight, and both face toward the left due to maximal pelvic rotation to the left (Fig. 19.2). During the right stance phase, the right innominate is rotating anteriorly and the left posteriorly (Fig. 19.3). At right midstance, there is maximal loading of the right hip and SIJ, and the sacrum between the innominates is rotating to the right, side-bending left, and moving into (anterior) nutational movement at the left sacral base. The lumbar spine is side-bent right and rotated left (Fig. 19.4). At left heel strike, the left innominate starts its anterior rotation, and as the right leg enters the swing phase, it begins to rotate posteriorly (Fig. 19.5). At this point, the sacrum has

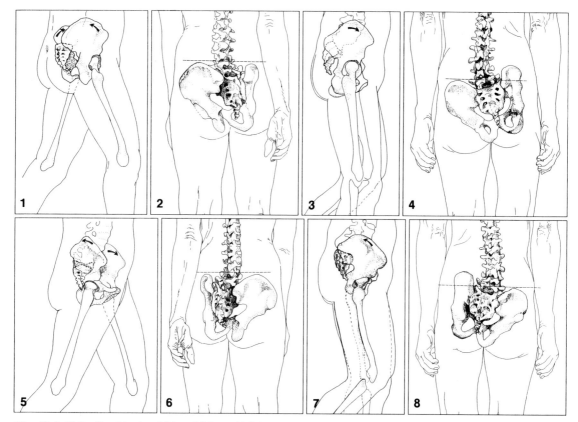

Figs 19.1–19.8 Combined activities of right and left innominates, sacrum, and spine during walking.
Figs 19.1 and 19.2 At right heel strike. (**Fig. 19.1**) Right innominate has rotated in a posterior and left innominate in an anterior direction. (**Fig. 19.2**). Anterior surface of sacrum is rotated to left and superior surface is level, while spine is straight but rotated to the left. **Figs 19.3 and 19.4** At right midstance. (**Fig. 19.3**) Right leg is straight and innominate is rotating anteriorly. (**Fig. 19.4**) Sacrum has rotated right and side-bent left, while lumbar spine has side-bent right and rotated left. **Figs 19.5 and 19.6** At left heel strike. (**Fig. 19.5**) Left innominate begins rotation anteriorly; after toe-off, right innominate begins rotation posteriorly. (**Fig. 19.6**) Sacrum is level but with anterior surface rotated to right. Spine, although straight, is also rotated to the right, as is lower trunk. **Figs 19.7 and 19.8** At left leg stance. (**Fig. 19.7**) Left innominate is high and left leg straight. (**Fig. 19.8**) Sacrum has rotated to left and side-bent right, while lumber spine has side-bent left and rotated right. (Reproduced with permission from Greenman 1990.)

returned to being level between the two innominates, the lumbar spine is straight, and the pelvis is rotated to the right (Fig. 19.6). During the stance phase on the left, the right innominate continues its posterior rotation during the swing phase and the sacrum now rotates to the left, side-bends right, and (anteriorly) nutates at the right sacral base (left-on-left sacral torsion). The lumbar spine is side-bent to the left and rotated right (Fig. 19.8). From there the cycle is repeated. With each succeeding step, each innominate alternately rotates anterior and posteriorly, the sacrum moves from right-on-right to left-on-left anterior torsion, and the lumbar spine side-bends

left and rotates right, and then side-bends right and rotates left. Regardless of the coupling at L5, it is clear that the upper lumbar segments and sacrum behave as described.

It is readily apparent that normal gait requires maximum symmetric movement of all of the lumbar vertebra, the two SIJs, and the symphysis pubis. This complex total body movement also requires maximal functional length and strength of the paired muscle groups of the lower extremity and trunk. Instability of the SIJs can have major consequences on gait. Strain of the joint can affect the osteoarticular ligamentous system (form closure), particularly with traumatic laxity of the strong posterior SI ligaments and of the myo-fascial system (force closure), with loss of muscle balance and control of the trunk and lower extremities (Lee 1995). Prolotherapy to strengthen the ligamentous structures of the SI region has been shown to improve the energy efficiency of a patient during walking (Dorman et al 1995). Manipulation of the lower back and pelvic region has been found to improve the symmetry of gait post treatment (Robinson et al 1987).

CONCLUSIONS

1. This discussion has been based upon current research knowledge available. Much more research needs to be done, particularly motion analysis of these complex motions in vivo.

A non-invasive method has yet to be developed and implemented.

2. It is apparent that normal gait is important for all patients, particularly those with lower back and lower extremity pain syndromes. The skilled clinician should assess the total musculoskeletal system for integrated function during gait.

3. The treating practitioner, whether employing surgical or non-operative care interventions, should have as a therapeutic outcome the maximal gait symmetry allowed by the anatomy.

4. The patient needs to be aware of his or her responsibility in exercising with appropriate stretching, strengthening, and motor control activities, to maintain a symmetric gait as so many of the activities of daily living revolve around it.

REFERENCES

Alderink G J 1991 The sacroiliac joint: review of anatomy, mechanics and function. Journal of Orthopedic and Sports Physical Therapy 13: 71–84

Beal M C 1982 The sacroiliac problem: review of anatomy mechanics and diagnosis. Journal of the American Osteopathic Association 81: 667–679

Bellamy N, Park W, Rooney P J 1983 What do we know about the sacroiliac joint. Seminar in Arthritis and Rheumatism 12: 282–313

Bowen V, Cassidy J D 1981 Macroscopic and microscopic anatomy of the sacroiliac joint from embryonic life until the eighth decade. Spine 6: 620–628

Chamberlain W E 1930 The symphysis pubis in the roentgen examination of the sacroiliac joint. American Journal of Roentgenology 24: 621–625

Colachis S C, Worden R E, Bechtol C O, Strohm B R 1963 Movement of the sacroiliac joint in the adult male: a preliminary report. Archives of Physical Medicine and Rehabilitation 44: 490–498

Dan B B 1988 Walk with your doc. Journal of the American Medical Association 259: 2743–2744

Dillingham T R, Lehmann J F, Price R 1992 Effect of lower limb and body propulsion. Archives of Physical Medicine and Rehabilitation 73: 647–651

Dorman T A 1994 Failure of self-bracing at the sacroiliac joints: the slipping clutch syndrome. Journal of Orthopedic Medicine 16: 49–51

Dorman T A, Cohen R E, Dasig D, Jeng S, Fischer N, DeJong A 1995 Energy efficiency during human walking before and after prolotherapy. In: Vleeming A, Mooney V, Dorman T, Snijders C J (eds) Second interdisciplinary world congress on low back pain. San Diego, CA, 9–11 November, pp 645–649

Gracovetsky S A 1995 Locomotion-linking the spinal engine with the legs. In: Vleeming A, Mooney V, Dorman T, Snijders C J (eds) Second interdisciplinary world congress on low back pain. San Diego, CA, 9–11 November, pp 171–173

Greenman P E 1990 Clinical aspects of sacroiliac function in walking. Journal of Manual Medicine 5: 125–130

Inman V T, Ralston H J, Todd F 1981 Human walking. Williams & Wilkins, Baltimore

Kirkaldy-Willis W H, Hill R J 1979 A more precise diagnosis for low back pain. Spine 4: 102–109

Lavignolle B, Vital J M, Senegas J et al 1983 An approach to the functional anatomy of the sacroiliac joints in vivo. Anatomia Clinica 5: 169–176

Lee D 1989 The pelvic girdle. Churchill Livingstone, Edinburgh

Lee D 1995 Instability of the sacroiliac joint and the consequences to gait. In: Vleeming A, Mooney V, Dorman T, Snijders C J (eds) Second interdisciplinary world congress on low back pain. San Diego, CA, 9–11 November, pp 473–484

Miller J A A, Schultz A B, Anderson G B J 1987 Load-displacement behavior of sacroiliac joints. Journal of Orthopedic Research 5: 92–101

Mitchell F L 1965 Structural pelvic function. Yearbook Academy Applied Osteopathy, Carmel 2: 178–199

Pitkin H C, Pheasant H C 1936 Sacroarthrogenetic telalgia. Journal of Bone and Joint Surgery (US) 18: 365–373

Rippe J M, Ward A, Haskell W L, Freedson P, Franklin B A, Campbell K R 1986 Walking for fitness. Physician and Sports Medicine 14: 145–159

Robinson R O, Herzog W, Nigg B N 1987 Journal of Manipulative Physiological Therapy 10: 172–176

Schmidt G L, McQuade K, Wei S H, Barakatt E 1995 Sacroiliac kinematics for reciprocal straddle positions. Spine 20: 1047–1054

Stevens A 1992 Sidebending and axial rotation of the sacrum inside the pelvic girdle. In: Vleeming A, Mooney V, Snijders C J, Dorman T (eds) First interdisciplinary world congress on low back pain and its relation to the sacroiliac joint. San Diego, CA, 5–6 November, pp 209–230

Strachan W F, Beckwith C G, Larson N J, Grant J H 1938 A study of the mechanics of the sacroiliac joint. Journal of the American Osteopathic Association 37: 576–578

Vleeming A, Stoeckart R, Volkers A C W, Snijders C J 1990a

A relation between form and function in the sacroiliac joint. Part I: Clinical anatomical aspects. Spine 15: 130–132

Vleeming A, Volkers A C W, Snijders C J, Stoeckart R 1990b Relation between form and function in the sacroiliac joint. Part II: Biomechanical aspects. Spine 15: 133–135

Vleeming A, Snijders C J, Stoeckart R, Mens J M A 1995 A new light on low back pain. In: Vleeming A, Mooney V, Dorman T, Snijders C J (eds) Second interdisciplinary world congress on low back pain. San Diego, CA, 9–11 November, pp 149–168

Weisl H 1954 The articular surfaces of the sacroiliac joint and their relation to the movements of the sacrum. Acta Anatomica 22: 1–14

Wilder D G, Pope M H, Frymoyer J W 1980 The functional topography of the sacroiliac joint. Spine 5: 575–579

20. Linking the spinal engine with the legs: a theory of human gait

S. A. Gracovetsky

INTRODUCTION

Human gait is unique from an evolutionary perspective, although the reasons for it and the advantages it brought are still a matter of conjecture. A mechanism to explain how the human spine evolved from our fish ancestors was proposed in 1985. This early theory of the spinal engine did not describe the specific interactions of the spine with the legs. The purpose of this chapter is to review and generalize the theory to merge spine and legs into a single machine, which achieves what is termed 'human gait'.

Lovett (1903) discovered that a lordotic spine, when bent to either side, induced an axial torque, a phenomenon dubbed 'coupled motion' and studied in detail by Panjabi and White (1971). Nachemson (1963) analysed the conditions under which the lumbar disc could be damaged by excessive compression. Farfan (1973) argued that excessive torsion was responsible for disc pathology. Following these leads, a considerable amount of experimental and theoretical work established that disc injury results from a combination of both compression and torsion, torsion being perhaps the more damaging element. Since lower back injuries are among the non-life-threatening diseases representing the greatest burden socially and economically, many were quick to interpret the experimental data to mean that compression and torsion indeed ought to be avoided in the workplace. However, administrative guidelines proposed by NIOSH (1981) to take these findings into account did not result in any kind of reduction or slow-down in the incidence of lower back injuries.

If torsion were indeed the primary source of disc pathology, why then did we acquire a spine that allows for high levels of torsion? Surely, the 33 vertebrae prone to disc disease ought to have been replaced through evolution by stronger components. The fact that we did not evolve in such a manner suggests that the high incidence of torsional injury ought to be compensated for by some fundamentally important advantage for our species.

It was essential to have access to more precise descriptions of dorsal and sacral musculature in order to relate spinal motion and the motion of the legs. By the early 1980s, Bogduk and Twomey (1987) had refined Gray's description of spinal musculature to a point at which it was possible realistically to analyse spinal motion through mathematical modeling. We proposed that the properties of spinal movement ought to be determined by the need to survive, i.e. to execute tasks in such a way that the stress within all structures ought to be minimized and equalized. This seemingly broad hypothesis led us to realize that the concept of the spine as a rigid 'column' was no longer tenable, not only that the human spine was capable of torsion and compression, but also that these properties of the spine are fundamental to its role in locomotion.

The theory of the 'spinal engine' (Gracovetsky 1988) incorporates these ideas. In essence, we have suggested that the evolutionary pressures for efficient locomotion on land forced the spine of our fish ancestors to evolve into our curved spine. The lordotic spine converts the primitive piscine lateral bend into an axial torque driving the pelvis. This theory neatly explained the need for spinal compression and torsion in locomotion. It also clarified the central role played by the earth's gravitational field in walking and running, and suggests that the human species exploits the constancy of that field to move anywhere on the planet with a minimum expenditure of energy. A prediction of the theory was that the legs were simply following pelvic motion. This suggestion was greeted with considerable scepticism by the gait-analysis community, who considered the trunk to be a passive unit carried by the legs.

The basic objection to the theory of the 'spinal engine' was the lack of understanding of the precise role of the legs. The solution eluded us until the early 1990s, when Vleeming (1992) and van Wingerden et al (1993) extended the anatomical dissections of Bogduk by exploring the layout of the ligaments across the sacroiliac joint (SIJ). Their descriptions supplied the necessary information to explain how the legs could interact with the spine in locomotion.

PELVIC ROTATION AND HUMAN GAIT

In its elementary form, human gait can be reduced to rotating the pelvis in the horizontal plane using a musculature that is more or less parallel to the spine (Fig. 20.1).

Two schools of thought have emerged over the years regarding this question. The first and older idea was that the legs played a primary role in human gait. Walking was simply a motion of the legs carrying its passive passenger, the trunk (Fig. 20.2A). In contrast, the theory of the spinal engine held that the spine was the predominant machinery involved with gait as inherited from our ancestor, the fish. Since both legs and spine are involved in locomotion, the problem is to elucidate their respective roles. This can be done by considering the logical implications of two basic hypotheses.

Hypothesis 1: the legs rotate the pelvis

The first hypothesis considers whether or not a leg can cause the pelvis to rotate. Suppose that the legs do rotate the pelvis. Conservation of the angular momentum requires that a counter-rotation be applied by the leg to the ground (Fig. 20.2B).

Force-plate data indicate that very little torque is applied to the ground during walking. Running on tiptoe excludes any significant torque transfer at the foot–ground interface. These observations suggest that the legs do not transmit torque to the ground; therefore, conservation of the angular momentum implies that no torque is transmitted to the pelvis either. Since the pelvis does rotate, the question is to determine what is responsible for pelvic rotation.

Hypothesis 2: the spine drives the pelvis to rotate

The spinal engine theory attempts to explain how the spine contributes to human locomotion. In substance, the lordotic spine converts a lateral bending movement into an axial torque driving pelvic rotation (Fig. 20.3A). This is the so-called coupled motion of the spine.

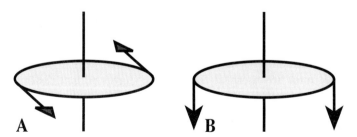

Fig. 20.1   (A) Efficient axial rotation of the pelvis requires the application of forces in the horizontal plane. Such an arrangement is not physiological. (B) Most forces acting on the pelvis are substantially parallel to the axis of rotation. Determining how the pelvis can be axially rotated with such an arrangement is the purpose of the spinal engine theory.

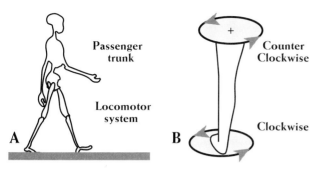

Fig. 20.2 (A) Classical theory of gait, in which the trunk is passively carried by the legs. (B) A counterclockwise torque applied to the pelvis must be balanced by an opposite clockwise torque to the ground. This is not observed. Hence, the leg cannot directly rotate the pelvis.

The theory predicts that legless individuals would 'walk' on their ischium by keeping a normal spinal motion and normal electromyograph (EMG) pattern for the trunk musculature. This has been verified on individuals, such as the young man shown in Fig. 20.3B (Gracovetsky 1988).

Kinematic and EMG studies demonstrated the striking similarities between his pattern of motion and that of a normal gait, except for the amplitude of the movements. The contribution of the spine was found to be consistent with the findings of Gregerson and Lucas in 1967 (Fig. 20.4).

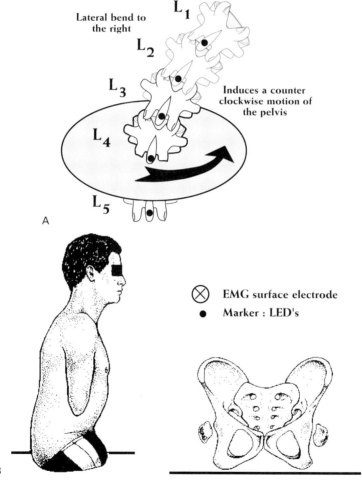

Fig. 20.3 (A) The spinal engine theory hinges on the concept of the coupled motion of the spine, whereby a lateral bend of the spine induces an axial torque driving the pelvis. (B) Lateral view of a subject with no legs and reduced upper extremities. Radiographic AP view of the pelvis showing clearly the absence of lower extremities.

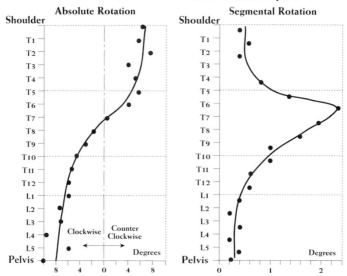

Fig. 20.4   Gregerson and Lucas implanted pins in the spinous processes of the thoracolumbar spine and measured their motion (axial rotation) during gait. Note the important contribution of the thoracic spine to the counter-rotation of pelvis and shoulder. *Absolute rotation*: measured rotation with respect to T7. *Segmental rotation*: rotation of each intervertebral joint with respect to its inferior neighbor.

Hence, there appear to be no contradictions between the proposed theory and the available data. This does not mean that the theory is correct. It simply means that it has not been proven wrong to date.

WHY THE LEGS?

Human bipedal locomotion can be achieved without legs. Indeed, we can 'walk' on our knees without any fundamental modifications to our spinal motion, except perhaps for an enhanced amplitude of movement; this demonstrates that the part of the leg below the knee is secondary in locomotion, a feature exploited by the makers of prostheses. However, besides amplifying the motion of the pelvis, there is a more fundamental reason for the evolution of the lower extremities.

Increasing velocity requires increasing the power available for locomotion. To increase power means to increase muscular mass. The expansion of erectores spinae is restricted by the contents of the abdominal cavity, so the increase in muscle mass must therefore be located outside the trunk,

such as with the hip extensors (Gracovetsky 1990). The hip extensors' power is returned to the spinal engine via the ligamentous structure described by van Wingerden et al (1993) in their study of the SIJ.

One problem remains: the unsupported spine collapses under a mass of about 2 kg. Yet, this apparent weakness allows fine movements requiring little energy expenditure to occur, a very desirable feature. However, in order to use the greater power produced by the hip extensors, the spine must first be strengthened, as will be seen later on.

MERGING THE CONTRIBUTIONS OF THE SPINE WITH THAT OF THE LEGS IN LOCOMOTION

In order to explain the contributions of the spine and legs in human gait, we must keep in mind the need to axially rotate the pelvis. This is achieved by a complex sequence of events, which can be summarized as follows:

In running or walking, the hip extensors fire as the toe pushes the ground. The muscle power is

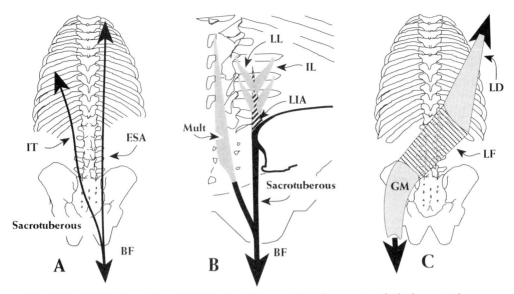

Fig. 20.5 (A) The biceps femoris (BF) is directly connected to the upper trunk via the sacrotuberous ligament, the erectores spinae aponeurosis (ESA), and iliocostalis thoracis (IT). (B) Enlarged view of the lumbar spine area showing the link between biceps femoris (BF), the lumbar intermuscular aponeurosis (LIA), longissimus lumborum (LL), iliocostalis lumborum (IL), and multifidus (Mult). (C) Relations between gluteus maximus (GM), lumbodorsal fascia (LF), and latissimus dorsi (LD).

directly transmitted to the spine and trunk via two distinct but complementary pathways:

1. For biceps femoris (BF): The sacrotuberous ligament extends the action of the biceps femoris all the way up the rib cage (Fig. 20.5A). In addition, this ligament crosses over the posterior superior iliac crest and continues on as the lumbar intermuscular aponeurosis (LIA) (Bogduk & Twomey 1987). The LIA has a direct link with the lumbar transverse processes via iliocostalis lumborum and longissimus lumborum (LL) (Fig. 20.5B), as well as the spinous processes via multifidus (Mult).

2. For gluteus maximus: gluteus maximus (GM) is connected to the lumbodorsal fascia (LF), itself linked with latissimus dorsi (LD) and the upper extremities (Fig. 20.5C).

As a consequence, firing the hip extensors extends and raises the trunk in the sagittal plane. The chemical energy liberated within the muscles is now converted, by the rising trunk, into potential energy stored in the gravitational field. When a person is running, so much energy needs to be stored that the necessary rise in the

center of gravity forces the runner to become airborne.

During flight (running) or single stance phase (walking), the force of compression applied to the spine is minimum (Fig. 20.6).

The spine can assume the proper lateral bending shape in preparation for landing (heel strike). To increase the stride, the acetabulum is brought

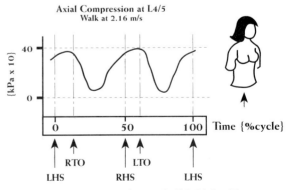

Fig. 20.6 Axial compression on the L4–5 joint. The compression is maximal after heel strike (pulse delayed as it travels upwards) and minimum during the double stance phase. LHS: left heel strike. RTO: right toe-off.

forward by the rotating pelvis. Little force is required to alter the spinal shape, and hence this
process is not taxing the erectores spinae. The
trunk now falls back towards the ground, and in
so doing converts its potential energy into kinetic
form.

At heel strike, a compressive pulse is generated
at the foot–ground interface. This compressive
pulse can be quite large. When running at 3.8 m/s,
pulses can reach 9.55 times the force of gravity
(Clarke et al 1985). This compressive pulse
recuperates the trunk's kinetic energy.

The pulse travels up the leg and pelvic SIJ into
the spine. To ensure synchronization with the
spinal motion, the pulse is reshaped and delayed
by the viscoelastic structure of collagen at the knee,
the hip joints, the sacrotuberous ligament, and the
lumbodorsal fascia. This filtering process is
essential to provide a perfectly matched pulse to
the spine kinematics regardless of ground surface
hardness, so that a maximum transfer of energy
occurs. The consequences of a mismatch can be
appreciated when running on soft sand: the kinetic
energy of the falling trunk is dissipated into the
shifting sand; the weakened pulse cannot be
properly reshaped by the knee and the resulting
mismatch with the spine further increases the
energy loss. To compensate for that loss, the
runner fires his (inefficient) abdominals to maintain the necessary pelvic rotation, rapidly resulting
in exhaustion. The relation between the elasticity
of a running surface and shoes is of particular
concern for high performance athletes who know
that some surfaces are 'faster' than others.

The energy carried by the compressive pulse is
sequentially delivered to each intervertebral joint
in ascending order so that no energy is left at the
upper cervical and head interface. It is widely
believed that the disc acts as a 'shock absorber',
attenuating the heel strike impact before it
reaches the head. This popular view is partially
true except that the pulse energy is not absorbed
(lost) into heat but is converted (used) by the
coupled motion of the spine to rotate the intervertebral joint.

Indeed, the timing is critical. The intervertebral
joint must first be bent laterally and fully rotated
axially to advance the acetabulum into the
direction of locomotion. Only then, as the spine

begins to unwind, can the pulse reach the spine.
Like a child on a swing reversing its motion just
before receiving a push, the unwinding spinal
motion is accelerated by the kick of energy it
receives from the compressive pulse. Improper
timing may be hazardous as the out-of-sync pulse
may increase the torque supported by the
intervertebral joint beyond physiological limits.
Such an event may occur when the ground
surface is either higher or lower than expected.

Gait experiments by Cappozzo in 1983
(Fig. 20.7) suggest that the torque through L4
can exceed the 20 Nm quasi static limit of lumbar
intervertebral joints (Farfan 1973).

By compressing the intervertebral joint, the
heel strike pulse stiffens the spine and increases
its torque strength beyond the critical 20 Nm limit.
The high level of torque is necessary to arrest and
reverse the lateral bending of the trunk, while
spinal lordosis induces the high axial torque
needed to drive the pelvis.

This sequence of events is repeated for each
intervertebral joint as the compressive pulse
propagates upwards, and the energy delivered to
the intervertebral joints of the thoracolumbar spine
is used to counter-rotate the shoulders and pelvis.
This provides the basic movement of locomotion,
which is amplified by the legs. Hence, the hip
extensors can be seen as axial rotators of the spine,
pelvis, and shoulders.

The weakened compressive pulse exits the
thoracic spine and travels into the cervical spine.

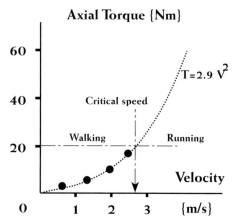

Fig. 20.7 The measured torque across L4–5 during walking
has been extrapolated for higher velocities.

Using the same principles as before, the pulse generates an axial torque. However, the peculiar shape and arrangement of the cervical facets reverses the direction of this induced axial torque. The net effect is to oppose and *de facto* cancel the motion of the shoulders so that the head remains steady. It is speculated that this arrangement evolved out of the necessity of stabilizing the motion of the head (semicircular canal and eyes sensors) during gait.

The legs have the required muscle mass to release enough chemical energy for running or walking. The legs also provide contact with the ground and modulate the timing, duration, and amplitude of the energy pulses generated at heel strike before transmitting them to the spine. The spine capitalizes on this energy to fuel its axial rotation, which in turn rotates the pelvis. Thus the legs perform these functions to assure gait modulation and velocity for a wide range of ground conditions.

DETAILS OF SPINAL MOTION DURING THE GAIT CYCLE

The leg and pelvic motion have been analysed at length in the literature. The specific movements of the spine are less well known and have been measured by a high-resolution optoelectronic system tracking the motion of 14 markers placed strategically over the spinous processes and other reference points (Fig. 20.8).

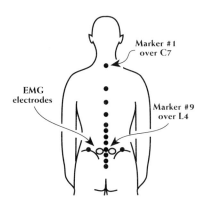

Fig. 20.8 Position of 14 skin markers, 12 above the spine and 2 above the iliac crest, and 2 EMG surface electrodes (bilateral at the L5 level over multifidus).

From this, the kinematics of lumbar intervertebral joints can be estimated (Gracovetsky et al 1995), as can the variations in lordosis during gait (Fig. 20.9). Also, the torque induced at the L4–5 level can be calculated; the relative contributions of the annulus fibrosus and facets to the total torque transmission are shown in Fig. 20.10.

Indeed, the torque is transmitted by the intervertebral joints via a dual (facets and annulus), but complementary, mechanism. The central feature of this arrangement is to spread the generation and transmission of torque over the entire gait cycle. Specifically, when the pelvic rotation is at its maximum, the interlocking facets transmit virtually all the available torque, while during the double stance phase, the facets are substantially aligned and cannot transmit any torque.

In contrast, the annulus fibrosus, made of viscoelastic collagen fibers, responds particularly well to changes in angular rotation velocity. Hence, the torque transmitted by the annulus is maximum when the velocity is maximum (double stance), which corresponds precisely to the instant when the facets' transmission is minimum. Conversely, at heel strike when the facets are most effective, the reversal in pelvic motion brings the angular velocity to zero and the annulus becomes inefficient.

Therefore, during gait, the torque needed to drive the pelvis is pulsating through both facets and disc, rhythmically and repeatedly as illustrated by their duty cycles in Fig. 20.10. This prevents the continuous loading of a single structure with the attendant high probability of failure.

This model of a dynamic role for the spine involving torsion and compression during locomotion has important ramifications for the diagnosis and treatment of spinal disorders:

• The spine must be impulse-loaded. Wearing soles that are too soft is not recommended because they absorb and dissipate the impulse intended for the spine to use for locomotion. The viscoelastic nature of biological material prevents it from sustaining constant loads for extended periods of time. A constant blood pressure would deform and damage the arteries, and prevent the heart from resting. Similarly, the regular sagittal

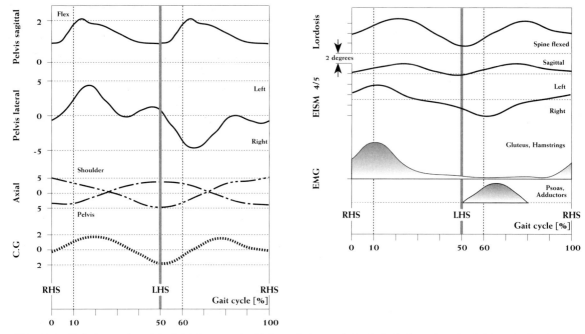

Fig. 20.9 Relative motion of the L4–5 intervertebral joint and changes in lordosis during gait cycle. *Pelvis sagittal and lateral*: rotation of pelvis in the sagittal and frontal planes. *Axial*: rotation of pelvis and shoulder in the horizontal plane. *C.G.*: vertical displacement of the center of gravity. *RMS*: right heel strike. *Lordosis*: variation of the estimate of the lumbosacral angle. *EISM4/5*: estimated rotation of the L4–5 in the sagittal and frontal planes. *EMG*: integrated EMG of muscles.

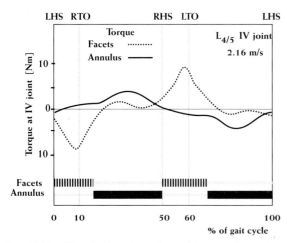

Fig. 20.10 Contribution of annulus and facets to the total torque transmitted through L4–5 during gait cycle (walk at 2.16 m/s). The duty cycles of facets and annulus illustrate the complementary nature of these structures in the generation and transmission of torque.

oscillating motion of the spine of the hiker carrying a backpack coupled with the anterior posterior motion of the pelvis prevents the

lumbodorsal fascia from continuously transmitting forces. During the double stance, the lordotic spine switches on the erectores spinae and slackens the posterior ligamentous system. Conversely, at heel strike, the posterior ligamentous system being tightened can transmit forces, thereby permitting the erectores to relax and rest. Hence, muscles and ligaments alternatively time-share the forces transmitted across the SIJ, delaying the onset of fatigue of the back.

• Surgery such as fusion or the implantation of metallic plates and screws intended to stabilize the spinal 'column' is not recommended, unless there are no good alternatives. The development of soft stabilization techniques without fusion appears to be a promising strategy for strengthening the spine.

• Diagnosis of spinal disorders ought to be dynamic and not static. In particular, static X-rays are of little use for functional assessment. Normality can be expected to be dependent upon the activity undertaken rather than an absolute decision across the board.

CONCLUSIONS

1. We propose that gait is the result of a sequential transformation of energy.

2. Beginning with the legs, muscular chemical energy is first used to lift the body into the earth's gravitational field where the chemical energy is stored in potential form.

3. When the body falls downwards, this potential energy is converted into kinetic energy, which is in turn stored into a compressive pulse at heel strike.

4. The pulse properly filtered by the knees and the massive ligamentous structure across the SIJ travels upwards.

5. The energy is then distributed to each spinal joint to counter-rotate pelvis and shoulder, while the head is stabilized by derotating the shoulders.

REFERENCES

Bogduk N, Twomey L T 1987 Clinical anatomy of the lumbar spine. Churchill Livingstone, New York

Capozzo A 1983 The forces and couples in the human trunk during level walking. Journal of Biomechanics 16: 265–277

Clarke T E, Cooper, L B, Hamill C L, Clark D E 1985 The effect of varied stride rate upon shank deceleration in running. Journal of Sports Science 3: 41–49

Farfan H F 1973 Mechanical disorders of the low back. Lea & Febiger, Philadelphia

Gracovetsky S 1988 The spinal engine. Springer–Verlag, New York

Gracovetsky S 1990 Musculoskeletal function of the spine. In: Winters J (ed.) Multiple muscle systems: biomechanics and movement organization. Springer–Verlag, New York, pp 410–436

Gracovetsky S, Pawlowsky M, Newman N et al 1995 Database for estimating normal spinal motion derived from non-invasive measurements. Spine 20: 1036–1046

Gregerson G G, Lucas D B 1967 An in vivo study of the axial rotation of the human thoracolumbar spine. Journal of Bone and Joint Surgery (US) 49(2): 247–262

Lovett A W 1903 A contribution to the study of the mechanics of the spine. American Journal of Anatomy 2: 457–462

Nachemson A 1963 The influence of spinal movements on the lumbar intradiscal pressure and on the tensile stress in the annulus fibrosus. Acta Orthopaedica Scandinavica 33: 183–207

NIOSH National Institute for Occupational Health and Safety 1981 Work practices guide for manual lifting. DHHS (NIOSH) Publication No. 81–122. NIOSH, Cincinnati, OH

Panjabi M, White A A III 1971 A mathematical approach for three-dimensional analysis of the spine. Journal of Biomechanics 4: 203–211

Van Wingerden J P, Vleeming A, Snijders C J, Stoeckart R I 1993 A functional anatomical approach to the spine-pelvis mechanism: interaction between the biceps femoris muscle and the sacrotuberous ligament. European Spine Journal 2: 140–144

Vleeming A 1992 Personal communication, and in First interdisciplinary world congress on low back pain and the sacroiliac joint. San Diego, CA, 5–6 November

21. Lower back pain as a gait-related repetitive motion injury

H J. Dananberg

INTRODUCTION

It has been known for some time that patients who injure their lower backs are often an 'accident waiting to happen'. Some types of repetitious stress act on the lumbosacral spine over a significant time, which results in an inherent fragility of one or more of its structural components. Once substantial change has occurred, an apparently inconsequential movement can then trigger an incapacitating event.

Walking is an activity of daily living. Assuming only 80 min per day of weight-bearing performance, an average adult will repeat 2500 stance/ swing cycles per limb. That equates to almost 1 000 000 steps per limb per year. By the age of 30, this number approaches 30 000 000 cycles. If the subject has a walking or standing job and/or participates in an exercise program, this number can easily double or triple. Should this gait practice be only slightly askew, the day-to-day cumulative effect is disguised by its subtle nature yet can be a hidden source that creates and/or perpetuates a pattern of chronic lumbosacral pain.

In the course of any particular step, many significant actions are interdependent, since the anatomy of the lumbosacral spine, upper torso, and lower extremity are all woven together. Muscle, tendon, ligament, and capsular components directly connect the medial column of the foot to the sacrum and lumbar spine (Vleeming et al 1995). While proper use creates a remarkable intrinsic stability, restrictions of motion at the foot level can adversely affect lumbosacral self-bracing and locking. Since this type of restriction is most often asymptomatic at the foot, there is rarely an association made between it and more proximal postural complaints. These mechanically inefficient motions, however, gradually create an environment for neurogenic hypersensitivity, myogenic overuse, and degenerative joint disease as the rotations necessary for secure support reverse themselves. For example, nutation of the sacrum, which is required for self-bracing of the sacroiliac joint (SIJ) during gait, demands that the biceps femoris, via its connection with the sacrotuberous ligament, relaxes during the midstance portion of the step as the pelvis rotates anteriorly. This is permitted by the ability of the weight-bearing limb adequately to extend out from under the hip joint during this point in the gait cycle. A previously described pathomechanical foot dysfunction known as functional hallux limitus has been shown to block this action (Dananberg 1986). Cyclic failure of adequate hip extension, coupled with concurrent flexion of the torso, causes a response of biceps femoris tightness, which restricts nutation and causes in its place counternutation. Self-locking, and therefore stability of the lumbosacral spine, fails to develop. Once intrinsically unstable at midstance, the ensuing motions required for walking add additional stress to this system.

In an average 70 kg adult, each lower extremity weighs approximately 15% of body weight, or 10.5 kg. At toe-off, the large iliopsoas muscles, which originate directly from the lower back, must fire to assist in the development of the swing phase of motion. Considering that this event is repeated at least 2500 times per day, the weight to be lifted equates to 26 250 kg per limb per day. Should the origin of these muscles fail to provide an adequately stable base from which to lift these limbs, cumulative stress must develop at this site of origin. This is felt directly as lower back pain. Should the muscle group responsible for this action become hypertonic, mechano-receptors sense this information and relay it to the CNS. The resultant spinal cord reflex gain directly lowers the pain sensor (nociceptor) threshold and can eventually cause secretion of inflammatory neuropeptides. Less and less motion creates greater perception of pain (Zimmermann 1989). Other compensatory motions then occur which assist in the limb lift process. These motions are visible as lateral trunk bends, which are created by the combination of actions of the contralateral quadratus lumborum and gluteus maximus/iliotibial band complex. These further add to the lower back pain syndrome (Dananberg 1993b).

Improper walking, as described above, causes a subtle but ever-present repetitive strain injury to the lumbosacral spine. Failure to lift each limb properly for the swing phase can essentially be seen as 'dragging the lower limbs' and is therefore a source of constant stress to the chronic lower back pain patient. Removing this deceptive origin can have a significant effect. In a previously published retrospective analysis of chronic postural pain patients considered at or near medical endpoint for long-term symptoms, 77% reported a 50–100% improvement when asymptomatic foot function was objectively addressed (Dananberg et al 1990). In a holistic approach to the back pain patient, the *application of this stress* would appear to be at least of equal consequence as the condition of the site to which it is applied. Objective gait analysis and treatment, as an addition to the physical examination and treatment of the lumbosacral spine, become an important adjunct of the therapeutic process.

This chapter will first provide a review of the process of taking a normal step. This will include a description of the generation of the power for movement as well as the actual biomechanical response to this power input. Following this, an approach to understanding the pathomechanical process is outlined. Specific pathologic movement that may lead to an overall postural decay over time along with lumbosacral stress are detailed. Markers for gait observation are also given, so that individual patients can be examined and proper treatment prescribed.

OVERVIEW OF GAIT MECHANICS

When the ancestors of our human species became bipedal millions of years ago, they needed an ambulation system that would function in a highly efficient fashion over long distances. Upright human walking is that efficient system. In order to appreciate its mechanics, some prior misconceptions must first be addressed.

It has been theorized that walking is the process in which muscles fire, creating force moments across joints, which in turn drive the weight-bearing limb to push the body forward (Inman 1981). This view cannot be supported by either logic or currently available information on muscle function. Muscles in the weight-bearing limb predominantly function eccentrically (Winter & Scott 1991). Eccentric contraction represents the resistance to motion. While this is highly efficient (1.5–6.0 times that of concentric contraction or muscle shortening) (Abbott 1952), it cannot create a pushing force. When concentric contraction finally occurs in the gastrocnemius, for example, both the knee and hip have already begun to flex forward. This would equate to the concept of pushing rope! Flexible systems cannot be effectively driven in this manner. Therefore, another model must be used to understand the mechanics of human walking.

Efficiency of the walking process

The human body can be viewed as a perpetual motion gait machine. The pendular actions of arms and legs act reciprocally, storing potential energy and returning kinetic energy in the process. These actions are visible as counter-rotations between the pelvic and shoulder girdles. Storage occurs in the ligamentous, muscular, and tendinous structures of the lower back (Dorman 1995). The cross-connections between the ipsilateral latissimus dorsi and contralateral gluteus maximus via the fascia thoracolumbocalis are ideally suited to this storage capacity. Each step prepares for the next one; the effect is to create a forward-directed rotation on the pelvic hemisphere as it coordinates with the limb that is about to begin the swing phase motion (Gracovetsky 1987).

During walking, there are periods of both single and double limb support (Fig. 21.1).

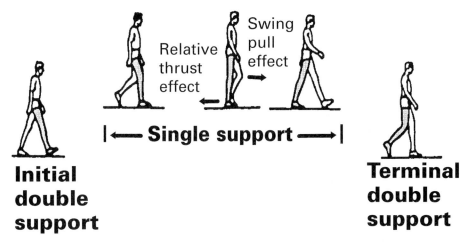

Fig. 21.1   Single and double support phases of gait.

Substantial forward motion can only occur in the approximately 400 ms of single support phase. As the weight-bearing limb supports the body, the contralateral limb acts to *pull* the center of mass forward (Claeys 1983). In essence, the free-swinging limb acts on the body and 'yanks' it over the weight-bearing side. As an analogy, imagine tying a 3 m rope between a rock and your waist. If the rock were picked up and thrown forward, a period would exist when the rope would lose its slack. Once sufficiently tightened, your body would suddenly be drawn forward towards the rock just as the rock would suddenly be halted in its forward progression. In walking, this is the action of the swing limb. It is 'thrown out' ahead of the body. As the swing limb is 'slowed' as it reaches its end range of forward motion, the center of mass is simultaneously pulled towards the forward position that the limb has attained. Gravity, continuing to act with momentum, pulls the center of mass towards the ground. Body weight, therefore, becomes the efficient prime mover (Dananberg 1993).

In order for forward motion to occur, ground contact must be present. This is the ultimate purpose of the weight-bearing limb. Through an elegant series of phasic, eccentric muscular contractions, the lower extremity is stabilized to accept the force created by the body advancing above. It can use this to create a relative 'push' or 'thrust' against the ground as the body is pulled over it. The length of the weight-bearing limb provides a mechanical advantage to the pull of the swing limb. It effectively serves as 'lever-like' structure to thrust the ground beneath the foot. Since the ground does not move, the subject advances.

Sagittal plane rotation of the load-bearing joints

It is a basic requirement in human gait for the torso and head to remain erect. For this to occur, there are two specific sites at which motion is obligatory: the hip and the foot. As the body passes over the weight-bearing foot (right limb viewed from the right side), the hip joint rotates in a clockwise direction while the foot simultaneously provides the same direction of motion. This permits the torso to remain erect as the leg and thigh extend at the hip. The foot's rotation permits advancement beyond a fixed point. Should one or the other not be present, the mechanics of walking are significantly altered (Fig. 21.2).

Rotation of the hip joint is simple to visualize. It is a ball and socket joint that permits sagittal plane extension during the single support phase. The foot, however, comprises 26 joints, which rotate in a complex yet interdependent manner. It must coordinate the effect of lower extremity internal rotation with the impact at heel strike. It must then reverse the direction of rotation by mid-step, and accommodate lower extremity external

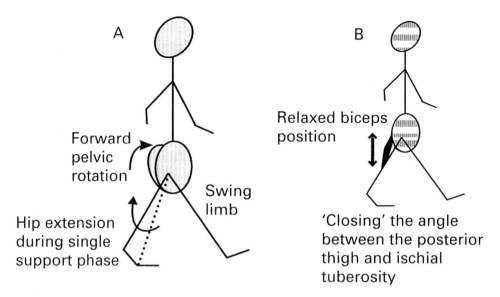

Fig. 21.2   The coordination of hip extension, forward pelvic rotation, and biceps relaxation.

rotation while simultaneously stabilizing itself to forces that can reach multiples of body weight prior to toe-off. Finally, it must maintain a portion of its structure in ground contact while permitting the entire body to pivot over it. These actions are repeated at least 2500 times per day, all within the time span of approximately 600–750 ms.

The foot as a sagittal plane pivot

The ability of the foot to permit the body to advance forward over it is a complicated action. There are three separate sites at which this pivotal response occurs (Dananberg 1995, Perry 1992). The initial location is the inferior, rounded under-surface of the calcaneus. This motion is completed following heel strike, once the forefoot touches the floor. With the heel and forefoot in contact with the ground, the ankle becomes the next site of rotation. It passively dorsiflexes as the pull of the swing limb advances the center of mass over it (Perry 1992). Dorsiflexion of the ankle is an intricate movement. The dome of the talus is shaped as a truncated pyramid, wider anteriorly than posteriorly. Therefore, as dorsiflexion occurs, the ankle joint must expand to accept the widening surface of the talar dome. This expansion is dependent on a translation motion of the fibula. It moves upward and laterally, reorienting the

fibers of the syndosmosis that connect it to the tibia. Not only does this permit continued dorsiflexion, but it also appears to store energy that will be used for ankle reversal into plantar flexion later in the step. The above two actions occur in a period of less than 200 ms.

The final pivotal 'hurdle' occurs in the second half of the single support phase. This represents the peak reactive ground thrust periods during the final 200 ms of one-leg support and further coordinates with the greatest forces concurrently being applied. Since the foot must act as both a shock absorber at heel strike and then reverse to be a rigid platform for propulsion at this time, a system must be present which regulates these events sequentially and establishes a stable structure from a flexible one. While this occurs, it must continue to permit the body to advance forward directly over it. This action has been shown to be dependent on the proper function of the first metatarsophalangeal (MTP) joint, the final pivotal site. In 1954, J. H. Hicks, a British research physician, proposed such a mechanism in the Journal of Anatomy (Hicks 1954). As recently as 1995, his concepts have been proven most accurate (Thordarson 1995).

This action, known as the windlass effect, is a purely mechanical (and therefore non-muscular) response. It uses the plantar aponeurosis as a tension band, altering its tightness as required by body and foot position. The plantar aponeurosis originates from the base of the calcaneus and inserts into the base of the proximal phalanx of the great toe (as well as providing smaller fibers to the lessor digits). As the MTP joint dorsiflexes to permit heel lift, the large, drum-like shape of the first metatarsal head–sesamoid bone complex serves as a mechanically advantaged cam, tightening the aponeurosis between the heel and toes. As the aponeurosis tightens, it secondarily close-packs the calcaneal cuboid joint on the lateral column of the foot. This action precipitates a stabilization of the tarsus, midtarsus and metatarsus, because the forces that would otherwise flatten the foot are rapidly escalating as the body advances forward (Bojsen-Møller 1979). The same movement that permits the body to pivot over the planted foot simultaneously stabilizes it to the cyclically applied stresses (Fig. 21.3).

The swing phase terminates with heel strike, and the entire process reverses, the trailing limb beginning its transition to swing movement. The passage from the stance to swing represents a mechanical challenge. It requires taking the 10.5 kg limb from an 'at rest' position to a full-speed, swing motion in 100 ms. The greater the efficiency in this transformation, the less the muscular input required.

Initiating swing phase

It appears that the body uses the actual weight of the limb itself to initiate this swing motion. As the former swing limb strikes the ground, the trailing limb immediately begins the 'pre-swing' activity. 'From its *extended* position', the knee joint 'collapses' into flexion. With knee flexion, there is a concurrent flexion of the hip joint above. Below, the ankle rapidly plantar flexes

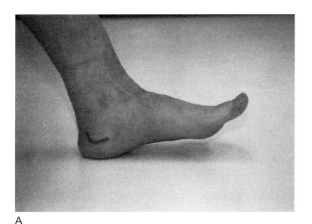

A

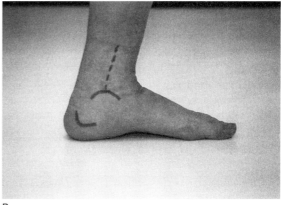

B

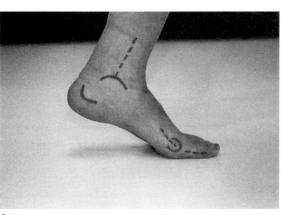

C

Fig. 21.3   (A) At heel strike, the round underside of the calcaneus serves as the initial pivotal site. (B) Once foot flat is achieved, sagittal motion is now accommodated by the ankle joint via dorsiflexion. (C) At heel lift, ankle motion reverses to plantarflexion as the MTP joint provides for the balance of the required sagittal plane motion.

while the MTP joint dorsiflexes at the same rate. The thigh therefore, based on the collapsing of the support joints, begins to accelerate rapidly forward until toe-off occurs. Just prior to toe-off, the gastrocnemius provides a brief burst of concentric contraction, propelling the limb into the swing phase (Dananberg, 1993a). (Since the knee and hip are flexing at this time, it would be impossible for this gastrocnemius activity to push the center of mass directly. It would, as described above, be analogous to 'pushing rope'. Instead, it provides the final thrust from below to initiate the swing phase.)

At the moment of toe-off, the now swing limb's motion is perpetuated by the hip flexors, the iliacus and psoas groups, which fire at this time. The iliacus originates from the crest of the ilium, whereas the psoas takes its origin from the lumbar spine, discs, and intervertebral septa. They insert via a common tendon to the lessor trochanter of the femur. Their action is complete by 50% of the swing phase cycle. The advancement of the swing limb coordinates with the energy return of the pelvis and shoulder girdle system (Dorman & Vleeming 1995). The pelvis of the swing side is now being propelled forward by the 'spinal engine' (see also Chapter 20), integrating the upper and lower body interactions. The now swinging limb pulls on the center of mass, drawing it over the weight-bearing limb as the cycle repeats itself time and time again (Fig. 21.4).

Changing from stance to swing: the pelvis–SIJ interaction

In order for the lower extremity and pelvic girdle to act in a synchronous fashion as rotations change directions rapidly, the SIJ acts as an intermediary, or 'clutch', permitting the transference of forces from the stance to the swing limb (Dorman & Vleeming 1995). For the clutch to close and create 'self-locking', the sacrum must undergo a forward rotation known as nutation. It is this motion which permits both a form and force closure of the SIJ and is critical in proper function.

The sacrum is interconnected to the lower extremity through a series of anatomic structures. The sacrotuberous ligament, originating from the coccygeal vertebrae, the SIJ capsule, and the posterior iliac spines, runs distally to the attachment of the biceps femoris on the ischial tuberosity. It has been shown that the biceps/sacrotuberous ligament is a continuous structure (see also Chapter 3). The distal connection of the biceps is to the proximal tibia, fibula, and fibers of the origin of the peroneus longus muscle on the lateral aspect of the leg (Vleeming et al 1995). Through this coupling, motion of the sacrum is integrally related to the function of the lower extremity.

Thurston and Harris (1983) have demonstrated that the sagittal plane motion of the pelvis coordinates with the motion of the swing limb.

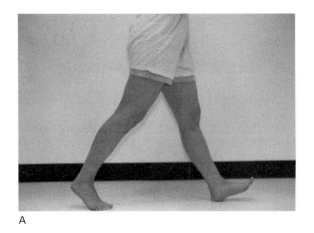

A

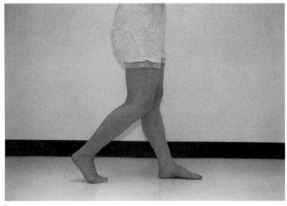

B

Fig. 21.4 (A) At the end of single support phase, the trailing limb reaches the peak amount of extension at the hip joint. The knee is fully extended and the foot has lifted off the support surface via motion at the MTP joints.

The pelvis is most posteriorly tilted just prior to toe-off, and is most anteriorly tilted just prior to heel strike. Sagittal plane motion of the pelvis during swing phase is therefore from posterior to anterior, or forwardly directed. This motion would directly coordinate with sacral nutation, which is a forward tilting of the sacrum and synonymous with SIJ self-locking (see Fig. 21.2).

Synchronizing the lower extremity and the pelvis

The synchronicity of motion of the lower extremity and the lumbosacral spine are essential for normal function. As any step occurs, the weight-bearing thigh will progressively extend at the hip joint until this motion terminates with opposite limb heel strike. With this extension motion, the angle between the posterior leg and the ischial tuberosity 'closes', thus keeping the biceps femoris in a relaxed position relative to its origin and insertion. This coordination of biceps relaxation and posterior-to-anterior pelvic motion is fundamental in maintaining the appropriate relationship between the pelvis and sacrum. Should the biceps fire prematurely, the forward rotation of the pelvis would be resisted. This would result in an inability to reach the necessary position required as single support terminates with the impact of the next heel strike.

Just prior to opposite limb heel strike, the biceps femoris becomes active (Basmajian 1974), which affects the direction of motion of the pelvis. Once heel strike occurs, the pelvis rapidly reverses its motion and moves from anterior to posterior (Lee 1995). Motion at this time is critical as the impact loads from heel strike must be either attenuated and/or stored as potential energy for use later in the step. The long dorsal ligament of the SIJ comes into significance at this time. As the pelvic rotation is reversed at this time, the ligament gradually becomes taut as the sacrum counternutates with posterior pelvic rotation. Failure to reach the full forward rotated position would mean that the available range of pelvic motion at heel strike would be lost. It would also create a situation in which the long dorsal ligament would be tightened prematurely, thus preventing its

gradual loading during the impact period. As double support phase completes and a new swing phase begins, the cycle of pelvic rhythm repeats again.

In summary, during normal function walking is a perpetual motion process. The active pull of the swing side provides a passive thrusting in the stance side against the ground. Pivotal motion of the hip and foot allow for the proper utilization of this power. Coordination of movement permits stabilization of the entire lower extremity/lumbosacral structure ideally suited for maximum efficiency. Cycles of stance and swing are repeated at least 2500 times per limb per day.

PATHOMECHANICAL PROCESS OF SAGITTAL PLANE BLOCKADE

Sagittal plane motion of the foot during the single support phase is critical to normal ambulation. It appears to coordinate both forward advancement with close-packing stabilization. A failure within this process would be repeated more than a million times a year. Wolfe, in the late nineteenth century proposed the axiom 'Form follows function'. This was shown to have validity by D'Arcy Thompson early in the twentieth century. It is now considered to be an absolute in understanding the reaction of the body to the stress applied to it over time. For a model of postural decay to be sound, it would therefore be logical to require that the forces applied during function would create the resultant form. It is the intent of this next section to demonstrate how failure of the sagittal plane pivotal action of the foot results in a cyclic breakdown in maintaining an erect posture and actually causes flexion deformity via a compensatory process.

The three sites of pivotal function at the foot were described earlier. The round, underside of the calcaneus, with essentially 'no moving parts', rarely fails to provide its initial pivotal action. The ankle and first MTP joints, however, are complex in their movements and, either singly or combined, can act to block normal progression.

Ankle equinus, or failure to achieve 10° of dorsiflexion while loaded, is a common pathomechanical entity. It has been shown to be an etiologic source of foot and postural pain in patients diagnosed as having it (Root et al 1977). Techniques of stretching the Achilles tendon and triceps surae complex, ankle manipulations, and even surgical intervention for lengthening have been conceived as methods to negate this pathomechanical influence. In and of itself, however, it would not impede forward progress provided that the last pivotal site, the first MTP joint, initiated its dorsiflexion motion early enough in the stance phase. It is the ability of the first MTP joint to react to the pull of the body over it which ultimately dictates the ability to advance the body over the bearing foot.

FUNCTIONAL HALLUX LIMITUS

Functional hallux limitus (Fhl) represents a complete locking of the primary sagittal plane pivotal site, the first MTP joint, strictly during all or portions of the single support phase of the gait cycle. This is true in spite of the fact that full range of motion occurs in the non-weight-bearing examination. As such, it is an entity that represents a paradox between those findings present during clinical examination and those found during function (gait). This contradiction defines Fhl. The functional abilities present during non-weight-bearing physical examination concerning range of motion are the opposite of those found during walking. Its capacity to permit forward advance-

ment while simultaneously creating close-packed alignment never materializes. The manifestations of its presence are most often visible at alternative sites that act to compensate for the failure of this joint to provide the motion necessary for forward progression. Clinically, the patient will rarely if ever exhibit symptoms of pain or swelling associated with this joint. The relationship between Fhl and more proximal postural symptoms has therefore not been readily apparent (Dananberg 1985, 1993, Wernick & Dananberg 1988) (see Fig. 21.5).

When driving a car, how hard one steps on the gas pedal is seen by the speed the car achieves. It is the motion of the automobile that serves as the manifestation of the input of power from the engine to the wheels. In walking, the bodily motions visible, for example hip extension, erect body position, knee extension, and ankle plantar flexion, are similar representations of the response to the input of power during the step. Should the site of primary sagittal plane motion be blocked at the time of maximum power input, an alteration of these movement patterns must occur. The total power input for any step (pull of the swing limb, momentum, gravity, elastic energy return) must be equal to body weight, or else speed of gait would decrease. The ensemble of energy to be dissipated is therefore quite significant. When these compensatory motions occur over a significant duration (more than 20 million

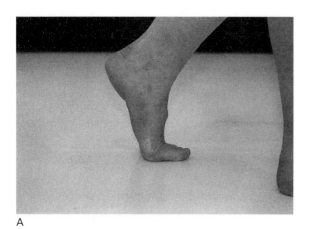 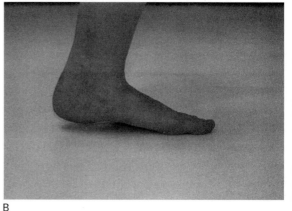

A   B

Fig. 21.5   (A) Normally, ROM of the 1st MTP joint when performed in a double support stance position. (B) During the 2nd half of the single support phase of the same foot, note the inability of the 1st MTP joint to exhibit any ROM. This paradox, that ROM of motion, while available in some positions, fails to occur during single support, defines Functional hallux limitus (Fhl).

times per decade), there is a substantial effect on postural integrity as dictated by Wolf's Law.

Clinicians are quite accustomed to seeing a variety of postural 'styles' in the course of daily practice. These may include forward head position, straight spine, round shoulders, knock knees, bow legs, abducted or adducted feet, or any combination of these 'structural' alignments. Certainly, osseous genetics plays some role in these various forms, but they also are known to worsen over time. For example, the classic appearance of a 'hunched over' elderly woman represents an age-related degeneration. The flexion deformity that she exhibits in her torso was not congenital, nor did it spontaneously occur on her eightieth birthday. Instead, there was a gradual change over a lifetime. Some mechanism (function), subtle enough to avoid obvious detection, must occur in a cyclic fashion over decades to produce this postural decay (form). The slow rate of this change and the subtle nature of the process has completely disguised it as an etiologic entity. This process in any individual's gait style can directly relate to Fhl. Although specific congenital or acute, trauma-induced changes may be etiologic for some of the classic presenting postures of chronic low back pain patients, Fhl can be partially or totally responsible and/or act as a perpetuating factor.

Foot mechanics have been known for decades to contribute to postural pain syndromes, particularly in the lower back. It has been difficult, however, accurately to connect the two processes. Excessive foot pronation was thought to contribute to alterations in pelvic position and thus create stress, but 4° or 5° of foot pronation was difficult to correlate with the magnitude of many postural deformities. Fhl is a unifying concept in understanding the relationship between foot mechanics and postural form. Since the sagittal motion required for pivotal function between the foot and supporting ground surface is 30–40° during the single support phase, the magnitude of this restriction at the foot requires compensatory action at a series of proximal sites. Excessive pronation of the medial longitudinal arch of the foot is one means by which these compensatory motions occur. Knee, hip, lumbar, and cervical spines represent additional locations at which this slow, repetitive deforming process takes place. Fhl, however, because of its asymptomatic nature and remote location, has hidden itself as an etiologic source of postural degeneration. Identifying and treating this can have a profound influence on the chronic lower back pain patient.

THE PROCESS OF SAGITTAL PLANE COMPENSATION

The elegance of the power of motion is to move the body forward efficiently through the sagittal plane. This is the process of forward walking. As the power is input for this purpose, the center of the body must advance over the planted foot. The general joint motions of the lumbar spine, hip, knee, and ankle are all in the extension direction. The MTP joints of the foot provide a dorsiflexion motion so as to permit forward advancement, while the joints above extend and maintain an erect torso. Failure of the MTP to provide this motion, at the time when the power is provided to create it, causes an immediate need for these proximal joints to 'give way' in the sagittal direction as an accommodation to this power (Fig. 21.6). This is the process of sagittal plane blockade. Tables 21.1 and 21.2 below will help in understanding the nature of this process. Table 21.1 describes the normal motion directions at the specific time they should occur. These are classified in terms of the single and double support phases of gait. This classification is clinically significant because it relates to the energy production versus energy storage process of gait. The double support phase equates with braking moments applied to the body by heel strike. This is also the period of energy storage. The single support phase applies to acceleration moments as the body advances forward during this period. This is essentially the period of energy return.

When Fhl is present, the entire period of single support phase movement is adversely affected. The ability of the joints proximal to the first MTP joint to undergo extension are directly related to the physical capacity of the first MTP joint to provide its normal range of motion. Should this pivotal action of the first MTP joint fail, the more proximal joints would now provide

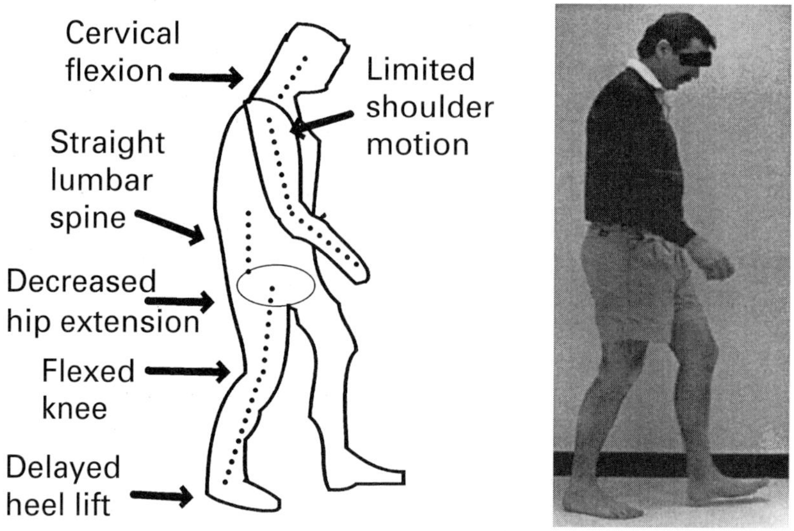

Fig. 21.6 Flexion compensation for Fhl during single support phase.

Table 21.1 Normal joint or segment motion

Joints or segments	Initial double support phase	Single support phase	Terminal double support phase
Ankle	Plantar flexion initially, then dorsiflexion	Dorsiflexion continues through heel-off, then reverses to plantar flexion	Plantar flexion to toe-off
Knee	Immediate flexion, then gradual extention	Continued movement to near-full extension	Rapid flexion to toe-off
Hip	Initial flexion, then gradual extension	Continued movement to full extension	Rapid flexion to toe-off
Pelvis	Rapid posterior rotation after heel strike	Begins at maximum posterior position and rotates anteriorly until end of single support	Rapid posterior rotation after contralateral heel strike

Table 21.2 Joint motion reversal as related to functional hallux limitus

Joints or segments	Initial double support phase	Single support phase	Terminal double support phase
Ankle	Plantar flexion initially, then dorsiflexion	Continues excessively with delay in initiating plantar flexion	Limited plantar flexion
Knee	Immediate flexion, then gradual extention	Delays or totally fails to achieve extension	Slowed flexion due to failure to achieve full extension
Hip	Initial flexion, then gradual extension	Delays or totally fails to achieve extension	Slowed flexion due to failure to achieve full extension
Pelvis	Rapid posterior rotation after heel strike	Stops anterior rotation or commences posterior rotation at midstance	Loss of posterior range of motion at heel strike

this motion. Therefore, movement will occur 180° opposed to the motion that should be taking place. For example, the thigh must extend on the hip, but failure to pivot sagittally at the foot negates the responsive hip joint motion. Flexion must replace extension as the accommodation to the power input for forward motion is now peaking. Table 21.2 above describes the motion reversals that occur. It is important to note that these motions may occur together or as individual compensatory movements.

THE EFFECT OF LIMITED HIP EXTENSION

When Fhl is present, the most evident marker is its effect on hip extension. During normal gait, the hip joint will extend approximately 15° by the end of single support phase. This action (1) permits the torso to remain erect, (2) allows for thrust against the support surface, (3) positions the limb appropriately in a position from which it can be lifted for the next swing phase, and (4) 'closes the angle' between the posterior aspect of the weight-bearing leg and the posterior aspect of the ischial tuberosity. Each of these is significant in understanding the process of lower back pain.

Facilitating an erect torso

As the thigh extends from under the torso, the rotary motion at the hip permits the lumbar spine to remain upright. Should hip motion abruptly stop, lumbar flexion occurs that creates disc compression as well as muscular overuse.

Undergoing extension for thrust

The extension of the leg and thigh permit the body efficiently to use the process of energy return to create forward motion. Failure of this motion then requires additional muscular input, resulting in fatigue.

Positioning the limb to initiate swing phase

The process for efficiently initiating the swing phase was described earlier. Should the thigh fail to extend adequately, this entire mechanism fails.

As the limb to be lifted weighs 15% of body weight, and it therefore represents a significant load on the iliopsoas structure. When the iliopsoas fires but the femur is fixed, Kapandji has shown that the lumbar spine will side-bend and rotate (Kapandji 1974). These pathomechanical actions will shear intervertebral discs and create an environment that has been shown to induce intervertebral disc herniation. Iliopsoas overuse will also produce both back and groin pain associated with this pathomechanical process.

'Closing the angle' between the weight-bearing leg and ischial tuberosity

The ability of the pelvis to rotate forward during single support was shown earlier to be related to the relaxed biceps femoris. Should hip extension fail to develop, the angle between the posterior thigh and the ischial tuberosity will instead 'open'. Torso flexion replaces hip extension, further exacerbating the situation. This will create tension in the biceps and, when sufficient, will cause Golgi tendon response and biceps firing. It will then force a premature halt of pelvic forward rotation, and if torso flexion is sufficient, pelvic rotation will reverse to an anterior-to-posterior movement. This action will create tightening of the long dorsal ligament as the reversal of motion creates a sacral counternutation. Motion which is necessary at the ensuing heel strike is prematurely exhausted. Patients with lower back pain as a rule exhibit tight hamstrings. This underlying mechanism should be noted, as the standard treatment of stretching the hamstrings will not alter the mechanics that bring about the tightness (Fig. 21.7).

THE ACCOMMODATION OF LATERAL TRUNK BENDING

When full extension of the weight-bearing limb ceases, the ability to create the following swing phase efficiently is lost. Obvious overuse to the iliopsoas results, but additional mechanisms are available to assist in developing the next swing phase motion.

A universal accommodation to this appears as the lateral trunk bend. Patients will routinely

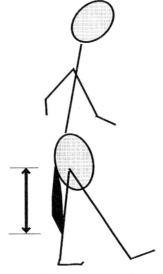

Angle between posterior leg and posterior ischial tuberosity 'opens', stressing the hamstrings

Fig. 21.7   Limited hip extension and hamstring contraction.

bend from the ipsilateral restricted side to the contralateral side at ipsilateral toe-off. This motion is generally created by two muscle groups: the contralateral quadratus lumborum and contralateral gluteus maximus/iliotibial band complex.

When activated, these structures create a lateral trunk-bending motion that 'drags' the trailing limb into the swing phase. Several pain patterns can be created by this mechanism: pain in the quadratus lumborum between the twelfth rib and iliac crest; greater trochanteric bursitis; lateral knee pain; and, owing to the quadratus lumborum's partial insertion into the iliolumbar ligament, disc compression pain related to rotation of the 5th lumbar vertebra (Dananberg 1993b).

OBJECTIVELY EVALUATING PATHOLOGIC GAIT

Completely covering gait analysis is far beyond the scope of this chapter. Specific markers will be described which can be helpful to the clinician treating the chronic lower back pain patient.

The principle of multiple viewpoints is important. When viewing X-rays of the patient, it is well known that a single view of the body is not acceptable. Generally, three views provide a far more accurate picture of a three-dimensional being. Viewing a patient walk is no different. Simply watching a subject walk back and forth in a hall-

Table 21.3   Joint motion/segment markers during multiview gait analysis

Level	Rear/front	Side	Treatment indication/option
Head	Look for left–right head tilt and timing of any tilting motion	Look for forward head posture	Consider heel lift to short side for tilting; treat Fhl for forward head posture
Shoulder/arm	Are shoulders level or does one lower during homolateral single support?	Do arms swing symmetrically; are they moving from the elbows or shoulders?	Lack of shoulder motion, particularly unilateral will usually indicate long limb functional accommodation
Pelvis/lumbosacral spine	Look for level of pelvic base; look for symmetry of rotation to left and right	Look for straight or lordotic spine; does the torso flex on the pelvis during SSP?	Elevation of ASIS/PSIS with concurrent lowering of homolateral shoulder indicates long limb function; waist flexion during SSP indicates Fhl
Hips/thigh	Not visible on rear view	Compare hip extension during SSP; asymmetry suggests leg length difference/Fhl	SSP hip extension is a critical marker. Treat for Fhl and re-examine
Knees	Varus or valgus alignment; watch for timing of internal/external rotations	Look for full extension during SSP; is this failure symmetrical?	Varus/valgus alignment indicates need for custom orthosis; lack of full extension may respond to Fhl treatment
Feet	Look for symmetry of heel lift; do the heels lift prior to contralateral heel strike?	Is Fhl visible; does the foot pronate?	Failure to raise heel during SSP indicates Fhl; unilateral presence indicates leg length unequal

SSP = single support phase; **ASIS** = anterior superior iliac spine; **PSIS** = posterior superior iliac spine.

way loses the entire sagittal plane view. Although most offices are not equipped for gait analysis, the use of a treadmill can be helpful in providing the multiple viewpoints necessary for accurate determination of cause and effect.

Table 21.3 above indicates the various levels of the body and the visible markers that would indicate a pathologic condition. Following this, a description of examination to identify Fhl will be given.

IDENTIFYING FHL

Aside from the visualization of Fhl during gait, there are two examination techniques for static recognition of this pathomechanical entity.

The first involves the patient in the seated position. For the right foot, the examiner places his or her right thumb directly under the first metatarsal head. A plantar-to-dorsal force is exerted. Then, with the left thumb placed on the underside of the great toe interphalangeal joint, a dorsiflexion force is placed on the toe. Failure to achieve 20–25° of dorsiflexion prior to resistance indicates Fhl.

The other method involves the patient standing. With the weight shifted predominately to the side to be examined, the examiner attempts to dorsiflex the great toe on the first metatarsal. A failure to raise the toe indicates Fhl (Fig. 21.8A–C).

TREATMENT OPTIONS FOR FHL

Since Fhl is a functional disorder, treatment must promote normal motion at the first MTP joint during the period in the gait cycle when this motion is required. Simply training and/or stretching muscle groups will not adequately

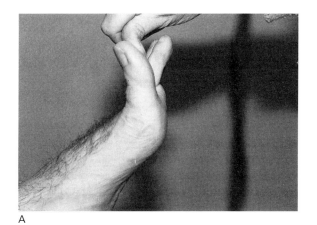

A

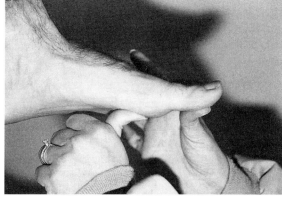

B

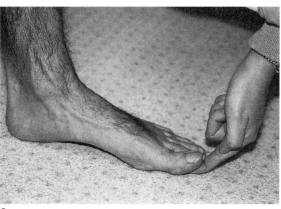

C

Fig. 21.8 (A) In the non-weight bearing analysis, ROM of the 1st MTP joint is available. (B) When examined clinically, pressure of the clinician's thumb under the 1st metatarsal head while simultaneously attempting to dorsiflex the hallux, reveals an absence of available ROM. This test is diagnostic of Fhl. (C) As an alternatively style of examination to (B), ROM of the 1st MTP joint can be examined with the patient standing on one foot. Failure to dorsiflex the 1st MTP joint 20–25° is also diagnostic of Fhl.

address this problem. Just as eyeglasses can correct a functional visual disturbance, so can functional, custom-made foot orthotic devices be effective in dealing with chronic postural complaints based on subtle gait disturbance.

The subject of custom orthotic fabrication is far beyond the scope of this chapter. Courses are available on which orthotic design and prescription writing techniques are taught. The Langer Biomechanics Group, Inc. (Deer Park, NY, USA) produces a patented, temporary orthotic device (licensed under US patents 4,597,195 and 4,608,988 and produced as Kinetic Wedge Orthotic; EPO, UK patents also apply), which is specifically designed to treat Fhl. This can be suitable as a test appliance to determine whether gait changes may be helpful to a particular patient. Accommodations for limb length difference as well as other functional aberrations can be made to this device. Actual custom orthotic fabrication is more complex than it would outwardly appear, and setting up relationships with podiatrists or others familiar with Fhl and its postural affect leads to a complete team approach to dealing with the postural pain patient.

SUMMARY

1. Viewing either recurrent acute or chronic lower back pain as a functional disorder is an advance in the current treatment process. The subtle alterations in an individual's gait when repeated over millions of cycles create overuse-type symptoms in the structures of the lumbosacral spine. The functional disorder may create abnormalities that, over sufficient time, become visible on either computerized tomography or magnetic resonance imaging. Just as often, however, the structures of the lumbosacral spine can be quite normal in appearance yet be painful in response to the cyclic stress placed upon them. The abnormal gait process causes repeated strain on the lower back by destabilizing the natural support mechanics at specific times in the gait cycle. This results is a series of mechanical inefficiencies that culminate in the failure to initiate competently the swing phase of motion. Since each limb weighs 15% of body weight, the stress load of lifting this limb improperly can be enormous

(over 20 tons per day). The cumulative burden of 'dragging a limb' into the swing phase can create the non-specific-type symptoms that are so common in the lower back pain population. These include:

- myogenic overuse symptoms of the iliopsoas group, quadratus lumborum, and gluteus maximus–iliotibial band complex
- structural symptoms at the origin of the iliopsoas (lumbar spine), insertion of the quadratus lumborum (L5 – via iliolumbar ligament), and SIJs via anatomic connection of the biceps femoris/sacrotuberous ligament.

2. The dysfunction of the foot plays a major role in preventing the body from passing over it efficiently during gait. The compensatory motions (listed below) are visible in the structures proximal to the foot, and can be thought of as 'gait markers' in observing the recurrent acute/chronic lower back pain patient:

- forward head position – cervical flexion
- straight lumbar spine – torso flexion
- decreased hip extension during single support phase
- flexed knee in midstance
- failure of heel lift during single support phase – visible foot pronation.

3. Since these can all be manifestations of asymptomatic functional aberrations at this pivotal site, examination of the biomechanics of the foot is essential in this patient population. When foot mechanics, Fhl, leg length discrepancy, and the overall style of walking were addressed as a primary stress-creating mechanism with properly fabricated custom foot orthotics, a retrospective outcome study of chronic, recurrent complaints demonstrated 77% near or complete resolution of symptoms.

CONCLUSIONS

1. Chronic or acute recurrent pain in the lower back may be related to style of gait.
2. Foot function plays a major role in gait mechanics.
3. The ability of the first MTP joint to dorsiflex during single support phase is critical.

4. Postural changes (flexion deformity of the lumbar and cervical spine) can be viewed as the form that follows the function.

5. Properly prescribed foot orthotics can be a successful measure in the long-term treatment of chronic or acute recurrent lower back pain.

REFERENCES

Abbott B C 1952 The physiological cost of negative work. Journal of Physiology 117: 380–390
Basmajian J V 1974 Muscles alive, 3rd edn. Williams & Wilkins, Baltimore
Bojsen-Møller F 1979 Calcaneocuboid joint and stability of the longitudinal arch of the foot at high and low gear push off. Journal of Anatomy 129(1): 165–176
Claeys R 1983 The analysis of ground reaction forces in pathologic gait. International Orthopaedics 7: 113–119
Dananberg H J 1986 Functional hallux limitus and its effect on normal ambulation. Journal of Current Podiatric Medicine, April
Dananberg H J 1993a Gait style as an etiology to chronic postural pain. Part I: Functional hallux limitus. Journal of the American Podiatric Medical Association 83(8): 433–441
Dananberg H J 1993b Gait style as an etiology to chronic postural pain. Part II: The postural compensatory process. Journal of the American Podiatric Medical Association 83(11): 615–624
Dananberg H J 1995 Lower extremity mechanics and their effect on lumbosacral function. Spine Review 9(2): 389–405
Dananberg H J, DiNapoli D R, Lawton M 1990 Hallux limitus and non-specific bodily trauma. In: DiNapoli D R (ed.) Reconstructive surgery of the foot. Podiatry Institute, pp 52–59
Dorman T 1995 Elastic energy of the pelvis. Spine Review 9(2): 365–379
Dorman T, Vleeming A 1995 Self locking of the sacroiliac articulation. Spine Review 9(2): 407–418
Gracovetsky S 1987 The spinal engine. Springer-Verlag, Vienna
Hicks J H 1954 The mechanics of the foot. Part II: The plantar aponeurosis and the arch. Journal of Anatomy 88: 25–30
Inman V 1981 Human walking. Williams & Wilkins, Baltimore
Kapandji I A 1974 The physiology of the joints, vol. 3, The trunk and vertebral column, 2nd edn. Churchill Livingstone, Edinburgh
Lee D 1995 Instability of the sacroiliac joint and the consequences to gait. In: Vleeming A, Mooney V, Dorman T, Snijders C (eds) Second interdisciplinary world congress of low back pain, San Diego, CA, 9–11 November, pp 471–484
Perry J 1992 Gait analysis: normal and pathologic function. Slack, Thorofare, NJ
Root M, Weed J, Orien W 1977 Abnormal and normal function of the foot. Clinical Biomechanics Corp., Los Angeles, CA
Thordarson D B 1995 Dynamic support of the human longitudinal arch. Clinical Orthopedics and Related Research 316: 165–172
Thurston A J, Harris J D 1983 Normal kinematics of the lumbar spine and pelvis. Spine 8(2): 199–205
Vleeming A, Snijders C J, Stoeckart R, Mens J M A 1995 A new light on low back pain. In: Vleeming A, Mooney V, Dorman T, Snijders C (eds) Second interdisciplinary world congress on low back pain. San Diego, CA, 9–11 November, pp 147–168
Wernick J, Dananberg H J 1988 Secondary active retrograde pronation as the ideology to overuse injuries in podiatry tracts, October. Data Trace Medical Publishers, Baltimore
Willard F 1995 The anatomy of the lumbosacral connection. Spine Review 9(2): 333–355
Winter D A, Scott S 1991 Technique for interpretation of electromyography for concentric and eccentric contractions in gait. Journal of Electromyography and Kinesiology 1(4): 263–269
Zimmermann M 1989 Pain mechanisms and mediators in osteoarthritis. Seminars in Arthritis and Rheumatism 18(4) (supplement 2): 22–29

PART II

Clinical aspects

SECTION 6

Differential diagnosis

22. Sacroiliac joint injection: pain referral mapping and arthrographic findings

J. D. Fortin   J. Pier   F. Falco

INTRODUCTION

The sacroiliac joint (SIJ) has regained interest as a primary source of low back pain (Bernard & Cassidy 1991, Brunner et al 1991, Schwarzer et al 1996, Solonen 1957, Vleeming 1989, Vleeming et al 1989). Recent studies reveal a 10–22% prevalence of SIJ dysfunction as the cause of low back pain (Bernard & Cassidy 1991, Bernard & Kirkaldy-Willis 1987, Schwarzer et al 1996). Confirming the diagnosis of SIJ dysfunction and pain, however, remains difficult. The recent use of provocative joint injections has begun to shed light on the tissue origin of low back pain (Dreyfuss et al 1994a, Fortin et al 1994a, Schwarzer et al 1994). Intra-articular SIJ injections have provided information on pain referral patterns (Fortin et al 1994b), detecting symptomatic joints in patients presenting with low back pain (Fortin & Tolchin 1993), and SIJ morphology (Fortin & Tolchin 1993). This information can now be used to improve our ability to diagnose and treat SI-related low back pain.

In the early part of the twentieth century, the SIJ was considered to be the primary structure responsible for sciatica (Brooke 1924, Goldthwaite & Osgood 1905). The enthusiasm for the SIJ as a cause of low back pain diminished following Mixter and Barr's report of the relationship between the herniated lumbar disc and back pain (Mixter & Barr 1934). Disc pathology, however, fails to explain many low back pain syndromes. The high incidence of herniated and degenerated discs noted on magnetic resonance imaging (MRI) in asymptomatic individuals promotes scepticism that discogenic and radicular pain are causally related to many presentations of low back and leg pain (Jensen et al 1994). Recent studies have focused attention on the role of the SIJ as a pain generator. The SIJ is a diarthrodial, synovial joint (Brunner et al 1991, Colachis et al 1985, Egund et al 1978, Frigerio et al 1974, Kuslich et al 1991) that has neural innervation (Solonen 1957) and is subject to mechanical stresses (Gunterbert et al 1976, Miller et al 1987, Vleeming 1989, Vleeming et al 1989, 1990) like any other joint. The fact that it can generate and radiate pain is not surprising. In fact, metabolic, inflammatory, infectious, traumatic, degenerative, and structural sources of SIJ pain have all been described (Ahlstrom et al 1990, Aprill et al 1990, Carrera et al 1981, DonTigny 1985, Fortin & Falco 1996, Kuslich et al 1991, Miskew et al 1979, Vleeming et al 1989, 1990a, 1990b). The consideration of SIJ dysfunction and pain as a cause of idiopathic low back pain has greatly improved our ability to diagnose and treat low back pain (Bernard & Cassidy 1991, Fortin et al 1994a).

The confirmation of SIJ pain has remained problematic. Imaging studies (X-ray, computerized tomography [CT], and MRI) do not demonstrate pain and therefore can not confirm whether an anatomic structure elicits pain. Clinical tests, although numerous and widely reported, have the potential for high interobserver variability and have not had a suitably high correlation with pain emanating from the SIJ (Dreyfuss et al 1994a, 1996). Likewise, predictive value as well as sensitivity and specificity of radiologic and clinical tests have not been determined for the SIJ.

Provocative analgesic injections provide an alternative approach to diagnostic confirmation and understanding pain referral patterns of somatic joints (Aprill et al 1990, Dreyfuss et al 1994a, Fortin et al 1994a, Schwarzer et al 1994). They have been used effectively to map pain referral patterns from the zygapophysial, atlanto-occipital, atlanto-axial, and now the sacroiliac (SI) joints (Dreyfuss et al 1994a, Fortin et al 1994a, Schwarzer et al 1994). The injections provide diagnostic confirmation of joint pain that has subsequently enhanced our knowledge of the anatomic origin of low back pain. The premise of diagnostic injections rests on four points:

1. determining a pain referral pattern of an anatomic structure by provoking that structure in asymptomatic individuals
2. utilizing known pain referral patterns to selectively inject anatomic structure in symptomatic patients
3. provoking a pain response concordant with a patient's typical pain pattern
4. eliminating pain with anesthetic injection.

The anatomic site of pain generation can be determined if these criteria are met with the provocative analgesic procedure.

SIJ REFERRAL PATTERNS

Until recently, there were no studies demonstrating that reproducible pain could be elicited upon stimulation of a normal SIJ. True intra-articular injections were considered difficult, and arthrography had only been described in cadavers (Bernard & Cassidy 1991, Hendrix et al 1982, Kissling 1992). The first description of SIJ injection was published in 1938 by Haldeman (Haldeman & Soto-Hall 1985) but did not gain widespread acceptance. Hendrix (Hendrix et al 1982) subsequently described the use of contrast medium to confirm intra-articular placement. In 1994 Fortin et al published the first report on pain referral maps in asymptomatic volunteers (Fortin et al 1994a).

In the study by Fortin et al (1994a), 11 subjects received a contrast injection into the right SIJ. The same SIJ was used in each patient to allow for comparison between patients. The subjects ranged in age from 21 to 47 years old. All individuals had no history of low back pain prior to the study. One subject was excused due to intolerance to provocation; therefore five men and five women were evaluated in the study.

The injection of contrast was used as the experimental stimulus in a protocol used effectively for other anatomic structures (Aprill et al 1990, Schwarzer et al 1994). the injection of contrast under fluoroscopy allows for visualization of the injection site, limiting the structures affected by injection. In this study, contrast material was injected into the SIJ until a firm endpoint was determined or extravasation of contrast was noted. A total volume of 0.8–2.0 cm^3 of injectate was instilled into each joint.

Pain upon injection of contrast can be fleeting and difficult to isolate to a specific, well-marginated area. Subsequent sensory changes rather than the initial distribution of pain can accurately represent referral patterns (Aprill et al 1990, Dwyer et al 1990, Feinstein et al 1954). The documentation of immediate pain complaints corresponds well with subsequent sensory examinations. This is consistent with previous reports that found hypesthesia induced by saline injection of deep spinal structures (Feinstein et al 1954). In a similar study of cervical facet joint injections, the area of hypesthesia corresponded to the subsequent pain referral patterns (Aprill et al 1990, Dwyer et al 1990).

The sensory diagrams compiled were grouped into three distinct categories. The first comprised six individuals who limited the distribution of sensory change to the medial buttock without further radiation. A second group of two individuals described a similar area, which was, however, extended to include the lateral aspect of the buttock and greater trochanter. Finally, two subjects further extended the area of sensory changes into the superior lateral thigh. Compiling the areas common to the entire group produced a pain referral map. This area was an approximate 3 × 10 cm area just inferolateral to the posterior superior iliac spine (PSIS) (Fig. 22.1). Based on the data gathered from this study, however, further radiation may occur (Fortin et al 1994a).

a blow to the lateral aspect of the pelvic ring; and a fall in a hole with one leg in the hole and the other extended outside (Fortin 1993). The diagnosis is further supported if the patient points to an area of pain just inferomedial to the PSIS, which is indicative of pain emanating from the SIJ. This exercise, described by the authors as the Fortin Finger Test, has been correlated with provocation position injections (Fortin & Falco 1996) and substantiated in an independent study (Dreyfuss et al 1996). All patients with suspect presentations should have the necessary laboratory and radiological work-up to exclude spondyloarthropathy, metabolic, or infectious causes of SIJ pain.

There are many clinical tests commonly employed during the physical examination to evaluate the SIJ. Aberrant motion can be tested with the seated flexion, standing flexion, or Gillet's test (Bernard & Cassidy 1991, Mitchell et al 1979). Patrick's or Gaenslen's maneuvers are used to detect ipsilateral SIJ pain (Bernard & Cassidy 1991, Bernard & Kirkaldy-Willis 1987). Tenderness over the ipsilateral SIJ, sacrotuberous ligament, piriformis muscle, and pubic symphysis can all implicate SIJ dysfunction (Fortin 1993, Solonen 1957, Vleeming 1989).

Screening imaging modalities such as bone and CT scanning may prove helpful (Goldberg et al 1978, Lawson et al 1982, Resnick et al 1975); however, studies have not yet confirmed their utility. A radionuclide scan may reflect misleading or indiscernible metabolic changes (Fortin et al 1994b), and asymmetric radioisotope uptake has not been a credible clinical indicator. Mild degenerative changes of the SIJ on CT scanning is a common sign in patients over 30 years of age (Resnick et al 1975). Characteristic morphological changes, however, can develop in response to stress (Vleeming et al 1990a, 1990b). Subtle CT changes, such as asymmetric joint width or sacral torsion, can manifest a greater clinical significance in the overall clinical context (Fortin 1993).

Diagnostic confirmation is attained when symptoms are reproduced upon distention of the joint capsule by provocative injection and subsequently abated with an analgesic block (Aprill et al 1990, Dreyfuss et al 1996, Dwyer et al 1990, Fortin et al 1994a, 1994b, Schwarzer et al

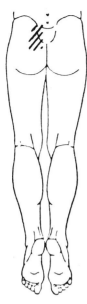

Fig. 22.1 SIJ pain referral composite map used for part II of the study design. (Reproduced with permission from Fortin et al 1994a.)

Much of the confusion regarding the diagnosis of SIJ dysfunction revolves around the inability to separate SIJ pain from pain originating from surrounding structures. Discogenic and facet pathology can have a clinical presentation similar to that of SIJ pathology. Not only are the pain distributions similar, but the clinical tests used in diagnosis are also well known to stress surrounding structures (Bernard & Cassidy 1991). Accordingly, this study was designed to cause pain in asymptomatic volunteers with no history of low back pain. The pain referred was therefore isolated to one specific structure, the right SIJ. The pain diagram generated can subsequently be utilized in the clinical setting.

DIAGNOSTIC CONSIDERATIONS

While the SIJ syndrome has gained acceptance, confirming the diagnosis can be difficult. SIJ syndrome is first suspected when a patient presents with a consistent mechanism of injury. Common mechanisms include: a direct fall on the buttock; a rear-end motor vehicle accident, with the ipsilateral foot on the brake at the moment of impact; a broadside motor vehicle accident, with

1994). The ligamentous integrity of the joint can be established arthrographically.

Because diagnostic injections are invasive, the procedure should be reserved for patients who fulfil the profile for a painful SIJ and who have failed to respond to aggressive functional restoration. Injections can also be helpful in patients who have reached a plateau in therapy (Dreyfuss & Michaelsen 1995). In these cases, SIJ injection can provide diagnostic affirmation as well as possible therapeutic benefit.

RADIOLOGIC EQUIPMENT AND MATERIALS

SIJ injections at or above the level of the PSIS are commonly performed as routine office procedures without the advantage of image intensifier control (Bernard & Cassidy 1991). These injections most probably result in ligamentous or subligamentous deposit of solutions owing to the thickness of the dorsal SI and interosseous ligaments as well as the tortuous opposing surfaces of the medial iliac wing and dorsal sacrum (Kissling 1992). Even at the relatively accessible inferior portion of the joint, a 'blind' injection is unlikely to find its way to the joint space. The needle is likely to be deflected by the irregular and convoluted joint surface or slip off the posterolateral margin of the iliac bone.

Fluoroscopic control is essential to ensure an intra-articular injection. Suitable equipment options include a routine fluoroscopy suite with an overhead tower or C-arm, a special procedures suite with a C-arm or angio unit, or an operating room with a C-arm. The C-arm has the advantage of allowing for adjustment of the X-ray beam without moving the patient.

A standard 25-gauge 3.5 in spinal needle with or without local anesthetic infiltration can be used in most cases. Skin and subcutaneous anesthetization with 1% lidocaine is recommended for larger-diameter needles. The tensile strength of a 22-gauge needle is occasionally necessary for narrow and tortuous joints. Rarely, a 6 in needle is required for larger individuals.

Luer-Lok 3 ml syringes allow the greatest sensitivity to change in resistance at the needle hub. Larger syringes require substantially greater pressure to inject, even without obstruction.

Contrast medium is used for needle position verification, provocation, and arthrography. Nonionic contrast agents are routinely used because they are less allergenic and irritating than are their ionic counterparts. A concentration of 240–300 mg/ml is recommended to ensure visualization of the arthrogram under fluoroscopy.

THE PROCEDURE

The patient is sterilely prepped and draped in the prone position (Fig. 22.2). Under image intensifier control, a 25- or 22-gauge 3.5 in spinal needle is directed into the inferior aspect of the SIJ using a posterior approach. The usual portal of entry is the inferior third of the joint. There is often a lucency in the inferior aspect of the joint that allows the least resistance upon needle passage.

There are usually two 'limbs' of the joint owing to the oblique orientation of the joint from posteromedial to anterolateral. The medial or posterior 'limb' is the site of cannulation. Rolling the patient or rotating the C-arm obliquely by 5–10° allows the technician a better three-dimensional perspective of the joint to select the 'window' for optimal needle trajectory. A small radiolucent zone in the inferior aspect of the joint is often visualized and is used as a target point for needle placement (Fig. 22.3A). A direct posterior approach

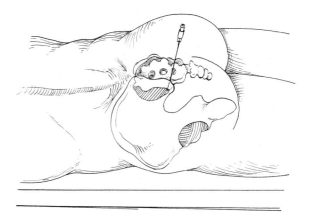

Fig. 22.2 SIJ injection. The patient is in a prone position and the needle has been guided into the inferior aspect of the joint using a direct posterior approach. (Reproduced with permission from Fortin 1995.)

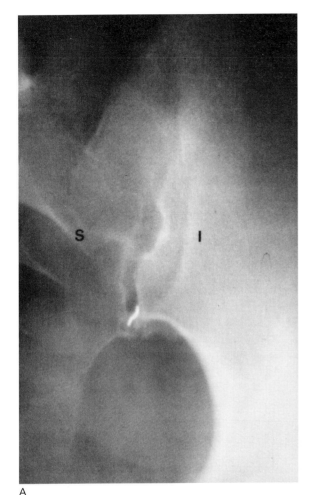

A

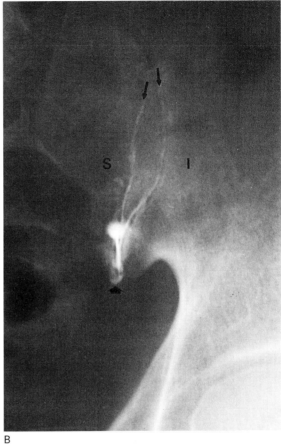

B

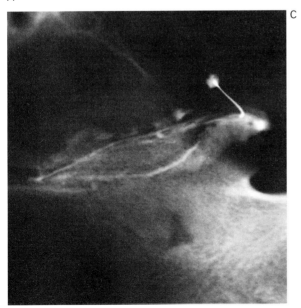

C

Fig. 22.3 SIJ arthrography. (A) Preinjection spot film documents the needle, with a characteristic bend, within the inferior aspect of the joint. Note the lucent area around the needle. (B) AP arthrogram of the right SIJ. Divergent joint surfaces appear as distinct beads of contrast (*arrows*) or 'separate' joint cavities. A 25-gauge $3\frac{1}{2}$-inch spinal needle is in the inferior aspect of the joint. Arrowhead, coin-shaped inferior recess; S, sacrum; I, ilium. (C) Oblique view of the right SIJ (LAO). This '*en face*' view delineates the auricular shape of the synovial joint (arrowheads). 4, pedicle of L4; 5, pedicle of L5; 1, pedicle of S1; arrow, diverticulum.

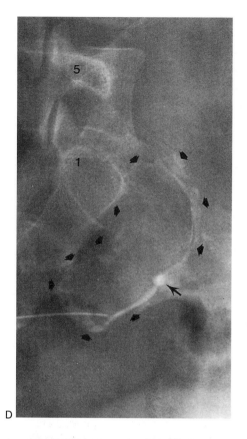

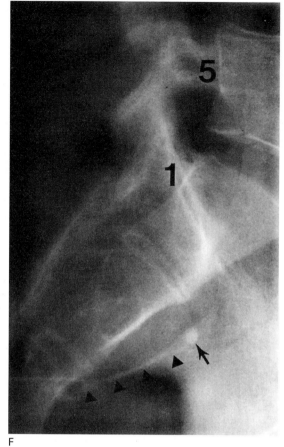

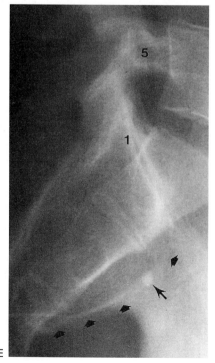

Fig. 22.3 (*Contd*) (D) 'Opposite' oblique view (LAO) of a left SIJ arthrogram. (E) Opposite oblique arthrogram (RAO) contiguously demarcates the vertical extent of the joint space. (F) Lateral view of the right SIJ capsular margin. The ventral capsular border is outlined by contrast medium (arrowhead). 5, pedicle of L5; 1, pedicle of S1; arrow, diverticulum.) (Reproduced with permission from Fortin 1995.)

can be used in most cases. Once the dorsal SI and interosseous ligaments are engaged, the needle often takes a characteristic bend as it conforms to the interdigitating contours of the diarthrodial joint. This phenomenon is often preceded by a subtle tactile sensation of a 'giving way' at the needle hub as the needle purchases and penetrates through the ligaments overlying the joint.

If bony resistance is met after the ligaments are engaged and the needle is not yet within the joint margin, the needle should be withdrawn slightly without becoming disengaged from the ligaments. Subsequent needle advancement while simultaneously rotating it around its own longitudinal axis will allow it to deflect and conform to the joint margins. The initial instillation of a small amount of contrast material should outline the coin-shaped inferior recess of the joint. This landmark on the anteroposterior (AP) projection (Fig. 22.3B) together with the auricular shape of the diarthrodial joint (as noted on the oblique view) (Fig. 22.3C) should allow definitive evaluation of proper needle position.

Following verification of initial needle position, additional contrast is instilled to a volume commensurate with firm endpoint or fluoroscopically visualized extravasation. Provocation responses are recorded at this time, followed by the administration of anesthesia. If arthrographic resolution is diluted by anesthesia, 0.2–0.4 ml additional contrast material will serve to enhance the image.

PROVOCATION/ANALGESIA RESPONSES

Provocation

Provocation of pain in a 'familiar' or 'unfamiliar' distribution can occur and should be recorded at the time of injection. Usual patterns include buttock, groin, and posterior thigh radiation. Occasionally, low back pain, anterior thigh pain, and radiation of pain below the knee in a L5–S1 distribution will occur. Although pain provocation alone has been used to confirm a positive test (Fortin et al 1994b), other studies utilize pain provocation and post-block anesthesia to indicate a positive response (Dreyfuss et al 1996, Schwarzer

et al 1994, 1996). If pain provocation is used as the sole criterion, the disparity between an asymptomatic 'pressure pain' upon injection must be distinguished from the 'intense, stabbing and concordant pain' seen in symptomatic joints.

Analgesia

Following a provocation positive injection, 0.6–2.0 ml anesthetic (2.0% lidocaine, 0.75% bupivacaine) is instilled into the joint. This can be incorporated in a 2 : 1 mixture of a long-acting corticosteroid such as betamethasone (Celestone). Volumes are small (less than 2.0 ml contrast material and anesthetic combined), commensurate with the joint's capacity. This ensures a focal anesthetic effect (i.e. a limited dispersal to adjacent structures). In a recent examination of 74 SIJ injections, the mean volume of contrast injected was 1.08 ml (standard deviation 0.29 ml) (Fortin & Tolchin 1993).

Patients should be evaluated 15–45 min after the injection (depending on the anesthetic agent) to determine the anesthetic response to injection. Visual analog scales or the percentage relief are commonly used to assess the anesthetic response. Positive anesthetic responses should result in at least a 75% reduction in pain (Schwarzer et al 1994, 1996).

POSTPROCEDURAL CARE

Patients are observed for 30–45 min following the procedure. Vital signs are obtained and the patients can be given fluids. If an arthrography/CT scan is indicated, the patient is transported to the CT scan within 1–2 h of injection.

Postprocedural instructions include education on the application of ice to the affected area and information on the usual postprocedural symptoms, such as increased local pain and/or stiffness. Occasionally, a 2-day supply of narcotic analgesics is judiciously dispensed. Driving, manual labor, and sports are discouraged on the day of the procedure. Physical therapy and even manipulation have been used on the day of the procedure to 'facilitate' mobilization (Dreyfuss & Michaelsen 1995). Care must be taken in these instances as an anesthetized joint is more prone to injury. Most patients resume their usual activities within 24 h. An instruction sheet provides emergency phone numbers and details the warning signs of infection. Patients may be safely discharged 30–60 min after the procedure. Physician follow-up should be within 1–2 weeks.

PLAIN FILM EVALUATION

The AP view demonstrates the inferior recess of the SIJ with contrast in the joint margins and any subligamentous or inferior recess extension (Figs. 22.3B, 22.4A, 22.5A). The oblique (*en face*) view is essential to precisely delineate the joint borders (Figs 22.3C, 22.4C). This view will reveal diverticula and ventral capsular tears. The lateral view also demonstrates posterior subligamentous or ligamentous extravasation, diverticula, or ventral tears (Fig. 22.3F). If bilateral arthrograms are obtained, an offset lateral (10–20° from a true lateral projection) will allow one to compare both capsular borders on the film (Fig. 22.4D). As a result of beam attenuation in the lateral projection, the ventral tears or diverticula are not as sharply resolved as in the *en face* view. At times, the opposite oblique view can add additional information, including a clear view of the contrast within the superior joint space, superior recess extravasation, outline of diverticula, and reaffirmation of extravasation from the inferior recess or anteroinferior capsule (Figs 22.3D, and 22.4).

UTILITY OF SI PROVOCATION ANALGESIA

The use of SIJ injections has begun to enhance our ability to diagnose the origin of 'mechanical low back pain'. Fortin et al were able to confirm SI joint pain in patients preselected from a group of 54 consecutive low back pain patients by using the pain diagram outlined in Fig. 22.1 above (Fortin et al 1994b). Provocative SI injections were positive in all 16 patients selected by the concordant pain diagram. Under expanded criteria for positive provocative analgesia (Schwarzer et al 1994) (positive provocative injection plus post-block anesthesia), 10 out of 16 patients were confirmed as having SIJ pain.

In a separate study, Schwarzer et al (1996) used SIJ provocation and postarthrography CT to confirm SI pain in 13 out of 43 patients who presented with pain unilaterally below L5–S1. There was a weak but statistically significant correlation between SI ventral capsular tears and the relief of pain upon anesthetization of the joint. In this study, the only pain pattern that correlated with successful provocation and post-block anesthesia was groin pain. No other pain distribution significantly correlated with confirmed SIJ pain.

In a recent study, Dreyfuss et al (1996) evaluated common SIJ provocative maneuvers and pain diagrams with provocation analgesic blocks of the SIJ. No physical examination maneuver was able consistently to predict a positive response to analgesic block. The Fortin Finger Test demonstrated a high specificity yet a low sensitivity. Although Laslett and Williams (1994) were able to show good inter-rater reliability of physical examination provocation tests, these have yet to be positively correlated with provocation analgesic blocks. In the study by Dreyfuss et al (1996), a composite of pain diagrams from patients with positive provocative analgesic blocks revealed a wide distribution of pain patterns. Pain diagrams predominantly started unilaterally below L5–S1 and extended down the posterior aspect of the leg, often below the knee. The cause of pain radiating below the knee (beyond that noted in asymptomatic volunteers) must be explored. A similar finding was reported by Mooney and Robertson (1976) when they compared pain patterns from intra-articular lumbar facet injections in asymptomatic and symptomatic volunteers. Possible hypotheses for referred SI pain may be extended when the arthrographic patterns of the joint are scrutinized under arthrography/CT.

PLAIN FILM AND CT ARTHROGRAPHIC FINDINGS

The arthrographic pattern of contrast medium spread can be determined following provocative injection of the SIJ. The morphologic characteristics of 74 SIJ arthrograms were recently

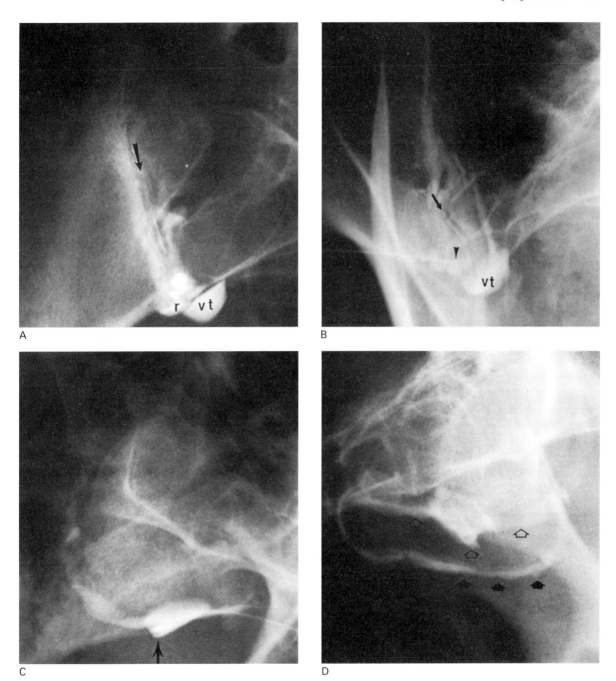

Fig. 22.4   The patient is a 37-year-old housewife whose motor vehicle was hit in the rear while her left foot was planted firmly on the brake. She presented with left hip, thigh, and groin pain. With the lumbosacral plexus immediately anterior to the SIJ, these findings may help to explain the lower extremity symptoms in some patients with SIJ pain. (A) An AP arthrogram. r, inferior recess; vt, collection of contrast escaping through a ventral tear, arrow, bead of contrast within joint margins. (B) Opposite oblique: confirms that the needle tip (arrowhead) is remote to the ventral tear (vt). Arrow, bead of contrast is within joint space. (C) Oblique view: smooth line of contrast medium outlining the capsular margins (arrow) is interrupted by an anterior capsular and anterior SI ligamentous rent. (D) Offset lateral: bilateral arthrogram discloses an intact right ventral capsule (closed arrowheads) in contrast to disrupted left capsule (open arrowheads).

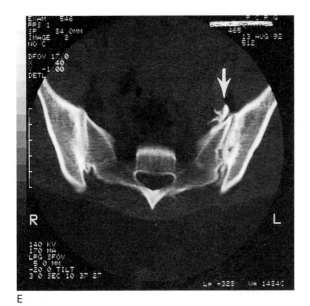

E

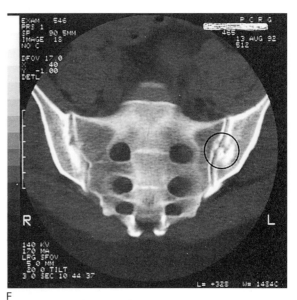

F

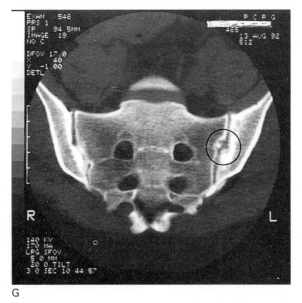

G

Fig. 22.4 (*Contd*) (E) Postarthrography axial CT at the proximal S2 level (bone window/level settings). Contrast medium is present within both SIJs. A presacral collection of contrast medium is clearly noted, evidencing a ventral tear (arrow). Contrast solution contacts the lumbosacral plexus elements. (F, G) Two coronal views through the SIJ joint in the same patient. Note the area of joint margin cortical irregularity on the left. These changes are similar to those of osteochondritis dissecans commonly seen in appendicular joints. The opposing areas of bony prominence on the iliac (most remarkable) and sacral surfaces suggest a partially detached subchondral fragment with a surrounding lucent area and adjacent iliac sclerosis (areas encircled). This combination of eburnation, macroporosity, and sclerosis may be the osseous footprints of stress hardening as a result of trauma. Similar changes may be occurring on the right to a lesser extent. (Reproduced with permission from Fortin 1995.)

described by Fortin and Tolchin (1993). They compared the findings of plain film arthrograms with postarthrography/CT. After scoring anterior, posterior, superior, and inferior aspects of the capsule, they found a significant correlation between the data recorded from each modality. Both plain film and CT arthrography, however, have specific diagnostic benefit. The plain film displays diverticula optimally and postarthrography/CT is superior in evaluating anterior capsular 'pathology'.

As with any other joint, SIJ arthrographic findings are very diverse. A variety of anterior capsular morphology has been disclosed, from discrete attenuated areas and schisms to frank tears. Diverticula have been isolated from all parts of the capsule and can vary in size, shape, and number. Attempts to determine the clinical significance of each of these findings needs further investigation.

Arthrographic findings also reveal three potential pathways of communication between the SIJ and the neural elements (Fortin & Tolchin 1993). These include (1) posterior subligamentous extension into the dorsal sacral foramina (Fig. 22.5), (2) superior recess extravasation at the alar level into the L5 epiradicular sheath (Fig. 22.6), and (3) leakage from a ventral tear to the lumbosacral plexus (see Fig. 22.4 above). Extravasation of inflammatory mediators from a dysfunctional SIJ to adjacent neural tissues may explain the radicular complaints of some patients and the varied pain patterns seen in previous studies. Electrodiagnostic correlation is needed; however, anecdotal cases of impaired nerve function in patients with SIJ pain have been observed (Fortin & Tolchin 1993).

The relevance of arthrographic findings, as they pertain to patient care, must still be established. At present, we are resigned to extrapolate findings on SIJ arthrography to what is 'normal' and 'abnormal' in other joints. For example, a full-thickness ligamentous tear often renders a joint unstable. In a weight-bearing joint, such instability is manifest as:

- intermittent and often 'painful' sounds, such as clicking, popping, grinding, or clunking
- sudden 'giving way',

- a sense of apprehension or being 'off-balance'
- an inability to bear weight fully on the affected side
- the inability to load the joint in a manner that stresses the involved structure.

As seen with patients with knee meniscal tears, these symptoms in a patient with a ventral capsular tear of the SIJ may be clinically significant. Conversely, asymptomatic patients may have incidental capsular tears of the SIJ that do not affect the clinical presentation.

SUMMARY

Imaging modalities provide detailed anatomic information but can not reveal whether or not these anatomic abnormalities are responsible for presenting pain complaints. Likewise, clinical evaluation has difficulty isolating positive and negative findings to specific tissue structures. Provocative examination maneuvers may stress multiple structures and pain may be localized or referred. Provocative analgesia with injections, therefore, remains the only direct method to distinguish symptomatic from asymptomatic joints. This has confirmed the SIJ as a pain generator in many presentations of low back pain (Fortin et al 1994, Schwarzer et al 1996).

Although provocation analgesic blocks have increased our understanding of spine pain, there are many questions that remain regarding these injections. Multiple pain generators, insufficient anesthetic block, diffusion of anesthesia away from primary site of injection, and unmasking secondary pain generators may all confound the results of provocation analgesia. An inflamed and irritated anatomic structure should be uniformly anesthetized post-injection; however, this is not always the case. A 'double block paradigm' (Schwarzer et al 1994), in which lidocaine and Marcaine are alternately used and the duration of pain relief is recorded, is an attractive means of increasing specificity, but the lack of uniform relief from this approach brings into question its validity. Pain relief frequently lasts longer than the duration of the local anesthetic even without steroid in the mixture. Further investigation is therefore needed fully to comprehend the mech-

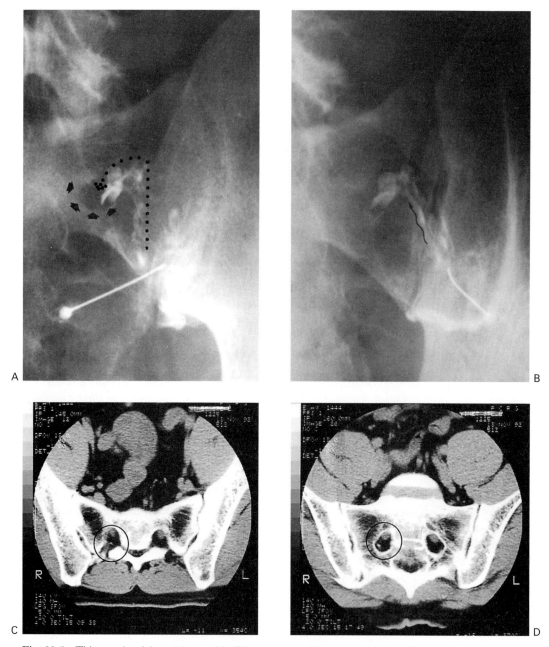

Fig. 22.5 This case, involving a 33-year-old offshore worker with a prolonged right H-reflex (on electrodiagnostics), illustrates a third arthrographic link between the SIJ and neural elements. Posterior subligamentous extension of contrast medium into the S1 dorsal foramina (arrowheads) is shown on the right, (A) AP arthrogram. Contrast medium from the joint margins into the S1 dorsal foramina (wavy arrow). (C–D) Axial and direct coronal postarthrography CT through the S1 dorsal foramina (soft tissue window settings). Contrast is visualized in the S1 dorsal foramina on both scans (areas encircled). Arrowheads, contralateral S1 anterior ramus. (Reproduced with permission from Fortin 1995.)

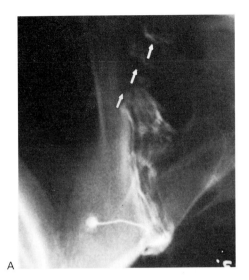

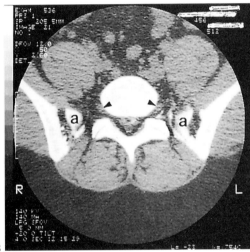

Fig. 22.6   Another putative pathway between the SIJ and the neural elements is visualized in this case of a 19-year-old clerk with a pain diagram suggestive of a left L5-radiculopathy. (A) Posteroanterior arthrogram demonstrates contrast medium extravasating from the superior recess (arrows). (B) Postarthrography axial CT at the level of L5–S1. Contrast medium has extended from the superior recess to the L5 epiradicular sheath at the alar level. a, sacral ala; arrowheads, anterior rami of L5. (Reproduced with permission from Fortin 1995.)

anism of action and the clinical results of provocation analgesia.

Improved understanding of SIJ anatomic morphology and neurophysiology may expand

our use of provocation analgesia. Future cadaveric studies may be able to discern the maturational capsular changes of the SIJ, allowing a perspective for viewing arthrographic data. Neurophysiologic investigations may hold answers to questions regarding the nerve fiber endings within the SIJ capsule and whether or not torn capsules lead to the release of inflammatory mediators. These findings will hopefully lend credence to the basis of provocative injections and help explain referred pain.

This is an exciting time in the diagnostic realm of the SIJ. Research utilizing provocative injections and diagnostic radiology, with therapeutic exercise and manual therapy, promise to expand our knowledge of SIJ dysfunction and pain. Treating practitioners will apply this research and assist patients previously believed to represent 'non-diagnostic' low back pain.

CONCLUSIONS

1. Imaging studies can not determine whether the SIJ or any anatomical structure is a pain generator.

2. Although physical examination does not correlate well with a symptomatic SIJ, the Fortin Finger Test and the use of a pain referral map can help identify those that are more likely to have pain emanating from the SIJ.

3. SIJ intra-articular injections can consistently be performed under fluoroscopic guidance.

4. Provocation analgesic injections reliably identify whether or not the SIJ is a pain generator.

5. Plain X-rays are best to evaluate for diverticula of the SIJ capsule whereas postarthrography-CT is superior to evaluate for anterior capsular pathology.

6. The relevance of SIJ pathology detected by plain films and postarthrography-CT requires further investigation.

7. Further studies are required to elicit the mechanism of action for provocation analgesic injections.

REFERENCES

Ahlstrom H, Feltelius N, Nyman R, Hallgren R 1990 Magnetic resonance imaging of sacroiliac joint inflammation. Arthritis and Rheumatism 33: 1763–1769

April C, Dwyer A, Bogduk N 1990 Cervical zygapophyseal joint pain patterns. II: A clinical evaluation. Spine 15: 458–461

Bakalim G 1966 Results of radical evacuation and arthrodesis in sacroiliac tuberculosis. Acta Orthopaedica Scandinavica 37: 375–386

Bernard T N, Cassidy J D 1991 Sacroiliac joint syndrome: pathophysiology, diagnosis and management. In: Frymoyer J W (ed.) The adult spine, vol. 2. Raven Press, New York, pp 2107–2131

Bernard T N, Kirkaldy-Willis W H 1987 Recognizing specific characteristics of non-specific low back pain. Clinical Orthopaedics 217: 266–280

Brooke R 1924 The sacroiliac joint. Journal of Anatomy 58: 299–305

Brunner C H, Kissling R O, Jacob H A C 1991 The effects of morphology and histopathology on the mobility of the sacroiliac joint. Spine 16: 1111–1117

Carrera G F, Foley W D, Kozin F et al 1981 CT of sacroiliitis. American Journal of Radiology 136: 41–46

Colachis S C, Worden R E, Bechtol C D et al 1985 Movement of the sacroiliac joint in the adult male. A preliminary report. Archives of Physical Medicine and Rehabilitation 44: 491–498

DonTigny R 1985 Function and pathomechanics of the sacroiliac joint. Physical Therapy 65: 35–44

Dreyfuss P, Michaelsen M, Horne M 1995 MUJA: Manipulation under joint anesthesia/analgesia. In: Vleeming A, Mooney V, Dorman T, Snijders C (eds) Second interdisciplinary world congress on low back pain. San Diego, CA, 9–11 November, pp 599–621

Dreyfuss P, Dryer S, Griffin J, Hoffman J, Walsh N 1994a Positive sacroiliac screening tests in asymptomatic adults. Spine 19(10): 1138–1143

Dreyfuss P, Tibiletti C, Dreyer S J 1994b Thoracic zygapophyseal joint pain patterns: a study in normal volunteers. Spine 19(7): 807–811

Dreyfuss P, Michaelsen M, Pauza K, McLarty J, Bogduk N 1996 The value of history and physical examination in diagnosing sacroiliac joint pain: a prospective study. Spine (in press)

Dunn E J, Byron D M, Nugent J T 1976 Pyogenic infections of the sacroiliac joint. Clinical Orthopaedics 118: 113–117

Dwyer A, April C, Bogduk N 1990 Cervical zygapophyseal joint pain patterns. I: A study in normal volunteers. Spine 15: 453–457

Egund N, Olsson T H, Schmid H et al 1978 Movements in the sacroiliac joint demonstrated with roentgenstereophotogrammetry. Acta Radiologica Diagnosis 19: 833–944

Feinstein B, Langton J N K, Janeson R M, Schiller F 1954 Experiments on pain referred from deep somatic tissues. Journal of Bone and Joint Surgery (US) 36: 981–997

Fortin J D 1993 The sacroiliac joint: a new perspective. Journal of Back and Musculoskeletal Rehabilitation 3(3): 31–43

Fortin J D 1995 Sacroiliac joint injection and arthrography with imaging correlation. In: Leonard T (ed.) Physiatric procedures in clinical practice. Hanley & Belfus, Philadelphia

Fortin J D, Falco F 1996 Enigmatic causes of spine pain in athletes. In: Fortin J D, Falco F, Jacob H (eds) Functional biomechanics and rehabilitation of sports injuries. Hanley & Belfus, Philadelphia (in press)

Fortin J D, Tolchin R 1993 Sacroiliac arthrograms and postarthrography CT. Archive of Physical Medicine and Rehabilitation 74: 1259

Fortin J D, Dwyer A, West S, Pier J 1994a Sacroiliac joint pain referral patterns upon application of a new injection/arthrography technique. I: Asymptomatic volunteers. Spine 19(13): 1475–1482

Fortin J D, Dwyer A, April C, Ponthieux B, Pier J 1994b Sacroiliac joint pain referral patterns. II: Clinical evaluation. Spine 19(13): 1483–1489

Frigerio N A, Stowe R R, Howe J W 1974 Movement of the sacroiliac joint. Clinical Orthopaedics 100: 370–377

Goldberg R P, Genant H K, Shimshak R, et al 1978 Applications and limitation of quantitative sacroiliac joint scintigraphy. Radiology 128: 683–686

Goldthwaite G E, Osgood R B 1905 A consideration of the pelvic articulations from an anatomical, pathological, and clinical standpoint. Boston Medical Surgeon Journal 152: 593–601

Greenman P E 1990 Clinical aspects of sacroiliac function in walking. Journal of Manual Medicine 5: 125–129

Grieve E 1981 Lumbopelvic rhythm and mechanical dysfunction of the sacroiliac joint. Physiotherapy 67: 171–173

Gunterbert B, Romanus B, Stener B 1976 Pelvic strength after major amputation of the sacrum. An experimental approach. Acta Orthopaedica Scandinavica 47: 635–642

Haldeman K O, Soto-Hall R A 1985 The diagnosis and treatment of sacroiliac condition by the injection of Procan. Journal of Bone and Joint Surgery (US) 67: 675–685

Hendrix R W, Lin P P, Kane B J 1982 Simplified aspiration or injection technique for the sacroiliac joint. Journal of Bone and Joint Surgery (US) 64: 1249–1252

Jensen M C, Brant-Zawadzki M N, Obuchowski N, Modic M T, Malkasian D, Ross J S 1994 Magnetic resonance imaging of the lumbar spine in people without back pain. New England Journal of Medicine 331(2): 69–73

Kissling R O 1992 Zur arthrographie des iliosacralgelenks. Zeitschrift fur Rheumatologie 51: 183–187

Kuslich S D, Ulstrom C L, Michael C J 1991 The tissue origin of low back pain and sciatica. Orthopedic Clinics of North America 22: 181–187

Laslett M, Williams M 1994 The reliability of selected pain provocation tests for sacroiliac joint pathology. Spine 19(11): 1243–1249

Lawson T L, Foley W D, Carrera G F, et al 1982 The sacroiliac joint: anatomic plain roentgenographic and computed tomographic analysis. Journal of Computer Assisted Tomography 6: 307–314

Mierau D 1992 Scintigraphic analysis of sacroiliac pain. Scientific program of the 7th annual meeting of the North American Spine Society

Miller J A A, Schultz A M, Anderson G B J 1987 Load-displacement behavior of sacroiliac joints. Journal of Orthopaedic Research 5: 92–101

Miskew D B, Block R A, Witt P F 1979 Aspiration of infected sacroiliac joints. Journal of Bone and Joint Surgery (US) 61: 1591–1597

Mitchell S L, Moran P S, Pruzzo N A 1979 An evaluation and treatment manual of osteopathic muscle energy procedures. Mitchell, Moran and Pruzzo, Manchester, MO

Mixter W J, Barr J S 1934 Rupture of the intervertebral disc with involvement of the spinal canal. New England Journal of Medicine 211: 210–215

Mooney V, Robertson J 1976 The facet syndrome. Clinical Orthopaedics and Related Research 115: 149–156

Norman G F, May A 1956 Sacroiliac conditions simulating intervertebral disc syndrome. Western Journal of Surgery 64: 461–462

Pitkin H C, Pheasant H C 1936 Sacrarthrogenetic telalgi. II: A study of sacral mobility. Journal of Bone and Joint Surgery 18: 365–374

Resnick E, Niwayama G, Georgen T G 1975 Degenerative disease of the sacroiliac joint. Investigative Radiology 10: 608–621

Schwarzer A C, Aprill C N, Derby R, Fortin J, Kine G, Bogduk N 1994 Clinical features of patients with pain stemming from the lumbar zygapophyseal joints. Spine 19: 1132–1137

Schwarzer A C, Aprill C N, Bogduk N 1996 The sacroiliac joint in chronic low back pain. Spine (in press)

Solonen K A 1957 The sacroiliac joint in the light of anatomical, roentgenological and clinical studies. Acta Orthopaedica Scandinavica (supplement) 27: 1–27

Vleeming A, van Wingerden J-P, Snijders C J, Stoeckart R, Stijnen T 1989 Load application to the sacrotuberous ligaments. Influences on sacroiliac joint mechanics. Clinical Biomechanics 4(4): 204–209

Vleeming A, Stoeckart T R, Snijders C J 1989 The sacrotuberous ligament: a conceptual approach to its dynamic role in stabilizing the sacroiliac joint. Clinical Biomechanics 4(4): 201–203

Vleeming A, Stoeckart R, Volkers A C W, Snijders C J 1990a Relation between form and function in the sacroiliac joint. I: Clinical anatomical aspects. Spine 15: 130–132

Vleeming A, Volkers A C W, Snijders C J, Stoeckart R 1990b Relation between form and function in the sacroiliac joint. II: Biomechanical aspects. Spine 15: 133–135

23. Pain provocation sacroiliac joint tests: reliability and prevalence

M. Laslett

INTRODUCTION

In spite of extensive research over recent years, the true cause of most episodes of low back pain is still unknown, although precipitating events are often clear. It is a complex undertaking to identify causes of pain in the low back region in that most of the structures and tissues found in the low back, hip, and pelvis are capable of producing symptoms. Thus it becomes a constant clinical challenge to make an anatomically accurate diagnosis. The sacroiliac joint (SIJ) is richly innervated by nociceptor receptors and is capable of producing pain (Bernard & Cassidy 1991, Fortin et al 1994). However, it is not known whether the SIJ does in fact contribute to common low back pain syndromes.

DIAGNOSTIC TESTS

The diagnostic value of tests may be assessed by research on interexaminer reliability, sensitivity and specificity. This process begins with interexaminer reliability: the consistency with which two independent examiners can arrive at the same conclusion when applying the same test to the same patient. If different examiners fail to agree on the result of a test, no agreement can be reached about a diagnosis based on that test.

One statistic, the kappa coefficient (Cohen 1960) effectively discounts the proportion of agreement that is expected by chance. This is important where tests give positive/negative results since there is a 50% chance of agreement were the examiners to make purely random judgements. The kappa coefficient ranges in value from -1 to $+1$, where positive values signify agreement better

Table 23.1 Guidelines of Landis and Koch (1977) for interpretation of the strength of agreement for the kappa statistic (K)

K	Strength of agreement
0.0–0.20	Slight
0.21–0.40	Fair
0.41–0.60	Moderate
0.61–0.80	Substantial
0.81–1.00	Almost perfect

than chance, a value of 0 denotes agreement no better than chance, and negative values signify agreement worse than chance. Landis and Koch (1977) have suggested guidelines for interpretation of the strength of agreement for the kappa statistic (Table 23.1).

Once acceptable interexaminer reliability of a test has been demonstrated, its ability to detect pathology has to be measured. The accuracy of a test is determined by measures of sensitivity and specificity. The sensitivity of a test is the proportion of cases with the pathology that test positive. The specificity of a test is the proportion of cases without the pathology that test negative (Nachemson 1992). If the test too frequently positively identifies pathology in patients without disease, these false positives invalidate the test because of poor specificity. If the test too frequently fails to identify the presence of pathology in patients with the disease, these false negatives invalidate the test because of poor sensitivity. Ideally, tests that have high levels of interexaminer reliability, sensitivity, and specificity should be chosen as clinical diagnostic tests.

TESTS OF MOBILITY OR POSITION USING MANUAL PALPATION

For a variety of reasons, palpation tests have been

shown to possess low levels of interexaminer reliability, in spite of claims to the contrary. For example, acceptable interexaminer reliability has been claimed for the Gillet motion palpation procedure, reporting 60% agreement between examiners (Herzog et al 1988, 1989). Percentage agreement is frequently reported as a measure of interexaminer reliability, but its use has limited utility in that it fails to compensate for agreements expected on the basis of chance alone. The kappa statistic was not reported in that study.

Cibulka et al (1988) claim to be able to detect SIJ dysfunction reliably using palpation tests to assess innominate tilt. Although these workers report a high level of interexaminer reliability (kappa = 0.88), their claim arises not from the analysis of individual tests but from the combined results of four different assessments. Patients were deemed to have SIJ dysfunction if three out of four tests were positive. Since kappa values for the individual tests were not reported, reliabilities for each separate test cannot be determined.

More recently, in a study of 45 patients using experienced manual therapy physicians, it was observed that interexaminer reliability of six commonly used palpation tests was fair, and in some cases worse than that which could be expected by chance (van Duersen et al 1990). The maximum kappa value achieved was 0.38, which is rated as slight agreement according to the criteria of Landis and Koch. Dreyfuss et al (1992) cast further doubt on palpation tests on assessment of the specificity of the Gillet, standing flexion, and seated flexion palpation tests. They found that 20% of asymptomatic individuals had false positive tests, and questioned the use of these tests in diagnosis.

The work of Potter and Rothstein (1985) on interexaminer reliability for selected clinical tests of the SIJ is probably the most widely quoted work in this area. Using therapists experienced in orthopaedic manual therapy and SIJ examination, these authors examined 13 tests of function on 17 patients and found that agreement fell below 70% in 11 tests that used palpation, leading the authors to classify them as unreliable. The kappa statistic was not reported.

The use of palpation to detect small variations of movement or position as a method of detecting SIJ pathology has significant inherent limitations.

It has poor interexaminer unreliability, produces high levels of false positives in an asymptomatic population and lacks specificity (Dreyfuss et al 1992, Potter & Rothstein 1985). Even if excessive or restricted movement could be reliably detected, no causal connection between an increased or decreased range of motion and the patient's symptoms has ever been identified. On the contrary, Sturesson et al (1989) have indicated that there is no significant difference in range of movement between the painful and non-painful sides in patients with unilateral low back pain who had been identified as possibly having SIJ pathology.

Until a causal relationship between low back pain syndromes and asymmetries of form, position or movement is established, such tests are at best experimental. In the same way that standard X-rays, computerized tomography (CT) and magnetic resonance imaging (MRI) scans do not in themselves demonstrate that observed anomalies are the sources of pain (Nachemson 1992), palpation tests of form, position, and mobility do not indicate the anatomic source of pain. Unfortunately, the popularity of these procedures far outweighs their validation and utility.

PAIN PROVOCATION TESTS

There are many tests that are used to detect SIJ pathology. Tests that mechanically stress the SIJ structures in order to reproduce the patient's pain may be called pain provocation tests. These tests do not claim to determine range of motion, position, or movement behaviour of the joints. Instead, these pain provocation SIJ (PPSIJ) tests aim to determine whether the SIJ is an anatomic source of pain, i.e. is a pain generator.

On the other hand, pain provocation tests have better potential as diagnostic tools since the symptoms that lead the patient to seek help are being used to indicate positivity or negativity of the tests. The results of research into the reliability of pain provocation tests are mixed. In one study, some provocation tests (distraction, compression, the Maitland test, pain on hip flexion, and pain on resisted hip external rotation) were shown to be unreliable (McCombe et al 1989). However, Östgaard et al (1992) have demonstrated that one PPSIJ test has high interexaminer reliability,

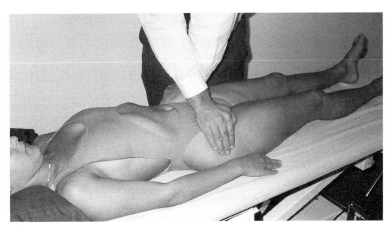

Fig. 23.1 Distraction or the 'gapping' test.

sensitivity, and specificity to a condition they call posterior pelvic syndrome, and is potentially useful for diagnostic purposes.

One recent study sought to determine the inter-examiner reliability of a selection of commonly used PPSIJ tests (Laslett & Williams 1994). In this study, 51 patients experiencing unilateral low back or buttock pain with or without radiation below the knee were examined. The following data were collected for each patient: age, sex, pain location using a pain drawing, and duration of symptoms.

The sacroiliac (SI) tests employed were:

1. *Distraction or the 'gapping' test.* This test applies pressure to both anterior superior iliac spines directed posteriorly and laterally, allegedly to stretch the anterior SI ligaments (Fig. 23.1).

2. *Compression.* This test compresses the pelvis with a pressure applied to the uppermost iliac crest, directed towards the opposite iliac crest. It allegedly stretches the posterior SI ligaments or compresses the anterior part of the SIJ (Fig. 23.2).

3. *Posterior shear or 'thigh thrust' test.* This test applies a posterior shearing stress to the SIJ through the femur. Excessive adduction of the hip is avoided since flexion and adduction combined are normally uncomfortable or painful (Fig. 23.3).

4. *Pelvic torsion, right posterior rotation* (sometimes called Gaenslen's test). Posterior rotation of the right ilium on the sacrum is achieved by flexion of the right hip and knee and simultaneous left

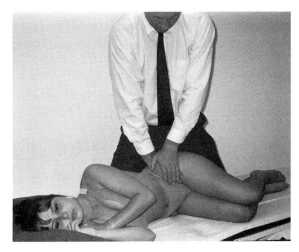

Fig. 23.2 Compresson test.

hip extension. Overpressure is applied to force the SIJ to its end range (Fig. 23.4).

5. *Pelvic torsion, left posterior rotation* (Gaenslen's test). Posterior rotation of the left ilium on the sacrum is achieved by flexion of the left hip and knee and simultaneous right hip extension. Overpressure is applied to force the SIJ to its end range (Fig. 23.5).

6. *Sacral thrust.* A pressure is applied directly to the sacrum while the patient lies prone. The force is directed anteriorly against the ilia, which are fixed against the examining couch (Fig. 23.6).

7. *Cranial shear test.* This test consists of a pressure applied to the coccygeal end of the sacrum,

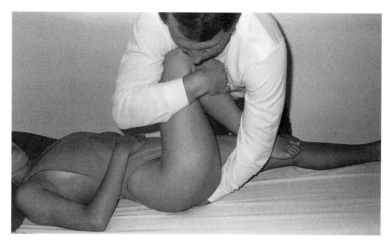

Fig. 23.3   Posterior shear or 'thigh thrust' test.

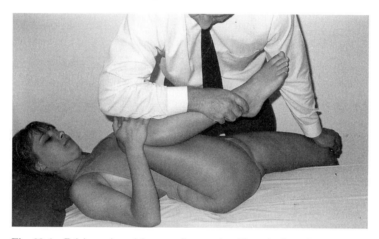

Fig. 23.4   Pelvic torsion, right posterior rotation (Gaenslen's test).

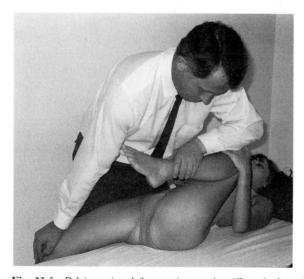

Fig. 23.5   Pelvic torsion, left posterior rotation (Gaenslen's test).

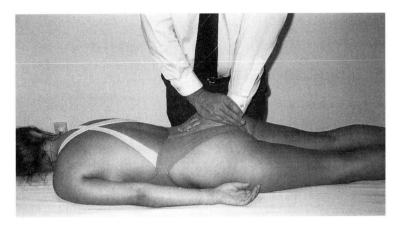

Fig. 23.6   Sacral thrust test.

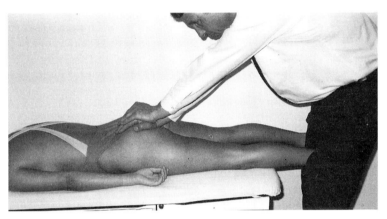

Fig. 23.7   Cranial shear test.

directed cranially. The ilium is held immobile through the hip joint as the examiner holds the leg firmly with a counterpressure in the form of a traction force directed caudad (Fig. 23.7).

Two examiners each performed all seven pain provocation tests on each patient. The second examiner was blinded to the results of the first examiner. A test was considered positive if one or more symptoms indicated on the pain drawing were aggravated or produced during the test.

The ordering of the seven tests for each patient and each examination session was randomized according to a computer-generated random number sequence. Such randomization was undertaken to control for sequencing or order effects.

For each SIJ test, the percentage agreement between examiners, the kappa agreement coefficient (*K*), and its standard error were calculated.

Results

Fifty-one patients (28 females and 23 males) with a mean age of 39.5 ± 13.4 years participated in the study. Patients had experienced their symptoms for a median duration of 60 days (range 1 day to 17.5 years). Twenty-three patients had pain in the low back/buttock area only, 12 had pain radiating to the knee, and 16 had pain radiating below the knee.

Table 23.2 shows the percentage agreement, kappa coefficients, their standard errors, and significance tests.

The percentages of positive signs obtained for each test by the first and second examiners are presented in Table 23.3.

The reliability of the SIJ tests for the total dataset (51 patients examined by one of five pairs of examiners), is presented in Table 23.2 below. Employing the criteria of Landis and Koch (1977),

Table 23.2 Interexaminer agreement for SIJ provocation tests for all patients ($n = 51$), showing kappa agreement coefficients (K), standard errors of the mean (SE) and statistical significance (p) (Reproduced with permission from Laslett & Williams 1994.)

SIJ test	Agreement %	K	SE	p
1. Distraction	88.2	0.69	0.12	< 0.001
2. Compression	88.2	0.73	0.10	< 0.001
3. Sacral thrust	78.0	0.52	0.13	< 0.001
4. Thigh thrust	94.1	0.88	0.07	< 0.001
5. Pelvic torsion (R)	88.2	0.75	0.09	< 0.001
6. Pelvic torsion (L)	88.2	0.72	0.11	< 0.001
7. Cranial shear	84.3	0.61	0.13	< 0.001

Table 23.3 Percentage of positive signs for SIJ pain provocation tests ($n = 51$) (Reproduced with permission from Laslett & Williams 1994.)

SIJ test	Examiner 1 %	Examiner 2 %
1. Distraction	27.5	23.5
2. Compression	35.3	27.5
3. Sacral thrust	34.0	36.0
4. Thigh thrust	43.1	45.1
5. Pelvic torsion (R)	37.3	41.2
6. Pelvic torsion (L)	27.5	31.4
7. Cranial shear	27.5	27.5

all tests used in this study are moderately reliable or better. The cranial shear and sacral thrust tests had the lowest kappa values (0.61 and 0.52 respectively). In a separate calculation based on a smaller subset of patients seen by two of the five examiners who saw 43% of the patients, the kappa value fell to 0.31 and 0.32 for sacral thrust and cranial shear tests respectively. The poorer performance of these two tests may be the result of the manual pressure applied to the sacral region. Tenderness in this area is common in low back syndromes and may have confused patients and examiners.

The findings confirm the reliability of the distraction and compression tests as suggested by Potter and Rothstein (1985) and also establish the reliability of the pelvic torsion and thigh thrust pain provocation tests. The sacral thrust and cranial glide tests are at least potentially reliable.

It is notable that McCombe et al (1989) report poor reliability for distraction and compression when the results from examinations performed by an orthopaedic surgeon are compared with the results from examinations performed by a physio-therapist. This poor reliability may have resulted from differences in technique of examination which, in the Laslett & Williams (1994) study, were minimized through employment of several training sessions.

While it seems reasonable that therapists should not rely on single tests for SIJ problems, only tests which have proven individual interexaminer reliability should be selected for diagnostic purposes. Furthermore, while tests may demonstrate good interexaminer reliability, this does not provide evidence for their validity. While further studies are required to assess the sensitivity and specificity of reliable tests, some work in this area has been completed. Östgaard et al (1992), in a blinded study of 72 pregnant women, found that concordance between the subjective complaint of pain and a positive pain provocation similar to the 'thigh thrust' test (see Fig. 23.3 above) was 81%. Positive and negative prediction values were 70% and 88% respectively. Sensitivity was 81% and specificity 80%.

PREVALENCE OF SIJ PAIN

The prevalence of the SIJ as a primary source of pain ranges from an extreme position claiming that 98% of common low back pain is caused by SI dysfunction (Shaw 1992) to outright scepticism (Nachemson 1992). Many standard texts on the subject of low back pain treat the SIJ as so unimportant that discussion on differential diagnosis fails even to mention the SIJ as a potential source of pain (Laros 1991). This 'invisibility' of SIJ pain is not uncommon.

Using a mixture of tests, including PPSIJ tests, Bernard and Cassidy (1991) estimated that the SIJ was the primary source of low back pain in 22.5% of 1293 patients. Using three PPSIJ tests for diagnosis, Cyriax (1975) stated that only 1 in 230, or 0.43%, of patients with lumbogluteal symptoms had the SIJ as the primary source of pain. Using pain provocation arthrography in 43 out of 100 chronic low back pain patients whose pain was centered below L5–S1, Schwarzer et al (1995a) estimated that between 13% and 30% had pain of SIJ origin.

Prevalence of the positive PPSIJ tests described by Laslett and Williams (1994) has been assessed.

Table 23.4 Percentage positives for each SIJ test ($n = 202$)

Test	Number positive	Percentage positive
1. Distraction	39	19.3
2. Compression	31	15.3
3. Sacral Thrust	68	33.7
4. Thigh thrust		
Right	43	21.3
Left	38	18.8
Both	19	9.4
Either	81	40.1
5. Pelvic torsion (R)	36	17.8
6. Pelvic torsion (L)	30	14.9
7. Cranial shear	30	14.9

In a study that is complete and in preparation for publication, Laslett and Grant (1996) have applied these seven PPSIJ tests to 202 chronic (mean duration of symptoms 85.3 weeks) low back pain patients to assess the prevalence of each positive test. The percentage of low back patients with positive tests ranged from 14.9% for cranial glide to 33.7% for sacral thrust tests. Values for each test are presented in Table 23.4. Sixty per cent of the low back pain population had at least one test positive. These PPSIJ tests stress structures other than the SIJ, and false positives are common. In an attempt to remove this area of confusion, a variety of other pain provocation tests were applied in order that the lumbar spine and hip joint could be assessed as potential pain generators. These tests included:

1. The dynamic mechanical evaluation of McKenzie (McKenzie 1981). This assessment evaluates the effect that repeated movements and sustained positions have on the intensity, frequency, and location of spinal pain. At the fourth McKenzie International Conference, Aprill presented preliminary evidence that McKenzie's conceptual model of disc pathology can predict the presence of symptomatic internal disc disruption (Aprill et al 1995). An important component of the evaluation is the recognition and use of the centralization sign (Donelson et al 1990, Long 1996). Cases identified as lumbar spine pathology by this method were considered non-SIJ in origin.

2. The 'spring' test was applied to L5, L4, L3, L2, and L1. This test applies an anteriorly directed pressure to the spinous process, and the pain response is recorded. If familiar pain was reproduced, a lumbar source of pain was presumed.

3. Passive medial rotation and abduction, and resisted lateral rotation of the hip, was performed to assess the possible involvement of the hip joint or piriformis muscle as pain generators. If these tests provoked the pain, the case was considered non-SIJ in origin.

4. Acute lumbar scoliosis or lateral shift cases are considered non-SIJ causes of pain since these are regarded as highly predictive of lumbar disc pathology (Porter & Miller 1986).

When all cases that were judged likely to have non-SIJ sources of pain were removed, only 17.3% had at least one test positive. My clinical experience mirrors that of others (Cibulka et al 1988) in that the diagnosis of painful SIJ pathology should only be made when at least three and preferably four of the PPSIJ tests are positive. If this criterion is applied, the SIJs are pain generators in 3.5–6.5% of this low back pain population.

DIAGNOSIS OF PAINFUL SIJ DISEASE

Using the PPSIJ tests as the foundation for building a clinical diagnosis of painful SIJ disease has potential. Validation of the specificity and sensitivity of these tests awaits appropriate research. In a recent study presented at the 1995 International Spinal Injection Society, Dreyfuss et al (1992) have tested four out of the seven PPSIJ tests and found them to be unable to predict familiar PPSIJ arthrography. In this study, no single item in the clinical history or physical examination could predict a positive or negative pain provocation arthrogram. This raises the question of whether the pain provocation arthrogram stimulates the same sensitive structures as the pain provocation stress tests. It may be argued that the arthrogram's stimulation is restricted to intra-articular tissues possessing nociceptor receptors, and capsular ligaments. In contrast, the pain provocation tests probably additionally stimulate extra-articular ligaments, yet perhaps do not stimulate much of the intra-articular structures at all. There is probably some overlap between the two forms of mechanical loading, but a failure of the PPSIJ tests to predict arthrogram outcomes may actually indicate that the different methods may be specific to different structures related to the SIJ.

CONCLUSIONS

1. The manual pain provocation tests of the SIJ described by Laslett and Williams (1994) are reliable and regularly provoke familiar symptoms in low back pain patients.

2. While 60% of chronic low back pain patients may have at least one PPSIJ test positive, only 3.5–6.5% are likely to have symptoms produced by a pain generator associated with the SIJ provided at least three positive tests are used as a minimum diagnostic criterion. Further research is needed to assess the sensitivity and specificity of this minimum criterion.

3. Where there is a lack of skilled image-intensifier-guided provocation injection facilities, and on the basis of the established interexaminer reliability of the PPSIJ tests, it is reasonable to propose the following criteria for stating that a SIJ is a pain generator:

a. Three but preferably four PPSIJ tests must provoke at least one of the symptoms that led the patient to seek medical advice.

b. Where other clearly defined pathologies, such as impingement of a spinal nerve, internal disc disruption (Schwartzer et al 1995b), neurogenic claudication, or symptomatic hip disease, are present, the SIJ is not considered a pain generator unless independent tests indicate SIJ disease. Independent indications of SIJ disease might include a pelvic fracture, septic arthritis, or an established diagnosis of ankylosing spondylitis with positive evidence of sacroiliitis visible on X-rays.

c. Evidence of lumbar spine pathology is absent or equivocal. I use a comprehensive McKenzie dynamic mechanical evaluation with repeated movements and positions for this purpose, with special emphasis on achieving centralization of the symptoms above the L5 level. If I am able to produce centralization above this level, a lumbar spine pathology is the likely pain generator.

d. There is no acute lateral shift (lumbar scoliosis).

REFERENCES

Aprill C, Medcalf R, Grant W 1995 Discographic outcomes predicted by the centralisation of pain and directional preference. Fourth McKenzie International Conference, Cambridge University, 19–22 October

Bernard T N, Cassidy J D 1991 The SIJ syndrome: pathophysiology, diagnosis, and management. In: Frymoyer J W (ed.) The adult spine: principles and practice. Raven Press, New York, pp 2107–2130

Cibulka M T, Delitto A, Koldehoff R M 1988 Changes in innominate tilt after manipulation of the sacro-iliac joint in patients with low back pain. An experimental study. Physical Therapy 68(9): 1359–1363

Cohen J 1960 A coefficient of agreement for nominal scales. Educational and Psychological Measurement 20: 37–46

Cyriax J 1975 Textbook of orthopaedic medicine, vol. 1, Diagnosis of soft tissue lesions, 6th edn. Baillière Tindall, London

Donelson R, Murphy K, Silva G 1990 Centralization phenomenon: its usefulness in evaluating and treating referred pain. Spine 15(3): 211–213

Dreyfuss P, Dreyer S, Griffin J, Hoffman J, Walsh N 1992 Positive sacro-iliac screening tests in asymptomatic adults: a prospective, blinded study. Poster presentation. In: Vleeming A, Mooney V, Snijders C J, Dorman T (eds) First interdisciplinary world congress on low back pain and its relation to the sacroiliac joint. San Diego, CA, 5–6 November, p II

Fortin J D, Dwyer A P, West S, Pier J (1994) Sacro-iliac joint pain referral maps upon applying a new injection/athrography technique. 1: Asymptomatic volunteers. Spine 19: 1475–1482

Herzog W, Nigg B M, Read L J 1988 Quantifying the effects of spinal manipulations on gait using patients with low back pain. Journal of Manipulative and Physiological Therapeutics 11(3): 151–157

Herzog W, Read L J, Conway P J, Shaw L D, McEwen MC 1989 Reliability of motion palpation procedures to detect sacro-iliac joint fixations. Journal of Manipulative and Physiological Therapeutics 12(2): 86–92

Landis R J, Koch G G 1977 The measurement of observer agreement for categorical data. Biometrics 33: 159–174

Laros G S 1991 Differential diagnosis of low back pain. In: Mayer T G, Mooney V, Gatchel R J (eds) Contemporary conservative care for painful spinal disorders. Lea & Febiger, Philadelphia, pp 122–130

Laslett M, Grant W 1996 The frequency of pain provocation tests of the sacroiliac joint in a back pain population (in preparation)

Laslett M, Williams W 1994 The reliability of selected pain provocation tests for sacroiliac joint pathology. Spine 19(11): 1243–1249

Long A L 1996 The centralisation phenomenon: its usefulness as a predictor of outcome in conservative treatment of chronic low back pain (a pilot study). Spine 20(23): 2513–2521

McCombe P F, Fairbank J C T, Cockersole B C, Pynsent P B 1989 Reproducibility of physical signs in low-back pain. Spine 14(9): 908–918

McKenzie R A 1981 The Lumbar Spine 1981 Mechanical diagnosis and therapy. Spinal Publications, Waikanae, New Zealand

Nachemson A L 1992 Newest knowledge of low back pain: a critical look. Clinical Orthopedics and Related Research 279: 407–410

Östgaard H C, Zetherström G, Roos-Hansson E, Svansberg B 1992 The posterior pelvic pain provocation test in pregnant women. In: Vleeming A, Mooney V, Snijders C J, Dorman T (eds) First interdisciplinary world congress on low back pain and its relation to the sacroiliac joint. San Diego, CA, 5–6 November, p V

Porter R W, Miller C G 1986 Back pain and trunk list. Spine 11(6): 596–600

Potter N A, Rothstein J M 1985 Intertester reliability for selected clinical tests of the sacro-iliac joint. Physical Therapy 65(11): 1671–1675

Schwarzer A C, Aprill C N, Bogduk N 1995a The sacroiliac joint in chronic low back pain. Spine 20: 31–37

Schwarzer A C, Aprill C N, Derby R, Fortin J, Kine G, Bogduk N 1995b The prevalence and clinical features of internal disc disruption in patients with chronic low back pain. Spine 20: 1878–1883

Shaw J L 1992 The role of the sacroiliac joint as a cause of low back pain and dysfunction. In: Vleeming A, Mooney V, Snijders C J, Dorman T (eds) First interdisciplinary world congress on low back pain and its relation to the sacroiliac joint. San Diego, CA, 5–6 November, pp 67–80

Sturesson B, Selvik G, Uden A 1989 Movements of the sacro-iliac joints: a Roentgen stereophotogrammetric analysis. Spine 14(2): 162–165

van Duersen L L J M, Patijn J, Ockhuysen A L, Vortman B J 1990 The value of some clinical tests of the sacro-iliac joint. Manual Medicine 5: 96–99

24. Measurement of sacroiliac joint stiffness with color Doppler imaging and the importance of asymmetric stiffness in sacroiliac pathology

H. M. Buyruk   H. J. Stam   C. J. Snijders   A. Vleeming
J. S. Laméris   W. P. J. Holland

INTRODUCTION

Low back pain is a very common complaint causing restrictions in the activities of daily living (Kelsey & White 1980). In the literature on low back pain, many possible causes are reported. It is commonly stated that low back pain is the result of spinal disorders, in particular internal or external disc hernias or lesions of the apophyseal joints. Idiopathic low back pain is described as a painful condition without diagnosed pathology such as lumbar disc hernias or spondylolisthesis. Although routine physical examinations (Hoppenfeld 1976; range of motion and other special tests) and laboratory investigations (Murray et al 1990; radiography, computerized tomography [CT], and magnetic resonance imaging [MRI]) provide information about the pathology of the lumbar spine, these techniques do not contribute to the understanding of abnormal pelvic biomechanics. Recently, a new theory has been introduced (Snijders et al 1993a, 1993b), according to which pelvic instability might play an important role in the development of low back pain. Pelvic instability is directly related to sacroiliac joint (SIJ) stiffness. There are different theories about the causes of hyper- and hypomobility in the SIJ. The restoration of SIJ stability can be delayed temporarily or permanently after childbirth (Snijders et al 1984). Pelvic instability during and after pregnancy has been described as a cause of peripartum pelvic pain (PPPP) (Mens et al 1996). In PPPP, the pain can be diminished in most cases with the application of a simple pelvic belt. In previous human specimen studies, the influence of such a pelvic belt on SIJ mobility has

been shown (Vleeming et al 1992). In that study, a custom-made belt was used. Therefore, in vivo assessment and follow-up of the SIJ stiffness during pregnancy is important.

Imaging techniques such as X-ray, CT, or MRI are useful for the diagnosis of pathology that may cause secondary SI instability, such as tumors or cysts. These static imaging techniques, however, cannot provide information on the stiffness levels of the SI joint.

In vivo assessment of the stiffness of pelvic joints remains a problem in clinical practice. In clinics, pain provocation tests of SIJ stiffness are done in several ways, such as using the Patrick or Fabere, Gaenslen, and pelvic rock tests (Hoppenfeld 1976). However, these methods are unreliable and subjective. The outcome depends entirely on the experience and skills of the observer. Furthermore, test results are not expressed as numeric data (Carmichael 1987, Mior et al 1990).

The need for a reliable and non-invasive assessment of SIJ stiffness initiated the question of whether a measuring technique could be developed to quantify SIJ mobility with the use of vibration. Such an approach has been reported on bones by Cunningham et al (1990). Testing the stiffness of materials with vibration was applied to the examination of bone stiffness and fracture healing. In traumatology, the healing stage of fractured bones has been tested with the signals generated by vibration and received by accelerometers. Such dynamic testing with excitation could possibly also be used for assessment of the stiffness of the SIJ. We hypothesized that the transmission of the vibrations through the SIJ would be proportional to joint stiffness.

A theoretical model for the description of the dynamic behavior of the different pelvic structures would be too complex. Therefore, a mechanical model that mimicked pelvic geometry was chosen, in which the effect of excitations in different directions could be measured by accelerometers (Buyruk et al 1996a). This approach allowed for reproducible measurements with the desired stiffness of the pelvic joints as the only parameter. The mechanical behavior of this mechanical model could be described by a multiple viscoelastic system (Fig. 24.1) simulating a patient in the prone position. During the transmission of vibration by these viscoelastic systems, change in stiffness affected the amplitude and shifted the peak point of the wave in time. From these in vitro laboratory experiments, it was concluded that vibrations can deliver information for accurate discrimination of stiffness levels of SIJ in frequencies without resonance. A foreseeable problem for the application of this technique in vivo was the registration of vibration using accelerometers because the SIJ is covered with thick ligament, muscle, fat, and skin layers. This diverted our choice to color Doppler imaging (CDI).

CDI, a combination of conventional gray-scale imaging and color Doppler ultrasound, is one of the major recent developments in medical imaging.

The clinical use of this apparatus has been restricted to blood flow examinations. Some of the combined Doppler apparatuses, such as Philips Quantum ADI (Philips Ultrasound Inc., Santa Ana, CA, USA), are sensitive to the vibrations under its transducer. This equipment can discriminate and quantify the amplitude of vibrations at different tissue sites and depths. The reaction of such an apparatus to vibrated soft tissues was studied earlier to identify tumors in liver and bladder (Parker & Lerner 1992). This technique is described in the literature as measurement of sonoelasticity or mechanical palpation. We called it Doppler imaging of vibrations (DIV).

To validate whether a testing method using vibrations and DIV would give reproducible and valid outcomes for SIJ stiffness measurements, we designed three studies: first, an in vitro study with 4 embalmed human pelvises; second, a study on 14 healthy subjects; and third, a comparative clinical study with 59 patients with PPPP and 45 healthy subjects.

STUDY ON EMBALMED HUMAN SPECIMENS

Stiffness measurements (Buyruk et al 1995a) were performed bilaterally on the SIJ of four embalmed

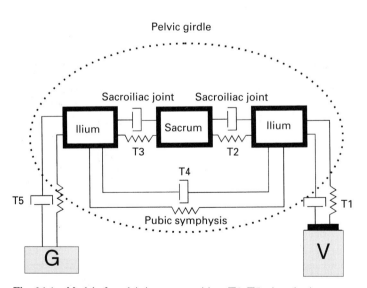

Fig. 24.1 Model of a pelvis in prone position. T1–T5, viscoelastic systems; M1–M3, masses; G, ground; V, vibrator. (Reproduced from Buyruk et al 1995a.)

female human specimens, of an age range 92–97 years. Pelvises were resected from L4 to mid-femur level, keeping all the superficial layers intact. To mimic the masses of the legs and trunk, 4 kg of metal masses were connected to metal rods, which were placed in the medulla of the femur and spinal canal and fixed with epoxy resin.

Vibrations were generated by a Derritron VP3 vibrator with a frequency range between 1.4 and 20 000 Hz and with variable output possibilities. A CDI scan, Philips Quantum ADI (Angio Dynagraph 1), was used to produce the DIV images. In all pelvises, the vibrations were applied unilaterally to the anterior superior iliac spine (ASIS). Since the angle between the vibration excitation direction and ultrasound propagation should be 0° for maximum Doppler shift, the excitations were received on the skin by a 7.5 MHz CDI transducer positioned perpendicularly on the dorsal region of the SIJ (Fig. 24.2). Before the examination, posterior superior iliac spines (PSISs) and sacral segments were marked on the skin for orientation points. For further evaluation, the DIV images were digitally recorded on the video, implemented in the apparatus.

Two pelvises were used to gain experience with the technique and to determine the optimal vibration frequencies. For further experiments,

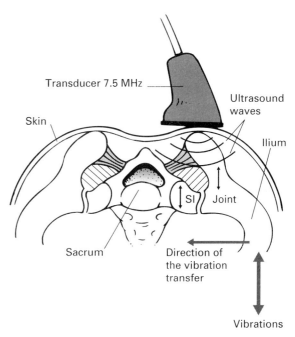

Fig. 24.2   Experimental set-up showing the direction of excitation of the pelvis resulting in vibrations picked up at both sides of the SIJ by a color Doppler ultrasound transducer. (Reproduced from Buyruk et al 1995a.)

we selected 200 Hz. The DIV images obtained from the sacroiliac (SI) region (Fig. 24.3) were evaluated for homogeneity of distribution of Doppler pixels, alternating Doppler threshold

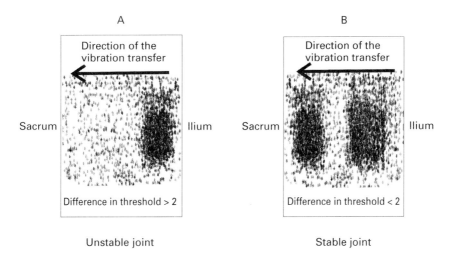

Fig. 24.3   Doppler densities obtained with different stiffnesses. (A) Unstiff (hypermobile) joint; no color Doppler pixels at the sacrum. (B) Stiff (hypomobile) joint, with high transmission of vibrations; Doppler pixels at both bones. (Reproduced from Buyruk et al 1995a.)

levels with different outputs, and superposition of grey scale image with Doppler effect.

Procedure for quantification of the DIV

The SI region was scanned (ilium and sacrum simultaneously). The vibrations propagate with a spheric distribution in the pelvis up to the SIJ area. These vibrations are picked up as moving reflectors by the CDI transducer, which covers both sides of one SIJ (see Fig. 24.2 above). The intensities of the vibration pixels of the sacrum and ilium appear simultaneously on the monitor at high threshold values. The threshold indicates the necessary signal power to display in color as motion. When the energy of the Doppler signal received back from the vibrating sacrum and ilium exceeds a certain level, these structures are displayed in red and blue on the CDI monitor. Below this level, conventional gray-scale B-mode images are displayed. The height of the level can freely be set by the operator by means of the threshold button present on the control panel of the CDI apparatus. Using the threshold button allows one to perform comparative vibrating energy measurements between the sacrum and ilium as follows. First, a threshold level is found at which the DIV of the vibrating sacrum disappears and changes to gray-scale. At the next step, a second threshold level is found for the ilium. Threshold unit is without dimensions, but the threshold levels are directly related to the vibration energies of the bone. A large difference between the threshold levels of the sacrum and ilium indicates a large loss of energy through the SIJ, which means an unstable joint. A small, or non-existent, difference is an indirect indication of a stiff SIJ.

Two pelvises were used for SIJ stiffness quantification. DIV of the sacrum and ilium was measured at three SIJ stiffness conditions: unaltered, artificially fixed, and artificially unstabilized (screws removed and the anterior and interosseous SI ligaments cut). All SIJs were imaged at least three times to test the repeatability of the DIV images. The results obtained from four SIJs at three different stiffness conditions were statistically assessed with the Sign test for reproducibility and significance of DIV measurements.

Results

From the pilot study on two cadavers, it appeared that a vibration of 200 Hz yielded optimal information from the images for discrimination of DIV levels; this frequency was also confirmed in the study on the physical model (Buyruk et al 1996a). In the successive study on two other specimens, it was possible to obtain reproducible DIV images. The SIJ presented different levels of stiffness during various stability conditions. The human pelvises showed a transmission block of vibrations (low stiffness) through the unstabilized SIJ (Fig. 24.3A), whereas the stabilized SIJ (Fig. 24.3B) showed an increase of vibration transmission (high transmission). Reproducibility is satisfactory, based on the proportion between the standard deviation and the mean of four repetitions. Figure 24.4 shows a clear difference between stable and unstable joints; from left to right: no intervention (A), stabilized with screws (B), and ligaments cut (C). In the unaltered pelvis position (Fig. 24.4A), it appears that both SIJs of specimen 2 showed almost no blockage of energy transmission. Fixation by screws resulted in a dramatic bilateral decrease in blockage in specimen 1 but not in specimen 2 (Fig. 24.4b). After removal of the screws and cutting the ligaments (Fig. 24.4c), all four SIJs showed a noticeable increase of blockage up to a level above the no-intervention position. The Sign test was applied separately for left and right and the differences between the 'screwed' and 'ligaments cut' situations were statistically significant (for both sides $p < 0.001$).

STUDY ON HEALTHY SUBJECTS

Fourteen healthy volunteers aged between 20 and 40 years were included in the study (Buyruk et al 1995b). All subjects were females who had not had lower back pain for at least 1 year, and none were regular users of alcohol and/or painkillers.

The experimental set-up was similar to the one used in the previous study on human specimens (Fig. 24.5). The subjects were asked to lay prone on the examination table with the muscles, especially gluteus maximus, biceps femoris, and erector spinae relaxed.

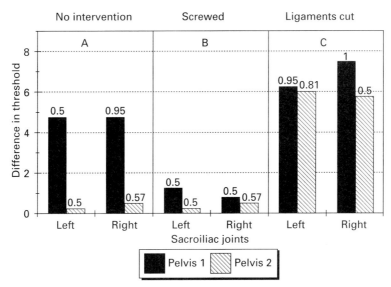

Fig. 24.4 The change in the Doppler threshold levels during the energy transfer through the SIJs at different stiffness conditions, are given with standard deviations. (Reproduced from Buyruk et al 1995a.)

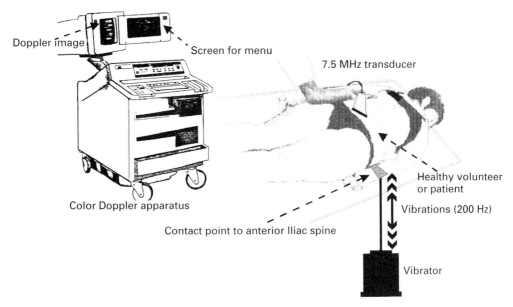

Fig. 24.5 In vivo experimental set-up. (Reproduced from Buyruk et al 1995b.)

Measurement of the left and right SIJ was repeated three times for each side at each session. Between each measurement, the subject had to stand up and perform some light exercises with the arms and legs. In total, three different sessions took place on different days and at randomly chosen times. The data collected from each pelvis were divided into two groups, i.e. the left and right SIJ. To test the measurement reliability, a one-way analysis of variance test was applied separately to both groups. The t-test for paired samples was applied to test the significance of differences between the two groups. For all tests a significance level of 0.05 was chosen.

Results

Table 24.1 presents the differences between the respective minimum thresholds recorded for all 14 subjects. The differences in threshold value reflecting SIJ stiffness range from 0 to 15. As an example, subject P1 showed no threshold difference (0) for both SIJ; this indicates high stiffness of both SIJs. Subject P6 shows large threshold differences, indicating an unstiff SIJ. In subject P10, the right SIJ appears to be stiffer than the left. One-way analysis of variance reveals that the reproducibility of the method is good; all left SIJs showed a reliability coefficient of 0.97 and all right SIJs one of 0.94 (97% and 94% respectively). The variation in reproducibility for the left side was intraindividually 0.39 and interindividually 11.85, and for the right side 0.45 and 6.83 respectively. Variance analysis showed that the method can significantly discriminate different interindividual stiffnesses. The t-test applied to the data from the left and the right sides showed no statistical significant difference ($p = 0.44$).

THE STUDY ON PPPP PATIENTS AND HEALTHY CONTROLS (Buyruk et al 1996b)

A group of PPPP patients ($n = 56$; ages 24–54 years) and a healthy control group ($n = 45$; ages 20–42 years) participated in the study. The patient group had an average of 1.46 ± 0.7 children, and the control group 0.11 ± 0.4. The inclusion criterion for the patient group was the existence of pelvic and/or lower back pain during at least the first three months after delivery. The clinical examination and the diagnosis were carried out by a physician who was not involved in this study. The clinical data were collected from the hospital files after the measurements were performed. The control group consisted of females without a history of idiopathic pain in the region of pelvis and lower back. Informed consent was given by the subjects.

The experimental set-up was similar to that used in previous studies on SIJ stiffness (Buyruk et al 1995a, 1995b, 1996a). The stiffness differences between the patient group and the control group were compared in four ways:

1. In the case of hypermobility of the SIJ, the mean joint mobility levels between the two groups were compared using Wilcoxon's two-sample test. This was done for the left and right SIJ separately, and in combination (the mean of left and right joints).

2. To assess whether there is a difference in the prevalence of hyper- or hypomobility between patients and controls, the data were grouped into three categories: threshold difference < 3, hypomobility; 3–7, intermediate mobility; > 7, hypermobility. The two groups were then compared using the chi-square test on the 2 × 3 table. Again this was done for the left and right joints separately, and in combination (the mean of left and right joints).

3. To test the prevalence of asymmetric SIJ stiffness, first the absolute difference in mobility between the left and right SIJs was computed. Then these differences were compared between patients and controls using Wilcoxon's two-sample test. The same tests were repeated using an age stratification of 10 years.

4. The relationship between the site of the pain and the unstiff SIJ was also tested using the student t-test in the patients ($n = 27$) who described one-sided dorsal pelvic pain (significance level set at 0.05).

Results

In both groups, low as well as high threshold levels were seen. In Fig. 24.6 (right SIJ) and Fig. 24.7 (left SIJ), it is possible to see the similar distribution of stiffness in PPPP and control groups. The mean (standard deviation) age for patients was 33.1 (5.7) years and for controls 27.6 (4.9) years. No statistical significant differences in mean mobility were found between patients and controls (left SIJ, $p = 0.78$; right SIJ, $p = 0.99$; left and right SIJ averaged, $p = 0.57$). The means for patients and controls respectively were 2.7 and 3.0 (left SIJ), and 2.8 and 2.8 (right SIJ). Furthermore, the patients did not show significantly more hyper- or hypomobility than did the controls (left SIJ, $p = 0.75$; right SIJ, $p = 0.82$, left and right SIJ averaged, $p = 0.27$). However, a highly significant difference was found between the groups with regard to the absolute difference of SIJ stiffness

Table 24.1 Differences in the threshold values seen in the left (L) and right (R) SIJ in the pelvises of 14 subjects (P1–P14), measured in threshold units

		Subjects																												
		P1		P2		P3		P4		P5		P6		P7		P8		P9		P10		P11		P12		P13		P14	
Session	Repetition	L	R	L	R	L	R	L	R	L	R	L	R	L	R	L	R	L	R	L	R	L	R	L	R	L	R	L	R
1	1	0	0	4	3	3	3	4	8	2	0	12	8	1	4	6	4	2	2	9	4	5	5	0	2	2	1	3	4
	2	0	1	4	3	4	3	4	9	1	0	13	11	0	3	6	4	2	1	8	4	4	4	1	3	1	0	2	3
	3	1	0	4	3	3	4	4	7	1	1	12	10	1	4	6	3	2	1	8	5	5	4	0	2	1	0	2	4
2	4	1	1	4	3	5	3	5	7	2	0	15	10	0	3	7	3	3	2	7	4	4	4	0	2	0	3	3	3
	5	1	0	4	3	3	4	5	5	1	0	13	11	0	3	7	3	3	2	8	4	5	4	0	3	1	1	3	3
	6	1	0	5	3	3	3	4	6	1	1	13	10	1	3	7	4	2	2	9	5	5	5	1	2	2	1	3	3
3	7	0	1	5	4	4	3	5	6	2	0	13	11	0	2	7	3	2	2	7	5	3	3	1	2	1	1	2	4
	8	2	1	5	4	5	3	4	7	2	1	13	10	1	2	7	3	2	3	7	4	4	4	1	3	0	2	2	4
	9	2	0	4	5	4	3	4	6	1	1	12	11	0	3	7	4	2	2	6	5	5	4	0	2	1	0	2	3
Average		0.8	0.4	4.3	3.4	3.5	3.2	4.3	6.7	1.4	0.4	12.9	10.2	0.4	3	6.6	3.4	2.2	1.8	7.6	4.4	4.6	4.1	0.4	2.3	1.2	0.4	2.4	3.4
Standard deviation		0.7	0.5	0.4	0.6	0.6	0.4	0.4	1.1	0.5	0.5	0.8	0.9	0.5	0.6	0.4	0.5	0.4	0.5	0.9	0.5	0.4	0.5	0.5	0.4	0.4	0.5	0.5	0.5

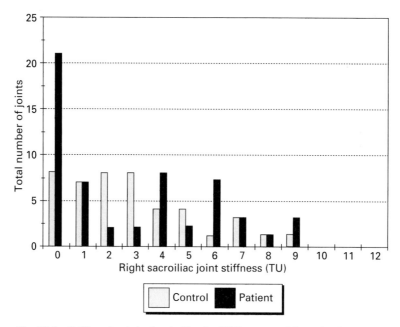

Fig. 24.6 Stiffness levels in threshold units (TU) measured from the right SIJ of control and patient groups.

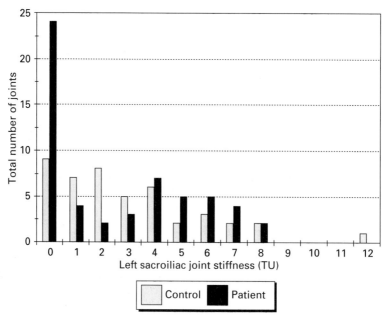

Fig. 24.7 Stiffness levels in threshold units (TU) measured from the left SIJ of control and patient groups.

between the left and right ($p < 0.00001$), patients showing much greater asymmetry of stiffness than controls (means 0.73 and 3.38 respectively; see Fig. 24.8). The same test with 10-year age stratifi-cation also showed a significant difference of $p < 0.00001$. There was no significant relation between the unstiff side and the site of the pain ($p = 0.22$).

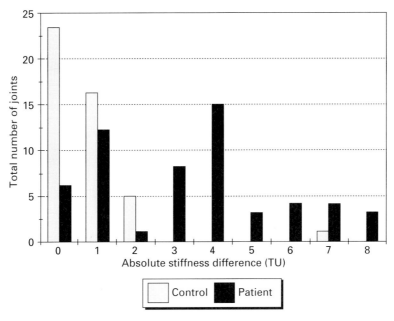

Fig. 24.8   The distribution of absolute stiffness differences in threshold units (TU) between the right and left SIJ.

DISCUSSION

Long-term exposure to vibrations with low frequency and high amplitude are harmful (Quandieu & Pellieux 1982). However, high frequencies such as 200 Hz with low amplitude, thus low energy, can be used safely in diagnosis (Buyruk et al 1995b, Cunningham et al 1990). At this frequency, the distribution of vibrations is spheric. This has the advantage that the transmission of vibrations through the SIJ is not sensitive to the direction of excitation. This is important because the positioning of the patients with respect to the vibrator may not be completely reproducible. In the earlier study on a pelvis model made of plastic, the frequency of 200 Hz appeared to be free of resonance.

DIV has several advantages compared with a technique using accelerometers: simultaneous measurement of two bones (ilium and sacrum) with one sensor, no damping influence of the skin, insensitivity to the thickness of soft tissue, and a lack of need for calibration. The intensity of the vibrations that appear at the screen was affected by the angle between probe and bone surface, while 90° is the optimal angle because of the Doppler shift theory. Because we use the relative difference of the threshold values at the sacrum and the ilium, this difference does not change, even if the probe was found not to be perpendicular to the bones.

The study on 14 healthy female subjects revealed that reproducibility of DIV is good. Reproducibility, however, seems to decrease with lower SIJ stiffness. An explanation may be that in subjects with low stiffness, change in muscle activity affects the SIJ stiffness (Snijders et al 1993a, 1993b). Chronic low back pain and pain sensitivity-decreasing addictions (e.g. regular alcohol consumption and painkillers) were designated as exclusion criteria since lowered pain threshold would cause the inclusion of false symptom-free subjects. The unexpected finding of a wide range of SIJ stiffness in the healthy volunteers indicates that the pathophysiology of the low back problem seems not to be connected to hyper- or hypomobility of the SIJ, as often stated in the literature. Thus unstiff joints may be free of symptoms, whereas some authors (Walheim et al 1984) mention SIJ hypermobility as a major cause of low back pain. Hypomobility is also regarded as pathological (Binkley et al 1993).

The DIV of two SIJs takes about 20 min (without repetitions) in the present procedure. It is expected that technical developments will lead to a reduction in time and costs. The position of the subject is currently restricted to the prone posture in order to ensure good contact with the vibrator and the biomechanically released SIJ. Testing in postures such as sitting and standing may provide a better understanding of the influence of passive structures (ligaments) and muscle activity on SIJ stiffness.

The main conclusion from this study is the different stiffness of the left and right SIJs of the PPPP group which is independent of age. An unexpected result was that a range from hyper- to hypomobility of both SIJs was found in the healthy controls. This does not meet the conclusions in the literature about SIJ problems. Some authors (Walheim et al 1984), in general and in PPPP in particular, mention hypermobility, i.e. instability of the SIJ and symphysis pubis, as a major cause of low back pain. Hypomobility is also regarded as pathological according to some reports in the literature (Binkley et al 1993, Grieve 1982, Vitanen et al 1995). The present finding with regard to asymmetry, however, does not match with the clinical reports that point to asymmetry in pain symptoms (Dreyfuss et al 1994, Myron 1982). The result of this study contradicts those authors who take the manually assessed mobility of one SIJ as a diagnostic tool. Equal stiffness of the SIJs, which was found in the control group, seems to be an important feature for normal functioning. Some authors refer to the mechanism of damping and shock absorption (Grieve 1982). However, this is especially required in, for example, walking, but most pain complaints are reported not during walking but during standing and sitting.

CONCLUSIONS

1. DIV is easy to apply and safe to use.
2. Stiffness measurements with DIV can make intra- and interindividual differences between SIJ stiffnesses visible and quantifiable.
3. This new method is objective and reproducible, which can be demonstrated with statistical significance by creating different stiffnesses in human specimens.
4. The prospective of future in vivo application is promising because technical and safety restrictions exist.
5. The in vivo SIJ stiffness measurements are reproducible.
6. Healthy subjects and patients experience no inconvenience with this non-invasive measurement procedure.
7. Clinical application of this new technique seems feasible, particularly because it is user-friendly.
8. This approach might contribute to the objective diagnosis of PPPP.
9. This tool does not require precise measures and intensive training.
10. In the healthy control group, the SIJ stiffness levels ranged from loose to stiff.
11. In the patient group, significant differences were found between left and right SIJ stiffness levels.
12. Asymmetry of stiffness is associated with lower back pain and pelvic pain, whereas the stiffness level of one particular SIJ is not.

ACKNOWLEDGEMENT

The authors would like to extend special thanks to Dr R. Stoeckart, Department of Anatomy, Erasmus University, Rotterdam, for his contribution to this project.

REFERENCES

Binkley J, Finch E, Hall J, Black T, Gowland C 1993 Diagnostic classification of patients with low back pain: report on a survey of physical therapy experts. Physical Therapy 73(3): 138–150

Buyruk H M, Stam H J, Snijders C J, Vleeming A, Laméris J S, Holland W P J 1995a The use of colour Doppler imaging for the assessment of sacroiliac joint stiffness: a study on embalmed human pelvises. European Journal of Radiology 21: 112–116

Buyruk H M, Snijders C J, Vleeming A, Laméris J S, Holland W P J 1995b The measurements of sacroiliac joint stiffness with colour Doppler imaging: a study on healthy subjects. European Journal of Radiology 21: 117–121

Buyruk H M, Stam H J, Snijders C J, Vleeming A, Holland W P J 1996a Assessment of sacroiliac joint mobility by dynamic testing of a pelvis model (submitted for publication)

Buyruk H M, Stam H J, Snijders C J, Vleeming A, Laméris J S, Holland W P J, Stijnen T H 1996b The measurements of sacroiliac joint stiffness in peripartum pelvic pain patients with colour Doppler imaging (submitted for publication)

Carmichael J P 1987 Inter- and intra-examiner reliability of palpation for sacroiliac joint dysfunction. Journal of Manipulative Physiology and Therapy 10: 164–171

Cunningham J L, Kenwright J, Kershaw C J 1990 Biomechanical measurement of fracture healing. Journal of Medical Engineering and Technology 14(3): 92–101

Dreyfuss P, Dryer S, Griffin J, Hoffman J, Walsh N 1994 Positive sacroiliac screening tests in asymptomatic adults. Spine 19(10): 1138–1143

Grieve E F M 1982 Mechanical dysfunction of the sacro-iliac joint. International Rehabilitation Medicine 5: 46–52

Hoppenfeld S 1976 Physical examination of the spine and the extremities. Appleton-Century-Crofts, Norwalk, CT

Kelsey J L, White A A III 1980 Epidemiology and impact of low back pain. Spine 5: 133–142

Mens J M A, Vleeming A, Stoeckart R, Stam H J, Snijders C J 1996 Understanding of peripartum pelvic pain, implications of a patient survey. Spine 21(11): 1363–1369

Mior S A, McGregor M, Schut B 1990 The role of experience in clinical accuracy. Journal of Manipulative Physiology and Therapy 13: 68–71

Murray R O, Jacobson H G, Stoker D J 1990 The radiology of skeletal disorders, 3rd edn. Churchill Livingstone, Edinburgh

Myron C B 1982 The sacroiliac joint problem: review of anatomy, mechanics, and diagnosis. Journal of American Orthopedic Associations 81: 667–679

Parker K J, Lerner R M 1992 Sonoelasticity of organs: shear waves ring a bell. Journal of Ultrasound Medicine 11: 387–392

Quandieu P, Pellieux L 1982 Study in situ et in vivo of the acceleration of lumbar vertebrae of a primate exposed to vibration in the Z-axis. Journal of Biomechanics 15(12): 985–1006

Snijders C J, Snijder J G N, Hoedt H T E 1984 Biomechanische modellen in het bestek van rugklachten tijdens de zwangerschap. Tijdschrift Sociale Gezondheidszorg 62: 141–147

Snijders C J, Vleeming A, Stoeckart R 1993a Transfer of lumbosacral load to iliac bones and legs. I: Biomechanics of self-bracing of the sacroiliac joints and its significance for treatment and exercise. Clinical Biomechanics 8: 285–294

Snijders C J, Vleeming A, Stoeckart R 1993b Transfer of lumbosacral load to iliac bones and legs. II: The loading of the sacroiliac joints when lifting in a stooped posture. Clinical Biomechanics 8: 295–301

Vitanen J V, Kokko M L, Lehtinen K, Suni J, Kautiainen H 1995 Correlation between mobility restrictions and radiologic changes in ankylosing spondylitis. Spine 20: 492–496

Vleeming A, Buyruk H M, Stoeckart R, Karamürsel S, Snijders C J 1992 An integrated therapy for peripartum pelvic instability: a study of the biomechanical effects of pelvic belts. American Journal of Obstetrics and Gynecology 166: 1243–1247

Walheim G G, Olerud S, Ribbe T 1984 Motion of the pubic symphysis in pelvic instability. Scandinavian Journal of Rehabilitation Medicine 16(4): 163–169

25. Psoas dysfunction/insufficiency, sacroiliac dysfunction and low back pain

R. M. Bachrach

INTRODUCTION

Low back pain is endemic in the US and other industrialized nations. It will involve between 80 and 90% of the population; 90% will recover from the initial episode with or without treatment within between 3 weeks and 3 months. Unfortunately, however, the single most important predictor of a low back pain event is a prior history of low back pain. An initial incident is usually followed by another, although the interval may vary from weeks to months or years. The episodes may increase in frequency, severity, and duration with each occurrence. In this chapter, I will present a possible explanation of the biomechanics and dynamics of most non-surgical or non-specific low back pain. This will provide therapists with a rational program for early diagnosis and timely treatment, and their patients with the tools for self-management and prevention.

THE PSOAS DYSFUNCTION/ INSUFFICIENCY SYNDROME

According to Wyke (1985), the proximate source of non-surgical low back pain is the depolarization of nociceptors in the soft tissues. Between 40% and 45% of this occurs in the joint capsules, either alone or in combination with the excitation of pain receptors in other tissues. Between 30% and 35% takes place in the thoracolumbar paravertebral intramuscular perivascular tissues. These exist either alone or in combination with joint capsule receptors.

Vleeming et al (1994) postulated the excitation of nociceptors in the posterior sacroiliac (SI) (particularly the long dorsal SI) ligaments, the

iliolumbar, and posterior longitudinal ligaments as a major source of low back pain. This is, in turn, related to SI dysfunction. In the absence of herniation, discogenic low back pain may result from distraction and/or chemical stimulation of nociceptors in the outer fibers of the annulus fibrosis.

This chapter takes the position that, in the presence of the ligamentous laxity related to aging, to gravity-assisted dysfunctional posture, and/or to repeated injury, these nociceptors are facilitated by biomechanical dysfunctions. These dysfunctions are often related to chronic contraction, shortening, and weakness of the psoas major. This, in conjunction with abdominal and gluteal weakness, perpetuates hyperlordosis of the lumbar spine: the psoas dysfunction/insufficiency syndrome (PDIS) (Bachrach 1991).

Psoas anatomy and mechanics

The psoas major arises from the bodies, intervertebral discs and transverse processes of the five lumbar and the twelfth thoracic vertebrae, and from the membranous septae between them. It courses downward, forward, and slightly laterally, crosses under the inguinal ligament, in front of the hip joint, and then passes posteriorly, joining the iliacus, to its insertion into the lesser trochanter of the femur. It is innervated by branches of the first, second, and third lumbar nerves, which pass through its substance (Hollinshead & Jenkins 1981). Overlying and adjacent to the psoas major at the level of the twelfth thoracic and first three lumbar vertebrae are the trunks of the sympathetic ganglia with their gray and white rami communicantes (Netter et al 1991). From above downward, the psoas acts to flex the hip, in conjunction with the iliacus and the rectus femoris (and, to a lesser extent, the pectineus, sartorius, and tensor fascia lata) (Fig. 25.1).

From below upward, with the lower extremities fixed, the paired psoas muscles act to pull forward on the lumbar spine, thereby flexing it on the pelvis. The forward pull of the psoas on the anterior aspects of the lumbar vertebrae increases the lumbar lordosis and lumbosacral angle (effectively extending the pelvis on the lumbar spine). Unilateral psoas contraction draws the lumbar spine downward. It is flexed forward and side-bent to the side of contraction. The lumbar spine is rotated to the opposite side (Michele 1962, Rasch 1989). The psoas acts also as an important stabilizer of the hip joint (Hollinshead & Jenkins 1981, Michele 1962, Rasch 1989).

Psoas major shortening

The sources of chronic psoas shortening are several, possibly including the age at which the erect posture becomes dominant (since bony growth outstrips muscle lengthening). Sleeping in the fetal position, repetitive hip flexion movements, as seen in aerobic exercise programs, and sedentary lifestyle with prolonged sitting may all contribute to psoas shortening. Most movement in sports, dance, and normal daily activity, including walking, is forward-oriented, thereby requiring repetitive or sustained psoas contraction or shortening without providing adequate offsetting stretching (Bachrach 1991).

Unloading and consequent increased fluid imbibition by the intervertebral discs during prolonged recumbency may produce anterior disc bulging. This is particularly likely in the presence

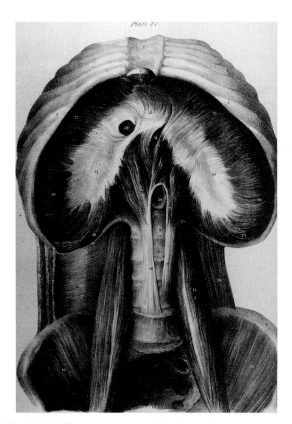

Fig. 25.1 The psoas major and its relationship to the diaphragm, iliacus, and quadratus lumborum.

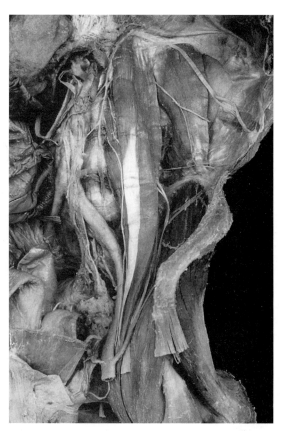

Fig. 25.2 Relationship of the autonomic nervous system to psoas major at the thoracolumbar junction. (Dissection and slide courtesy of Frank Willard, PhD.)

of degenerative changes of the annulus fibrosus. These, in turn, may be generated by increased shearing forces on the annuli of the middle and upper lumbar discs related to hyperlordosis. The anterior longitudinal ligament at the thoraco/lumbar transitional zone is stretched. Traction on the sympathetic and somatic motor fibers to the psoas overlying the anterolateral aspect of the vertebral column may ensue (Fig. 25.2) (Willard 1994). Thus psoas major contraction may be facilitated, accounting, at least in part, for many cases of low back pain and stiffness during the night and upon arising.

Anterolateral disc extrusion at L1–2 and/or L2–3 through invagination of the muscle belly itself may be a competent initiating and/or perpetuating cause of psoas major shortening (Fig. 25.3). Afferent fibers to the sympathetic ganglia are present in all anterior vertebral structures, including the anterior longitudinal ligament and the peripheral fibers of the annulus fibrosus, the vertebral body, and its periosteum. A major autonomic branch extends posteriorly from the sympathetic ganglion or gray ramus communicante to join the recurrent meningeal nerve (together forming the paravertebral autonomic neural plexus), (Jinkins et al 1989). In the presence of upper lumbar anterior disc extrusion, motor nerves innervating the psoas major can, quite possibly, be reflexively excited, with resultant contraction and shortening of that muscle. Certainly, the pathway for such a phenomenon is present. Similarly, then, anterolateral disc extrusion at the L5–S1 level might be expected to excite the sympathetic rami communicantes to the first three lumbar motor nerves, stimulating chronic contraction of the psoas major.

PDIS scenario

Facilitative alignment depends, to a great extent, on the balance between, on the one hand, the anterior pelvic rotation generated by contraction of the psoas major, the other hip flexors, and the erector spinae, and on the other, the posterior rotating effect of the abdominals, gluteals, and

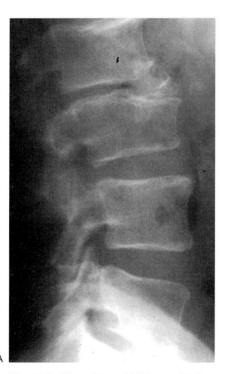
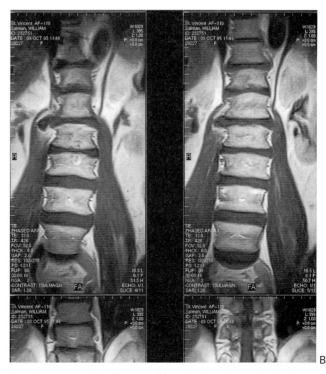

Fig. 25.3 X-ray (A) and MRI scan (B) demonstrating degenerative disc disease and invagination of psoas major by intervertebral disc protrusion at L1–2 and 2–3.

hamstrings (Fig. 25.4). Inadequacy of the compensatory mechanisms for contracture, shortening, or failure of adaptive lengthening of the psoas produces PDIS (Bachrach 1987). The following scenario presents. The lumbar lordosis is increased. The thoracolumbar paravertebral musculature and fascia are shortened. The distance between the pubic symphysis and the costal arch is increased, so the abdominal muscles are consequently overstretched and weak. There is a compensatory increase in the thoracic kyphosis. The head is forward and the cervical lordosis is frequently flattened (Fig. 25.5) (Bachrach 1988).

The intramuscular perivascular nociceptors in the paraspinal and accessory spinal muscles are facilitated by this malalignment. These pain

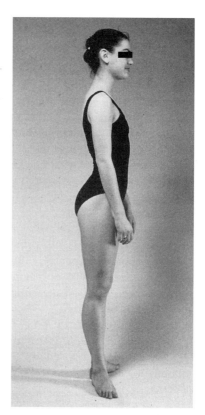

Fig. 25.5 Anterior weight-bearing postural mechanics related to PDIS in a dancer.

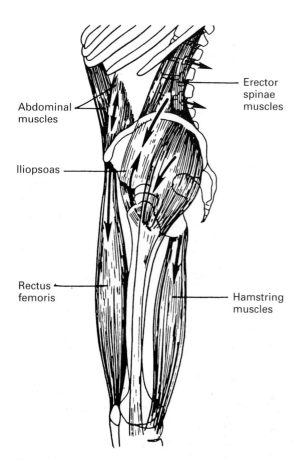

Fig. 25.4 Facilitative alignment: relationship of the hip flexors to the gluteals, hamstrings, and abdominals in the maintenance of posture. (Reproduced from Bachrach 1987.)

receptors are sensitive to stretching (and to crushing, twisting, or disruption), so that further muscle contraction, either to initiate or sustain forward movement, may depolarize them. The apophyseal joints are approximated, thus restricting extension. Furthermore, the leg, usually the right, on the side of predominant psoas tightness is long. The knee is often held in flexion, the foot in pronation (Bachrach 1991).

PDI sequelae

SI dysfunction

According to the 'tensegrity' model of Levin (1995), the SIJ and iliolumbar ligaments restrain the sacral base from anterior rocking while the sacrotuberous and sacrospinous ligaments restrain the apex from rocking posteriorly. Intact, and acting in concert, these ligaments serve to check gravity-assisted and psoas-insufficient posture-related sacral and anterior innominate rotation (counternutation; Vleeming et al 1992). With anterior weight-bearing postural mechanics, as seen in PDIS, the pelvis is rotated anteriorly; the sacrum sits relatively horizontally. In this position, the SI joints (SIJs) are relatively mobile. The line of gravity is displaced anteriorly in relation to the acetabulae. The sacrum, wider anteriorly than posteriorly, is wedged between the innominate bones, causing them to spread on the sacrum and flare out posteriorly. The posterior aspects of the iliac portions of the SIJ are approximated, thus relaxing the strong posterior SI ligaments. The weaker anterior capsular and ligamentous fibers are stretched, torn, and their pain receptors depolarized (Don-Tigny 1992). Additionally, as in anterolateral disc extrusion at L5–S1, the sacral autonomic plexus may be stimulated. Asymmetric (or predominately one-sided) psoas contracture or shortening produces additional downward and anterior rotation of the innominate on that side (Michele 1962). Dysfunction at L4–5 and L5–S1 may result through their attachment to the pelvis through the iliolumbar ligaments (Vleeming et al 1994, Willard 1994).

Acute psoas syndrome

Acute, prolonged, or repetitive flexion stress of the lumbar spine may result in spasm of the psoas major uni- or bilaterally. The trunk is forward flexed on the pelvis. The lumbar lordosis is flattened or reversed. A psoatic scoliosis convex to the side opposite predominant spasm presents. Certainly, the chronic psoas shortening is a competent predisposing and perpetuating factor for acute psoas spasm (Kappler 1973).

Relationship of PDIS to intervertebral disc disease

PDIS, through the generation and perpetuation of chronic lumbar hyperlordosis and dysfunctions of the lumbar vertebrae, may be a most significant source of lumbar disc disease. The resultant increase in torsional/shearing forces may be more important than compressive loading in producing failure of the annulus fibrosus (White & Panjabi

1978). In the upper and mid lumbar levels, near the apex of the lordosis, anterior disc extrusion may occur, with consequent stretching or compression of the neural plexus. Communication with somatic fibers innervating the peripheral annulus and the vertebral bodies may result in pain referred to the lower back, buttocks, and/or proximal lower extremities without accompanying neurological findings (Jinkins et al 1989). Compressive axial loading is more likely to produce vertebral endplate failure resulting in central or intrabody herniation (Schmorl's nodes), particularly in the mid to upper lumbar area (White & Panjabi 1978). Distortion of the nociceptor-containing outer fibers of the annulus may, as a result of irritation by glycosaminoglycan degradation products, for example phospholipase A2, generate discogenic low back pain without herniation and without neurologic findings (McCurron et al 1987). These changes, in turn, alter the mechanics of the apophyseal joints, ultimately resulting in osteoarthrosis and possibly contributing to eventual stenosis of the intervertebral foramina and spinal canal (Farfan et al 1970).

PDIS: CLINICAL PRESENTATION

The patient with PDI may present with thoracolumbar, lower lumbar, SI, anterior hip, or buttock pain. It may be unilateral or bilateral, alternating or consistently one-sided. It is never midline unless there is underlying median disk pathology (Bachrach 1991). There may be radiation to the lower extremity, typically not distal to the knee, although with increased tension and thus activation of trigger points in the sacrotuberous and sacrospinous ligaments, or with piriformis involvement, pain may extend into the calf. The patient may complain of low back pain on one side associated with pain in the contralateral upper back and shoulder. This may be related to decussation at the thoracolumbar junction of fibers of the gluteus maximus on one side with those of the latissimus dorsi on the other through the thoracolumbar fascia (Vleeming et al 1994). It may be provoked by forward or, more frequently, backward bending, or by side-bending toward or away from the side of pain. Pain in PDIS is not necessarily aggravated by sitting and is more frequently relieved in this position (Bachrach 1987).

There is commonly a history of recurrent painful attacks, increasing progressively in frequency, duration, and severity. The acute episode is often preceded by a recent history of prolonged sitting, lifting, or carrying heavy weights, for example at exam time, moving, and traveling. There may be a history of years of low-grade lower back pain not attributable to a specific cause. In many cases, the patient is unaware of significant prior back pain episodes (Bachrach 1991).

In my clinical practice, the patient is usually at either end of the spectrum of physical activity: almost totally sedentary or extraordinarily active, such as a dancer or an aerobics teacher or addict (8–10 or more classes per week) (Bachrach 1991).

Clinical findings

SI dysfunction

This is characterized by an anterior innominate (counternutation) on the side of primary dysfunction, usually the right. (This pertains even when symptoms are left-sided or bilateral.) There is sacral torsion, usually left on a right oblique axis (Kuchera 1995). The right forward flexion test is positive in the erect and/or seated positions. The right posterior superior iliac spine in the erect position is high, and forward bending is restricted, with pain at either or both SIJs. Patrick's test is positive on either or both sides. The right 'stork' is positive. One-legged standing on the involved side may evoke the pain of the chief complaint. There is dysfunction at the pubic symphysis (Bachrach 1991).

Pain provocation tests

1. Patrick's test (Fabere: **F**lexion, **a**bduction, **e**xternal **r**otation and **e**xtension). The hip and knee are flexed and the ankle is crossed just proximal to the opposite knee. The contralateral anterior superior iliac spine is stabilized and downward pressure is applied to the ipsilateral knee. Thus the SIJ is compressed. This test may also be positive in hip disease, but usually with pain elicited anteriorly or in the proximal posterior femur. In the presence of L4 or L5 disc disease, this motion may be markedly restricted.

2. Hip flexion/adduction. The hip is flexed to its full range of motion and then adducted. Axial compression of the femur is then applied. Pain at the SIJ is confirmatory. This is repeated at 90°, 65°, and then 45°. A positive reaction at those levels may indicate involvement of the iliolumbar and sacrotuberous ligaments.

3. Indirect SI distraction; direct and indirect SI compression.

4. Standing lumbosacral extension test.

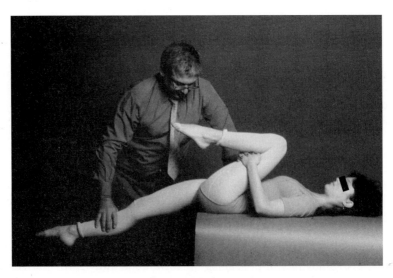

Fig. 25.6   Passive psoas stretch from Michele's test for psoas tension.

Therapeutic testing. The trochanter belt, through compression of the SIJs, provides at least temporary relief of pain (Vleeming et al 1994).

Psoas tightness

The lumbar lordosis is increased (or, less frequently, the trunk is flexed on the hips, the lordosis decreased or reversed). Psoas tightness as elicited through Michele's test (Michele 1962; Box 25.1) is present. Both psoas motor points are tender. If PDIS is present and etiologic, following psoas stretch there is a significant increase in the range of forward bending and a significant decrease in pain or discomfort. However transitory, this improvement is one of the most important confirmatory diagnostic signs of PDIS-generated low back pain (Fig. 25.6).

Psoas strength is determined by resisting hip flexion either at 90° with the patient in the seated or supine position, or, with the patient supine, at 15° of hip flexion with the knee extended. Asymmetric psoas major weakness often suggests L1–3 radiculopathy (Bachrach 1991).

Hamstring tightness

Tightness, particularly of the long head of the biceps femoris on the side of predominant psoas tightness, is probably the result of the relative increase in distance between the origin and insertion of the hamstrings owing to the anterior innominate rotation. Through transfer of this tension through the sacrotuberous ligament, nutation is suppressed, invoking the self-locking mechanism of the SIJ (Vleeming et al 1994). Hip flexion range is decreased, probably related to hamstring tightness and anterior iliac rotation. Low back or SI pain is elicited at the end of range. This pain is increased by adducting the femur. Hip extension (Yeoman's test) on the side of dysfunction is also restricted and there is pain, again owing to psoas tightness. The self-locking mechanism and hence stability of the SIJ is, in case of laxity of the sacrotuberous, sacrospinous, and interosseous ligaments, dependent on the maintenance of tension in the oblique abdominals, gluteus maximus, piriformis,

Box 25.1   Michele's test

> The patient assumes the knee-to-chest position at the end of the plinth. The left thigh is held with both hands just proximal to the popliteal fossa, flexing the femur at the hip *without discomfort*. The examiner extends the right knee and flexes the extended leg at the hip so the lower extremity is now as close to the perpendicular as hamstring tension will allow. The right leg is then extended on the hip supported by the examiner's right hand while the left hand monitors the ipsilateral anterior superior iliac spine. The point at which anterior rotation of the pelvis is palpated by the monitoring left hand, is noted. At that position, the angle the lower extremity makes with the horizontal is recorded as the degree of psoas tightness. Extension to 10° below table level should be attainable at the hip with the knee extended. Inability to extend one hip below 30° from the horizontal (without concomitant anterior rotation of the innominate) indicates significant hip flexor tightness. This is sufficient to cause asymmetric anterior pelvic rotation and consequent SIJ dysfunction. During the performance of this test, low back or lower extremity pain suggests disc disease at L2–3, 3–4, or, less commonly, 4–5 (DonTigny 1992).
>
> A patient with acute psoas spasm would be totally unable to position for this test. Any attempt to force the stretch would certainly result in severe exacerbation of the clinical picture.

thoracolumbar fascia, and biceps femoris (Fig. 25.7). In my clinical experience, I have found abdominal and gluteal muscle weakness to be extremely common in low back pain patients. Thus great care must be taken not to overstretch the hamstrings in situations in which the sacrum is counternutated lest the SIJs, and thus the lumbopelvic mechanism, be further destabilized.

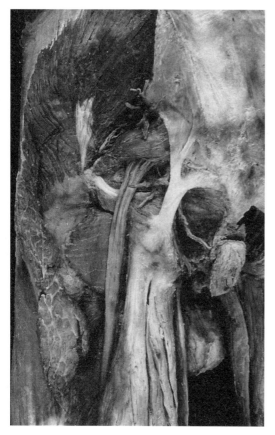

Fig. 25.7 Relationship of the long head of the biceps femoris tendon to the sacrotuberous ligament. (Dissection and slide courtesy of Frank Willard, PhD.)

Myofascial pain syndromes

Piriformis. Contra- and often bilateral piriformis tightness pertains. Piriformis pain is, in my clinical experience, one of the most obdurate myofascial pain syndromes associated with and perpetuating PDIS. I have found it particularly common in the presence of muscular imbalances stemming from hamstring, gluteal, and abductor weakness. These are often secondary to post L5 and S1 radiculopathies, the piriformis being recruited to substitute. Piriformis trigger points may be found both lateral to the sacrum and distally, proximal to its insertion into the greater trochanter of the femur. Stimulation of these points by stretching or pressure may reproduce pain at the SIJ, the proximal thigh, and through a satellite trigger point, occasionally into the calf (Travell & Simons

1983). The piriformis is an essential element in the 'rotator cuff' of the hip: the paired muscles act to brace the SIJ, enhancing the self-locking mechanism, just as does the trochanter belt (Vleeming et al 1994).

Quadratus lumborum. This is a deep abdominal muscle, which is actually the only one of the group acting as an extensor of the lumbar spine. Commonly, tightness of this muscle, also innervated by T12 and L1 nerve roots, is seen in PDIS. It is associated with psoas tightness, thereby augmenting the tendency to hyperlordosis and anterior rotation of the pelvis. Unilateral (or predominately one-sided) psoas contraction will result in contralateral rotation of the lumbar spine and ipsilateral side-bending. The ipsilateral costal arch and iliac crest are approximated. The quadratus lumborum on that side will be shortened and may develop trigger points. The contralateral quadratus lumborum will be overstretched and may also develop trigger points (Travell & Simons 1983).

X-ray findings

There are no hard rules, and diagnosis is never based on X-ray evidence alone. The standard protocol according to the Levitor Institute is followed with the patient erect, knees maximally extended, feet parallel, 100–150 cm apart. Posterior/anterior and lateral films are obtained. This subject is covered exhaustively in Chapters 9 and 39.

Diagnosis

Diagnosis is based on the accumulation of the above findings and is not exclusionary. The most important element in diagnosis is the response of the patient to the psoas stretch and correction of the SI dysfunction. This response may be immediate, but it certainly obtains within two or three treatments.

Differential diagnosis

Although L1–2, 2–3, 3–4 and occasionally 4–5 disc disease may produce low back pain with radiation to the hip and/or anterior thigh, the response to treatment and the absence of significant motor or sensory neurologic signs points toward PDIS as etiologic. Disc disease at these levels may be associated with PDIS as cause and/or effect. Anterior disc extrusion is not uncommon in the upper lumbar levels, with pressure on the anterior paraspinal afferent sympathetic rami at those levels. Articular pillar stress fracture (spondylolysis) is distinguished by a history of repetitive hyperflexion/extension injuries, as occurs in dance and gymnastics. It is found in a primarily younger age group. The pain is consistently reproducible with hyperextension of the lower back, and is confirmed, if necessary, by isotopic bone scanning. PDIS-generated lumbar hyperlordosis may predispose to it, and SI dysfunction may coexist with it (Bachrach 1991).

PDIS may, of course, through the consequent lumbar hyperlordosis, predispose to zygoapophyseal facet impingement. Depolarization of the nociceptors in the cancellous bone of the articular pillars and/or the apophyseal joint capsules may generate pain either of mechanical, chemical, or combined origin (Bachrach 1991). This pain is not reproducible other than by extension of the lumbar spine.

CONCLUSIONS

1. Lumbosacral and SI ligamentous laxity with anterior weight-bearing postural mechanics related to aging, gravity-assisted dysfunctional posture, and/or repeated injury is the probable source of progressive spinal disease.

2. This is perpetuated through chronic shortening, often asymmetric, of the psoas major muscle associated with weakness of that muscle and of the abdominals and gluteals, and with hamstring tightness.

3. Anterolateral disc extrusion or prolapse at L1, 2 and/or 3 may be a competent initiating and/or perpetuating cause of psoas major shortening through direct pressure on the muscle belly or through reflex excitation of motor nerves.

4. Anterolateral disc extrusion at the L5–S1 level may excite the sympathetic fibers of the sacral autonomic plexus, which, through the white rami communicantes may stimulate L1, 2 and 3 motor nerves, with resultant chronic contraction of the psoas major.

5. Low back pain due to erector spinae muscle strain and SI dysfunction may be an early consequence of PDIS-related muscle imbalances.

6. The increased shearing forces on the annulus fibrosus resulting from the PDIS-generated hyperlordosis may then produce intervertebral disc degeneration, with all its sequelae.

REFERENCES

Bachrach R M 1987 Injuries to the dancer's spine. In: Ryan A J, Stevens R E (eds) Dance medicine. Pluribus Press Chicago/Physician and Sports Medicine, Minneapolis, pp 243–265
Bachrach R M 1988 Relationship of low back/pelvic somatic dysfunction to dance injuries. Orthopaedic Review, October: 1037–1043
Bachrach R M 1991 The relationship of low back pain to psoas insufficiency. Journal of Orthopaedic Medicine 13: 34–40
DonTigny R L 1992 Anterior dysfunction of the sacroiliac joint as a major factor in the etiology of idiopathic low back pain syndrome. In: Vleeming A, Mooney V, Snijders C J, Dorman T (eds) First interdisciplinary world congress on low back pain and its relation to the sacroiliac joint. San Diego, CA, 5–6 November, pp 502–517
Farfan H F, Cossett J W, Robertson G H et al 1970 The effects of torsion on the lumbar intervertebral joints: the role of torsion in the production of disc degeneration Journal of Bone and Joint Surgery (US) 52: 468–497
Hollinshead W H, Jenkins D B 1981 Functional anatomy of the limbs and back. WB Saunders, Philadelphia

Jinkins J R, Whittemore A R, Bradley W G 1989 The anatomic basis of vertebrogenic pain and the autonomic syndrome associated with lumbar disc extrusion. American Journal of Neuroradiology, March/April: 219–231
Kappler R 1973 Role of psoas mechanism in low back complaints. Journal of the American Osteopathic Association 72: 794–801
Kuchera M L 1995 Gravitation stress, musculoligamentous strain, and postural alignment. Spine State of the Art Review 9(2): 463–490
Levin S 1995 The sacrum in three-dimensional space. Spine State of the Art Reviews 9(2): 381–388
McCurron R F, Wimpee M W, Hudkings P G, Laros G S 1987 The inflammatory effect of nucleus pulposus: a possible element in the pathogenesis of low back pain. Spine 12: 760–764
Michele A 1962 Iliopsoas. Charles C. Thomas, Springfield, IL
Netter F H, Mitchell G A G, Peterson B W, Mauro A 1991 The Ciba collection of medical illustrations, vol. I, The nervous system, part 1. Ciba-Geigy, West Caldwell, NJ
Rasch P J 1989 Kinesiology and applied anatomy. Lea and Febiger, Philadelphia
Travell J, Simons D G 1983 Myofascial pain and in

dysfunction. Ir
Wilkins, Baltir
Vleeming A, Var   ,
Stijnen T 199;
ligament: influ
Vleeming A, M
First interdiscij   nd
its relation to tl
November, pp
Vleeming A, Stoeckart R, Snijders C J (1994) A description
of the integrated function of the lower spine. A clinical
anatomical and biomechanical approach. Proceedings of
the American Association of Orthopaedic Medicine, The

Pelvis in Transition, Orlando, Florida, February
White A A S, Panjabi M M 1978 Physical properties and
functional biomechanics of the spine. In: Clinical
biomechanics of the spine. JB Lippincott, Philadelphia
Willard F H 1994 Human lumbosacral spine and sacroiliac
joint. Mechanical model of the sacroiliac joint and pelvis:
neurological model of the sacroiliac joint and pelvis.
Proceedings of the American Association of Orthopaedic
Medicine, The Pelvis in Transition, Orlando, Florida
February
Wyke B 1985 Clinical neurology of lumbo-sacral pain.
American Academy of Orthopedic Medicine, Los Angeles,
CA (audiotape)

26. Differential diagnosis of lumbar and pelvic pain

S. V. Paris

The differential diagnosis of sacroiliac from low back pain is difficult. (Stoddard 1959)

INTRODUCTION

It is said that the cause of low back and pelvic pain will never be found in a laboratory or on an X-ray, as back pain is not a disease, and X-rays have, in all but a few instances, lost their validity as a diagnostic tool, being used more to prove a bias rather than being a true investigative method. Back pain, when relieved, rarely if ever changes the X-ray. Now, of course, these two points are debatable, but they set the stage for realizing that the old paradigm of back pain as a medical complaint capable of being diagnosed and then treated medically has failed and will continue to fail. In its place, a better paradigm of back pain being caused by a summation of dysfunctions, each contributing to an accumulation of noxious stimuli, which, when the individual's level for appreciation is reached, will be interpreted by the individual as discomfort and, when sufficiently accumulated, will result in pain even in the stout-hearted, producing one more patient seeking assistance.

In back management, traditional medicine is invaluable for pain relief and for little else. Medical diagnosis is unable to find or agree on most causes of low back or, for that matter, shoulder pain. Again, the reason for this is that physicians are trained in disease, not in detecting dysfunctions, and dysfunctions are usually multiple rather than singular. Such a concept is alien to both the physician and the payer. This has to change.

There is no profession free of bias on this topic. Chiropractors traditionally considered the vertebrae as being out of alignment. Physicians, from Mixter and Barr to Cyriax, later saw the problem as arising from the disc. McKenzie (1996) also blames the disc, while others recognize the facet and debate its role. The truth is that all spinal structures are capable of producing noxious stimuli because all are either innervated or appear to be mediators for nociceptive nerve endings. Deciding on which structure is the cause is a waste of time – but trying to decide on which structures are involved is constructive. However, we must identify not only the structures, but also the causes, such as for poor posture or habits, which we must then seek to remedy by removing them when possible.

As to which structures of the spine may give rise to pain, it is recognized that the muscles are poorly innervated. However, when fatigued or deprived of adequate circulation, the muscles can cause discomfort of an aching nature. The outermost lamellae of the annulus (capsule) are both innervated and vascular, and there is good reason to believe that degenerative discs, invaded as they are by blood vessels, may also be pain-producing. Additionally, the disc appears able 'chemically' to produce pain by irritating its innervated capsule. Repetitive motion on the disc, which increases its water content (as viewed on a T2-weighted magnetic resonance imaging scan), appears to be relieved by temporarily changing the disc chemistry. The facet capsules, especially their medial expanse, are innervated, as are the ligaments of the back and, of course, the ligaments and capsules of the sacroiliac joint (SIJ). Even the dura mater has innervation, as does the sheath around the nerve roots. However, this is pointless to discuss other than to state that the pain can come from any source or, as this article would wish to convince, from an accumulation or summation of several sources.

We must not look for back pain as coming from a single structure or source. It also comes from behavioral, including postural, dysfunctions. I shall not present the behavioral factors, as they are well known even if not well understood. However, a simple example of how posture can be the cause of pain is to simply slouch into a forward head posture and then try to raise the arms as high as they will go above the head. What will be noticed is that their range is limited and that there is a 'hard' end feel in the glenohumeral region. In contrast, when sitting erect with the head back and chin in, the arms go much higher and there is less discomfort. Try it. Therefore, a forward head posture can be a cause of shoulder stress and strain. The later 'medical' diagnosis of, for example, supraspinatus tendinitis misses the point entirely and focuses attention on the dysfunctional result and not on the cause, which in this example is forward head posture. These principles are generally well understood by today's physical therapist practicing in the area known as manual therapy.

In this chapter, I shall briefly outline the principal contributing factors of low back pain. Standard diagnoses will be used and expanded, and the suggested treatments will address the dysfunctional aspects of those diagnoses.

Before doing so, I need to share the view that pain, a sensation arising more from suffering than from physical stimuli, needs to be managed in such a manner as not to in any way reward it. Rather, the patient should be focused on the fact that pain is not a warning sign but a useful indicator that the patient is doing something that stresses already sensitized tissues (and pathways), and that the patient, being responsible for his or her care, must learn to find those positions and behaviors that are pain-free. Only the patient, following adequate instruction, will know how to do this. The approach to pain is thus behavioral and very much existentialist.

CLASSIFICATION OF SYNDROMES AND THEIR TREATMENT

The title of this chapter begs the author to assist readers in enabling them to differentiate between lumbar and pelvic pain. Clearly, given the author's concept that pain results from a summation of nociception (pain) arising from several dysfunctions (as well as behavioral and postural), this distinction is not possible and not in the best interest of patient management. Rather, in the following pages, the various 'syndromes' will be presented, together with their signs, symptoms, and recommended treatments, so that the clinician will be better able to detect and treat the multiple causes of pain. The syndromes to be considered are:

- myofascial states
- facet dysfunction
- sacroiliac (SI) dysfunction
- ligamentous weakness and instability
- disc dysfunction
- spondylolisthesis
- central canal and lateral foraminal stenosis
- kissing lumbar spines (Baastrup's disease)
- thorocolumbar syndrome
- lesion complex.

Myofascial states

Changes in the myofascia will invariably accompany back pain, regardless of its origin. Not all myofascial changes, particularly those relating to changes in tone, require treatment, but they always require consideration. Tone is here defined as the normal elasticity of a muscle to stretch or touch. When we palpate a muscle and speak of its 'tone', we are actually speaking of its response to our touch as it contracts against our deforming palpation in order to protect its muscle spindles from deformation.

Spasm

When changes in muscle character are noted, clinicians are inclined to use the inappropriate term 'spasm'. Using spasm to describe any change in muscle behavior is like using the diagnosis of thoracic outlet syndrome – it is too broad and it fails to identify the numerous entities, from tight scaleni to cervical rib or hypertrophied subclavius muscle, that could be contributory. True spasm is defined as an 'uncontrolled involuntary jerking of muscles' ('Dorland's illustrated medical dictionary' 1985), and, while we may see this during active movement or in response to palpation, this is only one of the muscle dysfunctions that is critical to understand.

Treatment. Ignore the muscle behavior and address the causes.

Involuntary guarding

This is the most common of the hypertonic muscle states, usually involving the multifidus group, and will invariably coexist with most underlying joint dysfunctions. No doubt, the muscle response is an effort to either hold or guard the back from further stress. The resultant hypertonicity will often be noticed in standing or sitting, but will invariably disappear in lying if the patient is *adequately* supported. However, on occasions, a classic case of involuntary muscle holding is displayed when the patient, upon adopting a prone position and reporting to be comfortable, nonetheless displays muscle hypertonicity on one side of the back and hypotonicity on the other. This continued 'involuntary guarding' can be both seen and palpated. The patient confirms that he or she is comfortable, yet the muscles signal otherwise. Changing the position of the pillow under the abdomen will invariably restore a balanced tone.

When SI dysfunction is present, a common picture is hypertonicity on the same side (ipsilateral), which may or may not cease on adopting a prone position and can extend up into the lower thoracic spine. This would appear to be of the multifidi, which in the sacral region share attachment to the SIJ capsule.

Treatment. Ignore the muscle behavior and treat the causes.

Chemical muscle holding

When muscles have been overused, such as the quadriceps after an unaccustomed hiking expedition, the muscles will ache and feel doughy and tender to the touch. In the lumbar spine, this may again result from overuse, but is more commonly the result of the sustained involuntary guarding described above. The muscles ache. Stretching may give some temporary relief but 'self-cracking' of the back provides for a more immediate relief of both the hypertonicity and

discomfort, mediated perhaps by the type III facet articular mechanoreceptors or the Golgi tendon apparatuses of the attached multifidi.

Treatment. Heat, deep massage, stretching the muscle, and finding the causes. Discourage the self-cracking, as this usually takes place at a mobile or hypermobile joint, with ligamentous weakness (see below).

Voluntary guarding

Should nociception reach the threshold for pain, the patient may voluntarily hold the affected part fixed with voluntary muscle guarding owing to fear of creating more pain.

Treatment. Encourage movement based on the same principles expounded by Codman (1934) for the shoulder, i.e. repetitive motion. Of course, if the condition involves acute significant trauma, support, rather than movement, should be given initially.

Adaptive shortening

It is recognized that muscles undergo adaptive shortening and remodeling if maintained in a shortened position (Lieber 1992). This will also occur in the low back if the muscles, are either by involuntary, chemical or voluntary holding, kept in their shortened position. Such adaptive shortening will occur not only in the paraspinal multifidus muscles, but also in the iliopsoas, quadratus lumborum, and rectus femoris, to name but a few.

Treatment. Stretch the shortened muscles. Since stretching a muscle triggers an active contraction (the stretch reflex), the muscle must be first relaxed before being stretched, or stretched for a sufficient duration as to overcome the stretch reflex. Stretching, especially in the presence of dysfunction, is a skilled and poorly understood process.

Hypertrophy

This uncommon situation may occur in the presence of a moderate instability such as a spondylolysis or spondylolisthesis. It is noticed first in standing, where there is increased muscle bulk at the level of the instability.

Treatment. None is required.

Wasting and fibrosis

When the low back has been held rigid for some time, due initially to injury, pain, or the fear of pain, the muscles become shortened and fibrotic, losing their normal soft and extensible mass. A similar condition may accompany spine surgery, such as laminectomy and fusion, especially when the innervation via the medial branch of the posterior primary rami communicantes has been disrupted by the surgery.

Treatment. Heat and deep massage, along with exercises through the full available range of motion, will assist. Exercises should be for endurance, co-ordination, and strength, in that order.

Compartmental syndrome

When muscles in the lumbar spine hypertrophy, owing either to muscle guarding, instability, a change in the work environment, or body-building activities, they may become restricted in their fascial compartments, resulting in a chronic uni- or bilateral paravertebral back pain. The muscles will feel tender to the touch.

Treatment. Deep massage (Rolfing, connective tissue techniques) to the paravertebral area, plus sustained squats or sustained a knees-to-chest position to stretch the facial layers.

Myalgia (fibrositis)

In my view, fibrositis is not a clinical diagnosis. The term is incorrect as there is little evidence for inflammation of the muscle fibrils. Furthermore, the nodules that can be 'palpated' are non-existent until palpated, at which point the palpating finger creates a localized increase in fiber contraction, resembling a nodule, which may or may not be tender when rolled under the finger. Myalgia would be a better term for tender muscles that are probably fatigued with resultant secondary metabolic changes. In the cervical and thoracic regions, myalgia appears to be related to rheumatic conditions.

Treatment. Medication, heat, massage, and exercises may assist.

Facet dysfunction

The spinal facet joints, particularly their postero-medial aspect, are perhaps the most innervated structures in the spine (Paris 1984). Since the 1930s, they have been identified as a source of pain and have been the subject of a number of studies involving the reproduction of pain by injecting hypertonic saline (Mooney & Robinson 1976).

We can identify five separate clinical states in the spinal facets, which should not come as a surprise, as all five can exist in other synovial joints, such as the knee, which, in common with the spinal facets, have meniscal inclusions. These states are described below.

Facet synovitis/hemarthrosis (acute sprain)

Acute synovitis or hemarthrosis is perhaps the most common source of acute, usually transient, low back pain. Its cause appears to be a strain or nipping of the sensitive facet capsule and its synovial lining. Depending on the degree of noxious stimulation, it is accompanied by involuntary or voluntary muscle guarding. It is widely accepted that 80% of back pain resolves within 2 weeks; in my view, most of these cases are facet injuries.

Typically, the injury occurs when the spine is moved in a sudden motion or in recovering with a twist from a forward bent position. Although there are three structures designed to prevent capsular nipping, i.e. the elastic anterior capsule (ligamentum flavum), the intracapsular fibrous meniscoid, and the attachment of the multifidus muscle posteriorly, these mechanisms may fail, and a painful nipping can result. The joint swells and the nipping is relieved. The initial pain is sharp and often quite localized and, in the cervical spine, can be readily palpated.

The signs and symptoms are of localized low back pain and minimal radiation, perhaps to the iliac crest and buttock (further if there is a memory of sciatic pain from past problems). Movement, if limited, is from involuntary muscle holding and is not particularly uncomfortable. Loading the facet, as in backward bending and bending to the same side, is not painful at this stage.

In 2–3 days, the effusion would be expected to resolve and, similar to other joints, will leave behind some restrictions to movement. These restrictions help to splint the sensitive joint, thus enabling the muscle guarding to abate and the patient to move more freely. Such restrictions do, however, leave the joint less able to tolerate future insults, making it even more prone to reinjury, and resulting again in synovitis and hemarthrosis. Restrictions of facets also serve to limit nutrition to the intervertebral disc.

Treatment. None is really required. Medication for pain relief and assurance of a timely recovery are sufficient. Three days without strenuous work is sufficient. Ideally, the joint should be examined 10 days after injury, and any restriction resulting from the serofibrinous exudate may be manipulated.

Facet stiffness (restrictions)

Spinal facet restriction is very common and is a painless condition, as is initial stiffness in joints of the extremities. However, stiffness leads to loss of nutrition and hence aids degeneration. This may be true, especially in the spine, where stiff facets combined with adaptive muscle shortening (see above) may lead to interference with disc nutrition and precipitate disc degeneration and herniation.

Since stiff joints do not necessarily hurt, they are usually detected on examination for back pain from other causes. Segmental restrictions are detected with passive motion testing (motion palpation) (Bonella et al 1982), and adhesions have been demonstrated by the present author (Paris 1991).

Treatment. Manipulation directed specifically at the involved joint and in the direction of the restriction.

Facet painful entrapment

The patient reports with acute low back pain and postural deviation. Any effort to resume normal alignment is accompanied by a local and sharp pain on one side of the back. The pain does not radiate, but may, a day or so later, migrate up the spine owing to painful involuntary muscle guarding, leading to chemical muscle holding

The pathology of this diagnosis has never been demonstrated, but the logic of its presence is persuasive (Kraft & Levinthal 1951), especially given

the effectiveness of the treatment. Pathological specimens have shown enlarged facet capsules and intra-articular fatty cysts, which are believed to be innervated (Kirkaldy-Willis *c*. 1988).

The causative movement, as with most facet joint injuries, appears to be an awkward flexion with side-bending and rotation occurring at the initial moment of trying to assume the erect position. The onset of pain and the postural deformity are immediate.

Treatment. Manipulation is used, employing a lumbar rotary technique, which is, in effect, a distraction of the facet joint. Adequate relaxation of any muscle guarding due to the discomfort should be ensured (heat, massage, and acupressure) before attempting the manipulation. When the manipulation is successful, the relief is immediate but not complete. A synovitis hemarthrosis remains and should be treated accordingly for 10 days (relative rest and support). Any further manipulation to correct segmental stiffness should be delayed during this time.

Facet mechanical block

In contrast to painful block, a mechanical block is relatively painless. The patient quite simply becomes suddenly fixed in a laterally shifted position. Any attempt to straighten upward is met with difficulty, and the patient often reports being 'stuck' and in need of having it 'cracked'. The exact mechanism is speculative. However, since spinal facets contain menisci and on occasion loose bodies, and such joints elsewhere in the body (the knee, craniomandibular joint, and wrist) are known to become stuck or locked, it is surely possible that the spinal facets may also lock.

Treatment. Distraction manipulation as for a painful block.

Chronic facet dysfunction

This condition results from repeated strains and sprains to the facet joints and is no different from degenerative arthrosis affecting synovial joints elsewhere in the body. In the patient's history, the pain begins each day on one side of the lumbar spine and may then spread to the iliac crest and buttock. More severe cases will be felt in the posterior thigh and calf. The muscle guarding involves the leg, and a false positive straight leg raise (SLR) may result. This can be confirmed by a neuromuscular facilitation technique, which will immediately increase the SLR. A facet block is diagnostic.

Treatment. Postural to decrease the stress. Medial branch rhizolysis is also effective but damaging to the muscles.

Sacroiliac dysfunction

The SI is listed third in this classification as, in my opinion, it is the third most common cause of low back and pelvic pain, preceded only by muscular and facet syndromes.

The principal source of pain arising from the SI is, no doubt, the richly innervated, strong, deep posterior SI ligaments (Paris 1983), which are designed to resist vertical stresses, and perhaps even rotary stresses, should the sacrospinous and sacrotuberous ligaments become lax. This author was not successful in finding innervation of the scant anterior capsule of the SIJ. The iliolumbar ligament is also a key SI ligament. In the female, it attaches to the ilium and the transverse processes of both L4 and L5, but in the male only to L5 (Paris, unpublished data).

Since stiff joints do not, at least in their early stages, cause pain, and since stiffness of the SIJ, especially in middle-aged and older men, is the rule and SI pain the exception, it can be concluded that stiff SIJs are of no clinical importance unless they are 'locked' in some position beyond or at the end of their physiological range, thus giving rise to sustained ligamentous stress. Such a condition is most likely to occur, and does occur, in an unstable (hypermobile), young female SIJ. Such a patient would have a pre-existing history of one-sided low back pain.

For this author, there are only three conditions that need to be considered: acute sprain, hypermobility, and 'locked' or 'subluxed' SIJs. The nuances of positional faults, and the convoluted possibilities of subluxation and the numerous theories, are, in my opinion, just that. When interexaminer reliability on alleged position faults is as poor as it is, proponents of the SI as a source of low back pain need to be cautioned against appearing too sure of their theories, and should stick with fundamental principles common to joints elsewhere in the body.

Acute stain

Acute sprain is most commonly caused by a fall on one of the ischial tuberosities. If the ligaments are strong, they will resist a displacement, but it may be quite painful for a few days. The pain is local as is the tenderness.

Treatment. Modalities or medication for pain relief. If severe and persisting beyond a week, the joint should be re-examined for hypermobility and, if present, treated as recommended below.

Hypermobility

Hypermobility is, by contrast, caused by repeated sprains and strains, such as in falls, poor postural habits, as in one-leg standing, and vigorous positions in sexual intercourse wherein the thighs are repeatedly forced toward the chest – this is especially the case in those with restricted hip motion. All of the above activities cause the ilium to rotate posteriorly, i.e. the cephalic end (or top) of the ilium rotates backwards.

The onset of pain is usually gradual, is localized to *one side of the back, does not cross the midline*, and is usually relieved by supine rest, which, by its very nature, rotates the ilium forward, thus relieving the stress on the supporting ligaments. Being ligamentous in nature, the pain is usually most noticeable at the commencement of the menstrual flow. Involuntary muscle guarding of the ipsilateral spinal muscles and of piriformis may also be present.

Treatment. Begin with an explanation of the stresses that are causing the problem and how to avoid most, if not all, of them. If the hip joints are restricted, they should be manipulated. If the SI pain is acute or severe, a Skultetas binder or SI belt is recommended. Relief by either the binder or belt is generally confirmatory of the diagnosis.

Displacement (subluxation)

It is the hypermobile SI that is most likely to result in a displacement and a resultant lock of the irregular articular surfaces, giving rise to lower-level but more constant pain and disability than with hypermobility. The pain will be present in most postures, especially those that tend to increase the displacement, and is also present at night. Those postures that reduce the discomfort usually point to the direction of the corrective manipulation. There are numerous tests, most quite reliable, to determine whether the ilium is rotated posteriorly or anteriorly on the sacrum. Another situation, not uncommon, is an up-slip of the ilium (the same as a down-slip of the sacrum), and this interestingly enough appears more prevalent in men.

Treatment. Manipulation is in either forward or backward rotation or downward on the ilium for an up-slip. Once the manipulation has succeeded, the joint is usually found to be hypermobile and will benefit from support.

It should be noted that the previous three conditions are either aggravated or relieved by stress tests to the SI. Such tests are inconclusive if they are not specific to the supporting ligaments of the joint. Intra-articular injections have mixed results, as the anesthetic will fail to infiltrate the large posterior SI and the more distant iliolumbar ligaments, and will, quite probably, burst through a synovial recess in the anterior capsule mistaken by some as an SI tear (Neville et al 1996). Injections given by numerous releases into the posterior ligaments, especially at the upper pole of the joint at the level of S1 and S2, would appear to be more effective.

Ligamentous weakness and instability

Ligamentous laxity can be a source of pain in peripheral joints such as the knee, glenohumeral, and acromioclavicular joints. It is now accepted that the same situation is commonly present in the spine (Kirkaldy-Willis 1990, Nachemson 1985). The structures responsible for passive spinal stability are initially the ligamentous structures, including the outer annulus of the intervertebral disc. which is likewise made up of type I collagen. The facet joints also play a variable role in passive spinal stabilization, and their surgical removal may help to create instability. Additionally, the muscles of the spine are somewhat important in achieving stabilization, especially when ligamentous stability has been lost.

In the author's opinion, ligamentous weakness precedes segmental ligamentous instability, and instability is a precursor of the clinically apparent disc condition perhaps requiring surgery with or without fusion. A stable spine appears far less likely to present with a clinically obvious disc problem.

The pain of ligamentous weakness is characteristic. It begins with a dull ache in the back, which, as the day wears on, appears to spread to the muscles (the muscles are actually in involuntary guarding and the muscle pain comes from the chemical muscle holding; temporary relief can easily be provided by massage). This ache can be relieved by a change in position, movement or by 'self-cracking' of the back. The 'self–cracking', not to be recommended as it severely stresses the disc, leading to further instability, provides temporary relief as it causes muscle relaxation by firing the type III mechanoreceptors of the Golgi end organs of the tendon or, perhaps, even the disc itself (Roberts et al 1995). Walking is usually painless, and prolonged sitting, such as at a desk or while driving, is the most painful. Sitting with the back supported by a roll will relieve posterior ligamentous weakness, but less so of the intervertebral disc. The pain is dull and diffuse, at first localized to the lumbar spine.

Given that ligamentous weakness also involves the annulus fibrosus, transient neurological signs may occur, as may a transient lateral shift again toward the end of the day. Such a lateral shift may be considered to be a sign of instability, and is not unlike letting the air out of a car tire when parked on an incline: the car will shift sideways down the incline. Reinflation will set the car uphill once again, as will a night's rest straighten the spine – at least initially.

Causes of spinal instability are, no doubt, to be found in postural misuse and abuse, smoking, and athletics, such as springboard diving, weightlifting, and gymnastics, all of which are known to increase the incidence of spondylolisthesis. The clinical signs and symptoms of instability (Paris 1985) include:

- a visible or palpable step or rotary deformity, which is present on standing but which reduces on lying
- hypertonicity of the muscles on standing that disappears on lying
- hypermobility on motion passive palpation – grade 5 or 6 (Gonnella et al 1982)
- shaking or trembling of the lumbar spine on forward bending
- more difficulty in coming upright than going into forward bending
- a history of 'catches' and 'giving way'.

Treatment. Manipulation is often given to adjacent, restricted spinal segments and to any restriction in the hips, thus reducing the need for the unstable level to compensate. For the unstable segment, postural instruction and lifestyle changes will be necessary. 'Cracking' the back must cease as, although it may provide temporary relief, it is the unstable joint that appears to crack, and this wrenching of the disc will only add to the instability.

Disc dysfunction

In virtually all patients with a clinically evident disc protrusion or rupture, there is first a preceding history of ligamentous weakness and/or spinal instability. Without such a history, low back and leg pain must not be assumed to be from the disc, as both the facet and the SI may produce reference of symptoms into the leg. Some clinicians assume that if the pain does not go below the knee, its origin could be facet, but if below the knee, it is disc. This concept denies the fact that pain is referred, not only because of which structure is involved, but also because of the intensity of the stimulus. How pain in the posterior thigh can one day be considered facet and the next day, when it is more severe and in the calf, can be considered disc is beyond the comprehension of this author. Both facets and discs have referred pain into the calf, although I know of no study incriminating the SIJ in the same way. No doubt, however, if the patient is already experiencing low back and leg pain involving the discs and the SIJ, an irritant injection into the SI and, for that matter, any other segmentally related structure, will increase the already facilitated leg and calf pain.

For a clinical disc protrusion and/or prolapse to be diagnosed, there must be demonstrable neurological signs other than pain below the knee and limited straight leg raising. Objective muscle weakness and loss of skin sensation are indicative of nerve root involvement. Reduced or absent reflexes are less indicative.

The non-operative treatment will depend on the stage of the condition.

Immediate stage

This stage occurs when the patient, who has a history of ligamentous weakness and/or instability, performs an awkward or unguarded action and feels something 'give' or 'tear' in his or her back. The patient knows immediately that he or she has now received an acute injury on top of the already existing back problem. There exists a real possibility that the patient has just torn the outer annulus and that, should the tear be deep enough to communicate with the nucleus, an extrusion may soon result. Hopefully, these patients would have already been identified as being at risk (a history of ligamentous weakness and instability) and would have been instructed to go immediately into backward bending and to stay in that position should such an incident as that just described occur.

The theory behind the immediate assumption of backward bending, especially to the affected side, and to be supported by taping and corsetry, is to close down any disc tear or rupture that may have just occurred and thus prevent the nucleus, capable of expanding to three times its enclosed size, from oozing out. Just as a cut of the finger ceases bleeding if the sides of the tear are approximated, thus facilitating early healing, so it is with the neurovascular capsule of the disc (Paris 1990). Typically, however, the patient sits to rest and leans away from the side of the hurt. The sitting increases the load and the leaning away opens the tear. What usually occurs next is that, some 15–30 min later, the patient becomes aware of a vague deep leg pain. This is presumed due to the extruded disc causing pressure on the nerve root, resulting in ischemia. The patient may then try to move, but finds that this only increases the pain. Any attempt to straighten upward further pinches and extrudes the protrusion while narrowing the foramen, thus creating further nerve root pressure. The window of opportunity to keep it contained has been lost.

Acute stage

Here we presume that the disc is protruded/extruded and the nerve root is compromised. Any attempt to go into backward bending will only increase the pain, as all evidence points to such action as increasing the disc protrusion (McCall 1980, Spohr & Paris 1992). There is, in the present author's opinion, no physical therapy treatment other than to encourage a routine of rest, with minimal stress to the area, in order to allow any inflammatory response accompanying the protrusion to subside. Neurological signs will, in time, reverse, perhaps due to shrinking of the protrusion, but more probably due to the establishment of a collateral circulation to the nerve and reduction of the initial swelling. Active exercises, traction, and manipulation, especially rotary techniques, should be discouraged as it is all too easy to aggravate the condition by further extruding disc material.

Backward bending (extension) may be attempted but, in any true disc, it will most likely lateralize the pain by again pinching and protruding the disc and narrowing the foramen. It is the author's view that backward bending (extension routine) does not help a true disc protrusion but rather benefits all other types of back pain by introducing movement, however indiscriminate, which in turn helps to gate pain, aids in nutrition, and assists the patient in overcoming the fear of movement.

Treatment. Treatment is bed rest, the more complete the better, with analgesics, and a high-fiber diet and laxatives to enable the use of a bedpan. Bathroom privileges must be forbidden, as straining on a hard stool can only aggravate the condition, which, with rest, may settle quickly. The theory behind bedrest is that it is not so much the protrusion/herniation, but the soft tissue swelling that accompanies it, that is causing the symptoms. Imaging shows that the protrusion/herniation often remains, even though the symptoms have abated. We are thus nursing and reducing the swelling and should avoid any further aggravation of the site.

Settled stage

This stage begins about 3 weeks post onset. The patient is ambulatory.

Treatment. Backward bending to regain the lordosis and the erect position is the first priority should the lordosis have been lost.

Symptom relief and recovery may be effected by positional distraction, which seeks to open the foramen and gently pull the outer annulus flat, thus temporarily relieving the nerve root pressure. This treatment can be continued at home twice a day for 40 min each session. Emphasis then moves onto education, including what to do should an acute exacerbation occur (bend backward immediately), and more specific rehabilitation measures based on a thorough examination for dysfunction.

Chronic stage

This is at about 12 weeks, when all primary healing has taken place, and in a patient who still has symptoms.

Treatment. As for the settled stage, if it has not already been carried out. In addition, fitness training and work-hardening can be added. Emphasis should also be placed on behavioral modification techniques. Treatment is not very effective at this stage.

Spondylolisthesis

There are, of course, several types of spondylolisthesis. The most common is from a fatigue fracture of the pars interarticularis. In either event, a palpable 'step' and/or 'rotation' may be detected in the back upon standing. If the step or rotation disappears with lying, the slip may be considered to be unstable. X-ray confirmation should be taken at the end of the day, and perhaps with the patient standing, as unstable steps may disappear and, if of the degenerative type (no fracture), the diagnosis may be missed.

The symptoms are ligamentous and local. Only if the slip is advanced will neurological signs and symptoms result.

Treatment. This depends on whether or not the condition is stable or unstable. If it is stable, no treatment is called for, as the condition is unlikely to be the cause of any complaints. If it is unstable, posture, education, stretching (carefully) of the iliopsoas, and stabilization exercises of the deep spinal musculature are called for and are usually successful. When neurological signs and symptoms are present, surgical fusion must be considered.

Central canal and lateral foraminal stenosis

The typical patient is middle-aged to elderly, short, and heavy framed, with a history of a lifestyle physically stressful to the lumbar spine, and perhaps with obesity and smoking.

The signs and symptoms are extremely variable but include transient neurological signs and symptoms brought on by exercising, particularly in the afternoon. Neurovascular claudication occurs during walking, similar to vascular claudication, but is distinguished by the fact that forward bending tends to relieve the pain. The bicycle test is confirmatory. Riding a stationary bike with the back in lordosis will soon bring on leg pain, but riding the bike with the low back in kyphosis will delay or even prevent the onset of pain.

Treatment. This is an interesting challenge for physical therapy. In the early stages, or in the poor operative risk group, there are a number of mechanical approaches that can often help to manage the condition. Since the condition is a narrowing of the canal and/or foramen, the objective is to open these areas as much as possible. Attention should be paid to reducing the lumbar lordosis by both stretching out any tight lumbar myofascia and by manipulating the lumbar facets should restrictions be present, which they usually are. Additional consideration should be given to lowering the heels or using negative heels and, in the case of a male with a 'pot belly', advocating weight loss as this particular posture increases the lordosis. Reduction of impact loads associated with walking may be effected by using viscoelastic insoles and mobilizing any hip restrictions. Back exercises are of little value and lumbar traction of only temporary benefit.

For unilateral symptoms, placing a heel lift under the opposite leg is sometimes dramatically effective in that it produces side-bending to that side during standing and walking, thus opening the involved neural foramen. Again, use a viscoelastic polymer under each foot and a lift on the good side.

Another approach is to increase the individual's physical fitness with exercise on a treadmill while the spine is partially unweighted in a traction suspension device now being used extensively for gait rehabilitation. By increasing fitness, the patient should be able to walk with less effort, thus lessening the demands on the neurovascular system. Some good results have been reported (B. Svendsen, 1994, personal communication).

Kissing lumbar spines

In 1924 Baastrup described a condition in which the spinous processes of the lumbar spine impinge upon one another and give rise to arthritis and sclerotic changes, which can become quite painful (Baastrup 1933). The condition is most common in short, stocky males at middle life. It is in these individuals that the spinous processes tend to be large and the disc spaces small. With middle age and the natural shrinking of the intervertebral disc, the spinous processes impinge on one another, producing central low back pain relieved by forward bending or pulling the knees to the chest.

Treatment. Conservative treatment is limited beyond providing an explanation, stretching out any tight lumbar myofascia to lessen a static lordosis, pelvic tilt, negative-heel shoes, and abdominal strengthening, with perhaps counseling for weight loss. Surgical intervention to remodel the spinous process was recommended by Baastrup, while others have recommended sclerosing injections, and still others have had success with medial branch rhizolysis.

Thorocolumbar syndrome

This condition consists of pain in the lateral iliac crest and anterior thigh to the knee, with an occasional giving-way of the leg. The condition appears to originate from the T11–L1 levels, sometimes secondary to stiffness or surgical fusion of the lower levels.

Treatment. Manipulation of the lower levels when possible, and stabilization exercises for the thorocolumbar region, produces good results.

Lesion complex

The preceding sections have presented some of the more common dysfunctions that may cause pain in the spine. Although they have been presented as single entities and given names somewhat comparable with diagnostic terms, it is important to note that most of those who present with symptoms have signs and symptoms not simply of one syndrome but of several; therein lies the difficulty of a differential diagnosis.

ARRIVING AT THE DIAGNOSIS

For a patient with the complaint of low back, right buttock, and posterior thigh pain, Table 26.1 lists probable findings and their suggested treatments.

What is the diagnosis?

Given the findings in Table 26.1, my medical colleagues might state 'suspected disc protrusion', and if this is not found (I hate to suggest 'confirmed') on an X-ray, 'low back strain'. If asked for a diagnosis, I too am unable to give a precise, one-line diagnosis that carries a number or code for billing purposes. However, on the other hand, I do believe that what is outlined in Table 26.1 is a diagnosis, or at least a diagnostic description, of the objective physical findings, as it is my experience that, if this is all I can find, the very best I can do is to treat those findings – there is nothing else I can do and, I will argue, nothing else anyone can do or need do.

If we can correct the findings of poor posture and work habits, limited motion, instability, and shortened muscles, we are often able to provide for relief without ever being sure of the diagnosis.

Table 26.1 Findings in a patient with low back, buttock, and thigh pain

Clinical findings	Suggested treatment
Short left leg (this will narrow the right foramen)	Left heel lift
Restricted facet motion at L5/S1 on the right	Manipulation
Minimal hypermobility at L4/5	Ignore, otherwise stabilization routine
Positive Faber on both hips (capsular tightness)	Manipulation
Poor lifting and other postural bad habits	Back school

CONCLUSIONS

1. As stated in the introduction, it is important that we recognize that the old paradigm of back pain being a medical complaint capable of being diagnosed and then treated medically has failed and will continue to fail.

2. There is a better paradigm in its place, which is back pain as being caused by a summation of two or more dysfunctions.

3. Each dysfunction contributes to an accumulation of noxious stimuli, which, when the individual's level for appreciation is reached, will be interpreted by the individual as discomfort.

4. Discomfort may trigger entitlement behaviors and, when sufficiently accumulated, will result in pain even in the stout-hearted, producing one more patient seeking assistance.

5. As a result, it is not so important to treat the diagnosis or syndrome as to treat the objective physical findings deemed most likely to be responsible for the patient's symptoms.

REFERENCES

Baastrup C 1933 On the spinous processes of the lumbar vertebrae and the soft tissues between them, and on pathological changes in that region. Acta Radiologica 14: 52
Codman E A 1934 The shoulder. Boston, MA
Dorland's illustrated medical dictionary, 27th edn. 1985 WB Saunders, Philadelphia, PA
Gonella C, Paris S V, Kutner M 1982 Reliability in evaluating passive intervertebral motion. Physical Therapy 62(4): 436–444
Kirkaldy-Willis W H c. 1988 A slide from a collection of slides on lumbar spine pathology

Kirkaldy-Willis W H 1990 Segmental instability, the lumbar spine. WB Saunders, Philadelphia, PA
Kraft G L, Levinthal O H 1951 Facet synovial impingement. Surgery, Gynecology and Obstetrics: 439–444
Lieber R L 1992 Skeletal muscle structure and function. Williams & Wilkins, Baltimore
McCall I 1980 In: The lumbar spine and low back pain, 2nd edn. Pitman, London
McKenzie 1996 The lumbar spine, vol. II ch. 17
Mooney V T, Robinson J 1976 The facet syndrome. Clinical Orthopaedics 115: 149–156
Nachemson A 1985 Lumbar spine instability: a critical update and symposium summary. Spine 10: 254
Neville C, Graham-Smith A, Patla C E 1996 Sacroiliac joint

instability, diagnostically confirmed: a case study poster presentation. American Physical Therapy Association, Atlanta, GA

Paris S V 1983 Anatomy as related to function and pain. Orthopedic Clinics of North America 14(3): 484–485

Paris S V 1984 Functional anatomy of the lumbar spine. University Microfilms International, Ann Arbour, MI

Paris S V 1985 Physical signs of instability. Spine 10: 3

Paris S V 1990 Healing of the lumbar intervertebral disc. Proceedings of the Canadian Manual Therapy Association

Paris S V 1991 Physical therapy approach to facet, disc and sacroiliac syndromes of the lumbar spine. In: White A H (ed.) Conservative care of low back pain. Williams & Wilkins, Baltimore, ch. 22

Roberts S, Eisenstein S M, Menage J, Evans E H, Ashton K 1995 Mechanoreceptors in intervertebral discs. Spine 20(24): 2645–2651

Spohr C, Paris S V 1992 Discomyelogram, a flouroscopic study of disc protrusion. Proceedings of the Fifth IFOMT Congress, Vail, CO

Stoddard A 1959 Manual of osteopathic technique. Hutchinson, London

Visualization

27. Basic problems in the visualization of the sacroiliac joint

P. F. Dijkstra

The X-ray is a shadow of reality.

INTRODUCTION

Plain X-rays of the sacroiliac joints (SIJs) are often difficult to 'read'. It needs a thorough understanding of the anatomy of the SIJ and knowledge of how these images are made, to rebuild in our minds the flat image into a three-dimensional image. In order to understand the X-rays of the SIJ, we will describe the process that produces the final image, and discuss the problems inherent in interpreting the radiologic anatomy. Some pathologic conditions of the SIJ will be shown.

RADIOLOGIC ANATOMY

X-ray absorption

The photons of X-ray radiation are more or less absorbed in our body. In general, there are four different groups of body constituents in terms of radiation: air, fat, water, and bone. Air (as in the lungs or gut) has a low absorption value; bone has the highest absorption value, depending on its calcium content.

This differentiation allows us to 'see' the different parts of the body. Low absorption implies that many photons reach the photographic plate behind the body. That spot becomes black. Intermediate absorption gives shades of gray (as in body fat and muscles), and with high absorption, few photons reach the photographic plate, which remains white. There are several technical solutions to obtain a good image; these, however, will not be discussed here.

Projection of the object

There will always be a distortion of the object in the projection on the photographic plate. The X-ray tube can be seen as a point source from which the radiation leaves the tube as a fan beam in the direction of the object and the photographic plate. The further away from the tube, the broader the beam becomes. This means that on the edge of the beam, the enlargement of the object's projection will be greater than in the center (Fig. 27.1). Furthermore, parts of the object close to the tube will be projected larger

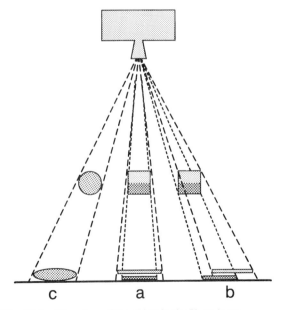

Fig. 27.1 The place of the object in the X-ray beam determines the object's projection. In the central ray (a), the top and bottom of the square are projected on top of each other, but the top is slightly larger than the bottom. At the right (b), top and bottom are shifted. The sphere on the left (c) is projected as an oval structure.

than parts close to the photographic plate. Therefore, international rules exist to produce X-ray pictures. The more complicated the structure of the object, the more difficult to understand the final X-ray image. Knowledge of the density (amount of radiation absorption) and the normal anatomic features of the object is a prerequisite to find pathological structures.

IMAGING TECHNIQUES

Plain X-ray

Plain X-rays should be used to get an overview of the sacrum and SIJ. We do not discuss the lateral view of the sacrum because it is not a helpful technique in investigating the SIJ. Several projections are possible, but anteroposterior (AP) and 25° cranial angulated views are the most informative (Dijkstra 1993). Oblique views should not be used: they look nice but, by superimposing the front and back of the SIJ, they will hide more detail than they reveal (see Fig. 27.3 below).

Tomography

This technique produces an image as a slice of the body of 2–5 mm thick. Because of the construction of the X-ray machine, these slices are in the coronal, oblique, or sagittal plane, depending on the position of the patient. Axial slices are usually difficult or impossible to make. This is in contrast to computerized tomography (CT), in which only axial slices can be made. The new spiral CT machines are able to reconstruct all imaging planes. Tomography is carried out using a multidirectional movement of the X-ray tube. This means a spiral or hypocycloidal movement of 25°; all other movements are insufficient for the SIJ. Both types of multidirectional movement have their pros and cons; when aware of the ghost images of the system, there is no problem. It is essential with tomography that the part of the joint under investigation is tangential to the movement of the X-ray tube. In a complicated joint such as the SIJ, one has to be careful to position the patient in the right way. The largest problem with reading tomograms concerns the ghost images;

these are, in fact, quite easy to interpret when one has a thorough knowledge of the normal anatomy and an understanding of the tomographic process (Firooznia et al 1984).

Computerized tomography

CT should be carried out using a 2 mm slice thickness, with a 5 mm interval and a high-definition filter. The angulation of the gantry is not important, being merely a question of taste, but slice thickness and filter are very important. In our experience, a window of 1600 and level of 400 with a high (software) filter are very satisfactory.

It is a misunderstanding that CT makes things easier: the pictures are just as difficult to read and to interpret as images obtained by other techniques. However, because of the high contrast in CT pictures, one is inclined to see more pathology. The borders of the joints are sharper, but the natural inclinations of the SIJs in the picture might fool one into thinking that erosions are present. Further discussion of CT scanning can be found in Chapter 28.

Magnetic resonance imaging

Magnetic resonance imaging (MRI) gives very promising results, and might eventually take over from most other imaging techniques. Up to now, the resolution of the images has been unsatisfactory with respect to small details in the SIJ cartilage.

MRI is very useful in the search for septic arthritis and is the only technique that can pinpoint the pathologic areas in bone and soft tissues.

Isotope studies

The possibility for discriminating between different diseases on the basis of isotope activity in the SIJ is very poor. In general, not more can be said than that some disease process is going on. It can be helpful in septic arthritis (leukocyte scan), when the origin of the disease is not clear, but in that case MRI is far more conclusive.

Choice

Plain X-rays are always taken, in order to get an overview of the patient's problems. Which other techniques are used depends on the sort of pathology anticipated. In the Old World, as opposed to the Americas, tomography is still largely used, although it is being more and more replaced by CT. In septic arthritis, MRI should be used. In spondylarthropathy, CT and tomography can be used.

In cases of trauma, the technique depends on the status of the patient, but CT is the method of choice. Because the patient usually has several iron plates in the bones and is difficult to handle, it is easier to carry out tomography, with less disturbance in the picture. Because of the metal artefacts, CT scanning is usually not possible.

RADIOLOGIC ANATOMY OF THE SIJ

The angulation of the joints is measured with respect to the sagittal plain. S1 has an angulation of 20–25° lateral. S2 usually has an angulation of 10–15° lateral. S3 has a more or less sagittal angulation (0–5° medial) (Fig. 27.2A,B). S1 is broader than S3 (Solonen 1957, Dijkstra et al 1989, Vleeming et al 1992).

Thus the joint has a double curvature: dorsoventral and craniocaudal. Obviously, in no single projection can all parts of the joint be viewed tangentially (Fig. 27.2C–E). With X-rays, we see a sharp edge only when it is perpendicular to our viewing direction; it is one of the problems specifically encountered in the SIJ. Figure 27.3 shows the different projections that are obtained when the supine patient is turned from right to left. As a mental exercise, understanding these projections is the first step necessary to be able to diagnose malformations or disease of the SIJ.

The general direction of the SIJ joint from posterior to ventral is about 25°. Thus if the patient is prone and the X-ray is taken in a posteroanterior direction, the joints seem to be covered in their entire length. This is the same when the joint is seen in the ventrodorsal direction with the patient turned 25°; this is called the oblique SIJ position. An oblique view seems nice,

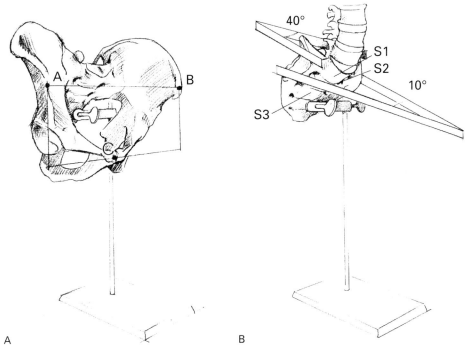

Fig. 27.2 (A,B) Drawings of the SIJ, showing the pelvis and the orientation of the SIJ. (A) shows a ventrolateral view of the pelvis in the erect posture. The angle between the sacral auricular surfaces of S1 and S3 is shown (B). (Reproduced with permission from Dijkstra et al 1989.)

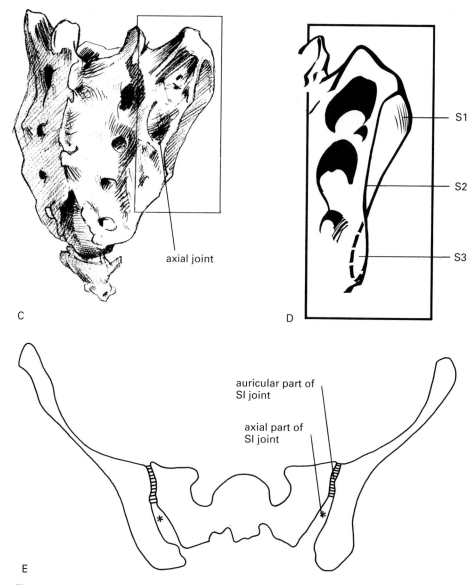

Fig. 27.2 (*Contd*) (C–E) A dorsolateral view of the sacrum shows the auricular surface (C). A schematic drawing of the auricular surface of the right SIJ depicts the general orientation and curvature (D). (E) shows a transverse section of the SIJ just above the ventral superior iliac spine and through the first pelvic sacral foramina. The hatched areas refer to the cartilage-covered auricular surface. The site of the axial joint, posterior to the auricular joint, is indicated by an asterisk.

but it is a superposition of all parts of the joint. To understand this more clearly, we have used a cadaver SIJ sawn into 5 mm slices. Figure 27.4 shows that the back and the front of one slice are quite different. In practice, the 25° cranial angled AP view gives the information to decide on further investigation.

In daily practice, the projections of the SIJ are those used for the lumbar spine, the pelvis, and the 25° cranial angled AP view. In CT scanning, transverse (Fig. 27.2C–E) or angulated transverse planes are used, but plain X-rays are taken in the coronal plane. Bearing in mind that the SIJ has a double curvature, we see in plain

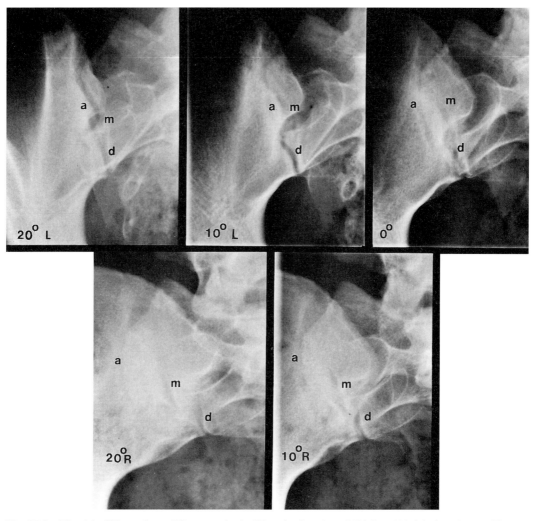

Fig. 27.3 The right SIJ seen from different angles in AP projection, from 20° left to 20° right in 10° steps. The ventral (a), middle (m) and posterior (d) parts of the joint are seen. In the 20° left directed projection, all parts are superimposed. This projection is a simulation of a posteroanterior projection or an AP projection with the patient turned 25° to the left, called the oblique position.

X-rays both the edges of the posterior and ventral parts of the joint as well as the middle part.

As an example, Fig. 27.5 shows a normal SIJ: Fig. 27.5A is the caudal part of the lumbar spine view, whereas Fig. 27.5B is a cranial angulated AP view. It is only in the second view that we can see the middle part of the joint. The posterior and the ventrolateral part of the joint is well seen in both views. Obviously, different projections influence the perception of the joint (Dijkstra 1993).

In Fig. 27.6 we introduce tomography as a means of evaluating the SIJ. The plain X-ray in Fig. 27.6A shows a superimposed projection of segments of the joint. Tomography of the posterior part of the joint (Fig. 27.6B) shows left–right asymmetry and a hook-like projection near the axial part of the joint located dorsal of the auricular part (see Fig. 27.2B above). The ventral part of the joint is well seen in Fig. 27.6C, and here we also see a persistent epiphysis in the joint. The epiphyses of the SIJ usually close at about 16 years of

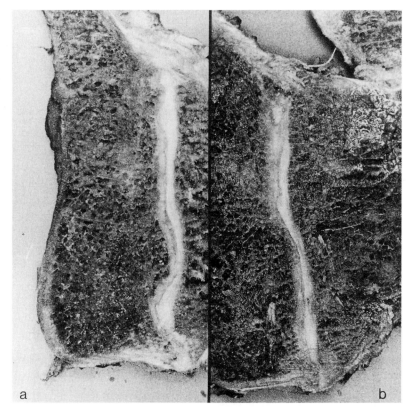

Fig. 27.4   Front (a) and back (b) of the same anatomic slice of a SIJ. Note the difference in configuration of the joint, notwithstanding a slice thickness of only 5 mm. This gives an impression of how difficult it is to show all parts of the SIJ on X-ray: most parts of the joint are hidden in a plain X-ray. (Reproduced with permission from Dijkstra et al 1989.)

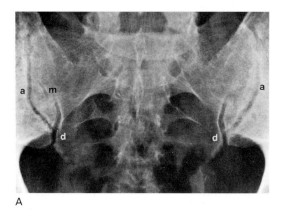
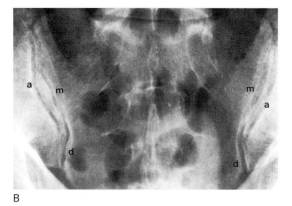

Fig. 27.5   A normal SIJ in two AP projections; a = ventral, m = middle and d = posterior parts of the joint. (A) The caudal part of a lumbar spine view. The SIJs are seen in the same projection as the lateral square in Fig. 27.1. The posterior part of S3 is more accentuated, and the middle part of the joint is usually not seen. (B) Cranial angulated AP view. The SIJs are in the center of the X-ray beam. Because the ventral and middle parts of the joint are closer to the X-ray tube, they are projected more to the lateral of the X-ray. The middle part of the joint is more easily seen.

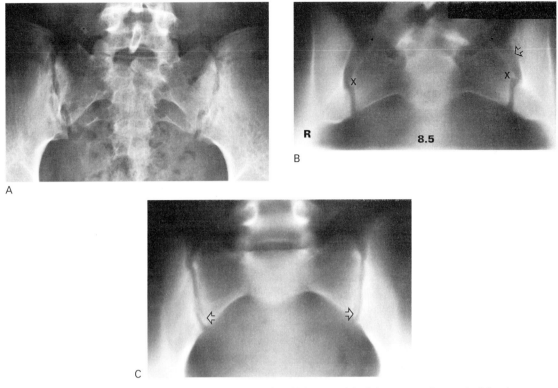

Fig. 27.6 (A) Plain X-ray of the SIJ in a 17-year-old boy in which parts of the joint are superimposed, giving the impression of irregularity on the left. The differential diagnosis was ankylosing spondylitis or closing epiphysis. Tomography revealed epiphyses and congenital irregularity of the joints. (B) Tomography of the posterior part of the left joint shows a hooklike (X) projection into the axial joint on both sides and a left–right asymmetry with bony exostosis (arrow) of the sacrum in the left axial joint. '8.5' depicts the distance of this slice from the table top. (C) Tomography of the ventral part of the joints. There is a slight sclerosis of the left joint, due to the closing of the epiphysis. In the caudal area, an epiphysis (arrow) is seen in the sacrum, especially on the right side.

age; because of their projection, they can be a source of confusion.

Congenital variations

There are many congenital variations. The sacrum can be more or less absent, which is usually accompanied by partial absence of the uterus and/or ureter and kidney. In several of the patients presented here, congenital variations are present, for example transitional vertebra (see Figs 27.7, 27.8 and 27.10 below), asymmetry (see Fig. 27.7 below) and persistent division between sacral segments (see Fig. 27.7 below), and also persistent epiphyses (Fig. 27.6). The axial part of the SIJ (see Fig. 27.2B above) can have a complex form and can give a confusing shadow (Fig. 27.6B). A non-closure of the

spinous process of L5 and S1 is sometimes associated with spina bifida, but in most people this variation is without clinical symptoms.

Symmetry

The SIJs often show left–right asymmetry. Many unnecessary X-rays can be avoided if one has some knowledge of this phenomenon. Figure 27.7 shows a persistent S1–2 joint on both sides, and also a left–right asymmetry. The left SIJ is somewhat smaller than the right. At the right side of this SIJ, there is also a fusion of the transverse process of L5 with S1.

Transitional vertebra

The first sacral vertebra can be more or less fused with the fifth lumbar vertebra. This fusion is

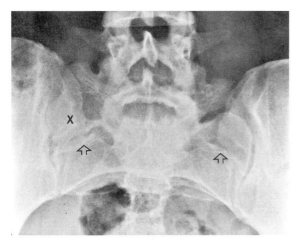

Fig. 27.7   An SIJ with congenital variations. There is a persistent S1–2 division (arrow) and a fusion of the transverse process of L5 with S1 at the right side (X). The S1 on the left is more rounded and smaller than usual. (Reproduced with permission from Dijkstra 1993.)

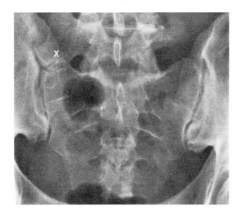

Fig. 27.8   A transitional vertebra L5–S1 is a congenital variation. There is a broad transverse process of L5 on the right, forming a joint with S1 (X). (Reproduced with permission from Dijkstra 1993.)

mostly asymmetric (Figs 27.7 and 27.8), but symmetric fusion can occur. There can be a joint between the transverse process of L5 and the body of S1 (Fig. 27.8 and see Fig. 27.10 below). These transitional vertebrae can be found in about 20% of those in whom L5–S1 is visible on X-ray.

DISEASES OF THE SIJ

Osteoarthritis (arthrosis)

Osteoarthritis is usually a disease of the elderly, but in the SIJ it can be found even at a young

age. The ventral ligaments, especially, calcify. The transitional vertebrae also have a tendency to become involved in osteoarthritis. In young adults, a localized form of osteoarthritis can be found in the form of iliitis condensans, occurring more often in women than in men. There is an oval area of bony sclerosis on the iliac side of the SIJ, with sclerotic margins of the SIJ, often with subchondral cysts. In Fig. 27.9 the iliitis condensans is located in the caudal area of the SIJ. The plain X-ray is difficult to evaluate, but the tomography reveals the true nature of this ailment.

In Fig. 27.10, we see a bony bridge in the ventral ligament of the SIJ and osteoarthritis of the transitional vertebra L5–S1. As in this case, other parts of the SIJ are often not involved.

Osteoarthritis can be mistaken for ankylosing spondylitis. In the patient seen in Fig. 27.11, the AP view shows complete ankylosis of the right SIJ; the frontal tomogram is not of much help either. However, the oblique tomogram shows a narrowed but otherwise normal joint. This oblique tomogram is an example of a tailored investigation of the SIJ. By choosing a direction of the tomogram deliberately tangential to the joint, much more information can be obtained. By its nature, the tomogram will blur non-tangential joint surfaces. Therefore we routinely perform oblique tomograms in areas where a non-tangential joint surface can be expected.

Very severe osteoarthritis is seen on the CT of the patient depicted in Fig. 27.12. The ventral SIJ ligaments are thickened into bony bridges, the joint surfaces show sclerosis, and intraluminal bony bridges are seen. This case shows that intraluminal bony bridges do not exclusively occur in ankylosing spondylitis, as this patient had no clinical signs of ankylosing spondylitis.

Trauma

In pelvic trauma, it is often difficult to delineate fractures of the SIJ. CT is the first choice in those cases, but when external and internal fixation are necessary to stabilize the fractures, only tomography is useful. In Fig. 27.13 the SIJs show multiple fractures, as do the pubic bones. There are, of course, ghost images of the metal plates, but they do not prevent diagnosis.

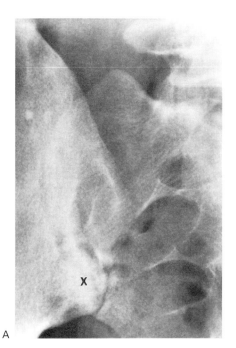
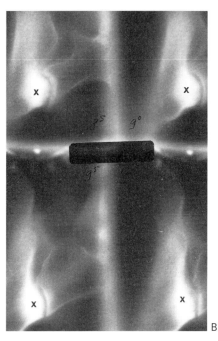

Fig. 27.9   Iliitis condensans. (A) Plain X-ray of the right SIJ with irregular and sclerosing changes in S3 (X). This type of sclerosis of the ilium can cause confusing plain X-rays. (B) Tomography of the posterior parts of the same SIJ. There is sclerosis of the ilium (X), with subchondral cysts and slight sclerosis of the sacrum, but normal joint width. The numbers 8.5 to 10 denote the distance from the table top.

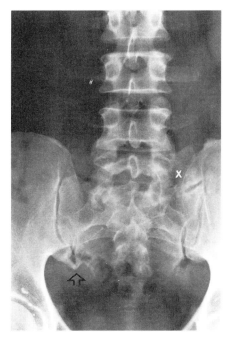

Fig. 27.10   Osteoarthritis of the right SIJ and left L5–S1 transitional vertebra (X). The figure shows bony bridge in the ventral S1 ligament (arrow) and a transitional vertebra L5–S1 on the left, with sclerosis of the joint.

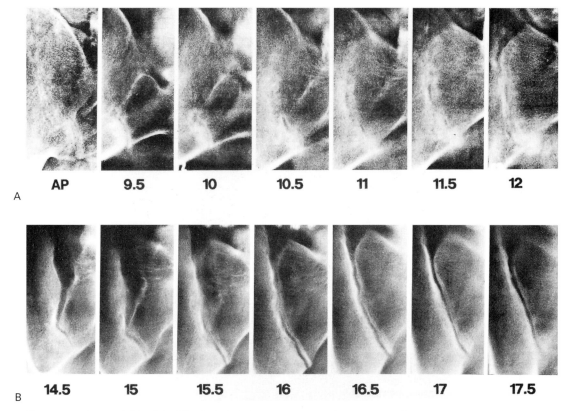

Fig. 27.11 Osteoarthritis of the SIJ. (A) Ankylosing spondylitis is often wrongly diagnosed in cases of osteoarthritis. In this patient, the plain X-ray (AP) shows barely discernable SIJ. Frontal tomography (slices 9.5 to 12) shows sclerosis of the joint margins and irregular joints, as in this patient the tomography is no longer tangential to the direction of the joint. (B) In this oblique tomography (slices 14.5 to 17.5), the middle and ventral parts of the joints appear small, but without erosions, and with slight sclerotic borders as found in osteoarthritis. (Reproduced with permission from Dijkstra et al 1989.)

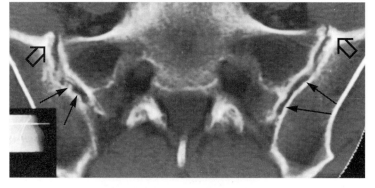

Fig. 27.12 Osteoarthritis with CT. In this patient (CT at the level of S2), severe sclerosis of the ventral SIJ ligaments and the joint margins was found. Even bony ankylosis (arrows) can be found.

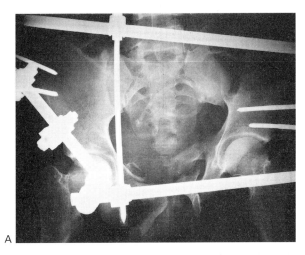

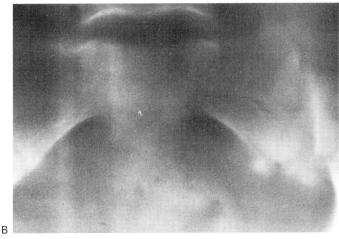

Fig. 27.13   (A) Severe pelvic trauma, stabilized with iron rods, can be difficult to X-ray. The precise extent of the fractures in the SIJ and pubic bones are difficult to establish in this severely traumatized patient. (B) In this patient, tomography shows severe luxation fractures of the left SIJ. Only mild ghost images of the iron rods are seen. Only the left SIJ is shown.

Ankylosing spondylitis

Erosions, intraluminal bony bridges, and often ankylosis of the SIJ can be seen in ankylosing spondylitis. Most often (Dihlman 1982), sclerosis, erosions, and irregular joints are seen (Fig. 27.14).

In a young patient with low back pain, ankylosing spondylitis must be considered as a possible diagnosis. However, the majority of these patients do not show the full clinical picture, and a plain X-ray is much too often used as proof of the disease. We have therefore investigated the X-rays and clinical data of 56 consecutive patients referred to our clinic with suspected ankylosing spondylitis (Dijkstra et al 1989). Based on plain X-rays, 8.3% were normal and 26.3% showed sacroiliitis; the others were non-diagnostic but were said to have 'probable arthritis'. Based on frontal tomography, more sacroiliitis was found, but it did not alter many of the diagnoses. Oblique tomography, tailored to the curvature of the joints, gave surprising results. Now 43% of the joints appeared to be normal (see Fig. 27.11 above) and 36% showed sacroiliitis.

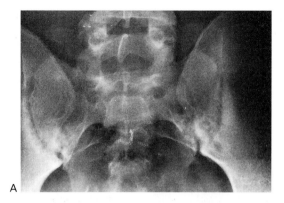

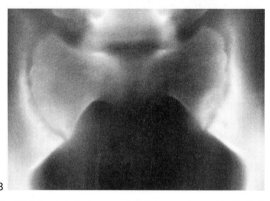

Fig. 27.14 Ankylosing spondylitis in a patient with Crohn's disease. (A) On X-ray, there are irregular joints with sclerotic borders and probably signs of ankylosis on the left side. (B) Tomography of the ventral part of the same SIJ. Erosions and sclerosis are clearly seen, but no ankylosis. The 'ankylosis' seen was, in fact, a superposition of parts of the joint.

The others showed features of congenital alteration and slight osteoarthritis. The importance of these observations is that they could be confirmed by clinical diagnosis. Especially in case of ankylosing spondylitis, it is of the utmost importance that the right diagnosis is found, since the wrong diagnosis can be devastating: no life insurance, no mortgage, and often no job. Much time in our clinic is now spent in altering the diagnosis given to these patients elsewhere, based on the criteria presented above.

Miscellaneous

Chondrocalcinosis is a disease of the elderly. Calcified cartilage can sometimes be seen in the SIJ (Fig. 27.15). Whether this is clinically

important is not known, as no systematic investigation has been carried out on this joint.

Hyperparathyroidism is seen in patients with severe kidney disease. In a clinical setting, this disease is not unexpected, but it can also be found without warning in the SIJ. It is the task of the radiologist to produce a reasonable differential diagnosis for these cases. In Fig. 27.16 we see a patient with kidney disease with severe

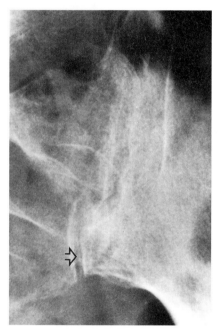

Fig. 27.15 Chondrocalcinosis can be found in any joint but is often not recognized in the SIJ. The faint sclerotic line (arrow) in the left SIJ is calcification in the superficial layer of the iliac cartilage.

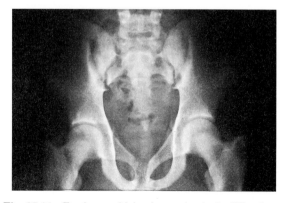

Fig. 27.16 Erosions and joint destruction in the SIJ and pubic symphysis due to secondary hyperparathyroidism in a patient with kidney disease.

destruction of the SIJ and osteolysis of the pubic symphysis.

CONCLUSIONS

1. It is essential to understand the normal plain X-ray.

2. Emphasis is placed on the use of (oblique) tomography tailored to the curvature of the SIJ.

Otherwise, CT scanning has to be used. With spiral CT the situation might change, provided this technique becomes more sophisticated.

3. MRI is the technique for the future but is still difficult to handle for the SIJ. It is superior in bacterial arthritis and tumorous conditions.

REFERENCES

Dihlman W 1982 Gelenke-Wirbelverbindungen. Klinische Radiologie. Thieme, Stuttgart

Dijkstra P F 1993 Radiology of the normal S. I. joint. Journal of Manual and Manipulative Therapy 1: 87–94

Dijkstra P F, Vleeming A, Stoeckart R 1989 Complex motion tomography of the sacroiliac joint. An anatomical and roentgenologic study. Fortschritte auf dem Gebiete der Röntgenstralen 150: 635-642

Firooznia H C, Golimbu C, Rofii M, Kricheft I, Marschall C,

Berenbaum E R 1984 Computer tomography of the sacroiliac joints: comparison with complex motion tomography. Journal of Computed Tomography 8: 31–34

Solonen K A 1957 The sacroiliac joint in the light of anatomical, roentgenological and clinical studies. Acta Orthopaedica Scandinavica 27 (supplement): 4–127

Vleeming A, Van Wingerden J P, Dijkstra P F, Stoeckart R, Snijders C J, Stijnen T 1992 Mobility in the S.I.-joints in the elderly: a kinematic and radiologic study. Clinical Biomechanics 7: 170–176

28. CT and MRI of the sacroiliac joints

E. Jurriaans   L. Friedman

INTRODUCTION

The most common indication for imaging the sacroiliac joints (SIJs) is for the investigation of inflammatory low back pain in patients thought to have sacroiliitis. The presence of sacroiliitis is an important criterion for the diagnosis of the seronegative spondyloarthropathies and in particular in those patients suspected of having ankylosing spondylitis (The et al 1985, van der Linden et al 1984). This is reflected by the current literature in which computerized tomography (CT) and magnetic resonance imaging (MRI) of the SIJs are almost exclusively described in terms of the investigation of sacroiliitis. This chapter will therefore deal primarily with sacroiliitis, only a brief mention being made of other disease processes that may involve the SIJs (see also Ch. 27).

Clinical assessment of the SIJ is difficult, and the diagnosis of sacroiliitis is dependent on imaging studies, particularly when using the New York or modified New York criteria (The et al 1985, van der Linden 1984). Unfortunately, the anatomy of the SIJ presents particular problems (Forrester 1990), which limits the ability of many imaging modalities to detect sacroiliitis, particularly in the early stages of the disease.

While plain X-rays remain the first and most widespread imaging modality employed in the investigation of sacroiliitis, studies have shown that CT (Carrera et al 1981, Fam et al 1985, Lawson et al 1982, Scott et al 1990, Taggart et al 1984) and MRI (Battafarano et al 1993, Docherty et al 1992, Friedman et al unpublished data, Murphey et al 1991) demonstrate improved sensitivity and specificity for the diagnosis of

sacroiliitis. Unfortunately, the determination of the exact sensitivities and specificities of these imaging modalities is severely hindered by the absence of a 'gold standard' investigation. Long-term follow-up studies are therefore required to confirm these results.

This chapter will describe CT and MRI of the SIJ, including the appearances of both the normal and the abnormal SIJ, and the role that these imaging modalities play in the investigation of sacroiliitis. In addition, we will propose a staging system based on MRI findings (Table 28.1 below), which is illustrated by a series of cases (Figs 28.1–28.10).

COMPUTERIZED TOMOGRAPHY

CT technique

A variety of CT techniques have been described in the evaluation of the SIJ. These include contiguous or non-contiguous axial and direct coronal (or oblique coronal) cuts. Initial studies (Carrera et al 1981, Lawson et al 1982) described a technique utilizing 5 mm thick contiguous cuts in an oblique coronal plane. The plane of section was determined by the lateral topogram, and the gantry of the CT scanner was angled to allow the slice to be as close to the coronal plane of the sacrum as could be permitted. Later studies (Fam et al 1985, Taggart et al 1984) utilized contiguous 5 mm or 4 mm thick axial slices without angling the gantry and with no apparent detriment.

Oudjhane et al (1993) have described a CT technique for the investigation of sacroiliitis in children. Coronal slices are utilized as this

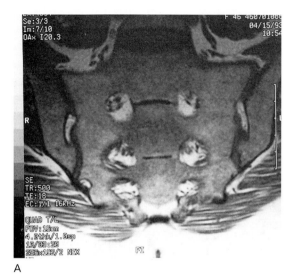 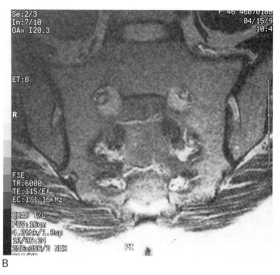

A   B

Fig. 28.1 Normal subject. (A) This T1-weighted coronal oblique image demonstrates the intermediate signal intensity cartilage interposed between the well-defined signal void of the adjacent cortical bone. Note the high-signal fat seen within the ligamentous compartment of the joint. The subchondral bone marrow is seen to be almost homogenous in signal intensity. (B) This FSE T2-weighted image illustrates the normal appearance of the SIJ. Note that the intermediate signal intensity cartilage cannot be as clearly visualized as in the T1 image (A).

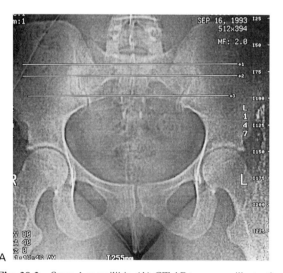 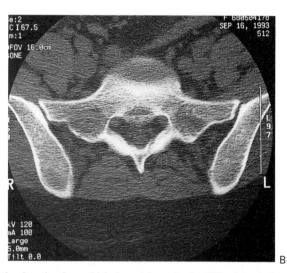

A   B

Fig. 28.2 Stage 1 sacroiliitis. (A) CT AP topogram illustrating the three levels at which the axial cuts in the 'CT miniseries' are obtained. See text for further details. (B) Axial CT cut at the level of the first sacral foramen – the 'sad face'. The anterior 25% of the joint represents the synovial compartment. Normal appearance.

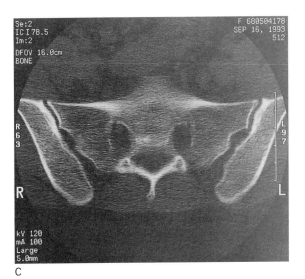

C

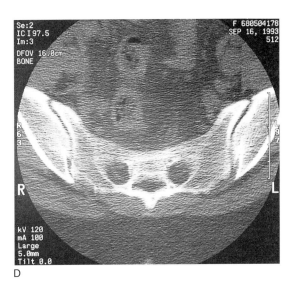

D

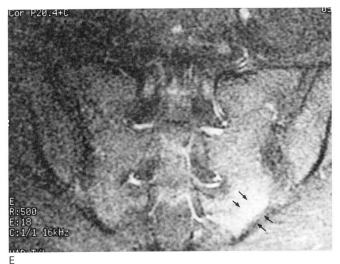

E

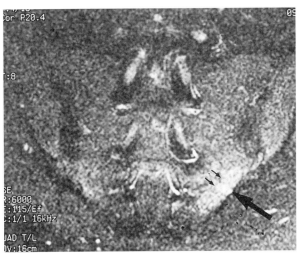

F

Fig. 28.2 (*Contd*) (C) Axial CT cut between the first and second sacral foramina, showing the 'happy face'. At this level, 50–75% of the joint is synovial. (D) Axial CT cut at the level of the third sacral foramina – the 'batman mask'. The whole joint at this level is synovial. There is no evidence of sacroiliitis on CT despite MRI changes. (E) T1 Gd-DTPA-enhanced image demonstrating enhancing subchondral edema (arrows) in keeping with stage 1 disease. (F) FSE T2 image demonstrating subchondral edema (large and small arrows) consistent with stage 1 sacroiliitis. These findings correspond to Ahlstrom's type I lesions. Note the changes are more prominent on the sacral side of the SIJ.

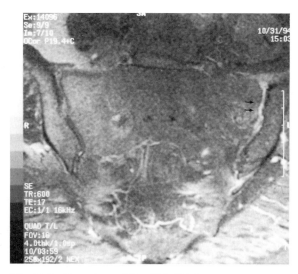

Fig. 28.3 Stage 1 sacroiliitis. This T1FS post-Gd-DTPA image demonstrates synovial enhancement (arrows). While synovial enhancement is usually seen in the presence of subchondral edema, this illustrates the only patient in our series in whom synovial enhancement was seen without subchondral marrow changes.

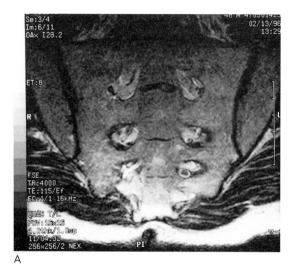

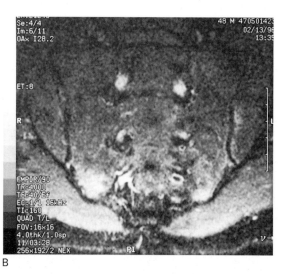

A

B

Fig. 28.4 Stage 1 sacroiliitis. (A) This FSE T2 image is essentially normal. The faint high signal seen within the sacral subchondral bone can easily be overlooked and can be attributed to inhomogeneous fat suppression. (B) This FMPIR sequence clearly identifies sacral subchondral edema and illustrates the sensitivity of this type of sequence in detecting Ahlstrom type I change.

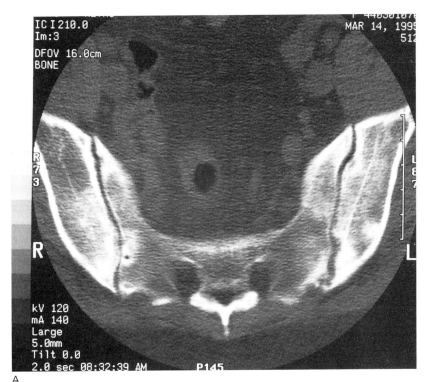

A

Fig. 28.5   Stage 2a sacroiliitis. (A) This axial CT cut at the level of the third sacral foramina demonstrates patchy, predominantly iliac, subchondral sclerosis. As described in the text, this can be seen in normal subjects. There is, however, also very faint irregularity of the joint space, with some loss of joint space width and early erosive change. This examination was reported by a general radiologist as being suspicious for metastatic disease, illustrating some of the problems that the non-musculoskeletal radiologist faces in the interpretation of examinations of the SIJ. (B) This T1FS post-Gd-DTPA image demonstrates marked enhancing subchondral bone marrow edema (small arrows) together with some synovial enhancement and one small erosion (large arrow). Note that the erosion is located on the iliac side of the joint while the subchondral edema is most prevalent on the sacral side. The predominance of the subchondral edema over the erosive change categorizes this as stage 2a disease.

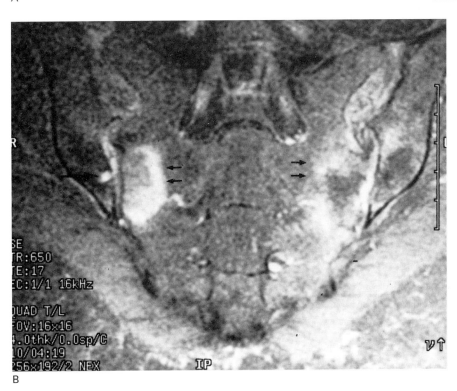

B

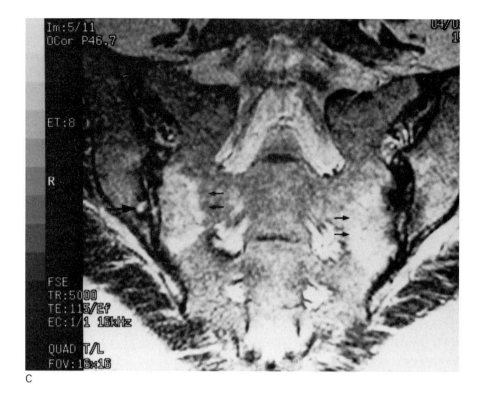

C

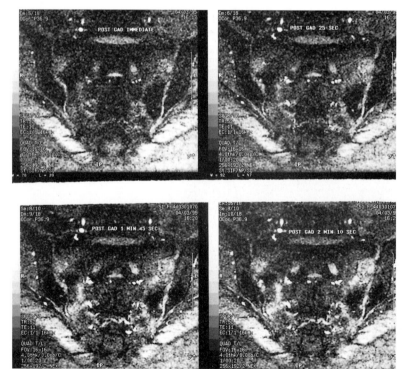

D

Fig. 28.5 (*Contd*) (C) This FSE T2 image demonstrates changes similar to those seen on the postcontrast T1 image (B). Subchondral edema (small arrows) and the erosion (large arrow) are clearly identified. While synovial enhancement obviously cannot be evaluated, this sequence can correctly identify stage 2a disease. Gd-DTPA is not required to make the diagnosis (see text). In addition to the changes seen on the T1 image (B), high signal is also seen within the synovial joint space consistent with joint fluid or inflammatory tissue. (D) These four images are taken from a dynamic SPGR study following Gd-DTPA. The images were acquired immediately following the intravenous bolus of Gd-DTPA and then at 25 s, 1 min 45 s, and 2 min 10 s respectively post injection. The abnormal enhancement of the subchondral bone marrow becomes more evident with time. Dynamic SPGR enables F_{enh} and G_{enh} to be calculated (see text).

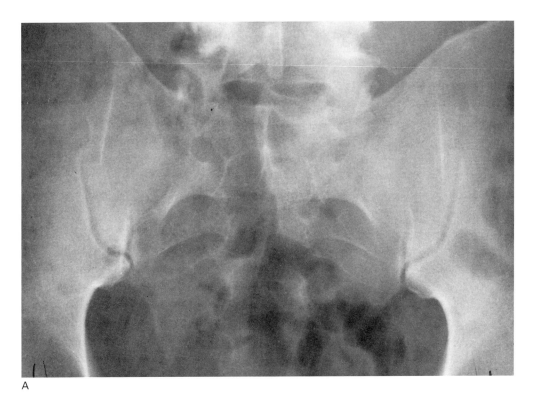

A

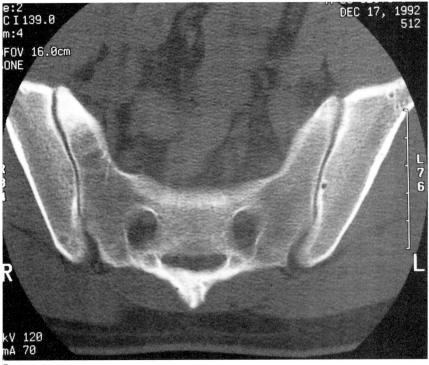

B

Fig. 28.6 Stage 2b sacroiliitis. (A) A conventional X-ray of the SIJ demonstrates no definitive abnormality. (B) Axial CT cut illustrates preservation of the joint spaces. The solitary finding of a small cystic lesion on the iliac side of the left SIJ is of uncertain significance.

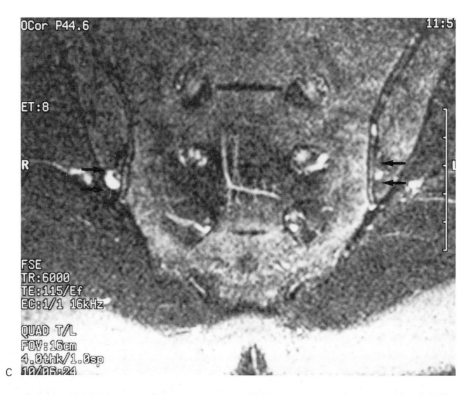

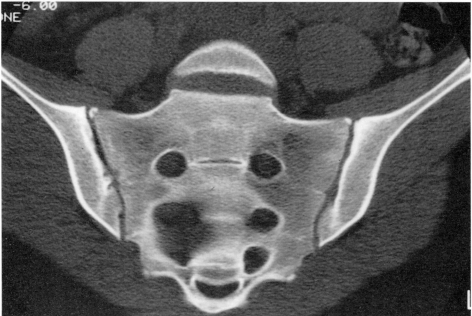

Fig. 28.6 (*Contd*) (C) FSE T2 image identifies bilateral erosions (arrows) on the iliac side of the joints together with slight increased signal within the synovial compartment, particularly on the left side. The presence of erosions with less marked or absent subchondral edema (as in this patient) is found in stage 2b disease. (D) A direct coronal slice of the SIJ of a different patient demonstrates the use of another CT technique (see text). Early erosive change is readily identified (case courtesy of E M Azouz, MD, Montreal, Quebec).

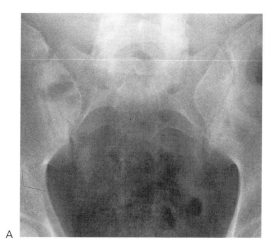

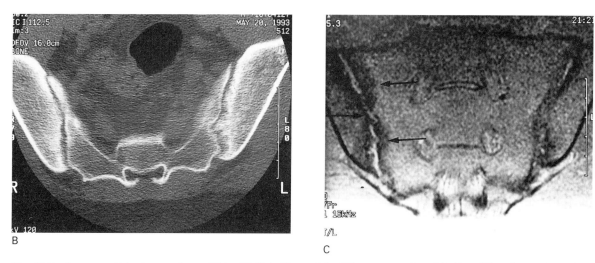

Fig. 28.7   Late stage 2b/early stage 3 sacroiliitis. (A) Plain X-ray of the SIJ presents equivocal findings. There is some loss of clarity of the left joint margins, with possible erosive change inferiorly. These findings warrant further investigation. (B) Axial CT slice demonstrates loss and irregularity of joint space bilaterally, in keeping with bilateral sacroiliitis. Note that the conventional X-ray represents grade 1 changes according to the modified New York criteria while the CT findings are consistent with grade 3 changes. This illustrates the increased sensitivity of CT over plain X-rays in detecting SI and the need for further investigation of equivocal plain radiographic findings. (C) T1FS image confirms the CT findings with irregular loss of joint space and erosive change. The periarticular subchondral low signal seen on this image, demonstrates similar signal characteristics on T2 weighting and represents sclerosis and/or fibrosis. This corresponds to Ahlstrom's type II lesions. This case represents late stage 2b/early stage 3 sacroiliitis.

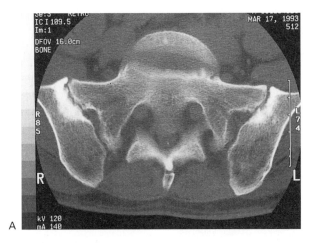

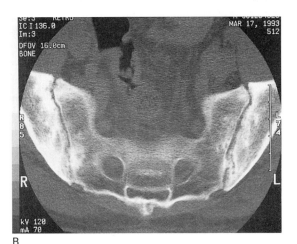

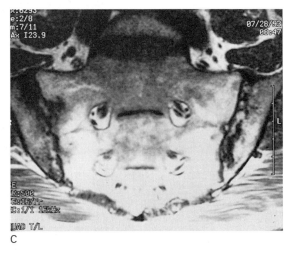

Fig. 28.8   Stage 3 sacroiliitis. (A) Axial CT cut at the level of the first sacral foramina (the 'sad face') showing loss of joint space of the anterior 25% of the SIJ together with erosions. The pathological involvement of the synovial compartment rather eloquently demonstrates the differentiation between the ligamentous and synovial compartments. (B) Axial CT cut at the level of the third sacral foramina (the 'batman mask') reveals evidence of extensive sacroiliitis, with joint space narrowing, erosions, and sclerosis. Again, the pathological involvement of the synovial compartment illustrates the anatomic description that 100% of the joint is synovial at the level of the third sacral foramina (see text). The degree of fatty infiltration is not appreciated on CT. (C) T1 image without fat saturation or Gd-DTPA reveals extensive subchondral high signal in keeping with fatty infiltration. In addition, erosions and irregularity and loss of joint space are noted. Stage 3 disease includes fatty infiltration and sclerosis/fibrosis. Fatty infiltration can be readily differentiated from sclerosis/fibrosis by the signal characteristics on non-fat saturated sequences. The findings of stage 3 disease correspond to Ahlstrom's type II lesions.

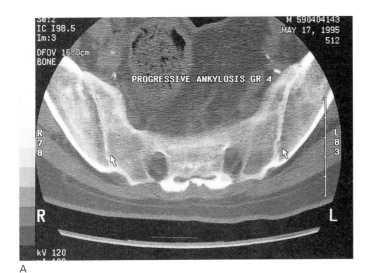

A

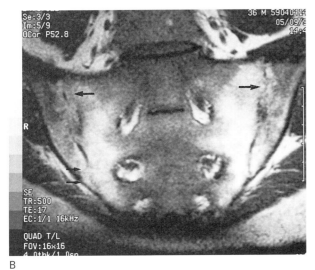

B

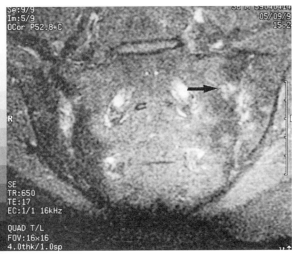

C

Fig. 28.9 Stage 4 sacroiliitis. (A) Axial CT slice at the level of the third sacral foramina demonstrates progressive ankylosis. This corresponds to grade 4 disease using the modified New York criteria. (B) T1 image without fat saturation illustrates bridging of the SIJ by high signal fatty marrow in keeping with ankylosis. (C) T1FS image reveals subchondral and periarticular low signal in keeping with saturation of the signal from fat (compare with B). Note that bridging of the joints by fatty marrow (and hence ankylosis) cannot be as clearly seen on the fat-saturated images compared with normal T1 images (B).

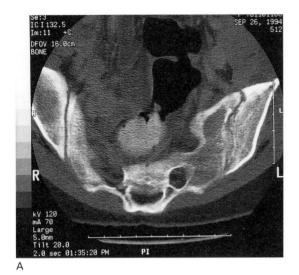
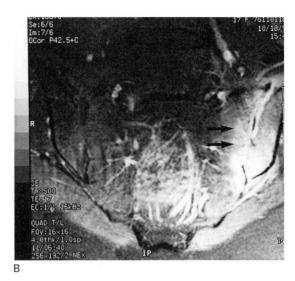

A   B

Fig. 28.10 Unilateral pyogenic sacroiliitis. (A) Axial CT reveals loss of joint space of the left SIJ with early destruction of the cortical bone. The right joint is normal. *Staphylococcus aureus* was isolated from blood cultures. (B) T1FS image post-Gd-DTPA reveals a unilateral sacroiliitis with both synovial and subchondral bone marrow enhancement in keeping with a pyogenic sacroiliitis. While the unilaterality of these findings is suspicious for infection, these are non-specific changes and correlation with clinical findings is imperative. Note that the contralateral normal joint demonstrates no visible synovial or subchondral bone marrow enhancement.

provides visualization of the entire surface of the SIJ. A pillow is placed under the patient's lumbar spine to increase the lordosis. Maximum gantry angle (+20°) is employed and 3 mm thick contiguous coronal slices are then obtained through both SIJ. The average number of scan slices is 12. Apart from visualizing the entire SIJ in the coronal plane (Fig. 28.6D), this method has the added advantage of preventing direct exposure of the ovaries to radiation. There is also a decrease in the number of slices required to visualize the entire SIJ when compared with the axial plane. This is a further consideration in the reduction of radiation exposure.

We use a 'CT miniseries' for the investigation of sacroiliitis, as described by Friedman et al (1993). Three non-contiguous 5 mm thick axial slices are taken through the SIJ at three levels determined from an anteroposterior (AP) topogram. These are selected at the level of the first sacral foramina, between the first and second sacral foramina, and at the level of the third sacral foramina (Fig. 28.2A–D). These levels ensure adequate visualization of the synovial component of the SIJ and are easily reproduced by the technologist. No gantry angulation is applied.

The exposure factors were altered so that the minimal acceptable milliamperes × seconds (mAs) level was determined. By limiting the number of scan slices to three and by cutting down on the mAs level, there was a marked reduction in both the radiation exposure as well as the total scan time. This study found that there was no loss of sensitivity in the detection of sacroiliitis.

While this 'CT miniseries' has been shown to be an excellent means of investigating sacroiliitis, contiguous 5–10 mm thick slices in either the axial or coronal plane are necessary in the investigation of possible tumor or infection as well as trauma.

Further important technical factors to consider are the utilization of a high-resolution bone algorithm as well as suitable window settings to optimize visualization of the SIJ. Our preferred window width is 2000 Hounsfield units, centered at 600 Hounsfield units. These are altered if soft tissue visualization is required.

Normal CT appearance

The anatomic description of the SIJ is very complex (Bowen & Cassidy 1981). In simple terms, the joint consists of a smaller postero-superior ligamentous compartment and a larger anteroinferior synovial compartment. As the joints have an oblique orientation on the frontal (AP) plane, there is considerable overlap of the ligamentous and synovial compartments on plain X-ray. Cross-sectional imaging using either CT or MRI in the axial or coronal planes affords the best differentiation of these compartments.

The two compartments can be readily identified on axial CT slices. Using the 'CT miniseries' described by Friedman et al (1993), the synovial compartment is easily recognized at the prescribed three levels by the 'three faces of the SIJ'. The synovial compartment is found to represent the anterior 25% of the SIJ at the level of first sacral foramina (the 'sad face'), approximately the anterior 50–75% of the joint midway between the first and second sacral foramina (the 'happy face'), and all of the SIJ at the level of the third sacral foramina (the 'batman mask') (Figs 28.2A–D, 28.8A–B).

On coronal scanning, the synovial compartment has a relatively vertical orientation. From the posterosuperior aspect, 25% of the joint surface is synovial, from the middle aspect, 50–75% is synovial, and from the anteroinferior aspect, 100% is synovial (Friedman et al 1993).

The normal SIJ demonstrates considerable variance, particularly with increasing age (Vogler et al 1984). Thus there is symmetry of the joints in normal subjects under the age of 30, but asymmetry is seen in 77% of subjects over the age of 30, and in 87% of subjects over the age of 40. The width of the normal SIJ varies from 2 to 5 mm (Lawson et al 1982, Vogler et al 1984). Certain findings that were thought to be indicative of sacroiliitis may be seen in normal subjects (Vogler et al 1984). These include non-uniform iliac sclerosis, focal joint space narrowing in patients over the age of 30, and ill-defined areas of subchondral sclerosis, particularly on the iliac side. These findings were seen in 83%, 74%, and 67% of normal subjects respectively. These CT findings are therefore poor discriminators of sacroiliitis.

The same study describes other findings thought to be indicative of sacroiliitis which are indeed very uncommon in normal subjects. These include increased sacral subchondral sclerosis in subjects under the age of 40, bilateral or unilateral joint space of less than 2 mm, erosions, and intra-articular ankylosis. These were found in only 11%, 2%, 0%, 2%, and 0% of the normal subjects respectively. These findings may therefore be useful in the diagnosis of sacroiliitis.

CT in sacroiliitis

The CT findings that suggest sacroiliitis are the same as those described for conventional X-rays. The plain radiographic criteria for the diagnosis of sacroiliitis are included in the modified New York criteria (The et al 1985). The CT findings include subchondral sclerosis on both sides of the joint, erosions, irregular joint space narrowing or widening, and ankylosis (Borlaza et al 1981, Carrera et al 1981, Fam et al 1985, Lawson et al 1982, Scott et al 1990, Taggart et al 1984) (Figs 28.5A, 28.6D, 28.7B, 28.8A–B, 28.9A, 28.10A).

Borlaza et al (1981) found a good correlation between plain radiographic and CT findings in patients with sacroiliitis and concluded that CT offered no advantage over plain X-rays in the hands of an experienced radiologist. Subsequent studies (Carrera et al 1981, Fam et al 1995, Lawson et al 1982, Scott et al 1990, Taggart et al 1984) found that CT identified changes of sacroiliitis in patients with normal and equivocal plain X-rays (Fig. 28.7A–B). The improved accuracy of CT in these later studies may reflect technical advances in the scanners with an improvement in image quality.

CT is currently used to evaluate further those patients suspected of having sacroiliitis in whom the plain X-rays are normal or equivocal. In our practice, CT has completely replaced plain tomography. CT is now readily available in most centers and, using the 'CT miniseries' described above, the technique offers a marked reduction in radiation exposure compared with conventional radiography and tomography. The radiation risk of the three non-contiguous scans is less than that of one single X-ray (Friedman et al 1993). In addition, there is likely to be less interobserver variability in the interpretation of CT of the SIJ compared with conventional radiography, although this has not been documented in the literature. When the plain X-rays demonstrate unequivocal evidence of sacroiliitis, CT is not warranted.

CT in other conditions affecting the SIJs

CT is useful in diagnosing SIJ infection and may identify unilateral changes suggesting the diagnosis (Fig. 28.10A). Review of the examination on soft tissue windows is essential lest soft tissue abnormalities be missed. Changes involving the adjacent bone may occur only later, and CT may appear normal in the early course of infective sacroiliitis. Therefore in the relevant clinical setting, more sensitive imaging modalities such as radioisotope bone scan or MRI should be employed (Abbott & Carty 1993, Haliloglu et al 1994). However, radioisotope bone scan and MRI (Fig. 28.10B) are non-specific, and CT-guided joint aspiration may confirm the diagnosis and may also be crucial in planning appropriate antimicrobial therapy.

CT is invaluable in assessing and staging tumors at or about the SIJ. Bone destruction and soft tissue masses can be readily identified. The differentiation between benign and malignant bone lesions is usually possible.

Schwarzer et al (1995) have found CT useful following SIJ arthrography. In their investigation of a group of patients with chronic low back pain, they found a weak but statistically significant association between ventral capsular tears of the SIJ and relief of pain upon anesthetizing the joint. The extent and site of the capsular tears were well shown on CT, as were diverticula of the capsule. The significance of these findings and the role of CT sacroiliac (SI) arthrography remains to be determined.

CT has a well-established role in the management of patients with pelvic trauma. It is the preferred imaging modality for assessing soft tissue injury. While a correct pathoanatomic classification of pelvic fractures is best obtained by plain X-ray, CT provides additional information regarding acetabular fractures, involvement of the posterior pelvic ring, intra-articular fracture fragments, and fractures of the femoral head (Albrechtsen et al 1994). Recently, CT-guided insertion of iliosacral screws has been

used to reduce pelvic fractures (Ebraheim et al 1987, Nelson & Duwelius 1991).

Finally, CT may be invaluable in the diagnosis of insufficiency fractures. These fractures most commonly occur in elderly females with osteoporosis. The osteopenia makes assessment of plain X-rays difficult. The diagnosis can be confirmed by CT, which demonstrates patchy sclerosis, often with fissure-like fractures and no associated soft tissue mass (Rogers 1992). The absence of an associated mass makes it possible to differentiate an insufficiency fracture from a metastatic lesion, which is often a clinical dilemma in these patients (Rogers 1992).

MAGNETIC RESONANCE IMAGING

MRI technique

A variety of MRI techniques have been described in imaging of the SIJ. For the purposes of this discussion, we will describe our preferred technique.

Our examinations are conducted on a 1.5 Tesla superconducting magnet (Signa, General Electric, Milwaukee, WI, USA) using a Quadrature thoracolumbar spine surface coil (General Electric). We use a T1 sagittal localizer followed by a combination of oblique coronal sequences. These sequences include T1, T1 with fat saturation (T1FS), fast spin echo (FSE) T2 with fat saturation, short tau inversion recovery (STIR) (fast multiplanar inversion recovery (FMPIR)) and T1FS following the administration of intravenous gadolinium diethylenetriamine pentaacetic acid (Gd-DTPA). In addition, we occasionally use a dynamic spoiled gradient echo (SPGR) sequence during Gd-DTPA enhancement (Fig. 28.5D).

The contraindications to MRI include cardiac pacemakers, cochlear implants, and ferromagnetic intracranial or intraorbital surgical clips and foreign bodies. Occasionally, patients experience claustrophobia, which is usually overcome by sedation (lorazepam 1–2 mg orally or benzodiazepine 2–10 mg intravenously).

Normal anatomy

The normal appearance of the SIJ on MRI has been described by several authors (Ahlstrom et al

1990, Bollow et al 1995, Docherty et al 1992, Murphey et al 1991, Wittram & Whitehouse 1995). As with CT, MRI is also able to identify the ligamentous and synovial compartments and their orientation and position (see above). MRI has the advantage of affording direct visualization of the cartilage of the synovial compartment.

On both T1 and T2 images, the normal cartilage of the SIJ appears as a zone of intermediate signal bounded on either side by the signal void of the cortical bone of the adjacent sacrum and ilium (Fig. 28.1A–B).

Murphey et al (1991) found that the normal synovial cartilage has a maximum thickness of 4–5 mm posteriorly and is slightly thinner anteriorly and inferiorly. The adjacent cortical bone is well defined. On T1FS, the cartilage is of intermediate-to-high signal. Following the suppression of the high fat signal, the altered gray scale of the T1FS sequence improves visualization of the cartilage and adjacent cortical bone and is therefore superior to T1 sequences in assessing the synovial compartment (Wittram & Whitehouse 1995). In a study of patients with clinical evidence of sacroiliitis as well as a group of normal controls, Docherty et al (1992) found that proton-density (PD) weighted images offered the best visualization of the cartilage. T1FS images were not assessed in this study. In keeping with the findings of Wittram and Whitehouse (1995), we have found the T1FS sequences best in imaging the cartilage (Friedman et al, unpublished data). Standard T1 sequences are, however, invaluable in assessing the subchondral bone marrow and, in particular, in differentiating between subchondral sclerosis and fat, which both appear as a low signal on T1FS.

Cortical erosions and subchondral sclerosis were not identified in a study of normal patients (Wittram & Whitehouse 1995). A partial volume artefact between the anteroinferior synovial compartment of the SIJ and the posterosuperior ligamentous compartment should not be mistaken for an erosion (Wittram & Whitehouse 1995) (Fig. 28.1A–B). In addition, prominent sacral irregularities and marrow defects at the attachment of the interosseous ligaments, termed insertion pits, may be seen in normal subjects (Murphey et al 1991). The characteristic site of

the above described findings, the intact signal void of the adjacent cortical bone and the presence of fat within the ligamentous compartment (readily identified on a combination of T1 and T1FS sequences) resolves any potential dilemma. Anatomic variants, such as an accessory articular facet of the SIJ, are easily identified by MRI (Wittram & Whitehouse 1995).

In general, the adjacent bone marrow has a homogenous intermediate signal intensity (Fig. 28.1A). In adults, the subchondral bone may have a heterogeneous signal due to non-uniform fatty replacement of hemopoietic bone marrow (Levine et al 1994). A patchy distribution of fat within the subchondral bone marrow was found in some normal patients and is of no significance in the absence of cortical erosions or subchondral sclerosis (Wittram & Whitehouse 1995). On fast short tau inversion recovery (Fast STIR) images, a well-defined para-articular band of subchondral high signal may be identified in normal patients (Wittram & Whitehouse 1995), and this should not be mistaken for subchondral edema, which is less well defined and more diffuse.

The normal pattern of enhancement following the administration of intravenous Gd-DTPA is controversial. A region of interest (ROI) can be drawn over a particular part of the synovial compartment of the SIJ or adjacent subchondral bone. Enhancement can be assessed by a delayed T1 or T1FS sequence, or by a dynamic SPGR sequence following an intravenous bolus of Gd-DTPA. The increase in signal intensity can then be calculated and expressed an an enhancement factor (F_{enh}) (Bollow et al 1995, Braun et al 1994, Wittram & Whitehouse 1995):

$$F_{enh}\% = \frac{(SI_{max} - SI_0) \times 100}{SI_0}$$

Where: SI_0 = signal intensity pre-Gd-DTPA
SI_{max} = maximum signal intensity post-Gd-DTPA

Alternatively, using a dynamic sequence, an enhancement gradient (G_{enh}) can be calculated (Bollow et al 1995, Braun et al 1994):

$$G_{enh}\%/minute = \frac{(SI_{max} - SI_0) \times 100}{SI_0 \times T_{max}}$$

where: T_{max} = time interval (minutes) from injection of Gd-DTPA to SI_{max}.

Wittram and Whitehouse (1995) found the F_{enh} of the synovial compartment in five normal subjects to be between 20% and 49%. Braun et al (1994) found values of 3 (SD ± 5%) and 1 (SD ± 2%/min) for F_{enh} and G_{enh} respectively in a control group of 12 patients with non-inflammatory spinal pain. Bollow et al (1995) describe no increase in signal intensity following Gd-DTPA in 53 control patients with non-inflammatory back pain and suggest that an F_{enh} of less than 20% represents no SI inflammation, an F_{enh} greater than 20% represents latent SI inflammation, and an F_{enh} greater than 90% represents florid inflammation. There is thus no clear consensus with regard to the enhancement pattern seen in the normal SIJ. The number of controls in the studies of Braun et al (1994) and Bollow et al (1995) clearly exceeds that of the five normal subjects studied by Wittram and Whitehouse (1995) and may therefore favor the results of the former studies. The discrepancy between the studies may in part reflect the positioning of the ROI. If the ROI is placed over a vessel, the enhancement factors will be erroneously high. Furthermore, there must be consistency with regard to the position of the ROI on both the pre- and post-Gd-DTPA images in order to obtain meaningful results. In our experience with a small control group (five patients), there is no visible enhancement in normal subjects (Friedman et al, unpublished data). Only minor enhancement, similar to that recorded by Braun et al (1994) and Bollow et al (1995), is identified using a ROI measurement.

Outside the synovial compartment, Wittram and Whitehouse (1995) found the normal subchondral bone marrow to enhance considerably, with an F_{enh} of up to 85% on a T1 image and 94% on a T1FS image. We have found no significant enhancement of the subchondral bone marrow in our small group of five controls (Friedman et al unpublished data). The spectrum of normal enhancement and the best means to standardize the measurement of enhancement remains to be determined.

MRI in sacroiliitis

In the first description of MRI in sacroiliitis, Ahlstrom et al (1990) found striking changes in the subchondral bone marrow. These abnormalities were classified as type I and type II lesions. Type I lesions were described as low signal intensity on T1 and high signal intensity on T2, and were located in patchy areas close to the joint space and/or diffusely distributed in the periarticular bone marrow (Figs 28.2E, 28.4B, and 28.5C). These lesions were associated with erosions seen by CT in 4 out of 5 patients. Type II lesions were more common and were characterized by low signal intensity on both T1 and T2 weighting (Fig. 28.7C). These abnormalities were associated with erosions and more or less extensive sclerotic changes seen on CT. Ahlstrom et al (1990) suggested that the difference in signal characteristics of these lesions is due to a difference in water content, type I lesions representing inflammatory edema and type II lesions portraying fibrotic tissue or sclerosis. This is supported by the work of Shichikawa et al (1985) in which histopathological findings suggest that the early changes of sacroiliitis occur in the subchondral bone.

In addition to the type I and II lesions, Ahlstrom et al (1990) describe the presence of periarticular high signal on both T1 and T2 weighting, suggesting subchondral fatty accumulation (Fig. 28.8C). This differed from the patchy distribution of subchondral bone marrow fat seen in some normal subjects. The authors suggest that the fatty accumulation seen in sacroiliitis reflects a later stage in the inflammatory joint disease since it was associated only with type II lesions. This is supported by similar changes seen in the marrow of the vertebral bodies associated with degenerative disc disease (Modic et al 1988).

In their initial study, Ahlstrom et al (1990) found that discrete erosions seen on CT were not visible on MRI. While they found the sensitivity of MRI to be similar to that of CT or conventional radiography, they emphasized the unique ability of MRI to demonstrate abnormalities in subchondral bone and periarticular bone marrow. They conclude that the early inflammatory changes in sacroiliitis are likely to occur in the subchondral structures of the SIJ. This is a topic that will subsequently be further addressed.

Murphey et al (1991) described somewhat different findings in their study, in which the predominant abnormalities were felt to involve the synovial compartment of the joint rather than the subchondral structures. Their findings included the following: replacement of the thin band of intermediate signal intensity cartilage by areas of heterogeneous mixed signal intensity tissue, thought to represent cartilage destruction by pannus; thickening of the cartilage, with the presence of increased linear signal intensity attributed to synovial proliferation; erosions that were more prominent anteroinferiorly and on the iliac side of the synovial compartment; and increased signal intensity within the synovial compartment on T2 weighting, thought to reflect acute inflammatory tissue or fibrous proliferation with pannus. Beyond the synovial compartment, high signal intensity was seen within the adjacent bone marrow on both T1 and T2 weighting, suggesting the presence of fatty accumulation. Ankylosis was identified by a bridge of marrow signal intensity crossing the SIJ in the absence of normal cartilage or inflammatory tissues (Fig. 28.9B–C). No further observations of the subchondral bone marrow were made. In this study, MRI was found to be superior to CT for the evaluation of cartilage and the detection of erosions. This was ascribed to direct visualization of the cartilage and the high contrast resolution afforded by MRI.

The next study to assess MRI in sacroiliitis (Docherty et al 1992) identified abnormalities within both the synovial compartment and the subchondral bone. Their findings included erosions, joint space narrowing or widening, and changes in the subchondral marrow presumed to be due to fat deposition or edema. They did not detect synovial fluid within the SIJs of any of their patients, nor of their controls. The most consistent finding in their group of patients was the presence of erosions. More abnormalities were detected by MRI than plain X-rays. Using the modified New York criteria (The et al 1985), normal or equivocal findings on plain X-ray (grades 0–1) matched definite abnormalities on MRI (grades 2–4) (Fig. 28.7A–C). MRI was

slightly better at detecting erosions than were plain X-rays. There was little difference in the detection of changes in joint width or sclerosis. MRI was worse at identifying ankylosis or abnormalities of the ligamentous compartment. The sensitivity and specificity of abnormal articular cartilage were 95% and 90% respectively, and the sensitivity and specificity of abnormal bone marrow signal were 30% and 100% respectively.

The increased sensitivity of MRI in detecting sacroiliitis was not associated with a corresponding increase in the false positive identification of similar abnormalities in normal controls. In fact, Docherty et al (1992) showed that more reported abnormalities were seen on plain X-rays of normal controls than on corresponding MRI studies. The same study also assessed inter- and intraobserver variability, and the variation within and between observers was comparable for both plain X-rays and MRI. High interobserver variation in the interpretation of plain X-rays of the SIJ has been reported and has been suggested as a possible cause of apparent sacroiliitis in certain disease states (Yazici et al 1987). The comparable interobserver variation of MRI and plain radiography in the detection of sacroiliitis described by Docherty et al (1992) is therefore disappointing. They suggest that this variability may become less marked with time as the observers gain more experience with this imaging modality.

Docherty et al (1992) are uncertain whether abnormalities in the subchondral bone reflect early or late changes of the disease. Contrary to the study of Ahlstrom et al (1990), Docherty et al (1992) found that subchondral marrow changes were present only in association with advanced radiographic evidence of sacroiliitis. They therefore postulate that the subchondral changes may have occurred secondary to inflammation of the articular cartilage rather than as the primary pathogenic event as suggested by the MRI findings of Ahlstrom et al (1990) and the histopathological analysis of Shichikawa et al (1985). Docherty et al (1992) emphasize the importance of establishing the relationship of the subchondral abnormalities to the natural history of the disease. In their view, this will determine the clinical importance of these MRI findings and possibly the pathogenic mechanisms involved in sacroiliitis. This is addressed by our study (Friedman et al, unpublished data) which will be discussed below. Docherty et al (1992) conclude that MRI is best reserved for those patients with a clinical history suggesting sacroiliitis who have normal plain X-rays.

Battafarano et al (1993) compared radio-isotope bone scan, CT, and MRI in the diagnosis of active sacroiliitis. They demonstrated that the type I lesions described by Ahlstrom et al (1990) are found in patients who have active sacroiliitis on clinical grounds and that these abnormalities are indicative of subcortical bone marrow edema. The Ahlstrom type II lesions were found to represent old postinflammatory changes. Battafarano et al (1993) further characterized the type II lesions according to their T1-weighted signal – high T1-weighted signal representing fatty replacement, low T1-weighted signal being consistent with sclerosis and/or fibrosis. Type I and II lesions may be found together, suggesting active inflammation in a patient with long-standing and established disease. CT alone or in combination with other tests was not found to be a reliable predictor of active sacroiliitis. MRI, which had 100% predictability, was the best single test for confirming active inflammatory sacroiliitis. The authors emphasize that conventional X-rays and CT of the SIJ represent static images and detect only pathological changes that have already been produced by the disease process. Unlike MRI, plain X-rays and CT are not able to determine disease activity. While radio-isotope bone scan is able to detect active disease, it lacks the specificity of MRI.

Battafarano et al (1993) stress the importance of STIR images in detecting bone marrow edema. These images suppress fat signal and are very sensitive in identifying increased water content or inflammation (Fig. 28.4A–B). The authors draw attention to one trap that may ensnare the unwary: findings on STIR images consistent with bone marrow edema (and hence active sacroiliitis) may also be seen in degenerative changes. Modic et al (1988) describe these signal findings in the vertebral body marrow adjacent to degenerative discs; subsequent histopathological examination found that these changes repre-

sented fibrovascular replacement. Clinical history together with the location, nature, and extent of the MRI findings should readily permit distinction between the presence of active sacroiliitis and degenerative changes on STIR sequences. Under the description of the MRI appearance of the normal SIJ, mention has been made of one further potential hazard in interpreting the STIR images, namely the well-defined, para-articular high-signal band described by Wittram and Whitehouse (1995), which should not be attributed to subchondral edema.

In a study comparing MRI and single photon emission computed tomography (SPECT) in the recognition of early sacroiliitis (Hanly et al 1994), 57% of patients with subchondral edema did not have evidence of abnormalities involving the articular cartilage. This was contrary to a previous study by the same group (Docherty et al 1992) but in keeping with other studies already mentioned. This finding supports the impression that subchondral edema represents one of the earliest manifestations of sacroiliitis. Hanly et al (1994) report the sensitivity and specificity of MRI in detecting sacroiliitis in their patient population as 54% and 67% respectively, and the sensitivity and specificity for SPECT as 38% and 100% respectively. They conclude that MRI and SPECT bone scanning provide objective and complementary evidence of sacroiliitis in the absence of plain X-ray changes. The relatively poor sensitivity and specificity of MRI are contrary to their previous study (Docherty et al 1992). As mentioned above, the determination of the sensitivity and specificity of imaging modalities in the diagnosis of sacroiliitis is problematic in view of the absence of a 'gold standard'.

The uncertainty regarding normal post-Gd-DTPA enhancement patterns has already been described. Interpretation of enhancement in sacroiliitis is therefore difficult. Braun et al (1994) found that dynamic MRI post-Gd-DTPA was able to demonstrate acute sacroiliitis in all 15 of their patients. These patients had clinical evidence of early ankylosing spondylitis but had normal plain X-rays and only minor changes on CT or non-constrast-enhanced MRI. They are cautious in determining the sensitivity and specificity of dynamic MRI in view of the previously noted absence of a standard reference test.

The same group further evaluated the role of dynamic Gd-DTPA-enhanced MRI (Bollow et al 1995). Large erosions (more than 2 mm diameter) were detectable without Gd-DTPA. In patients with undifferentiated spondyloarthropathy and normal plain X-rays, small erosions (less than 1 mm diameter) were seen in 72% of the joints only following Gd-DTPA enhancement. Juxta-articular enhancement was seen in 82% of these patients and thought to represent Ahlstrom's type I lesions. Bollow et al (1995) suggest that the precontrast MRI reveals a grade-dependent increasing tendency toward subchondral sclerosis, periarticular fat accumulation, and irregular joint spaces. Their study also calculated the sensitivity and specificity of dynamic MRI on the supposition that enhancement of the inner joint space is reliable evidence of sacroiliitis, while at the same time acknowledging the limitations of these calculations in the absence of the previously mentioned reference standard. Thus the sensitivity of 10% for precontrast MRI compared with a sensitivity of 100% for both pre- and post-contrast MRI in the detection of early sacroiliitis.

Our initial experience with MRI in sacroiliitis revealed the importance of the changes within the subchondral bone marrow. We therefore sought to substantiate the histopathological findings of Shichikawa et al (1985), which suggested that the early changes of sacroiliitis were those of inflammation localized to the subchondral bone. We also wished to assess the role of Gd-DTPA enhancement and hoped to develop a staging system based on the MRI findings. While this study has not yet been published, it was presented at the Second Interdisciplinary World Conference on Low Back Pain (San Diego, CA, November 1995) and awarded a certificate of merit at the Annual Meeting of the Radiological Society of North America (Chicago, November 1995). In addition, it supports the findings of several of the studies already described and a brief synopsis of our findings therefore seems justified (Friedman et al, unpublished data).

We have assessed 33 patients with low back pain and the clinical diagnosis of seronegative spondyloarthropathy as well as five normal controls. MRI was compared with plain X-rays and CT examinations. In normal subjects, the synovial compartment was not found to enhance visibly, although there was a small increase in signal intensity using a ROI measurement. Subchondral edema was the most prevalent finding in the early stages of sacroiliitis and was seen without abnormality of the joint space. While Gd-DTPA-enhanced MRI demonstrated both subchondral and synovial enhancement, synovial enhancement in the absence of subchondral edema was seen in only one patient (Fig. 28.3). Subchondral edema is therefore a very sensitive discriminator of early sacroiliitis. Subchondral edema was more prevalent on the sacral side of the joint, while erosions were found to be more prevalent on the iliac side (Figs 28.5B–C, and 28.6C). The latter finding has been described previously by Murphey et al (1991) and may reflect the presence of thicker hyaline cartilage on the sacral side compared with thinner fibrocartilage on the iliac side of the SIJ (Bowen & Cassidy 1981).

We propose a staging system based on MRI findings which is summarized in Table 28.1 and illustrated by Figs 28.2–28.9. This staging system is in keeping with the histopathological study of Shichikawa et al (1985) and the MRI findings of Ahlstrom et al (1990), Battafarano et al (1993), Hanly et al (1994), and Bollow et al (1995).

The exact temporal relationship between subchondral edema and synovial enhancement has yet to be established. Based on the evidence provided, it is tempting to postulate that the

Table 28.1   Proposed MRI staging system

Stage	Findings
1	Early subchondral bone marrow edema with synovial enhancement (grade 1–2NY) (Ahlstrom type I lesion)
2a	Marked subchondral bone marrow edema; erosions less prevalent (Ahlstrom type I lesion) (grade 3NY)
2b	Erosions more prevalent; subchondral bone marrow edema less marked (*)
3	Fatty infiltration ±-sclerosis; synovial enhancement variable (grade 3NY) (Ahlstrom type II lesion)
4	Ankylosis (grade 4NY)

NY = modified New York criteria.
*Depends on the presence/absence of active inflammation.

disease process commences in the subchondral bone with secondary involvement of the synovial compartment. However, it is not possible to exclude the alternative – that the disease process commences in the synovial compartment with a prompt inflammatory response in the subchondral bone before the development of definitive architectural changes of the synovial joint compartment. While our study of 33 patients cannot confirm the proposed order of the pathologic changes, we believe that the earliest changes seen on non-contrast MRI are those of subchondral bone marrow edema; this is followed by changes within the synovial compartment, subsequently by fatty infiltration and/or sclerosis, and finally by ankylosis. As suggested by Battafarano et al (1993), subchondral edema (Ahlstrom type I lesions) may occur together with the more advanced changes of fatty infiltration and/or sclerosis (Ahlstrom type II lesions). This is felt to represent active inflammation superimposed on long-standing changes of sacroiliitis.

In our study, 5 patients had stage 1 disease, 7 patients had stage 2 disease, 3 patients had stage 3 disease, and 1 patient had stage 4 disease. In the 5 patients with stage 1 disease, both plain X-rays and CT were normal (Fig. 28.2A–F). In view of the limitations previously described, we have not calculated the sensitivity and specificity of MRI in the diagnosis of sacroiliitis. Nonetheless, in common with other studies already quoted, we believe that MRI is the most sensitive imaging modality in the detection of early sacroiliitis. Based on our experience, we now employ a screening MRI protocol which consists of T1, T1FS, and FMPIR coronal oblique images. Scanning time is under 20 min. If there are positive findings or the examination is normal without strong clinical evidence of sacroiliitis, no further images are obtained. If the findings are equivocal or normal in the presence of a highly suspicious clinical history, Gd-DTPA-enhanced imaging is undertaken.

CONCLUSIONS

1. The wide availability of conventional radiography and the marked cost advantage makes it the screening examination of choice in the investigation of sacroiliitis. The main disadvantages of conventional X-rays are the lack of sensitivity in detecting early sacroiliitis, the false positive rate, and the use of ionizing radiation. Furthermore, inter- and intraobserver variation in the interpretation of these examinations is high. When plain X-rays reveal definite evidence of sacroiliitis, further investigation is not necessary unless specifically indicated.

2. MRI is fast emerging as the optimal method of imaging the SIJ in patients with suspected sacroiliitis who have normal or equivocal conventional X-rays. This can probably be attributed to the unique ability of MRI to directly visualize both the synovial cartilage and the subchondral bone marrow, and thereby identify early sacroiliitis. MRI may also be indicated in circumstances in which conventional X-rays reveal sacroiliitis but additional information is required. These indications may include the determination of disease activity and the therapeutic response to treatment regimes. In the latter context, dynamic Gd-DTPA-enhanced MRI may be particularly helpful. Apart from the increased sensitivity in detecting early sacroiliitis, the advantages of MRI include the absence of ionizing radiation. This is a very important consideration in view of the young age of most of the patients investigated for sacroiliitis. MRI offers a multiplanar ability, although in our experience only a single plane, the oblique coronal, is required. The disadvantages of MRI include cost and availability. The examination may be contraindicated in a very small minority of patients, and some patients may experience claustrophobia.

3. In those situations in which further imaging is required but the cost or availability of MRI limits the use of this modality, CT has been shown to be extremely helpful. By utilizing the 'CT miniseries' described by Friedman et al (1993), the radiation exposure and the scan time can be kept to a minimum. CT also has a very important role in the investigation of conditions other than sacroiliitis.

4. Future research will no doubt address some of the uncertainties described in this chapter. These include the role of Gd-DTPA-enhanced MRI and the pathogenesis of the disease. The use of positron emission tomography (PET) has

yet to be described. A long-term follow-up study is required to determine the exact sensitivities and specificities of the imaging modalities that are available and that are currently utilized in the investigation of sacroiliitis.

REFERENCES

Abbott G T, Carty H 1993 Pyogenic sacroiliitis, the missed diagnosis? British Journal of Radiology 66: 120–122

Ahlstrom H, Feltelius N, Nyman R, Hallgren R 1990 Magnetic resonance imaging of sacroiliac joint inflammation. Arthritis and Rheumatism 33(12): 1763–1769

Albrechtsen J, Hede J, Jurik A G 1994 Pelvic fractures: assessment by conventional radiography and CT. Acta Radiologica 35: 420–425

Battafarano D F, West S G, Rak K M, Fortenbery E J, Chantelois A E 1993 Comparison of bone scan, computed tomography, and magnetic resonance imaging in the diagnosis of active sacroiliitis. Seminars in Arthritis and Rheumatism 23(3): 161–176

Bollow M, Braun J, Hamm B et al 1995 Early sacroiliitis in patients with spondyloarthropathy: evaluation with dynamic gadolinium-enhanced MR imaging. Radiology 194: 529–536

Borlaza G S, Seigel R, Kuhns L R, Good A E, Rapp R, Martel W 1981 Computed tomography in the evaluation of sacroiliac arthritis. Radiology 139: 437–440

Bowen V, Cassidy J D 1981 Macroscopic and microscopic anatomy of the sacroiliac joint from embryonic life until the eighth decade. Spine 6(6): 620–628

Braun J, Bollow M, Eggens U, Konig H, Distler A, Sieper J 1994 Use of dynamic magnetic resonance imaging with fast imaging in the detection of early and advanced sacroiliitis in spondylarthropathy patients. Arthritis and Rheumatism 37(7): 1039–1045

Carrera G F, Foley W D, Kozin F, Ryan L, Lawson T L 1981 CT of sacroiliitis. American Journal of Roentgenology 136: 41–46

Docherty P, Mitchell M J, MacMillan L, Mosher D, Barnes D C, Hanly J G 1992 Magnetic resonance imaging in the detection of sacroiliitis. Journal of Rheumatology 19: 393–401

Ebraheim N, Rusin J, Coombs R, Jackson W, Holiday B 1987 Percutaneous computed-tomography stabilization of pelvic fractures: a preliminary report. Journal of Orthopaedic Trauma 1: 197–204

Fam A G, Rubenstein J D, Chin-Sang H, Leung F Y K 1985 Computed tomography in the diagnosis of early ankylosing spondylitis. Arthritis and Rheumatism 28(8): 930–937

Forrester D M 1990 Imaging of the sacroiliac joints. Radiologic Clinics of North America 28(5): 1055–1072

Friedman L, Silberberg P J, Rainbow A, Butler A 1993 A limited, low-dose computed tomography protocol to examine the sacroiliac joints. Canadian Association of Radiologists Journal 44(4): 267–272

Haliloglu M, Kleiman M B, Siddiqui A R, Cohen M D 1994 Osteomyelitis and pyogenic infection of the sacroiliac joint. Pediatric Radiology 24: 333–335

Hanly J G, Mitchell M J, Barnes D C, MacMillan L 1994 Early recognition of sacroiliitis by magnetic resonance imaging and single photon emission computed tomography. Journal of Rheumatology 21: 2088–2095

Lawson T L, Foley W D, Carrera G F, Berland L L 1982 The sacroiliac joints: anatomic, plain roentgenographic and computed tomographic analysis. Journal of Computer Assisted Tomography 6(2): 307–314

Levine C D, Schweitzer M E, Ehrlich S M 1994 Pelvic marrow in adults. Skeletal Radiology 23: 343–347

Modic M T, Steinberg P M, Ross J S, Masaryk T J, Carter J R 1988 Degenerative disk disease: assessment of changes in vertebral body marrow with MR imaging. Radiology 166: 193–199

Murphey M D, Wetzel L H, Bramble J M, Levine E, Simpson K M, Lindsley H B 1991 Sacroiliitis: MR imaging findings. Radiology 180: 239–244

Nelson D W, Duwelius P J 1991 CT guided fixation of sacral fractures and sacroiliac disruptions. Radiology 189: 527–537

Oudjhane K, Azouz E M, Hughes S, Paquin J D 1993 Computed tomography of the sacroiliac joints in children. Canadian Association of Radiologists Journal 44(4): 313–314

Rogers L F 1992 Radiology of skeletal trauma, 2nd edn. Churchill Livingstone, New York

Schwarzer A C, Aprill C N, Bogduk N 1995 The sacroiliac joint in chronic low back pain. Spine 20(1): 31–37

Scott W W, Fishman E K, Kuhlman J E et al 1990 Computed tomography evaluation of the sacroiliac joints in Crohn disease. Skeletal Radiology 19: 207–210

Shichikawa K, Tsujimoto M, Nishioka J, Nishibayashi Y, Matsumoto K 1985 Histopathology of early sacroiliitis and enthesitis in ankylosing spondylitis. In: Ziff M, Cohen S B (eds) Advances in inflammation research, vol. 9, The spondyloarthropathies. Raven Press, New York, pp 15–24

Taggart A J, Desai S M, Iveson J M, Verlow P W 1984 Computerized tomography of the sacro-iliac joints in the diagnosis of sacro-iliitis. British Journal of Rheumatology 23: 258–266

The H S G, Steven M M, van der Linden S M, Cats A 1985 Evaluation of diagnostic criteria for ankylosing spondylitis: a comparison of the Rome, New York and Modified New York criteria in patients with a positive clinical history screening test for ankylosing spondylitis. British Journal of Rheumatology 24: 242–249

van der Linden S, Valkenburg H A, Cats A 1984 Evaluation of diagnostic criteria for ankylosing spondylitis. Arthritis and Rheumatism 27(4): 361–368

Vogler J B, Brown W H, Helms C A, Genant H K 1984 The normal sacroiliac joint: a CT study of asymptomatic patients. Radiology 151: 433–437

Wittram C, Whitehouse G H 1995 Normal variation in the magnetic resonance imaging appearance of the sacroiliac joints: pitfalls in the diagnosis of sacroiliitis. Clinical Radiology 50: 371–376

Yazici H, Turunc M, Ozdogan H, Yurdakul S, Akinci A, Barnes C G 1987 Observer variation in grading sacroiliac radiographs might be a cause of 'sacroiliitis' reported in certain disease states. Annals of Rheumatic Diseases 46: 139–145

29. Visualization of pelvic biomechanical dysfunction

T. Ravin

INTRODUCTION

Radiography and imaging of the lumbosacral spine for evaluation of biomechanical dysfunctions are more important now than ever. Since the beginning of the twentieth century, radiologists have tried to identify bony and soft tissue alterations that might help to explain the cause of low back pain on images of the spine. Over these years, many useful observations were forgotten or misplaced as technology changed our capabilities to image the pelvis and spine. The relentless pursuit of the 'disc' as a cause for back pain diverted radiographers and clinicians away from assessing images that could help to identify the functional causes of the pain.

There is now a renewed interest in spinal imaging, with an emphasis on functional assessment. Imaging makes it possible to diagnose several congenital and acquired biomechanical dysfunctions that significantly impact on treatment. The clinician interested in identifying the cause of low back pain can find considerable support in the careful evaluation of images. This chapter will review some of the more important congenital abnormalities that affect low back and pelvic function, such as the unlevel sacral base, mixed lumbosacral joint orientation, steep lumbosacral angle, and a high L5 vertebral body. There are also some important acquired problems that can create low back and pelvic pain. These include mechanical joint dysfunctions that cause a short-curve scoliosis, pubic dysfunctions, sacral torsions, coccygeal displacements, and ligamentous laxity

that allows retrospondylolisthesis. The impact of gravity on our posture can be evaluated radiographically as changes in spinal position.

The treatment of low back and pelvic pain with manipulation, postural training, and injection therapy is increasing the importance of images in the assessment of the lumbosacral spine. Standing lumbar spine films are returning to their rightful position as benchmark studies in the evaluation of low back pain.

TECHNIQUE

Plain-film imaging of the lumbosacral spine should be taken standing. The basic examination consists of an anteroposterior (AP) film of the lumbar spine and pelvis, and a lateral film of the lumbosacral spine. The feet are shoulder width apart and the weight is equally distributed between the two legs. Lateral X-rays in flexion and extension are also useful. These images can, in some cases, define the nature of mechanical joint dysfunctions. The film of the pelvis should be taken so that the central ray of the beam, or where the cross-hairs point, is at the L4 level. This will reveal a good view of most of the structures of the lumbar spine and pelvis as well as a view of the femoral heads, coccyx, and symphysis pubis. On the lateral lumbar film, the patient should be positioned so that the horizontal beam is at L4 and the vertical beam is centered on the spine. In the lateral view, the technique should be adjusted so that good detail of the lumbosacral junction, coccyx, and symphysis pubis can be well visualized. The third set of films that may occasionally be obtained are the oblique films for the evaluation of spondylolisthesis.

CONGENITAL ABNORMALITIES AND MECHANICAL DYSFUNCTIONS

The relationship between congenital abnormalities and mechanical dysfunctions is perhaps the single most important reason to image the spine. The reported incidence of clinically significant congenital abnormalities ranges from a maximum of 50% (Ferguson 1934) to a minimum of 6% (Frymoyer 1984). In the 1930s, O'Reilly, Ferguson, Mitchell and others began to notice the relationship between congenital abnormalities and low back pain (Mitchell 1934, O'Reilly 1921). They observed that several common congenital anomalies, particularly those of the lumbosacral joints, were frequently associated with low back pain. These radiographic observations and their clinical corollaries became separated over the years. Now in the twilight of the twentieth century, with a rising interest in non-surgical care of the back and renewed interest in functional assessment, it is again time to read these gems of clinical imaging literature. For example, Ferguson wrote in 1934:

Our spines were developed for the four-footed position and are not yet adapted to the erect, so mechanical weakness at the lumbosacral area is usual rather than exceptional. We must consider the lumbosacral area not as normal or abnormal but as mechanically sound or mechanically unsound.

The lumbosacral facets

The relationship between congenital alignment of articular surfaces and mechanical dysfunctions is best demonstrated at the lumbosacral junction. The clinical impression that lumbosacral joint asymmetry may be associated with a higher incidence of low back pain has some basis in fact dating back to the early part of the twentieth century. The normal lumbosacral facet joint is in the coronal plane (Van Schaik 1985) (Fig. 29.1).

If the lumbosacral joints are more sagittal in nature, there will be greater stress on both the ligaments anteriorly and the lamina posteriorly (Sharma et al 1995) (Fig. 29.2). A sagittal facet orientation significantly increases the stress on the iliolumbar ligaments because in this joint orientation only these ligaments can resist lumbar flexion.

X-rays of the lumbosacral spine reveal many variations of the lumbosacral joints, including

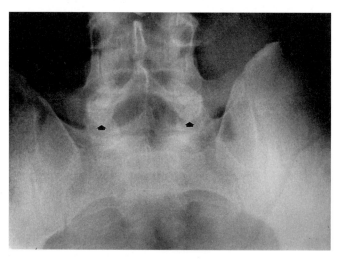

Fig. 29.1 The normal lumbosacral facets should have a coronal orientation (closed arrows). This orientation allows for flexion, extension, and some side-bending, but little rotation.

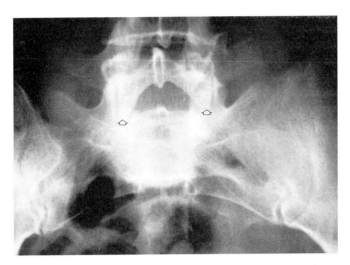

Fig. 29.2   Lumbosacral joints that are in the sagittal plane allow for excessive movement and are inherently unstable (open arrows). This orientation creates strain in almost all the soft tissue structures adjacent to the lumbosacral junction, particularly the ligaments.

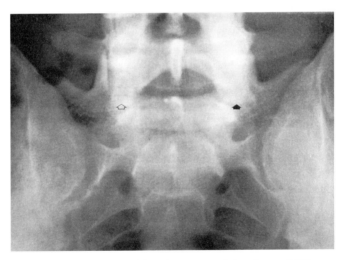

Fig. 29.3   The lumbosacral junction commonly has facets of different orientation: one joint has a coronal orientation (closed arrow) and the other is in a more sagittal plane (open arrow).

inclined, rudimentary, irregular, and defective joints (Jonsson et al 1989). Asymmetric lumbosacral joints, one being coronal and one sagittal, are some of the most common abnormalities in the low back (Fig. 29.3). This situation is a functional disaster; and it is easy to envision how this situation could lead to a mechanical joint dysfunction. For example, if an individual has this lumbosacral facet alignment and lifts from the side, there will be a real possibility that one of the joints will malfunction. There is good reason for carrying out plain-film imaging of the lumbar spine for assessment of joint orientation, as it can be helpful in explaining persistent complaints of pain (Farfan 1967). Ferguson concluded that 'practically every person with a severe degree of asymmetry of these facets has symptoms referable to the lower part of the back'.

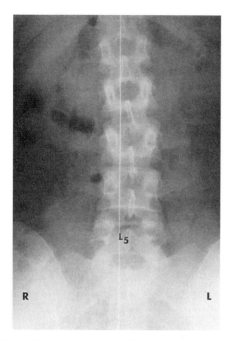

Fig. 29.4   The 'high L5 vertebra' is an important congenital variant. In this figure, notice that the transverse processes of the L5 vertebra are separated by a considerable distance from the medial side of the hip bones. The iliolumbar ligament spans this space. The white vertical line is a true vertical wire.

The high L5 vertebra

The presence of an L5 vertebra that is high, relative to the iliac crest, can also be a cause of low back pain. The increased length of the iliolumbar ligament in this anatomic variation increases its vulnerability to ligamentous strain when resisting nutation of the sacrum or flexion of the lumbar spine. Figure 29.4 shows how this looks on the AP film of the pelvis. This congenital problem is not a frequent finding but, when present, is often associated with low back pain that will respond nicely to both prolotherapy (Klein et al 1993) and postural corrections (Kuchera & Jungmann 1986).

Leg length and the unlevel sacral base

The importance of unequal leg lengths on mechanical dysfunction and back pain has waxed and waned for nearly a hundred years (Kerr 1913). The height of the ankle, and the length of the tibia and femur are just a part of this abnormality. The size of the ipsilateral hip bone and sacral ala also affects what really matters. Is the sacral base level? (Kappler 1983) – that is the real question. It is not unusual to find all of the structures in one of the rear quarters slightly smaller, so that leg length will be only one of the components of the unlevel sacral base. The impact of this anomaly on mechanical dysfunctions of the back seems to be directly related to the degree of tilt of the sacral base (Denslow 1983) (Fig. 29.5). The unlevel sacral base creates sacroiliac joint

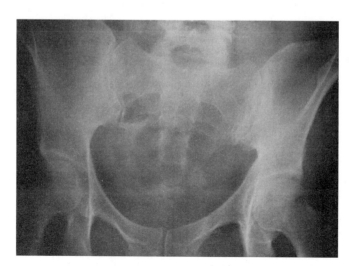

Fig. 29.5   Is the sacral base level? It is important to assess this on the standing AP pelvis film (see text).

(SIJ) dysfunctions in the pelvis, such as sacral sheers and torsions, and in the axial skeleton with the creation of long- and short-curve scoliosis (Kuchera 1995b) (see also Ch. 9).

The next question is, 'Does an unlevel sacral base and treatment with foot lifts alter low back pain?' The results of this type of treatment have been unpredictable. Several authors have pointed out that in some individuals the treatment of leg length differences is an effective, simple, and inexpensive way to decrease low back pain (Heilig 1983). The mechanical correction of the unlevel sacral base can be carried out using 'foot lifts'. Figure 29.6 illustrates how to calculate the amount of lift necessary to achieve a level sacral base.

An unlevel sacral base needs and demands a corrective curve in order to keep the eyes level with the horizon. These corrections often occur at the level of the lumbosacral junction and L4. If the sacrum is unlevel to one side, there will be a compensatory side-bending and rotation of L4 or L5 relative to S1, which will help to correct the sacral base tilt. As one can see from Fig. 29.7, identifying the side-bending and rotation is often not as difficult radiographically as one would imagine.

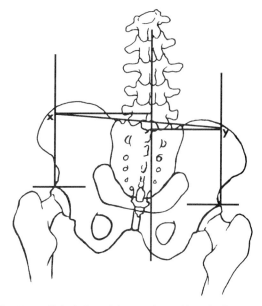

Fig. 29.6 Calculation of degree of sacral base inclination. First find the lateral sacral notches, draw a connecting line and extend it across the innominate bones – line x–y. Draw two vertical lines from the apex of the femoral heads to meet the x–y line representing the sacral base inclination. Next draw two horizontal lines across the film that intersect the sacral baseline at the femoral heads. The amount of foot lift necessary to correct the sacral base inclination is the distance in millimeters between these solid lines in the midline.

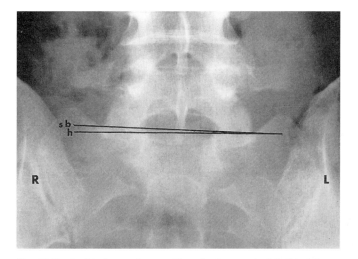

Fig. 29.7 In this figure, the sacral base inclines to the left (black line sb, line h being the horizontal). Notice that the L5 vertebra appears to be side-bent to the right. This compensatory right side-bending of L5 effectively straightens the lumbar spine and there will be little remaining scoliosis. In this situation, the L5 vertebra will not function in a completely normal manner as some of its normal ranges of motion are used to correct the unlevel sacral base.

Ferguson's angle

The lumbosacral junction is uniquely individual and, when assessed on lateral radiography, contains considerable information about lumbar spine function. The angle created by a line that is horizontal and the cephalad surface of the first sacral vertebra is known as 'Ferguson's angle'. It is seldom measured but it is worth the effort. In 1934 Ferguson documented that this angle changed between standing and supine imaging (Fig. 29.8). He noted that the sacrum moved with gravitational stress and, in individuals with painful backs, that this movement was paradoxical. The fact that the angle became less when standing in patients with painful low backs has been clinically confirmed many times by individuals using the Levator (Jungmann 1992), an orthotic that aids the spine in resisting gravitational strain. The normal horizontal lumbosacral angle is about 42°. If the angle is greater than 52°, the sheer stresses at the lumbosacral junction become significant (Frisch 1994). Steep angles combined with abnormal lumbosacral joints are functionally unstable and significantly increase facet joint forces.

Frymoyer noted that some of these abnormalities are often present in individuals who do not have any back pain at all and that these radiographic findings cannot be used to predict the presence of back pain (Frymoyer 1984). Clinical experience in treating the painful back, however, has shown that the finding of congenital abnormalities and sacral base unleveling on X-ray films often influences treatment protocols.

ACQUIRED SOMATIC JOINT DYSFUNCTIONS

The lumbar spine and pelvis are the most manipulated regions in the body. The presence of acquired somatic joint dysfunctions, created by trauma and ligament laxity, are often demon-

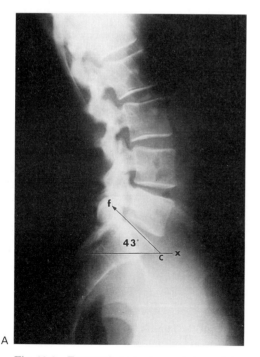
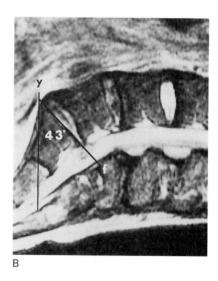

Fig. 29.8 Ferguson's angle changes between lying and standing and is not a static angle. It can, in fact, help to establish the presence of low back pain. In the normal individual, the angle should increase between lying supine and standing. In the standing image (A), line x is horizontal. In the supine image, line y is true vertical. (B) This is an MRI image, which is one way to get a supine measurement of Ferguson's angle. The lines f are drawn along the cephalad surface of S1 in both images. This patient is abnormal because the angle did not increase between the supine and standing images.

Table 29.1 Vertebral motion

	Position	Motion restriction
L4 on L5	Extended	Flexion
	Left side-bent	Right side-bending
	Right rotated	Left rotation
	Left side-bent	Right side-bending

strated in lumbosacral spine X-rays. X-rays can aid the clinician in identifying manipulable lesions. Radiographic description of the lesions should follow palpatory findings. The position of the lumbar vertebra noted on physical examination can be described using the guidelines of Greenman (1995).

The current convention of describing vertebral motion is either from the perspective of the position in which the segment is stuck in or by the restrictive motion of the segment. Therefore, a segment that is backward bent (extended), right rotated and right side-bent has restriction of motion in forward bending (flexion), left side-bending and left rotation. Table 29.1 summarizes the changes. In radiography of the spine, the position description is the only one that can be used.

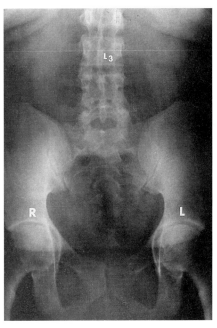

Fig. 29.9 'Short-curve scoliosis' in the AP projection is often a sign of mechanical dysfunction. In this lumbar spine, L3 is side-bent to the left and slightly rotated to the left. Notice that the L3–4 disc space tapers to the left. In the lumbar spine, there is relatively more side-bending than rotation because of the sagittal orientation of the facets.

Lumbar vertebra

The radiographic evaluation of the pelvis and lumbar spine for somatic joint dysfunctions has remained a challenge since osteopaths and chiropractors began evaluating these structures in the early 1900s. The difficulty has been the correlation of the physical examination of a specific mechanical joint dysfunction with a specific radiographic finding. This has been and will remain a challenge to both the hand and the eye.

Mechanical dysfunctions of the pelvis and lumbar spine can generate numerous radiographic findings. The persistently side-bent and rotated lumbar vertebra, 'the short-curve scoliosis', is often seen on both plane-film and computer-aided images. Side-bending is easy to see on radiography as the transverse processes are closer together on one side than the other (Fig. 29.9). Side-bending often comes with rotation, either towards or away from the side of the side-bending, as these spinal joint movements are coupled together. Due to

the orientation of the zygoapophyseal joints at L4–5, which are nearly sagittal, there is limited rotation, but there will be a noticeable amount of side-bending.

Lateral flexion and extension views demonstrate movement of the lumbar vertebra in the sagittal plane. These views allow the complete description of vertebral functional restrictions (Fig. 29.10). In the clinic, the specific manipulation needed to correct the problem should be determined by palpatory findings rather than radiographic ones. Clinically, the upper lumbar vertebrae are frequently involved in mechanical dysfunctions probably related to the attachments of the psoas muscles. These muscles can both extend and flex the upper lumbar vertebrae, but when in spasm they tend to cause extension.

Ligamentous spondylolisthesis

Ligamentous laxity allows increased motion of the lumbar vertebrae on each other. This finding

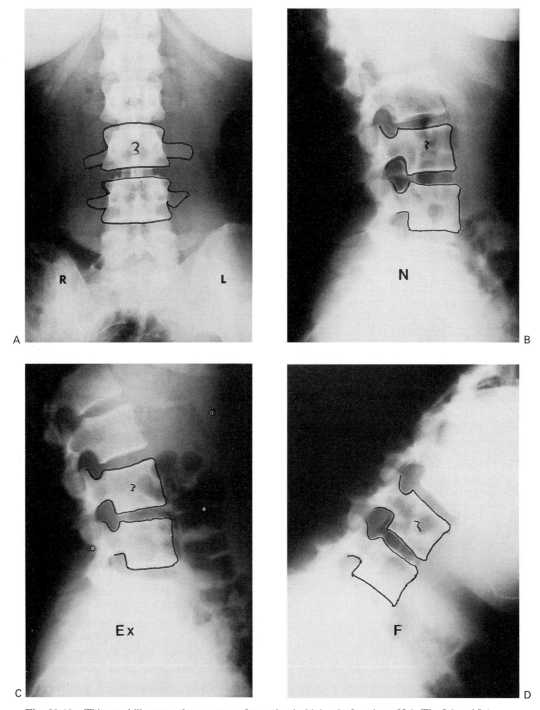

Fig. 29.10 This panel illustrates the presence of a mechanical joint dysfunction of L3. The L3 and L4 lumbar vertebra are outlined in order to illustrate the vertebral motion. (A) An AP film. (B) A standing lateral pelvis and lumbar spine in neutral (N). (C) In extension (Ex). (D) In flexion (F). Notice that the L3–4 disc space does not appear to increase in size or shape when the patient tries to extend. This is because the L3 vertebra is already extended and cannot extend further. The L3 vertebra can still move into flexion so that when the patient bends forward, the L3 vertebra moves and makes the disc space nearly normal looking. This vertebral body is extended, side-bent right, and slightly rotated right.

can be identified on lateral films. Anatomic studies show that ligamentous laxity of the supraspinous, interspinous, and even facet joint capsules need to be present for spondylolisthesis to occur. The presence of ligamentous laxity is best demonstrated on the extension films, where the retrospondylolisthesis can be easily identified (Putto & Tallroth 1990). The radiographic changes range from subtle in neutral to considerable anterior spondylolisthesis on flexion films and obvious retrospondylolisthesis on extension films. Significant anterior spondylolisthesis is considered by some to be a reason for spinal fusion.

Figure 29.11 is an example of the retrospondylolisthesis. This abnormal movement can lead to spinal nerve root compression, cause pain, alter nerve root function, and be misinterpreted as disc disease (Garfin et al 1995). The disc disease that accompanies the spondylolisthesis changes is often more obvious radiographically than is the spondylolisthesis itself. The static and horizontal

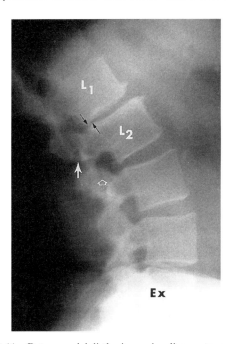

Fig. 29.11 Retrospondylolisthesis requires ligamentous laxity of almost all the ligaments surrounding the vertebra. This lateral lumbar spine was taken with the patient in extension. The white arrow points to the gap in the zygoapophyseal joints at the L1–2 level. Notice that this joint space is much larger than the joint space at L2–3 (open white arrowhead). The black closed arrows point to the posterior displacement of the L1 vertebral body. Notice the degenerative disc disease of the L1–2 disc space.

magnetic resonance imaging (MRI) or computerized tomography (CT) images are often relied upon to explain back pain, but they seldom demonstrate the functional causes of lumbar and pelvic pain.

The sacroiliac joints

Degenerative joint disease of the SIJs seen on radiographic images is not usually thought of as reflecting mechanical dysfunction. The presence of periarticular osteophytes, subarticular sclerosis, or osteitis condensans and joint space narrowing are, however, good indicators of abnormal joint mechanics (Dilhmann 1980, Dreyfuss 1994) (Fig. 29.12). The developing consensus is that these findings represent the presence of mechanical joint dysfunctions and ligamentous laxity. These findings on all forms of imaging should be clues that mechanical dysfunctions might be present and are excellent documentation when correlated with the clinical findings (Greenman 1992).

Sacral torsion is the one major somatic dysfunction of the sacrum that can be identified on MRI/CT scanning. This is an osteopathic descriptive term and can be thought of as a sacrum that has rotated about an oblique or diagonal axis. This twisting is sometimes called 'asymlocation' (Dorman & Ravin 1991). It is possible because of the unique nature of the SIJs and the lumbosacral junction. The basic model of spinal mechanics leads us to believe that side-bending and rotation are integral parts of spinal and sacral motion. The normal sacrum lying horizontal in a gantry should be nearly parallel with the floor.

If there is a side-bent lesion anywhere in the spine, the most likely place for this spinal twist to be exhibited is at the level of the vertebra involved. However, it can occasionally manifest as rotation at either end of the spine – the sacrum or the atlas. This process is documented in 'The spinal engine' (Gracovetsky 1988). The sacral twisting component is often evident in MRI/CT scans. In a normal patient without mechanical joint dysfunctions, the spine is straight, but if there are vertebral somatic joint dysfunctions that are side-bent and rotated, there will be some scoliosis of the spine. This curve or 'kink' in the spine will create a twisting that will travel to the sacrum.

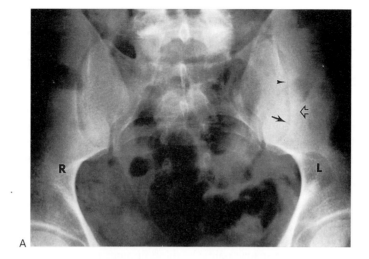

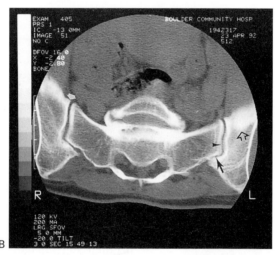

Fig. 29.12 Degenerative SIJ disease creates numerous radiographic changes. In panel (A), a standing AP film, and in panel (B), an MRI, the degenerative joint disease is manifest as a narrowed joint space (black arrowheads), irregular joint contours (black arrows), subchondral sclerosis of cancellous bone (open black arrows), and marginal osteophyte formation (white arrow). Note the left sacral rotation on this MRI.

The visualized twisting of the sacrum is not created by malposition of the patient by the technician but by mechanical dysfunction in the spine. If this sacral torsion is mechanically corrected by forcing the sacrum into horizontal, the patient will quickly become uncomfortable because the spine will be forced to side-bend and the imaging table will not allow the patient to do so.

Sacral torsion is clinically quite common in individuals with back pain, and the MRI/CT will quite often demonstrate some degree of sacral torsion. At present, the normal range of sacral torsion seen on MRI/CT is unknown, but the gross changes noted on many scans would clearly be abnormal (Fig. 29.13).

Symphysis pubis

Mechanical dysfunction of the symphysis pubis is a common clinical diagnosis and can frequently

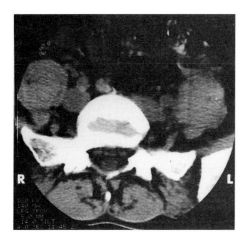

Fig. 29.13 This CT demonstrates significant left rotation of the sacrum. This much rotation is another finding of abnormal spinal joint mechanics.

joints of the pelvis work in unison; dysfunction of one joint leads to instability in the entire structure just as in the uncoupling of one angle in a triangle. That is why treatment of pelvic dysfunctions often begins with treatment of the pubes.

The radiographic manifestation of mechanical dysfunctions of the symphysis pubis is simply a malalignment of the two bones. This finding is sometimes considered to be positional but is most often the result of a true mechanical dysfunction of the pelvis. These pubic displacements, when combined with SIJ degenerative joint disease, are further evidence of the presence of pelvic mechanical dysfunction (Fig. 29.14).

be identified radiographically. The relationship of the pubes is critical in the clinical diagnosis and treatment of mechanical dysfunction of the pelvis. Innominate up-slips, down-slips, and rotations are easily identified clinically. They can, and do, create radiographic changes in this joint space (see Fig. 29.14). Evaluation of the symphysis pubis on AP pelvic images can aid in the documentation of displacement and is of considerable help to the treating clinician. It is critical that these images be obtained standing. The three bones and three

Coccyx

This small bone is often ignored on imaging but is a vital link between the bony pelvis and the soft tissues of pelvic floor. The coccyx is directly attached to the sacrotuberous ligaments (Barral 1988) and to the dural sac by the filum terminale. It is also the posterior bony anchor of the pelvic floor muscles. Mechanical dysfunctions of this small bone can impact directly upon the axial skeleton by way of the dura. It can create visceral dysfunctions by straining all the muscles and ligamentous structures of the pelvic floor. The

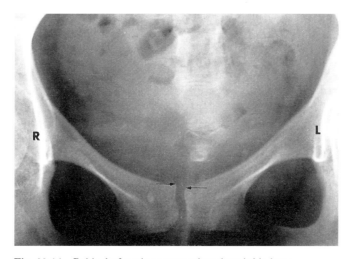

Fig. 29.14 Pubic dysfunctions occur when there is hip bone dysfunction. The black arrows point to the malalignment of the pubes on this standing AP pelvis. Notice the bony sclerosis of the left pubic bone, which reflects the early changes of osteitis involving the pubes.

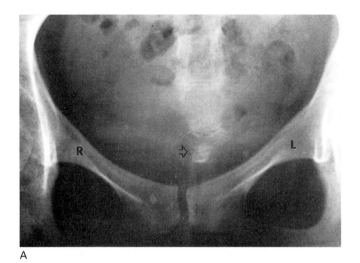

A

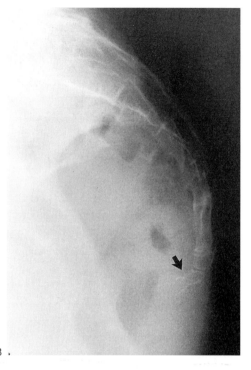

B

Fig. 29.15   The coccyx is easily seen on the AP pelvis films (A). However, it may be hard to identify on the lateral film (B). It is usually forced into abnormal flexion (black closed arrow) and in this case side-bent to the right (open arrow in A).

coccyx is a vulnerable structure in many thin individuals, particularly those without gluteal muscle mass. Some individuals may literally be sitting on one of the most critical bones in the body. The coccyx is usually forced into excessive flexion and the somatic joint dysfunctions create symptoms that include low back pain, headaches, and even incontinence in females.

Mechanical displacements of this bone are often clinically hard to identify and frequently overlooked, so their radiographic demonstration is particularly helpful (Fig. 29.15). Plane-film imaging is one of the best ways to identify displacements (see also Chapter 30 in this volume).

Pelvic index and weight-bearing axis

Measurements of the pelvic index and the weight-bearing axis are helpful in defining how an individual is coping with the effects of gravity. The ideal posture is one in which gravitational force is directed along the structures adapted for weight-bearing. This normal situation requires a minimum of energy for its maintenance. As the alignment of these structures changes with poor or abnormal posture, the gravitational force is redirected and creates additional stress on the muscles, tendons, and ligaments. The importance of gravitational stress on the bony, musculotendinous, and ligamentous structures of the lumbosacral junction is reflected in changes that can be measured on lateral films. These films reflect changes in posture created by the constant and underestimated stress of gravity. The ability of the musculoligamentous structures to maintain effectively both static and dynamic stability in the face of gravity can be estimated with the calculation of the pelvic index.

The pelvic index is a valuable measurement for the objective evaluation of the relative position of the sacrum with respect to the innominate bones. The importance of this measurement as a gauge of gravitational stress was first proposed by Jungmann in 1963. Changes in this index correlated with increasing age suggest that these alterations might be the result of gravitational strain. These measurements are obtained from the lateral lumbar–pelvic X-ray and can be helpful in identifying individuals whose bad posture is one of the primary causes of their back pain. This index can assess increased myofascial and ligamentous strain created by bad posture (Janda 1986). The use of this index is currently

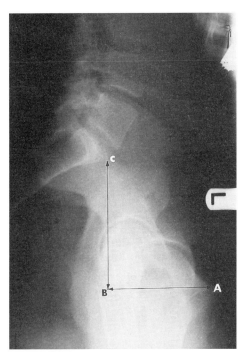

Fig. 29.16   The pelvic index is calculated by first finding point A, which is the crest of the pubes. Then find point c, which is at the sacral promontory. Draw a horizontal line from point A across the film, and then a vertical line from point c downwards until it intersects the horizontal line, which is point B. The pelvic index is the width in millimeters of line A–B divided by the height in millimeters of line B–c.

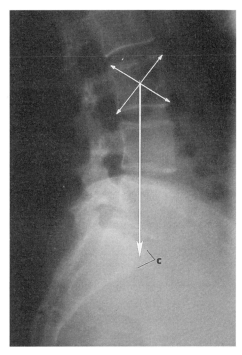

Fig. 29.17   The gravitational line should pass through the middle of the L3 vertebra and in front of the sacral promontory (point c in this figure). In this patient, the weight-bearing line is abnormal because it is posterior to the sacral promontory.

increasing in the clinical setting as it also can aid in the identification of the muscle imbalances described as the 'Unterkreuz' by Janda (Kuchera 1995a) (Fig. 29.16).

The lateral image also contains information about the weight-bearing axis. This line is calculated by drawing a vertical line through the midpoint of the L3 vertebral body. This provides information regarding the sagittal plane balance of the individual (Fig. 29.17). This theoretical line passes through the external auditory canal, the lateral head of the humerus, the anterior body of L3, the head of the femur, the anterior third of the sacrum, and the lateral malleolus. This 'ideal' alignment requires a minimum of energy expenditure by the postural muscles. Displacement of this line anteriorly or posteriorly significantly increases muscle energy expenditure and ligamentous strain, particularly in the regions of the neck and pelvis.

The importance of calculating the pelvic index and the weight-bearing axis for diagnosis and therapy is further developed in Chapter 39 in this volume, and the reader is encouraged to integrate these chapters.

CONCLUSIONS

1. There are many reasons to image the lumbar spine and pelvis for biomechanical dysfunctions. There are several important congenital abnormalities that can influence the stability of the lumbosacral spine:

   a.   Imaging demonstrates the orientation of the lumbosacral facets. The normal coronal facets are associated with fewer clinical problems than are facets of other orientations. Congenital anomalies of the facets are commonly associated with clinical problems.

   b.   The presence of an unlevel sacral base demonstrated on the AP pelvic film can explain the resistance of a mechanical joint dysfunction to manipulation. The correction of the unlevel sacral base can be determined by measurements made from the X-rays.

c.   Ferguson's angle, often thought of as a static measure, is really a dynamic angle; the angle will be smaller in the painful back.

d.   The presence of a 'high L5' can explain persistent iliolumbar ligamentous pain. This radiographic finding implies a long iliolumbar ligament and one that might respond to prolotherapy.

2. Lumbosacral spine radiography can also reveal the presence of acquired biomechanical dysfunctions:

a.   'The short-curve scoliosis' created by a side-bent and rotated lumbar vertebra. These are frequent findings on all types of images of the spine. These biomechanical dysfunctions are common causes of back, pelvic, and leg pain. The identification by imaging is important, as the treatment may depend on this form of documentation of their presence.

b.   The presence of a malaligned symphysis pubis. The radiographic signs are clear and can help to explain persistent lumbosacral instability.

c.   SIJs showing changes of degenerative disease may reflect the presence of long-standing mechanical dysfunction. The recognition of degenerative joint disease can be of considerable aid to the clinician struggling with an 'unstable back' by directing him or her to the primary cause.

d.   A coccyx in an excessively flexed position noted on X-ray can help to explain pelvic and low back pain that seems to have 'no explanation'.

e.   Sacral torsion or rotation and degenerative joint disease on computerized imaging can identify mechanical dysfunctions and the presence of long-standing instability.

f.   The pelvic index and the weight-bearing line that are calculated from the standing lateral images can explain how gravity effects biomechanical stability.

3. As our clinical understanding of the biomechanics of the lumbar spine and pelvis increases, we are forced to review these areas of imaging. Observations of mechanical dysfunctions collected over the last century are now finding a new place in contemporary spinal diagnostic and therapeutic literature. The past emphasis on imaging the discs and the SIJs without integrating congenital and acquired dysfunctions is passing, as this book reveals.

REFERENCES

Barral J P 1988 Visceral manipulation. Eastland Press, Seattle
Denslow J S 1983 Mechanical stresses in the human lumbar spine and pelvis. In: Peterson B (ed.) Postural balance and imbalance. American Academy of Osteopathy, Indianapolis, pp 144–151
Dilhmann W 1980 Diagnostic radiology of the sacroiliac joints. Georg Thieme Verlag, New York
Dorman T A, Ravin T H 1991 Diagnosis and injection techniques in orthopedic medicine. Williams & Wilkins, Baltimore
Dreyfuss P 1994 The sacroiliac joint: a review. International Spinal Injection Society 2: 22–58
Farfan H F 1967 The relationship of facet orientation to intervertebral disc failure. Canadian Journal of Surgery 10: 179–185
Ferguson A B 1934 The clinical and roentgenographic interpretation of lumbosacral anomalies. Radiology 22: 548–588
Frisch H 1994 Systematic musculoskeletal examination. Springer-Verlag, New York
Frymoyer J W 1984 Spine radiographs in patients with low-back pain. Journal of Bone and Joint Surgery (US) 66: 1048–1055
Garfin S R, Rydevid B, Lind B 1995 Spinal nerve root compression. Spine 20: 1810–1820
Gracovetsky S 1988 The spinal engine. Springer-Verlag, New York
Greenman P E 1992 Sacroiliac dysfunction in the failed low back pain syndrome. In: Vleeming A, Mooney V, Snijders C J, Dorman T A (eds) First interdisciplinary world congress on low back pain and its relation to the sacroiliac joint. San Diego, CA, 9–11 November, pp 329–352
Greenman P E 1995 Principles of manual medicine, 2nd edn. Williams & Wilkins, Baltimore
Heilig D 1983 Principles of lift therapy. In: Peterson B (ed.) Postural balance and imbalance. American Academy of Osteopathy, Indianapolis, pp 113–118
Janda V 1986 Muscle weakness and inhibition (pseudoparesis) in back pain syndromes. In: Grieve G P (ed.) Modern manual therapy of the vertebral column. Churchill Livingstone, Edinburgh, pp 113–118
Jonsson B, Stromquist B, Egund N 1989 Anomalous lumbosacral articulations and low-back pain – evaluation and treatment. Spine 14: 831–834
Jungmann M 1992 The Jungmann concept and technique of anti-gravity leverage, 2nd edn. Institute for Gravitational Strain Pathology, Rangley, Maine
Kappler R E 1983 Postural balance and motion patterns. In: Peterson B (ed.) Postural balance and imbalance. American Academy of Osteopathy, Indianapolis, pp 6–12

Kerr H E 1913 Observations on anatomical short leg in a series of patients presenting themselves for treatment of low-back pain. Journal of the American Osteopathic Association 42: 437–440

Klein R G, Eek B C, DeLong B W, Mooney V 1993 A randomized double-blind trial of dextrose–glycerine–phenol injections for chronic, low back pain. Journal of Spinal Disorders 6: 23–33

Kuchera M L 1995 Gravitational strain pathophysiology and 'Unterkreuz' syndrome. Manuelle Medizin 33(2): 56

Kuchera M L 1995 Prolotherapy in the lumbar spine and pelvis. Spine: State of the Art Reviews 9(2): 463–490

Kuchera M L, Jungmann M 1986 Inclusion of levitor orthotic device in the management of refractive low back pain patients. Journal of American Osteopathic Association 86: 673–678

Mitchell G A G 1934 The lumbosacral junction. Journal of Bone and Joint Surgery (US) 16: 233–254

O'Reilly A 1921 Backache and anatomical variations of the lumbosacral region. Journal of Orthopedic Surgery 3: 171–187

Putto E, Tallroth K 1990 Extension–flexion radiographs for motion studies of the lumbar spine – a comparison of two methods. Spine 15: 107–110

Sharma M, Langrana N A, Rodrequez J 1995 Role of ligaments and facets in lumbar spinal stability. Spine 20: 887–900

Van Schaik J P J 1985 The orientation of laminae and facet joints in the lower lumbar spine. Spine 10: 59–63

30. Lateral dynamic X-rays in the sitting position and coccygeal discography in common coccydynia

J.-Y. Maigne

INTRODUCTION

Common coccydynia is poorly understood. Numerous hypotheses have been proposed for the origin of the syndrome, including pain from the pericoccygeal soft tissues, spasm of the muscles of the pelvic floor, referred pain from lumbar pathology, arachnoiditis of the lower sacral nerve roots, local post-traumatic lesions, and somatization (Howorth 1959, Jurmand 1976, Nelson 1991, Postacchini & Massobrio 1983, Stern 1967). Thus far, there has been no sound confirmation of any of these, nor have there been any controlled studies.

Because patients often mention a fall on the buttocks or a delivery as precipitating event, a mechanical basis for the pain is likely. In addition, in the majority of cases, the pain occurs only in the sitting position. These factors led me to develop a protocol to document the painful coccyx with dynamic films and coccygeal discography (Maigne et al 1994). Dynamic films are defined as X-ray films in the lateral sitting position (the painful position), compared with standard lateral X-rays. Since 1992, 189 patients with coccygeal pain have undergone this protocol.

ANATOMIC STUDY OF THE SACROCOCCYGEAL AND INTERCOCCYGEAL DISCS

There is a paucity of information regarding this topic. According to Williams (1995), the sacrococcygeal joints are thin intervertebral discs of fibrocartilage. Occasionally, the intercoccygeal joints are synovial.

By examining nine aged coccyges from fresh cadavers, we found that the sacrococcygeal joint was a disc in one case, a synovial joint in four cases and a third type in four cases, the joint being an intermediate structure made of a disc containing a more or less extensive cleft, parallel to the endplates, and bordered by annular fibers or synovial cells (Maigne et al 1992). This intermediate state was not found in the intercoccygeal joints. It is not known whether young individuals show the same distribution or not, i.e. if a sacrococcygeal joint can be transformed from one form to another during a person's lifetime.

A fourth type of connection exists, in the form of ossification, which may involve only the sacrococcygeal joint. Studying two different populations, the frequency of this type was found in 22 and 68% of the cases by Saluja (1988). In some of our patients, the whole coccyx was ossified.

The movements of the coccyx are restricted to flexion and extension. Flexion (movement in a forward direction) is performed by the levatores ani and the sphincter ani externus muscles. Extension (movement in a backward direction) is due to relaxation of these muscles and to the increased intra-abdominal pressure that occurs during defecation and parturition (Smout et al 1969). Surprisingly, the movements of the coccyx in the sitting posture have never, to our knowledge, been reported in the literature.

TECHNIQUE OF DYNAMIC FILMS

The standard way to X-ray the coccyx is to take the film in the standing position. I coin the word 'dynamic exploration' for the comparison between a standard film and a 'dynamic film', in a sitting (painful) position. The first (standard) film is taken in the lateral standing position. In order for the coccyx to be in a neutral position, it is very

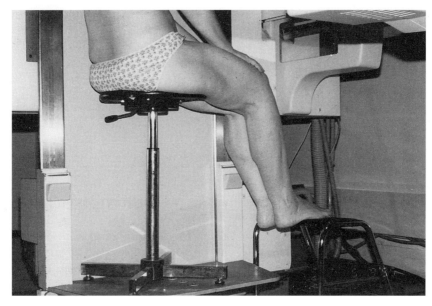

Fig. 30.1   The correct position to X-ray the coccyx in a sitting posture. Note the foot rest.

important for the patient to avoid sitting for the 15 minutes preceding the X-ray examination, otherwise, in some cases of hypermobility, there is not enough time for the coccyx to come back into the neutral position. The second (dynamic) film is taken laterally while asking the patient to sit on a hard stool with the back slightly extended from a sitting position, in a posture in which the pain is most pronounced (Fig. 30.1). It is mandatory to wait a few minutes for the pain to occur. If the pain is not present, no sound conclusion should be drawn.

Both films are superimposed over a bright light in order to compare and measure movement of the coccyx. This movement is measured in degrees of flexion or extension (Fig. 30.2).

In a first study (Maigne et al 1994), the films of 51 patients and controls were compared and read by two independent observers at two different time intervals, the second reading performed 1 month after the first. The final value used was the average of the four separate readings. Inter- and intraobserver variations of the angle measurement were 12.5% and 15.3% respectively, and the accuracy of the measurement technique was ± 2.6°. This is therefore a reliable technique, in particular in view of the definition of hypermobility (see below).

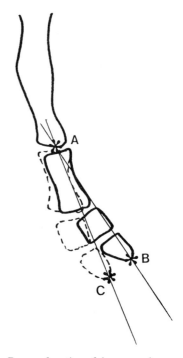

Fig. 30.2   Range of motion of the coccyx is measured in degrees (angle ABC). Bold line: standard film. Dotted line: coccyx in the sitting position. A: apex of the angle located at the caudal part of the sacrum (or of the first coccygeal vertebra if the sacrococcygeal disc is ossified).

THE MOBILITY OF THE NORMAL COCCYX

In a control group consisting of 47 pain-free volunteers with no history of local trauma and no more than two pregnancies (Maigne et al 1994), the mean mobility (flexion or extension) was 9.3 ± 5.7° (range 0–22°). Thirteen coccyges (27.6%) had an extension of between 5° and 15° and eight (17%) a flexion of between 5° and 22°. Twenty-four (51%) others had a very limited mobility of between 0° and 5°. In two cases, there was a slight (asymptomatic) backward slipping of less than 20% (one fifth of the anteroposterior diameter of the vertebra).

Allowing for a certain degree of non-pathologic variation, I therefore consider that flexion greater than 25° represents hypermobility and slipping greater than 25% represents luxation. Theoretically, extension greater than 15° should be pathologic, but this has never in my experience been encountered.

Whether coccyges flex or extend in the sitting position (in controls and in patients) is based upon their position relative to the horizontal plane of the seat at the very moment when the pelvis reaches the seat. If the coccyx is near a vertical position (related to the seat), the increase of the pelvic pressure will push it backward (extension). However, if the coccyx is near the horizontal position (i.e. parallel to the seat), the pelvic pressure will have no effect on it. It is the direct pressure exerted by the seat which pushes it forward (into flexion). This is illustrated in Fig. 30.5 below. The angle between the mobile coccyx and the horizontal is the 'basic angle'. An approximative value of this angle can be calculated on the dynamic film (Fig. 30.3). If this angle is larger than 35°, the coccyx is likely to extend when sitting; under 12°, it will flex. Between 12° and 35°, 61% of the coccyges showed flexion, and 39% extension.

COMMON COCCYDYNIA

Standard and lateral sitting X-rays of 189 patients suffering from common coccydynia for at least 6 weeks duration have been made since 1992. This report concerns the last 91 patients (Maigne 1996).

This group of patients consists of 76 women and 15 men, with an average age of 47.7 ± 13.5 years, who had suffered for more than 2 months (average 31 ± 31.9 months). They were referred

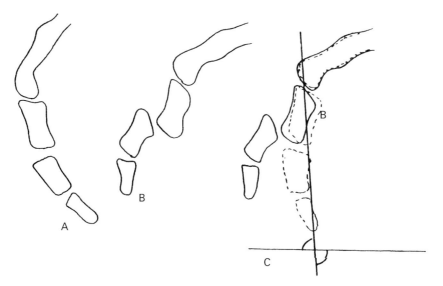

Fig. 30.3 Measurement of the 'basic angle'. (A) Standing film. (B) Sitting film, showing a luxation. (C) Measurement of the angle. This angle reflects the theoretical position that the mobile part of the coccyx would take if the subject were 'sitting without the seat', that is without any force acting on the coccyx.

to our Spine Center in the Hotel-Dieu Hospital after failure of the usual treatments. A history of direct and recent trauma was found in 44 of the cases. The diagnosis 'idiopathic' was made only after a thorough clinical examination (including rectal examination), standard radiography, computerized tomography of the pelvis, and routine blood tests that showed no particular abnormalities (fracture, tumor, infection).

Luxation and subluxation

Sagittal luxation of all or part of the mobile portion of the coccyx while in the sitting position is the most striking abnormality observed (Figs 30.4 and 30.5). It was noticed in 26 cases (28.6%). In all but three cases, it was a posterior luxation, these three showing an anterior luxation. The sacrococcygeal disc and the first intercoccygeal disc were equally affected. This luxation was spontaneously reduced in lateral decubitus, except in three cases, where it was permanent.

Patients with luxation had certain characteristics that set them apart from those with normal dynamic films. Their body mass index was statistically higher. A history of direct and violent trauma to the coccyx prior to the pain was more frequently found. An acute pain while passing from the sitting to the standing position, more intense than the usual pain felt in the sitting position, was found in 21 out of the 62 patients in whom it was sought. These were patients presenting with luxation (14 cases) or hypermobility (7 cases); this never occurred in normals. This clinical symptom (acute pain when standing up) had a specificity of 100%, a sensitivity of 60%, a positive predictive value of luxation or hypermobility of 100%, and a negative predictive value of 65.8%

Hypermobility

Hypermobility is defined by flexion of the coccyx of more than 25° in the sitting position (Fig. 30.6). It was found in 18 cases (19.8%). The extreme and mean values in this subgroup were 25–70° and 35° respectively. Hypermobility always occurred in flexion and never in extension.

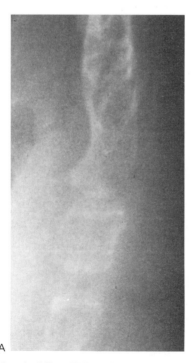 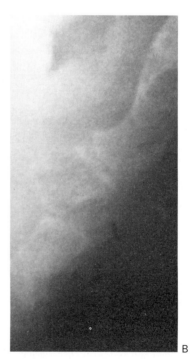

A   B

Fig. 30.4 (A) Standard film. (B) Luxation in sitting position, reversible when the patient stands up.

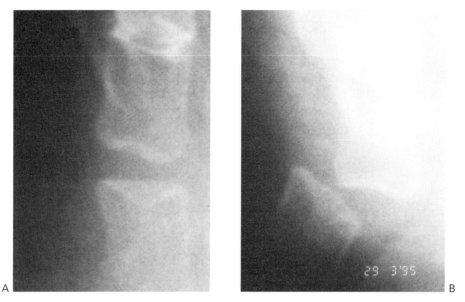

Fig. 30.5   Luxation of the first mobile vertebra in the sitting position (B). (A) shows the standard film.

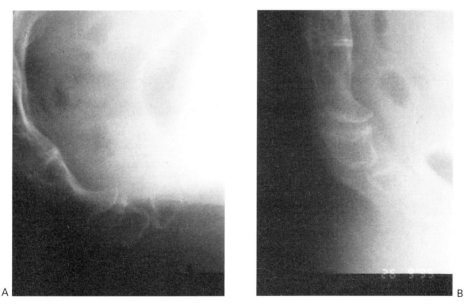

Fig. 30.6   Hypermobility. (A) Standard film. (B) Film in the sitting position.

Luxation and hypermobility can be interpreted as coccygeal instability similar to lumbar instability. It is of interest that, contrary to the degenerative lumbar disc, the coccygeal disc does not sustain any compressive load that would lead to osteophyte formation, considered to act as restabilizing processes.

Contact between two adjacent vertebrae

In two cases, the only abnormality seen was a collapse of an intercoccygeal space in the sitting position, leading to contact and encroachment between the two adjacent vertebral endplates (Fig. 30.7). The bone around the contact area

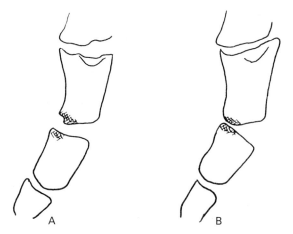

Fig. 30.7 Contact of two coccygeal vertebrae in the sitting position. At the contact surface, the bony sclerosis indicates osteoarthritis (drawn from an X-ray).

was sclerotic. This particular lesion looks like osteoarthritis of peripheral synovial joints. Such a contact could also occur in case of hypermobility and luxation.

Normal coccyges

The remaining 47 cases (51.6%) exhibited a normal range of mobility (0–25°) in the sitting position. Lack of mobility was considered normal, even when the coccyx was completely ossified (4 cases). These 47 cases with normal dynamic films represent the actual 'idiopathic' coccydynia. The question raised by this finding (normal dynamic exploration in patients with coccydynia) concerns the source of their pain. I can just give some indications and hypotheses.

The presence of a rigid coccyx could sometimes lead to a phenomenon of chronic bursitis between the tip of the coccyx and the skin, this latter being compressed between the bone and the seat when sitting. Injection of the subcutaneous tissues with anesthetic may suppress symptoms, thus confirming the diagnosis.

In some cases, the pain is located at the sacral insertion of the sacrotuberous ligament. This could be compared with a local sprain and treated with steroid injections.

Pain referred from other structures is another possibility. The sacroiliac joint or lumbosacral area is sometimes advocated as a possible origin of coccydynia. These diagnosis should be evoked only if the coccyx appears normal after the dynamic exploration.

Psychogenic pain (hysteria or depression) has been felt to be a very common etiology. In my series, however, I considered this diagnosis in only a few cases.

TREATMENT OF COMMON COCCYDYNIA

Treatment of common coccydynia should be considered according to the diagnosis.

Luxation and hypermobility

In a recent study (Maigne 1996), we established that patients with luxation or hypermobility were much better responders to a local intradiscal corticosteroid injection than were patients with normal coccyges. About 2 months after the injection, 45% of the patients with luxation or hypermobility were improved or healed, whereas only 27% of the patients with normal coccyges improved. The difference is significant (Chi square = 4.53, $p = 0.033$).

The technique of coccygeal discography is simple. The patient is asked to lie on his or her left side with the hips flexed. The skin is carefully disinfected. Each disc or synovial joint is entered with a 25 gauge, 25 mm needle under aseptic conditions, using a posterior approach through the midline to avoid small blood vessels. I inject a very small amount of dye, to control the position of the needle, and a steroid (Fig. 30.8). The injection is generally effective within 1 week. In cases of partial relief, another injection can be given 1 month later. The abnormal mobility, if present, remains, but ceases to be painful.

Another treatment for unstable coccyges is prolotherapy. Although I have no experience in this method, the rationale for its use is convincing (Dorman 1995, personal communication).

In case of failure, I suggest a total coccygectomy, including the sacrococcygeal disc (Pyper 1957). At the present time, we have operated on more than 25 patients with very good results. We are waiting for a longer follow-up before publishing these.

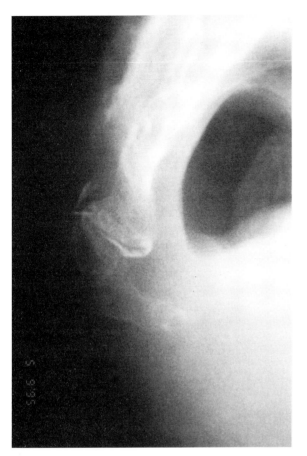

Fig. 30.8 Coccygeal discography. The figure shows a synovial joint.

Normal coccyges

Coccyges exhibiting a normal mobility are treated according to the suspected diagnosis. In cases of bursitis or suspected ligamentous sprain, I locally inject a steroid. Some cases are treated by coccygeal manipulations. I do not recommend surgery for these patients.

CONCLUSIONS

1. Common coccydynia is related to coccygeal instability in almost half of all cases.

2. The diagnosis should be documented with dynamic X-ray films to show evidence of luxations and hypermobility, which may need specific treatment.

REFERENCES

Howorth B 1959 The painful coccyx. Clinical Orthopedics 14: 145–150

Jurmand S H 1976 Les injections péridurales dans le traitement de la coccygodynie. Revue du Rhumatisme et des Maladies Ostéoarticulaires 43: 217–220

Maigne J Y 1996 Standardized radiological protocol for the study of common coccydynia. Characteristics of the lesions observed in the sitting position. Clinical elements differentiating luxation, hypermobility and normal mobility. Spine (in press)

Maigne J Y, Molinie V, Fautrel B 1992 Anatomie des disques coccygiens. Revue de Medecine Orthopedique 28: 34–35

Maigne J Y, Guedj S, Straus C 1994 Idiopathic coccygodynia: lateral roentgenograms in the sitting position and coccygeal discography. Spine 19: 930–934

Nelson D A 1991 Idiopathic coccygodynia and lumbar disk disease: historical correlations and clinical cautions. Perspectives in Biology and Medicine 34: 229–238

Postacchini F, Massobrio M 1983 Idiopathic coccygodynia: analysis of fifty-one operative cases and a radiographic study of the normal coccyx. Journal of Bone and Joint Surgery (US) 65: 1116–1124

Pyper J B 1957 Excision of the coccyx for idiopathic coccygodynia. Journal of Bone and Joint Surgery (UK) 39: 733–737

Saluja P G 1988 The incidence of ossification of the sacrococcygeal joint. Journal of Anatomy 156: 11–15

Smout C F, Jacoby F, Lillie E W 1969 Gynaecological and obstetrical anatomy, 12th edn. Oxford University Press, Oxford

Stern F H 1967 Idiopathic coccygodynia among the geriatric population. Journal of the American Geriatric Society 15: 100–102

Williams P 1995 Gray's anatomy, 38th edn. Churchill Livingstone, Edinburgh

Pregnancy and peripartum pelvic pain

31. Quadrupedalism, bipedalism, and human pregnancy

M. M. Abitbol

INTRODUCTION

The transformation from quadrupedalism to bipedalism necessitated a complete reorganization of the orthostatics and orthodynamics of the human body. Actually, any non-human mammal, specifically any non-human primate, can stand on its hind limbs. The fundamental difference, and in fact the definition of human erect posture, is that it is effortless. Any non-human mammal standing on its hind limbs wastes a tremendous amount of energy, while humans who stand erect tire much less (Abitbol 1988). How humans manage erect posture effortlessly is achieved through complete reorganization of the anatomy, specifically the bony anatomy. It is in the vertebral spine and pelvis that reorganization is most noticeable, although it is also noticeable in the lower limbs (hip joint rotation) and other parts.

THE VERTEBRAL SPINE CURVATURES

An erect vertebral spine does not mean a straight vertebral spine – far from it. The vertebral spine may appear to be straight when seen from an anterior–posterior (AP) view, but it presents numerous vertebral curvatures (Fig. 31.1) when viewed laterally.

Essentially, for the body to stand without effort, the center of gravity (CG) of each segment of the human body has to fall within the base of support formed by the segment immediately underneath. This requires displacement (moving back and forth) of various segments of the vertebral column in order for the CG in each segment of the trunk to align vertically. For the body to be erect without effort, the vertebral

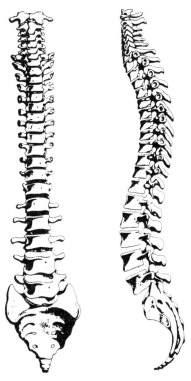

Fig. 31.1 In a frontal view, the vertebral column is perfectly vertical, but on lateral view the vertebral curvatures become evident.

column has to undergo four AP curvatures: cervical, thoracic, lumbar, and sacral. The direction of each curvature depends on the part of the body involved. The second, third, and fourth curvatures are not genetically (ontogenetically) determined and are acquired as the human infant and young child is progressively acquainted with proper erect posture (Abitbol 1993b). The reason the human infant is slow in acquiring its final erect posture is because spinal curvatures have

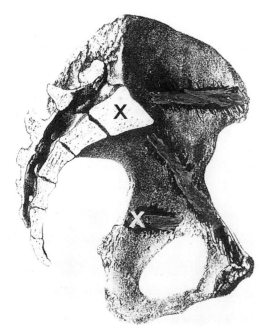

Fig. 31.2 Effortless erect posture in humans supposes vertical alignment of the biauricular line (above) and biacetabular line (below). In such a posture, the weight of the trunk is transferred to the biacetabular line without any muscular effort.

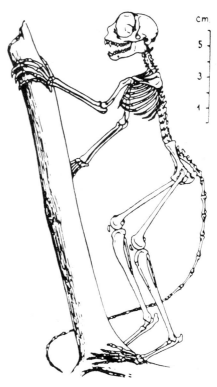

Fig. 31.3 When a monkey or ape attempts an erect posture, the biauricular line is well in front of the biacetabular line.

not yet taken their final forms (Abitbol 1987). It is only progressively that the curvatures are formed and posture becomes more or less effortless (Abitbol 1988).

The first curvature starts to form at the lumbo-sacral region because proper (effortless) erect posture requires that the biauricular and biacetabular lines be in the same vertical plane for alignment of the CG of the upper and lower body (Fig. 31.2). If the biauricular line is located ventrally in relation to the biacetabular line (Fig. 31.3), as happens in pongids when they use erect posture, the entire body has to bend forward to re-establish an orthostatic equilibrium. If the biauricular line is located ventrally in relation to the biacetabular line (Fig. 31.4A), as happens in young children first attempting an erect posture, a marked lordotic curvature is necessary to re-establish the orthostatic equilibrium. Under these two conditions (pongids and human infants attempting erect posture), tremendous energy is necessary to maintain erect posture. It is no wonder that the pongid or the human infant cannot

stay erect for a long time (Abitbol 1988). It is only in human adults that erect posture becomes effortless, since the biacetabular and biauricular lines are almost in the same vertical plane. Indeed, on a lateral X-ray film of an erect human, the center of the sacroiliac joint (SIJ) and the acetabulum more or less form a vertical line (see Fig. 31.2 above). This vertical alignment is an important factor contributing to effortless erect posture. Of course, this is also helped by the biauricular and biacetabular lines getting close to each other.

The anatomical consequence of the biauricular-biacetabular vertical alignment is the anterior displacement and rotation of the sacrum in the SIJ, necessary for the biauricular line to align vertically with the biacetabular line. The SIJ rotation results in compensatory curvatures at other levels of the vertebral spine (see Fig. 31.1 above).

Formation of the sacral curvature is followed by multiple anatomic changes. The upper sacrum becomes almost horizontal, while the lower sacrum, which is retained in its original position by various ligaments, remains almost vertical. The upper sacrum widens and the opposite auricular surfaces of the two SIJs increase in size better to support the load from above. The auricular surface becomes L-shaped instead of elongated. Therefore, the base of the sacrum (superior surface of the first sacral vertebra) is no longer horizontal as it is in pongids (or any other non-human mammal) who use an erect posture. The angle of the sacral promontory becomes acute (less than 90°) instead of forming a right angle as it does in non-human primates.

The second curvature is the formation of a lumbar lordosis to make up for the sacral rotation. This lordosis is barely present in non-human mammals who use an erect posture.

The third curvature is at the cervical spine. It takes a lordotic shape because the human head has to be kept in equilibrium over the atlas–axis complex. Also, the Frankfurt horizontal (that joining the external acoustic meatus to the inferior border of the orbital cavity) has to be kept horizontal for the eyes to look straight ahead. In terms of energy, another difference between humans and animals who use an erect posture is that the human head is in more or less effortless equilibrium over the cervical spine.

The fourth curvature is at the thoracic spine. It is 'caught' between the lumbar and cervical lordosis, resulting in the formation of the thoracic 'kyphosis' to keep the body in equilibrium.

Essentially, the curvatures are interdependent: any kind of physiologic (e.g. bending) or pathologic (e.g. hyperlordosis) alteration in one curvature initiates a chain reaction altering all other curvatures. The double sinusoid curve formed by the vertebral column is really dynamic rather than static.

All the vertebrae have joints between each other. The only exception is the sacral vertebrae, which have fused together in all mammalian species to present a solid body to the iliac side of the SIJ (Abitbol 1987). The immobilization of the sacral vertebrae was 'replaced' by limited mobility of the SIJ, as described by Dorman (1992, 1993). He has demonstrated that synarthrosis joints accumulate energy during compression and, in view of their elasticity, release this energy during the relaxation period. Dorman applied this principle to the SIJ and it can be extended to the intervertebral joints, as previously demonstrated (Abitbol 1995).

THE ORTHOPEDIC INSTABILITY OF THE HUMAN BODY

The orthopedic problems associated with pregnancy are simple to follow if one keeps in mind that they are the consequence of our orthopedic evolution. The basic facts are:

1. Phylogenetically speaking, our animal ancestors were quadrupedal, and it is only secondarily that we became bipedal. Our quadrupedal ancestry has been well established for hundreds of millions of years, while our bipedal ancestry is at most three million years old (Stern & Susman 1983).

2. The orthostatics and orthodynamics of the human body are, therefore, originally and essentially quadrupedal. The transition was progressive. It started about three million years ago with the australopithecines (Stern & Susman 1983) and, even with the Neanderthals 40 000–100 000 years ago, the transition was not entirely complete (Rak & Arensberg 1987). It is only with modern *Homo sapiens* that erect posture and bipedal stride became what they are today.

3. In view of the above, one can conclude that our bipedal achievement is only 'skin deep' and is easily subject to imperfections, misadaptations, and regression. These problems can occur at any age but become more and more frequent past maturity and are predominant in old age. It is essential to stress that old age exists only in humans and in some animals living in contact with humans. Evolution has never 'perfected' or prepared humans for old age (Abitbol 1996a). There is a strong likelihood that our ancestors of 10 000 years ago died in full maturity (Aries 1992) and therefore with fewer orthopedic defects. Of the systems or organs of the human body to fall apart when aging, bipedal posture and locomotion are among the first. Animals are spared most orthopedic defects because they have no old age. Incidentally, another problem of very old age in humans is a diminution of mental faculties because these also are a recent acquisition from the evolutionary point of view.

With old age, vertebral curvatures have a tendency to fail: the cervical curvature diminishes as the head has a tendency to fall forward, and the thoracic curvature increases in a compensatory manner; the lumbar curvature has a tendency to decrease, the SIJs and hip joints are strained, the lumbar spine slides over the sacrum (the latter can occur at any age), and backache (a universal human complaint) appears (Burton 1995). Backache appears because the center of erect posture is at the lumbosacral level, and this level is the first to suffer. The result – backache – can occur at any age but is more frequent with advanced age. Backache is the price humans pay for the combination of erect posture and advanced age, both very recent in human evolution.

Another disturbance to the stability of human erect posture is during pregnancy.

OUR QUADRUPEDAL ANCESTRY

Mammalians and, in fact, most terrestrial vertebrates except humans, have a vertebral spine that is more or less horizontal. This is how terrestrial vertebrates functioned for a billion years, from the most primitive vertebrates to the higher primates. The higher primates have flirted with erect posture, but they are essentially still quadrupeds. All mammals keep this posture when pregnant and when giving birth. Schultz (1969) has doubted that human erect posture has reached its final stage and has suggested that there is more evolution to come.

Erect posture is not only an unstable equilibrium, but also a succession of unstable equilibria that manage to balance and correct each other. The main reason for instability of erect posture is that, in quadrupedal posture, the CG is low and the base of support is wide, whereas in bipedal posture the opposite occurs, with a high CG and a narrow base of support. How fragile and unstable erect posture is can be demonstrated in different ways.

Homo sapiens takes the longest time to acquire and perfect posture. The process starts at between 1 year and 18 months of age, but is not perfect until 6–7 years of age (Abitbol 1988). During the last few months of the first year of life, the child practices both quadrupedalism and bipedalism.

Since erect posture is acquired and practiced before complete ossification, one can conclude that erect posture tremendously influences (in fact, determines) the anatomy of the human body, and specifically the anatomy of the pelvis and spinal column, during the time erect posture is being acquired (Abitbol 1987).

The whole orthostatics and orthodynamics of the mammalian body became altered when the trunk rotated 90° around the hip joint (Fig. 31.4) and the pelvis had to support the whole trunk. The repercussions on parturition are tremendous.

In conclusion, erect posture is not only a phylogenetic (genetic) inheritance, but also ontogenetic (Abitbol 1993b). The whole anatomy and physiology has had to readapt to erect behavior; this readaptation is not always perfect, and even less so during parturition. The typical example I like to quote is the position of the heart within the chest. In a quadrupedal posture, this organ rests peacefully on the sternum for an entire lifetime, while in erect posture it 'floats' in the middle of the chest with practically no strong

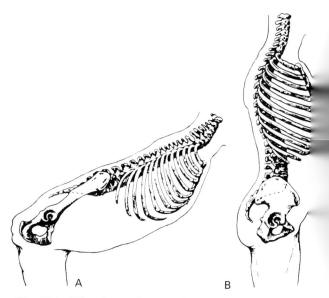

Fig. 31.4 When the trunk rotates (in an evolutionary respect) around the biauricular line from horizontal (A, pongid) to vertical (B, human), the main anatomical events are (1) shortening of the innominate bone; (2) vertical alignment of the biacetabular and biauricular lines; and (3) formation of the spinal curvatures.

anatomic support. The impression one gets from a review of the forms that preceded *Homo sapiens* is that present erect behavior is unstable and easily subjected to defects. There is hardly any organ or function in the human body that has not readapted, or rather that has not poorly readapted, to erect posture and locomotion. The two organs that underwent the most readaptation, or sometimes misadaptation, to erect behavior are the pelvis and the vertebral spine. The readaptation–misadaptation of the pelvis to erect behavior has been the subject of much research. The readaptation–misadaptation of the spinal column to erect behavior, mainly as far as the spinal curvatures are concerned, has previously been discussed (Abitbol 1995).

The main manifestation of imperfect erect locomotion is wobbling. Lateral wobbling is observed easily in frontal view. It occurs in non-human mammals attempting erect locomotion, in human infants starting bipedal locomotion, in women with advanced pregnancy, in a human walking while very tired, and in old age. In these cases, the gluteal muscles do not function, or function less, as abductors. The graceful appearance of the human stride is lost.

ENCEPHALIZATION OR ENLARGEMENT OF THE HUMAN BRAIN

Complete reorganization of the pelvis by erect posture is only half of the problem facing human parturition. The other half is the tremendous enlargement of the fetal head at term. The fetal head of the australopithecines was not much different in size from that of a chimpanzee (Leutenegger 1972), but the pelvis presented an accentuated platypelloidy associated with erect posture (Tague & Lovejoy 1986). With *Homo erectus*, the fetal head was most likely midway in size between that of the chimpanzee and the present human condition (Walker and Leakey 1993), and it is only with Neanderthal man that the fetal head most probably reached the present human size and became (as it still is) a serious obstetric problem. As a practicing obstetrician, I can definitely state that the relationship between the narrow human pelvis and the enlarged fetal head is disproportional or at least a tight fit.

Humans have adapted so much to this disproportion that it is now considered natural.

I will discuss the readaptation–misadaptation of the human female body to pregnancy, birth, delivery, and the postpartum period, in relation to erect posture and locomotion.

ORTHOPEDIC PROBLEMS IN PREGNANCY

Over the last three million years, hominids (including humans) have managed to find a *modus vivendi*, or workable arrangement, for efficient bipedal behavior. For the largest segment of their lives, humans are adapted to erect behavior. During pregnancy, however, this arrangement, which is already unstable to begin with, falls apart. The pelvis and the vertebral spine do not adapt well to human parturition because postural and obstetric requirements make demands in opposite directions on the pelvis (Abitbol 1993a, 1993b). Contrary to parturition, erect posture would benefit from lumbar lordosis, triangular and narrow pelvis, and protruding epiphyses (sacral promontory, ischial spines, and sacral apex) (Fig. 31.5).

Erect posture took precedence over pelvic obstetric requirements from a phylogenetic as well as an ontogenetic point of view (Abitbol 1993a, 1993b).

Human intervention can either 'ease' obstetric demands on the pelvis or completely bypass them, and this can make obstetric demands less imposing from an evolutionary point of view (Abitbol 1993a).

The final impression is that the human female body (specifically the vertebral spine and pelvis) is not entirely and perfectly adapted to human parturition. The human female practices erect posture all her life, while advanced pregnancy concerns only a short period. In that respect, erect posture is more important than parturition. The demands of erect posture and locomotion on the lumbar spine and pelvis have created the following obstetric problems.

Mechanical problems during pregnancy

First, the abdominal cavity is already, relatively speaking, smaller in a superior–inferior direction

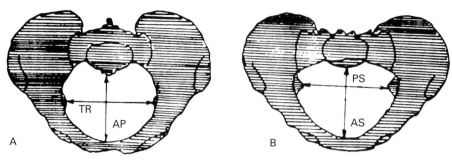

Fig. 31.5 The male pelvis (B) satisfies the requirement of an erect posture, with a protruding promontory, protruding ischial spines, and a triangular shape. The female pelvis (A) is more circular, with less protrusion of ischial spines.

(see Fig. 31.4 above) in view of the sacralization of the last two lumbar vertebra (L6 and L7) and their integration into the sacrum (Abitbol 1987), and smaller in an anterior–posterior direction in view of the formation of the lumbar lordosis. Human pregnancy barely has adequate space in the abdominal cavity, and this results in compression on all surrounding organs, such as the major abdominal vessels (Abitbol 1976), anterior abdominal wall, vertebral and pelvic joints, muscles, ligaments, etc. (Fig. 31.6). This is contrary to the quadrupedal condition in which the pregnancy rests comfortably over the anterior abdominal wall with the necessary space available and with no undue pressure on any organ.

Second, the human fetus grows in a ventral direction and, at or near term, the CG of the human body no longer falls over the base of support formed by the feet. To regain her equilibrium, the pregnant woman at term has to lean backwards, and this results in important orthostatic and orthodynamic consequences. Spinal curvatures are completely disorganized. The lumbar curvature moves dorsally and may or may not be accentuated (Snijders 1995), the thoracic curvature has to compensate accordingly, and the equilibrium of the body has to be maintained in an unusual (painful) position. Because of the dorsal displacement of the trunk, the rectus abdominis muscles have to increase their tension and the intra-abdominal pressure is increased, producing elevation of the diaphragm. The cardiopulmonary consequences are numerous.

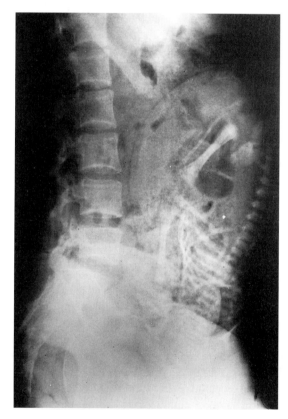

Fig. 31.6 In a primiparous woman in a standing position, the pregnant uterus is held against the lumbar curvature by the muscles of the abdominal wall.

Third, from the orthodynamic point of view, the situation is even worse. Because of the backward position of the trunk in relation to the pelvic girdle, the glutei lose some of their abductor function (Warwick & Williams 1973) and the pregnant patient at term now wobbles, as previously described. The elegant striding walk, the pride of human erect behavior, is all but gone in advanced pregnancy.

Obstetric problems during labor

During labor, the fetal head and body have to find passage at the level of the three pelvic planes through a bony pelvis that has been adapted to and distorted by erect posture and locomotion.

1. *Pelvic inlet.* The sacral promontory has moved forward, thus restricting the AP diameter of the pelvic inlet. When the fetal head presents at the pelvic inlet (Fig. 31.7), it pushes the sacral promontory dorsally, thus producing a backward rotation of the upper sacrum around the SIJ.

2. *Midpelvis.* The ischial spines have moved inward, thus restricting the transverse (TR) diameter of the midpelvis. When the fetal head presents at the midpelvis, it attempts to widen the TR diameter of this pelvic plane, and thus stretches the SIJ wide open (see Fig. 31.5).

3. *Pelvic outlet.* The bi-ischial diameters and the subpubic angle are narrower when the pelvis is android (30% of cases; Berman 1955, Warwick & Williams 1973), thus restricting the diameters of the outlet. When the fetal head presents at the outlet, it pushes the sacral apex dorsally and therefore produces a backward rotation of the lower sacrum around the SIJ (see Fig. 31.5 above).

In conclusion, the obstetric complications resulting from fetal body–maternal pelvic distortion produced by erect posture are numerous and far-reaching.

Soft tissue problems in human pregnancy

Bony readaptations–misadaptations are not the only anatomic consequences of erect posture. Soft tissue structures are also altered and adapted–misadapted. In quadrupedal posture, all the abdominal viscera, including the pregnant uterus, are supported by the anterior abdominal wall, but in erect posture all these organs pound against the pelvis (Fig. 31.8). Adequate and strict control

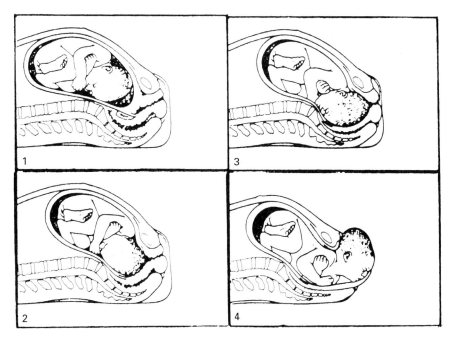

Fig. 31.7   A fetus traversing the birth canal at the time of delivery. (1) The pelvic inlet is stretched and the sacral promontory is pushed dorsally. (2) At midpelvis, the pelvic ligaments are stretched to the maximum. (3) At the pelvic outlet, the pelvic diaphragm and the pelvic floor are stretched to the maximum. (4) All pelvic structures are thinned out and sometimes even torn.

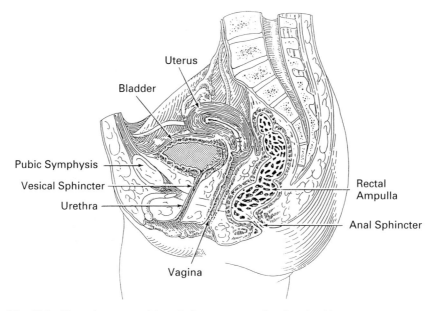

Fig. 31.8   Normal anatomy of the soft tissue structures in a female taking erect posture. Practically all the bony and soft tissues are displaced, stretched, thinned out, and sometimes torn during labor and delivery. The 'damage' is usually temporary but can become permanent.

of the rectal and bladder sphincters becomes imperative (Mostwin 1991). To carry out these new functions, the pelvic floor and the perineal body have become stronger and firmer. In addition, the sphincter of the uterine cervix has become hypertrophied in order to close the cervical canal tightly. The result is a build-up of the soft tissues. All these anatomic changes are directly or indirectly connected with the demands of erect posture and locomotion (Abitbol 1996b).

All these soft tissue structures that have been built to perform a support function in erect posture are markedly stretched during labor and delivery and may even become obstructive. In this case, they are literally torn apart to allow the passage and birth of the fetus. The stretching may be temporary but, more often than not, it takes on tearing proportion. The permanent scars of these tears may be serious unless they are properly handled (Droegemueller et al 1987). Incompetent cervical os is a congenital or acquired weakness of the cervical sphincter in which the cervix opens in midpregnancy and the fetus is expelled. Postpartum relaxation of the pelvic floor results in urinary and even fecal incontinence and prolapse of the bladder, rectum, and uterus. All these defects require surgical correction.

The hormones of pregnancy, specifically relaxin, are produced during gestation and contribute to relaxation of all the body joints, including intervertebral and pelvic joints (Birnberg & Abitbol 1959).

There is a need to resume erect posture and locomotion immediately or as soon as possible after giving birth, to avoid complications of excessive bedrest such as phlebitis and thromboembolism. This early resumption of erect posture and locomotion may impose some stretching of the pelvic joints before they return to their normal prepregnancy condition because they have been softened by hormones of pregnancy (progesterone and relaxin, among others). The damage may be permanent (leading to backaches, etc.).

My personal impression is that, as previously mentioned, the human body has more or less adapted to erect posture and locomotion, and has modified its anatomy accordingly (Fig. 31.9). However, the body of the female human has not entirely adapted to parturition. Parturition, rather,

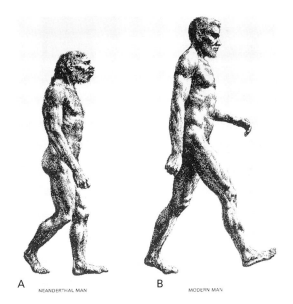

Fig. 31.9   (A) Neandertal man: the head is not in equilibrium over the cervical spine and therefore requires more energy to be held properly. (B) Modern man: the head is in equilibrium over the cervical spine.

suffers somehow from the anatomic modification resulting from erect posture. Pregnancy, labor, and delivery are meant to be carried more by a quadrupedal than by a bipedal body. If it were not for progressive interference of *Homo sapiens* with its own birth process (labor and delivery attendance, primitive then modern midwifery, assisted and directed labor, oxytocin stimulation, cesarean section, for example), the survival of the human species would have been difficult, and this is what might have happened to the other hominid species (now extinct) that preceded modern *Homo sapiens* (Abitbol 1993a) and who

might have become extinct for various reasons, among which are difficulties of giving birth.

CONCLUSIONS

1. Erect posture is a recent (three million-year-old) acquisition in human evolution. The equilibrium in erect posture is not as stable because the CG is high and the base of support is narrow, in contrast to quadrupedal posture, in which the CG is low and the base of support is wide.

2. On lateral view, the vertical alignment of the biauricular and biacetabular lines is necessary for an almost effortless erect posture, and this is associated with spinal curvatures.

3. To carry her pregnancy to or near term, the human female has had to lean backward in order to keep her equilibrium. This results in disequilibrium of the vertical alignment of the body, with a reorganization of the spinal curvatures. This may be associated with a partial loss of abductor function of the gluteal muscles and wobbling.

4. The hormone relaxin stretches all the lumbar and pelvic joints, and makes erect locomotion and even erect posture painful and tiring.

5. The distortion and narrowing of the three planes make labor and delivery painful, prolonged, and traumatic.

6. The soft tissues of the pelvis are temporarily stretched or permanently damaged by the passage of the fetus.

7. Erect posture and encephalization, therefore, make human parturition particularly difficult (Abitbol 1996b).

REFERENCES

Abitbol M M 1976 Aortic compression by the pregnant uterus. New York State Journal of Medicine 76: 1470–1475

Abitbol M M 1987 Evolution of the sacrum in hominoids. American Journal of Physical Anthropology 74: 65–81

Abitbol M M 1988 Effect of posture and locomotion on energy expenditure. American Journal of Physical Anthropology 77: 191–199

Abitbol M M 1993a Adjustment of the fetal head and adult pelvis in modern humans. Human Evolution 8(3): 167–185

Abitbol M M 1993b Quadrupedalism and the acquisition of bipedalism in human children. Gait and Posture 1: 189–195

Abitbol M M 1995 Energy storage in the vertebral column. In: Vleeming A, Mooney V, Dorman T, Snijders C J (eds)

Second interdisciplinary world congress on low back pain, San Diego, CA, 9–11 November, pp 259–290

Abitbol M M 1996a Overcoming the fear of death (unpublished manuscript)

Abitbol M M 1996b Birth and human evolution: anatomical and obstetrical mechanics in primates. Bergen & Garvey, Westport, CT

Aries P 1992 The hour of our death. Vintage Books, New York

Berman R 1955 Obstetrical roentgenology. FA Davis, Philadelphia, PA

Birnberg C, Abitbol M M 1959 The use of cervilaxin in term labor. Obstetrics and Gynecology 75: 1016–1022

Burton K 1995 Natural history of low back pain in adolescents. In: Vleeming A, Mooney V, Dorman T,

Snijders C J (eds) Second interdisciplinary world congress on low back pain, San Diego, CA, 9–11 November, pp 775–777

Dorman T A 1992 Storage and release of elastic energy in the pelvis: dysfunction, diagnosis and treatment. Journal of Orthopaedic Medicine 14: 2

Dorman T A 1993 Pelvic mechanics and dysfunction. Review article. San Luis Obispo, California

Droegemueller W, Herbst A, Mishell D Jr, Stenchever M 1987 Comprehensive gynecology. CV Mosby, St Louis MO

Leutenegger W 1972 Newborn size and pelvic dimensions of Australopithecus. Nature 240: 568–569

Mostwin J L 1991 Current concepts of female pelvic anatomy and physiology. Urologic Clinics of North America 18(2): 175–195

Rak Y, Arensburg B 1987 Kebara 2 neanderthal pelvis: first look at a complete inlet. American Journal of Physical Anthropology 73: 227–231

Schultz A H 1969 The life of primates. Universe Books, New York

Snijders C J, Vleeming A, Stoeckart R, Kleinrensink G J, Mens J M A 1995 Biomechanics of sacroiliac joint stability: validation experiments on the concept of self-locking. In: Vleeming A, Mooney V, Dorman T, Snijders C J (eds) Second interdisciplinary world congress on low back pain, San Diego, CA, 9–11 November, pp 75–91

Stern J T, Susman R L 1983 The locomotor anatomy of australopithecus afarensis. American Journal of Physical Anthropology 60: 279–317

Tague R G, Lovejoy C O 1986 The obstetric pelvis of Al 288-1 (Lucy). Journal of Human Evolution 15: 237–255

Walker A, Leakey R E F 1993 The postcranial skeleton. In: Walker A, Leakey R E F (eds) The Nariokotome Homo erectus skeleton. Harvard University Press, Cambridge, MA, pp 227–233

Warwick R, Williams P L 1973 Gray's anatomy, 35th British edn. Churchill Livingstone, Edinburgh

32. Epidemiology of pelvic pain and low back pain in pregnant women

E. Heiberg   S. P. Aarseth

PELVIC PAIN IN PREGNANCY: AN AMBIGUOUS CONDITION?

Pain in the area of the pelvic girdle in pregnancy, commonly labeled peripartum pelvic Pain (PPP) and/or low back pain (LBP), has in recent years been considered to be a great problem for Scandinavian women (Berg et al 1988, Endresen Heiberg 1995, Östgaard et al 1988). There are, however, some ambiguities inherent in the terminology, diagnosis, and classification of PPP and LBP. Even though these uncertainties have been repeatedly discussed (Endresen Heiberg 1995), no definition or criteria have been agreed upon for PPP. Various terms, such as pelvic girdle relaxation (MacLennan 1991), pelvic joint instability (Saugstad 1991a), posterior pelvic pain (Östgaard et al 1994), and peripartum pelvic pain (Mens et al 1992), have been suggested as identifying labels. The variety of terms probably reflects a heterogeneous group of patients. This chapter attempts a discussion on this phenomenon from a joint epidemiological and sociological perspective.

In recent Norwegian literature, a distinction has been made between, on the one hand, 'pelvic girdle relaxation' as a physiological condition during pregnancy and, on the other, 'symptom-generating pelvic girdle relaxation', when there is considerable pain and dysfunction. The latter includes, for example, the need to use crutches for walking. If the pain persists for more than 6 months after childbirth, the condition is labelled 'pelvic joint syndrome'. This may involve an inability to care for the baby or do housework, or even the necessity for a wheelchair for transportation.

Interesting hypotheses have been put forward by Saugstad (1991b) considering biological factors, such as early menarche, and the use of oral contraceptives as being crucial to development of PPP. An inquiry among patients of the Norwegian association for women with PPP revealed an excess of post-term deliveries, an increased proportion of infants of 4000 g or more, more female births and an increased rate of congenital hip dysplasia, consistent with elevated estrogen and relaxin levels (Saugstad 1991b). MacLennan (1991) and Kristiansson (1995) have also found associations between pelvic pain/back pain in pregnancy and serum levels of relaxin.

PREVALENCE IN THE LIGHT OF INSUFFICIENT CRITERIA

Studies from Norway, Sweden, and Great Britain report a prevalence of 'back pain' in pregnancy of 25–50%, of which between 5–10% of cases are said to be severe (Berg et al 1988, Endresen Heiberg 1995, Mantle et al 1977, Östgaard et al 1988). Östgaard et al (1988) make the essential distinction between women suffering from back problems before pregnancy and those who develop back pain during pregnancy. The incidence of the latter was 25–30% in their study. However, the data on prevalence are difficult to assess as the extent to which PPP and LBP can be seen as separate conditions has not been systematically studied.

In some studies, both PPP and LBP in pregnancy show a relationship to occupation. Physically strenuous work that involves frequent bending forward and heavy lifting has been found to be a factor that increases the risk of developing both PPP and LBP. The same holds for jobs tied to the sitting position, as well as an inability to take breaks at will during the working day (Berg et al 1988, Endresen Heiberg 1995, Östgaard et al 1988).

PREGNANT WOMEN IN THE PUBLIC ARENA

Throughout history, work has traditionally been gendered and related to the inborn biological as well as culturally patterned norms prescribed for women and men. After the industrial revolution, production and reproduction were split, pregnancy, childcare and work within the household becoming a strictly private business not to be connected with other areas of production belonging to the public arena.

In the 1970s and early 1980s, Norway, like most other Western societies, experienced a substantial growth in the labor force participation of married women. From the mid-1970s to the mid-1980s, the percentage of married women in paid employment increased for all birth cohorts of working age, except for those close to retirement. The increase was strongest for the younger women with children still at home (Skrede 1989). This means that Norwegian women work through their first pregnancy and stay economically active between subsequent births. Thus, the pregnant state represents a new situation in salaried work. Possibilities of adjusting the workload to the demands of pregnancy vary both with respect to type of work and type of workplace. The high rate of sick leave for pregnant women may serve not only as an example of illness *per se*, but also as an expression of the conflict between pregnancy and work (Strand et al 1992).

EPIDEMIOLOGY AND SOCIOLOGY – TWO STUDIES

The studies to be presented are an epidemiological and a sociological analysis. Both are correlation analyses on PPP, the epidemiological one also including LBP. The basis for both analyses is a comprehensive questionnaire aimed at exploring interrelations between pregnancy, work, and the workplace by identifying factors associated with how women relate to their employment on realizing

they are pregnant and throughout their pregnancy (Endresen Heiberg 1995, Strand et al 1992).

Under the auspices of the Department of Preventive Medicine (University of Oslo), self-administered questionnaires were presented at maternity wards to all women giving birth in Norway during a 6 week period in the fall of 1989. In total, 5438 women responded between 1 and 4 days postpartum. This represented 87.2% of the total population giving birth during that period. The questionnaire had a total of 118 questions, all of which had been extensively pilot-tested (Strand et al 1992).

The following questions regarding LBP and PPP were selected for an epidemiological analysis of the relationship between the two phenomena.

1. *Did you in the course of pregnancy suffer from low back pain?*
   - ☐ YES, quite often
   - ☐ YES, rarely
   - ☐ NO, never

2. *Did you suffer from pelvic pain during this pregnancy?*
   - ☐ YES, I experienced it for the first time in month

     1.2.3.4.5.6.7.8.9

     (circle number of month)
   - ☐ No
     Did you have difficulties managing your housework because of pelvic pain?
     - ☐ YES, to a large extent
     - ☐ YES, to some extent
     - ☐ NO

Both questions had a high response frequency. The question regarding PPP was answered by 96% of the women, suggesting that young Norwegian women are familiar with the concept. The LBP question was answered by 90%. In spite of the fact that many women reported having suffered from both conditions, their answers indicated that they distinguished between the two conditions. This was later confirmed in a series of explorative interviews conducted by one of the authors (Heiberg, unpublished data).

The main purpose of the *epidemiological* analysis, apart from a simple prevalence description, was to answer the following questions:

• Do PPP and LBP have different relationships to potential risk factors such as age, parity, education, occupation, and lifestyle habits, for example smoking and alcohol intake?

• Do such differences, if they exist, imply differences in etiology that may suggest methods of prevention?

The purpose of the *sociological* analysis was to investigate PPP in wage-earners, housewives, and students, by means of biological variables as well as selected lifestyle habits and various working conditions in the wage-earner group.

About 5200 women were included. In the epidemiological analysis, the statistical analysis was carried out as stepwise multiple linear regressions with p for inclusion <0.05 and p for exclusion >0.1. A number of independent variables from the questionnaire study were included (Endresen Heiberg 1995).

The category of wage-earner included the women who were occupationally active at the time of realizing that they were pregnant. In total, 4205 women (77.3%) were wage-earners. The number of work hours spent weekly in paid employment was used to estimate the amount of salaried work. More than 60% of the women worked full time, which in Norway is 35 hours or more per week. Only 16% worked less than 20 hours per week.

RESULTS AND DISCUSSION

Although 42% of the women reported suffering from PPP (Table 32.1), only 9% reported great difficulties in managing their housework. Comparing women without previous children with those with one child, the percentage of both women with PPP and those with great difficulties with housework increases strongly. With a second child, these percentages are higher still. In women with no previous children, the onset of PPP occurred later in pregnancy than in women who had given birth before.

Table 32.2 shows the distribution of PPP in wage-earners, housewives, and students. There is little or no difference between the wage-earners and the housewives, whereas only one-third of the student group reported PPP. This may have to do with the students more often being primipara

Table 32.1 Degree of pelvic pain (PPP) by age and number of previous children

	Number	Percentage reporting PPP	Percentage reporting PPP and great difficulties with housework
Age			
Under 19	330	37.9	4.8
20–24	1483	43.7	9.3
25–29	1871	43.4	8.6
30–34	1146	41.4	10.6
35–39	348	40.8	10.3
40+	37	37.8	13.5
Total	5215	42.4	9.2
Number of previous children			
0	2419	32.9	5.3
1	1636	47.7	11.1
2	845	54.4	15.3
3+	265	55.8	14.3
Total	5165	42.3	9.2

Table 32.2 Distribution of PPP for wage-earners, housewives, and students; all parities

	Number	Percentage with PPP
Age 16–24		
Wage-earners	1046	45.3
Housewives	361	42.4
Students	168	32.7
Age 25–29		
Wage-earners	1493	44.6
Housewives	331	46.5
Students	80	31.3

than the other two groups. This we do not know for sure, as the student group was not divided by parity at the time of making the analysis. It may also indicate that being a student gives more opportunity to adjust work in accordance with personal needs.

In Table 32.3, the answers to the questions on PPP and LBP in relation to parity are dichotomized, using the following groups:

• PPP yes, LBP often
• PPP yes, LBP rarely or never
• PPP no, LBP often
• PPP no, LBP rarely or never.

It was noted that many women reported having suffered from both PPP and LBP. Of the primipara,

Table 32.3 PPP and LBP percentage distribution by parity ($n = 3789$ wage-earners only)

Number of previous children	Number	PPP yes LBP yes	PPP yes LBP no	PPP no LBP yes	PPP no LBP no
0	1928	21.0	14.6	13.5	50.9
1+	1861	30.7	21.4	14.5	33.4
All parities		25.8	17.9	14.0	42.3

21% had experienced both, whereas 51% had experienced neither. The figures for multipara were 31% and 33% respectively. After stratification by parity, perhaps paradoxically, the frequency of both types of pain decreased with increasing age. Women aged 20–24 years reported most pain.

A number of multiple linear regression analyses were carried out. PPP was graded from 0 to 3 according to difficulties experienced with managing housework. LBP was graded from 0 to 2 according to the frequency reported: 0 was none, 1 was rarely, and 2 was often. Two alternatives were used throughout: with and without the other type of pain among the independent variables. For both types of pain, the other type was found to be the most prominent independent variable.

In the final regressions, the dependent variables were PPP in women reporting no LBP, and LBP in women reporting no PPP. Among the independent variables, parity on the scale of 0–2 (where 2 was two or more previously born children) came out as highly significant for both types of pain. However, the coefficient was more than twice as high for PPP as for LBP. Age in years was negatively associated for both conditions and here the coefficients were almost equal. Thus, the prevalence of both PPP and LBP was higher in younger women, with simultaneous statistical adjustment for parity. Smoking, measured as the number of cigarettes smoked per day, was highest in the youngest women (less than 30 years of age), both before and during pregnancy. Smoking came out as significant only for PPP, and highly so.

Among the variables on working conditions, frequent (more than 5–10 times per day) lifting of 10–20 kg, twisting and bending, as well as having to bend forward or work above shoulder height turned out to be correlated with both PPP and LBP. It was, however, more strongly associated with LBP than with PPP. The variable 'economic dependence', denoting whether the economy of the household was dependent on the woman's income, was correlated to indices of heavy physical work and was significant only for LBP. Education was a protection against both PPP and LBP. The findings may suggest that LBP is more closely associated with a lower socioeconomic status than is PPP.

Primipara had more physically demanding work, more working hours per week, and thus a greater risk in their workplace. The largest 'population attributable risk', i.e. that part of the prevalence which would not have arisen had the effect associated with the risk factor been absent, was seen in those who had daily work that involved twisting and bending many times per hour. The multivariable analysis showed, however, that the different working conditions independently 'explained' PPP or LBP only to a limited extent.

FURTHER FINDINGS ON PPP AND WORKING CONDITIONS

Even if working conditions explain PPP to a limited extent, it may be at the workplace that strategies for prevention might be applicable. Thus, to assess the degree of physically strenuous work, an additional index of 'extensive physical work' was developed in the sociological analysis; this included the following variables:

- twisting and bending many times per hour
- daily work with the body bent forward
- daily work standing or walking.

To fulfil the criteria of the extensive physical work index, a woman had to work daily with tasks involving all three situations. The data were then dichotomized in women with and without such work. The data were also bisected in two other ways: lifting 10–20 kg more than 5–10 times daily, and having a job tied to a sitting position without the possibility of taking a break at will.

In relation to PPP, both extensive physical work ($n = 1287$) and heavy lifting ($n = 1177$) came out as statistically significant. Fifty-one per cent of both groups reported PPP, compared with 43% in the total group of women. The distribution within each of these indices must, however, be further considered, as the sample shows an accumulation of extensive physical work as well as of heavy lifting in the youngest age groups. The accumulation among these women can be seen in relation to education: being a very young wage-earner probably also implies a poor education. The most striking findings of the socio-logical analysis were that young (under 25 years old), poorly educated, multipara smoking 10 or more cigarettes daily, and women in what are traditionally seen as women's jobs (for example, service and sales work, nursing assistantships, and cleaning) were most strongly exposed to PPP.

PPP AND EXPERIENCE OF PREGNANCY

Being social scientists, we feel it necessary to direct attention to the women's personal experience of pelvic pain. The last question analysed in our investigation was posed as follows: 'How do you think you will remember this pregnancy?' The following response alternatives were available:

- I will remember this pregnancy mostly with joy.
- I will remember this pregnancy with mixed feelings.
- I hope I never experience such a pregnancy again.
- I do not know.
- None of the answers fit.

The 5041 women who replied (97%) were divided in two groups: those who had and those who had not experienced PPP.

Table 32.4 shows a strong association between PPP and a woman's attitude to her pregnancy. It can be reasonably assumed that it is PPP which affects the attitude, rather than the other way around. However, by focusing on personal experi-ence, it must not be concluded that PPP is seen as only a private matter. PPP should be viewed as

Table 32.4 PPP related to how pregnancy was experienced

Experience	Number	Percentage with PPP
Mostly with joy	3161	37.8
Mixed feelings	1498	50.3
Never again	255	66.0
Do not know	127	52.0
Total	5041	43.0

both a private and a public issue, and both need to be considered. Pregnancy in itself, and PPP in particular, is an issue that reflects the personal troubles in the occupational and/or family en-vironment as well as the public issues of social structure. One may say that women today are pregnant in a public arena that is, in many ways, not adapted to the personal needs of pregnant women.

In our opinion, the outcome of the present study also calls for a broader investigation of the relationship between the physical sensation of pain, its subjective perception, and the sociocultural factors surrounding the symptoms. It is known from other fields in the medical realm that reported symptoms should not be viewed only as straightforward reflections of biological realities. Socialization into a particular culture exerts strong influence on the general recognition as well as the labeling of somatic sensations. Physical symptoms are culturally patterned, and making a diagnosis is a multifaceted social process.

CONCLUSIONS

1. This presentation is based on a cross-sectional analysis of self-reported pain, so it can only be seen as a first step in the study of the epidemiology of PPP on a population basis.

2. Summarizing the findings on the relation-ship between PPP and LBP, there is a clear statistical association between the two conditions. PPP was found to be more closely associated with parity, weight of the newborn, and smoking than was LBP. In conclusion, the data from the epidemiological analysis indicate that what the women called PPP and LBP are really different conditions, with different etiologies, although they often occur together and are probably often confused.

3. Objections toward the two studies may be raised to the inclusion of extremely different variables (parity, smoking, occupational stress of a physical and mental nature, education, economic needs, etc.). Which is the underlying variable in the chain of causation, and which variables are merely intermediate, we still do not know.

4. The data presented correspond well with those of other studies that also indicate prevalences between 25 and 50%, of which 5–10% are considered severe (Berg et al 1988, Endresen Heiberg 1995, Mantle et al 1977, Östgaard et al 1988).

5. The question remains of where now to go from here. We are still a long way from a satisfactory descriptive epidemiology, namely good data on how incidence and prevalence vary by time, place, and person. In addition, we need to investigate personal and cultural aspects embedded in different diagnostic and therapeutic procedures, and the possible lack of comparable routines in some societies. Eventually, we want to arrive at randomized, controlled prophylactic as well as therapeutic trials. The clinical expertise of physiotherapists in the field should be utilized in both diagnosis and the measurement outcomes of different treatment regimes.

ACKNOWLEDGEMENTS

We would like to thank Professor Tor Bjerkedal, Dr Ebba Wergeland, and Dr Kitty Strand for the use of data from the investigation 'Pregnancy and work' carried out in the Department of Preventive Medicine, University of Oslo. We also thank Alex Line for correcting the English.

REFERENCES

Berg G, Hammar M, Möller-Nielsen J, Lindèn U, Thorblad J 1988 Low back pain during pregnancy. Obstetrics and Gynecology 71: 71–75

Endresen Heiberg E 1995 Pelvic pain and low back pain in pregnant women – an epidemiological study. Scandinavian Journal of Rheumatology 24: 135–141

Kristiansson Å, Svärdsudd K, von Schoultz B 1996 Serum relaxin, symphyseal pain and back pain during pregnancy. In: Kristiansson P (ed) Back pain and symphyseal pain during pregnancy. Doctoral thesis, Uppsala University, Sweden

MacLennan A H 1991 The role of the hormone relaxin in human reproduction and pelvic girdle relaxation. Scandinavian Journal of Rheumatology (supplement) 88: 7–15

Mantle M J, Greenwood R M, Currey H L F 1977 Backache in pregnancy. Rheumatology and Rehabilitation 16: 95–101

Mens J M A, Vleeming A, Stoeckart R, Stam H J, Snijders C J 1996 Understanding peripartum pelvic pain. Implications of a patient survey. Spine 21: 1363–1370

Östgaard H C, Andersson G B J, Karlsson K 1988 Prevalence of back pain in pregnancy. Spine 16: 549–552

Östgaard H C, Zetherström G, Ros-Hansson E, Svanberg B 1994 Reduction of back and posterior pelvic pain in pregnancy. Spine 19: 894–900

Saugstad L F 1991a Persistent pelvic pain and pelvic joint instability. European Journal of Obstetrics, Gynecology and Reproductive Biology 41: 197–201

Saugstad L F 1991b Is persistent pelvic pain and pelvic joint instability associated with early menarche and with oral contraceptives? European Journal of Obstetrics, Gynecology and Reproductive Biology 41: 203–206

Skrede K 1989 Work, family and life-cycle squeezes. Working paper. Institute for Applied Social Research, Oslo

Strand K, Wergeland E, Endresen Heiberg E, Bjerkedal T 1992 Factors associated with work status of pregnant employees in Norway, 1989. In: Wijma K, von Schoultz B (eds) Reproductive life – advances in research in psychosomatic obstetrics and gynaecology. Parthenon Lancashire, pp 617–622

33. Lumbar back and posterior pelvic pain in pregnancy

H. C. Östgaard

INTRODUCTION

Pelvic change in pregnancy is a well-known problem and has been documented since the Hippocratic period. It was believed that the pelvis expanded during the first pregnancy and thereafter remained permanently enlarged throughout life. In the sixteenth century, it was maintained that delivery was possible only because of enormous yielding of the female pelvis. Cantin (1899), at the end of the nineteenth century, found palpable evidence of movement of the pubic symphysis among all but 2% of 500 women late in pregnancy. He believed that increased motion in the pelvic joints was a problem in itself. He also believed that it was the most common and most overlooked problem in pregnancy.

In modern times, pelvic changes in pregnancy have been described by several authors (Berg et al 1988, Farbrot 1952, Kristiansson 1996, MacLennan et al 1986, Östgaard et al 1994a, Walde 1962, Young 1940). Widening of the symphysis pubis has been illustrated on X-rays from the 8th week in normal pregnancies (Genell 1949). There is no correlation between the degree of symphyseal widening and pain in the pelvis during pregnancy, and pain can not be related to any radiographic finding. In spite of the development of imaging, including computerized tomography (CT) and magnetic resonance tomography (MRT), we still have to rely on a thorough clinical examination and a good history when diagnosing pelvic pain among pregnant women.

EPIDEMIOLOGY

Back pain is frequent among pregnant women (Berg et al 1988, Endresen 1995, Fast et al 1987, Grünfeld & Qvigstad 1991, Hauge-Lundby et al 1991, Mantle et al 1977, Östgaard et al 1991a, 1994a, Sydsjö et al 1989) and is often accepted as an unavoidable complaint of normal pregnancy. Several studies have found that more than 50% of all pregnant women have some kind of back pain during pregnancy. Fortunately, the majority of women with back pain during pregnancy recover spontaneously shortly after delivery. Back pain in pregnancy has been regarded as a self-healing condition. Therefore, no effective treatment of these problems or early identification of at-risk patients has been developed. Unfortunately, some women with pain during pregnancy do not get well spontaneously. These women often encounter little understanding when they seek medical advice for their pain. They are often misunderstood and treated as psychosomatic cases. Sometimes pain from the lumbar region of the back is confused with pain from the posterior pelvis, or vice versa. Therefore, treatment for back pain in pregnant women often fails (Dumas et al 1995a, 1995b).

Back pain is reported by more than one out of every two women for longer or shorter periods during pregnancy (Berg et al 1988, Endresen 1995, Fast et al 1987, Grünfeld & Qvigstad 1991, Hauge-Lundby et al 1991, Östgaard et al 1991a, 1994a, Sydsjö et al 1989), and the number of pregnant women complaining of some kind of back pain seems to have increased over the past few decades (Grünfeld & Qvigstad 1991, Hauge-Lundby et al 1991, Sydsjö et al 1989). The reason for this increase is multifactorial and to a large extent unknown. Nowadays, more women are at work, often on low wages and with ergonomically badly planned work places. In most jobs, the working day cannot be planned around the capacity of a pregnant woman, who often also has to take care of the house and children. All these factors are known to increase the number of complaints of back pain in a non-pregnant population, and there is no reason to believe that pregnant women should respond differently. Furthermore, pregnant women are being told that pregnancy is not a disease, so normal working capacity is expected. Some pregnant women can initially fulfil these demands, but no woman can do it throughout pregnancy. Pregnancy is not a disease, but it produces a very large and growing burden on the female body.

Pain intensity has been reported to average 4.3 on a 0–10 visual analog (VA) scale, with large variations and a maximum pain intensity around the 30th week of pregnancy. Two studies showed that 70% of all working pregnant women in Sweden took sick leave for some reason at some time during their pregnancy (Hauge-Lundby et al 1991, Sydsjö et al 1989). This sick leave period amounted to on average, 7 weeks, unspecified 'back pain' being by far the most prevalent diagnosis (Östgaard & Andersson 1992). Other studies from Scandinavia have shown the same trend (Grünfeld & Qvigstad 1991, Hauge-Lundby et al 1991), indicating that back pain in pregnancy is also a large socioeconomic problem.

DEFINITIONS

The concept of back pain in pregnancy is not well defined, and the anatomic origin of the pain is unknown.

Earlier studies have shown that it is important to define two types of back pain during pregnancy (Endresen 1995, Östgaard et al 1991a, 1994a, 1996b): pain from the lumbar area and pain from the posterior part of the pelvis. Those two types of pain should be treated differently, as inappropriate treatment may increase pain. The two types of pain may occur simultaneously or at different times in the same individual during pregnancy and after delivery. Pain in the pubic symphysis is not an isolated phenomenon but is normally found in women with posterior pelvic pain (Östgaard et al 1991a, 1994a, 1996b).

THE POSTERIOR PELVIC PAIN PROVOCATION TEST

The posterior pelvic pain provocation test is very useful in distinguishing between the two types of pain. It is performed with the patient supine and her hip flexed to 90°. When the woman's femur is gently pressed posteriorly by the examiner, simultaneously stabilizing the patient's pelvis, the test is said to be positive when the woman feels a pain that she recognizes in her posterior pelvis (Östgaard et al 1994a, 1994b) (Fig. 33.1). The test is not specific for any anatomic structure, but it does help to identify women with posterior pelvic pain. Evaluation of the test has shown that in this aspect the test has a specificity of 80% and a sensitivity of 81% (Östgaard et al 1994b).

PAIN DRAWINGS

Pain drawings are useful when back pain in a non-pregnant population is classified (Ransford et al 1975), and they are also a great help among pregnant women. The drawings can be completed by the patient before the consultation; the markings are different for lumbar pain and posterior pelvic pain. Furthermore, pain drawings will help to identify women with non-physiologic pain patterns.

Lumbar back pain

Lumbar back pain is common in the general population as well as among pregnant women. The condition is not specific for pregnancy but is often found among pregnant women who have had lumbar back pain earlier in life. The same

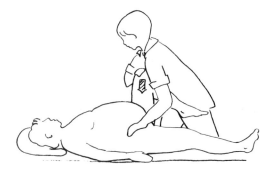

Fig. 33.1   The posterior pelvic pain provocation test. (From Östgaard et al 1994b © Springer-Verlag, with permission.)

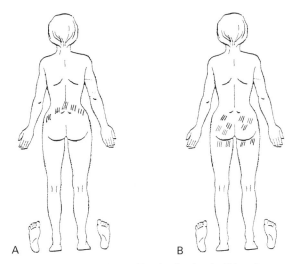

Fig. 33.2 Pain drawings of lumbar back pain (A) and posterior pelvic pain (B).

women will often have lumbar back pain after delivery. The pain intensity during pregnancy is less than among women with posterior pelvic pain. Some increase of pain intensity may occur because of the extra load on the spine caused by pregnancy. These women will mark the lumbar area above the pelvis on pain drawings (Fig. 33.2A).

Posterior pelvic pain

Pregnancy may also predispose to a different type of pain (Mantle et al 1977). This type is described by a large number of pregnant women and is located in the posterior part of the pelvis distal and lateral to the lumbosacral junction. It is felt deep in the gluteal area and is often described as stabbing. The pain may radiate to the posterior thigh and may extend to the knee. There is a history of time- and weight-bearing-related pain, as well as pain-free intervals with sudden pain attacks. There is free range of motion in the back and hips. Twisting and asymmetric loading of the pelvis is most painful, for example when vacuum cleaning. Overloading of the pelvis will often cause more pain the following day. The condition may be uni- or bilateral and is often misinterpreted as sciatica, facet joint syndrome, or lumbar back insufficiency. The condition is, however, different from sciatica in that it is less specific

than the nerve root syndrome in distribution and does not extend down into the foot. It is different from facet joint syndrome and lumbar back insufficiency because it does not emerge from the lumbar area and does not include a reduced range of motion in the spine. Furthermore, there is no initial muscle weakness or sensory impairment, and reflexes are normal. Therefore, the condition should not be treated as lumbar back insufficiency, facet joint syndrome, or sciatica (Mantle et al 1977, Östgaard et al 1994a). On the contrary, women with posterior pelvic pain may feel more pain if treated with back-strengthening exercise. Pain drawings will be marked distal and lateral to the lumbosacral junction (Fig. 33.2B).

Some 10% of all pregnant women suffer from more than one of these conditions, which complicates the problem of back pain in pregnancy (Berg et al 1988, Endresen 1995, Östgaard et al 1994a).

Symphysiolysis

An increased range of motion and pain from the pubic symphysis is often registered in pregnancy but is not an isolated phenomenon. There are three joints in the pelvic ring, and it is therefore not possible to have an increased range of motion isolated to just one joint. To accomplish symphysiolysis, the range of motion must also be increased in at least one of the sacroiliac joints (SIJs). Consequently, anterior pelvic problems are caused by posterior pelvic malfunction. A thorough examination of the pelvis will detect that pain from the pubic symphysis is always combined with posterior pelvic pain (Östgaard et al 1991a, 1994a).

SUMMARY OF CHARACTERISTICS FOR LUMBAR BACK AND POSTERIOR PELVIC PAIN

Lumbar back pain:

- a history of lumbar back pain even before pregnancy
- a pain drawing with markings cranial to the sacrum
- pain and a decreased range of motion in the lumbar spine

- pain on palpation of the erector spinae muscle
- a negative posterior pelvic pain provocation test.

Posterior pelvic pain:

- no history of back pain before the first pregnancy
- a pain drawing with markings in the gluteal area
- time- and weight-bearing-related pain
- pain-free intervals with sudden pain attacks
- a free range of motion in the hips and spine and no nerve root syndrome
- a positive posterior pelvic pain provocation test.

BIOMECHANICS

Posterior pelvic pain may be caused by a disturbance of the requested coordination of ligaments, muscles, and joints in the posterior part of the pelvis. The problem is probably caused by the combined effect of the pregnancy hormones relaxin, estrogens, and progesterone on the large ligaments in the posterior part of the pelvis. The result is an increased laxity, allowing a small but important instability in the pelvic joints. This is a speculation based on scattered scientific findings, and there is no thorough proof for the theory. However, there is a well-documented increased range of motion in the pelvic joints, which may compromise pelvic stability. Instability in the pelvis is inconsistent with normal body motion. Increased muscular tension in the large muscles of the posterior pelvis and lumbar spine may follow, as an attempt to re-establish pelvic stability. If left untreated, longlasting increased muscle tension will cause pain, leading to secondary muscle insufficiency, and a vicious circle has started. Recent studies have shown a higher incidence of pain in the posterior pelvis among women with elevated levels of relaxin in blood samples taken during pregnancy (Mantle et al 1977, Kristiansson 1996).

It has been postulated that the pain should derive from the SIJs, themselves, but there is no strong scientific proof for that. These joints appear normal on X-rays, CT scans, and MRT, so no known skeletal characteristic can be detected in these women. Furthermore, there are no specific tests for SIJ dysfunction. Several studies have found an intraexaminer variation of around 50% for most commonly used tests of dysfunction of the SIJ, indicating that these tests are highly unspecific (Laslett & Williams 1994). Apparently, all we know is that pain is found in the area of the posterior pelvis, so this is the expression we have chosen to describe the condition.

The anatomic details of SIJ pain are dealt with in other chapters in this book.

RISK FACTORS

It cannot be clearly anticipated which women will later develop pain in their pregnancy or, if they do, where the pain will present. As different areas may be involved in the same women at different times it is important to identify the areas of pain correctly and treat the women with respect to this. Some women will change pain type during pregnancy. It is not known in detail from which anatomic structures pain emerges, either among women with lumbar back pain or among women with posterior pelvic pain. This ignorance is generally accepted as far as pain in the lumbar spine in a non-pregnant population, i.e. lumbago, is concerned. Likewise, it must be accepted for the pelvis among women in relation to pregnancy.

Women with a history of lumbar back pain earlier in life run a 2.1 times higher risk of getting lumbar back pain in a subsequent pregnancy, and women who are physically fit have a lower (0.7) risk of getting lumbar back pain in pregnancy (Östgaard & Andersson 1991b). Furthermore, such vocational factors as heavy lifting, monotony at work, and low job satisfaction have an unfavorable impact on developing lumbar back pain in pregnancy, as do many social factors. In these aspects, pregnant women follow the same pattern as in a non-pregnant population (Östgaard et al 1991a). The known risk factors for lumbar back pain in pregnancy cannot be summated in a simple way, so we still know little about which women will develop lumbar pain in a future pregnancy (Östgaard & Andersson 1991b).

No prepregnancy risk factors for posterior pelvic pain are known. During a first pregnancy, the pelvis is in a totally new condition, and we can only speculate about how it will react. There is evidence that physical exercise before pregnancy is not beneficial, as even well-trained athletes may get serious posterior pelvic pain, although lumbar pain is not as common in this group of women (Östgaard et al 1994a). Posterior pelvic pain may begin very early in pregnancy, but it begins on average in the 18th week, long before any increase in weight has occurred. This indicates that hormonal changes, rather than increased weight, are connected with this type of pain. Furthermore, there is no correlation between pain and body weight before pregnancy nor between pain and weight increase during pregnancy (Östgaard et al 1991b). The theory of an early hormonal effect on the ligaments of the body is supported by the correlation between high concentrations of relaxin in the first trimester of pregnancy (MacLennan et al 1986) and a general increase in ligament laxity from the 12th to the 24th week of pregnancy (Östgaard et al 1993). As no risk factors are known, no prophylaxis against posterior pelvic pain in pregnancy is possible. However, after posterior pelvic pain during pregnancy, there is a small trend for the same pain to recur in subsequent pregnancies.

Apparently, only little is to be gained from known risk factors with respect to lumbar pain and almost nothing for posterior pelvic pain. The solution is to wait for the pain to appear and then to classify and treat it as soon as possible. All pregnant women should be informed early during pregnancy on what to expect from their backs and pelvises later in pregnancy and to seek help promptly if pain appears. A thorough examination should then be made to initiate the correct treatment, be it of the back, the pelvis, or a combination of the two.

DEVELOPMENT OF PAIN

When using the above-mentioned criteria, the types of pain will be distributed in incidence during pregnancy as shown in Fig. 33.3, and the two groups will respond to physiotherapy. Some 10% of the women will have symptoms from the pelvis as well as from the lumbar back. The majority of these women will have had a lumbar back pain problem before pregnancy and have developed posterior pelvic pain later during pregnancy. Pain intensity during pregnancy is higher among women with posterior pelvic pain. After delivery, pain in the lumbar back is more intense. Furthermore, after delivery, women with posterior pelvic pain will improve more than women with lumbar pain (Östgaard et al 1996b).

TREATMENT

The majority of women with locomotor problems in pregnancy have posterior pelvic pain. The cause of pelvic pain is primarily hormonal changes

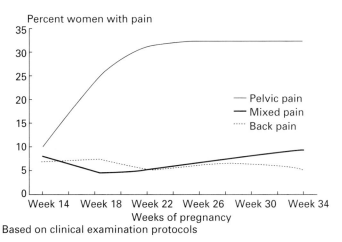

Fig. 33.3 Frequencies of pain types during pregnancy. (From Östgaard et al 1994a, with permission)

induced by pregnancy, which, of course, cannot be eliminated without great danger to the fetus. The condition itself cannot be cured during pregnancy, but secondary muscle pain may be prevented. There is evidence that, provided no secondary muscle pain develops, posterior pelvic pain will, largely speaking, always disappear soon after pregnancy. However, muscular pain may become chronic when once established. One study showed that persisting lumbar back and posterior pelvic pain 18 months after delivery existed in more than 35% of all women who had received no treatment during pregnancy. Most of the women, however, experienced some type of regression of symptoms, but 7% had no regression of pain at all (Östgaard & Andersson 1992). In a study of women who had been treated with physiotherapy and given information about their condition during pregnancy, only 11% had persisting pain 5 months after delivery and only 3% had no regression at all (Östgaard et al 1996b). In other words, much is to be gained by treating these women during pregnancy.

Lumbar back pain

Treatment of pregnant women with simple lumbar back pain, where muscular insufficiency is predominant, is not complicated. Serious lumbar back disease presenting for the first time during pregnancy is rare. Disc herniations appear in 1 in 10 000 pregnancies (Heliovara et al 1987) and hardly any of these women need an operation during pregnancy. Other degenerative back diseases are rare at the time of life when pregnancy takes place. There is no evidence that scoliosis gets painful or increases in painfulness during pregnancy. However, severe spondylolisthesis may cause increased pain late in pregnancy because of the increased load on the lumbar spine in combination with the hormone-induced ligament laxity.

The treatment of lumbar back pain among pregnant women is basically the same as in a non-pregnant population: for example, education in anatomy and kinesiology, back-strengthening exercises, training in range of motion, and body posture correction to avoid hyperlordosis, which is common among pregnant women (Snijders et al 1976). Later in pregnancy, there is a relative insufficiency of the abdominal muscles because of the normal elongation and separation of the two rectus abdominis muscles caused by the expanding uterus. The muscles of the abdominal wall should be trained specifically to reduce this insufficiency, which cannot be totally avoided. Furthermore, being physically fit before pregnancy reduces the risk of lumbar pain, of which all women should be informed before they become pregnant. It is much easier to become physically fit before getting pregnant than to begin training after pregnancy has started to influence the body.

Posterior pelvic pain

There is no cure for posterior pelvic pain while pregnant. The challenge is to teach these women how to live with a pelvis that is insufficient to serve as the stable center of normal body motion. For simple biomechanic reasons, daily demands of walking, lifting, sitting, housekeeping, or taking care of children may become overwhelming problems. It is possible to increase stability in the pelvis by muscular force, but only for a limited period of time. If the large ligaments in the posterior part of the pelvis are insufficient, the muscles will invariably soon fail, which is why these women can do most things only for a short period of time. After a while, however, they have to change body position, for example from walking to sitting, standing to lying, or vice versa, as even these simple everyday actions become painful. Even in sitting, normally functioning ligaments and muscles are required to keep the sacrum from rotating in relation to the iliac bones. The forces on the pelvis are as large in sitting as in standing, the only difference being that the weight shifts from the hip joints to the ischial tuberosities. However, this small change may be a temporary relief for tense muscles. Education in anatomy and kinesiology is the key for these women to handle their situation. Furthermore, relaxation training is important to release tense muscles.

It is crucial to understand that vigorous exercise will increase pain, as such exercise demands a stable pelvis. Ligament insufficiency cannot be overcome by exercise, a painful lesson many well-trained women with posterior pelvic pain have learned. Most musculoskeletal pain disappears without exercising being discontinued, but this is unfortunately not the case with posterior pelvic pain. Typically, the pain increases after exercise and presents on the following day. The insufficiency of the pelvis must be respected, and all exercise performed within the limits of this insufficiency; it must be remembered that normal muscle function is not possible around a malfunctioning joint anywhere in the body.

If the pelvis is unstable, it must be accepted that locomotion is impaired. Avoiding stairs, one-leg standing, an extreme range of motion in the hips and back, overloading the pelvis, and physical monotony is good advice. A pelvic belt will help 80% of the women (Östgaard et al 1994a), and in severe cases walking sticks may be needed.

Following the above advice will not restore normal function but it will reduce pain. A wheelchair should always be avoided, as it will increase muscular insufficiency. This makes rehabilitation more difficult later on, when the ligaments have returned to normal functioning shortly after delivery. For the same reason, prolonged bedrest is not recommended.

Manipulation of the pelvis is a matter of debate. If used, it must be with great care and always in combination with muscle training, relaxation and increased muscle control. Manipulation alone will not help in the long run. A further description of this method is found elsewhere in this book.

Cesarean section is never indicated for lumbar back pain, and hardly ever for cases of posterior pelvic pain. Providing that adequate physiotherapy is available, no woman should ever develop a situation in which caesarean section is discussed for these reasons.

Sick leave because of lumbar back and posterior pelvic pain can be reduced during pregnancy by physiotherapy and information. In a study from Sweden, sick leave for lumbar back and posterior pelvic pain during pregnancy amounted to 54 days per woman among controls, while women who were treated with physiotherapy and given information took sick leave for 30 days during pregnancy, a statistically significant difference (Östgaard, 1996a). The true reasons for the

reduction of pain and sick leave are not known. An education and training program may reduce pain and anxiety by teaching the women how to handle their problems better, but the mere effect of being cared for *per se* cannot be neglected.

THE MODEL

One model for taking care of pregnant women with back or pelvic pain is as follows (Fig. 33.4). At her first visit to the midwife or obstetrician, the pregnant woman should be informed about possible future back and pelvic problems and where to get help, as well as the usual obstetric topics. A physiotherapist with a special interest in pregnancy problems is often preferable in this discussion. Helping a pregnant woman with such problems calls for teamwork to widen the skills available, as no obstetrician, midwife, or physiotherapist alone possesses all the necessary interdisciplinary knowledge. Whenever back pain occurs, the woman should have a thorough back and pelvic assessment and the problem should be identified as being lumbar back, posterior pelvic, or a combination of the two. An educational and training program should be developed with individual variations depending on the type of pain, and vocational and daily life demands. It has been shown that changes in ergonomics at the workplace are useful in reducing pain even during pregnancy (Östgaard et al 1994a). If needed, a pelvic belt should be provided. Initially, it is

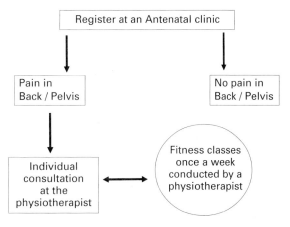

Fig. 33.4 Flowchart for pregnant women with back pain.

important that women are given at least one individual consultation with the physiotherapist, but later on they may join fitness classes for pregnant women with the same pain type. However, some 15% of the women may change from one pain type to another during pregnancy, and they should also change training program. Furthermore, some women may get worse and may have to return to individual therapy for a time.

Using this model, half the women with back or pelvic pain will need only one individual consultation. One-third of the women will need two individual consultations, and no women will need more than four individual consultations. The subsequent problems can be managed in weekly fitness classes, with special emphasis on pain type, conducted by a physiotherapist (Östgaard et al 1996a). This means that one physiotherapist is needed for every 1000 pregnant women. From a socioeconomic point of view this is a very good investment. In Sweden, a physiotherapist working in this way saves Social Insurance 10 times her own salary because of the reduction in sick leave among pregnant women (Östgaard 1996a). How much the costs are reduced by earlier return to work after pregnancy is not known. Furthermore, the increased well-being and reduced pain cannot be expressed in economic terms.

AFTER DELIVERY

After delivery, posterior pelvic pain disappears in the majority of women within 3 months (Östgaard & Andersson 1992). Some women may have developed a chronic posterior pelvic pain, which will persist even after the pelvis has regained its normal stability. These women should be referred to a physiotherapist for specific training of the muscles of the pelvis, abdomen, and back. It is important that the pelvic muscles are attended to first in order to stabilize the pelvis, and only thereafter should training of the back muscles be initiated. This rehabilitation is slow, 6–12 months, and always contains periods of serious relapse, which is very discouraging. It is important that the women are informed about this at the beginning of rehabilitation.

A small group of women may get well spontaneously shortly after delivery and return to a physically demanding daily life only to experience severe posterior pelvic pain some months later. Unfortunately, this is a bad omen. These women can be difficult to treat, and their rehabilitation may extend over several years. The treatment program is the same, but it should be started at a very low level and increased very slowly, with careful observation of relapses. Some of these women are so handicapped that they can start doing exercises only in a weightless condition in warm water. To avoid this problem, it should be emphasized that after delivery, although pain has disappeared, strenuous work should be avoided for at least 6 months if a woman has had posterior pelvic pain during pregnancy. There is a strong correlation between high pain intensity during pregnancy and persisting problems after delivery (Östgaard & Andersson 1992, Östgaard et al 1996b).

Painkillers seldom have any substantial effect and are best avoided during pregnancy and breastfeeding. Among women who have been treated by us during pregnancy, we have not seen severe prolonged postpartum problems. It should therefore be possible to avoid these longlasting pain problems in the future.

Women with pain during pregnancy often worry about their own future, harm to the fetus, and their ability to take care of a newborn child when they are so handicapped. However, there is scientific evidence that problems with the child or the delivery itself in no way correlates to lumbar or posterior pelvic pain suffered during pregnancy (Östgaard et al 1991b). Furthermore, the pain normally reduces substantially directly after delivery, often within a few days, so taking care of the newborn baby is seldom a great problem.

In looking for an explanation for posterior pelvic pain, the question of oral contraception is often raised. However, one published (Östgaard et al 1991b) and several unpublished studies have shown that no correlation exists. This indicates that, from an orthopedic point of view, oral contraception can be used as wanted, both before and after pregnancy, by all women.

Because posterior pelvic pain is induced by hormones, speculations about breastfeeding have arisen. Breastfeeding is supposed to change normal hormone levels and block ovulation to prevent a new early pregnancy. This might have an impact on the ligaments of the pelvis and thus on pain. One study (Östgaard & Andersson 1992) has shown no correlation between breastfeeding and the regression of lumbar or posterior pelvic pain after pregnancy, so this is not a reason to stop breastfeeding. Furthermore, it is not a logical that breastfeeding that blocks a new pregnancy should increase pregnancy-induced problems.

If more children are planned, one can speculate about the timing of the next pregnancy. There is no study on this issue, but even severe posterior pelvic pain often disappears within 1 year, provided that treatment is correct. Therefore posterior pelvic pain should not be the limiting factor when timing the next pregnancy. On the contrary, women well educated in the locomotor problems of pregnancy do not have to wait until all symptoms have disappeared before becoming pregnant again. Increased awareness of symptoms and early treatment will be sufficient in most cases.

In some centers, chronic posterior pelvic pain is treated by fusion of the SIJs (described elsewhere in this book). This is, in my opinion, seldom necessary.

CONCLUSIONS

1. Women with any type of back pain should be identified as early as possible and enrolled in a special program.

2. Back pain in relation to pregnancy should always be divided into two types, depending on the pattern of pain: pain in the lumbar area, and pain in the posterior part of the pelvis.

3. Differentiation into the two types of pain can be made by means of a short history-taking and a simple back and pelvis examination, including the posterior pelvic pain provocation test.

4. The two groups of women should be provided with individual information about their specific condition, and a program for muscle-training and relaxation should be developed.

5. The program must respect individual needs at home and at work, and any change in pain

pattern should be assessed and followed by changes in the program.

6. A pelvic belt is recommended for women with posterior pelvic pain.

7. Teamwork with an obstetrician, a midwife, and a physiotherapist is necessary to cover the skills needed for these obstetric–orthopedic problems.

8. Most women will need only a few individual consultations, and later training can be performed in groups.

9. It is important that the exercise groups include only women with the same pain type, and changes in the type of pain must be looked for. Some women will need to go back to individual therapy for a short period.

10. With this planning, the intensity of lumbar back and posterior pelvic pain can be reduced during pregnancy and after delivery. The number of women with lumbar back pain can be reduced, and the number of women with chronic back pain after delivery can be diminished. Furthermore, the population of women with persisting posterior pelvic pain after pregnancy can be almost eliminated.

11. The abundant prescription of rest as the only treatment will do few women any good but will complicate rehabilitation because of general muscle wasting. Taking care of a newborn infant is a demanding job, and women who have been resting excessively because of undefined back pain are not best fit to fulfil the task.

12. After pregnancy, posterior pelvic pain should disappear spontaneously within 3 months. If it does not, the woman should consult the physiotherapist who helped her during pregnancy in order to avoid developing a chronic pain condition. Attention is often focused on the newborn, and the problems of the mother are either easily missed or are expected to disappear spontaneously along with other problems of pregnancy. Although newborn babies are fascinating, we ought to pay more attention to their mothers: they may not be as well as they pretend.

REFERENCES

Berg G, Hammar M, Möller-Nielsen J, Lindén U, Thornblad J 1988 Low back pain during pregnancy. Obstetrics and Gynecology 71: 71–74

Cantin L 1899 Relouchement des symphysies et artralgies pelviennes d'origne gravidique. Thesis, Paris
Dumas G, Reid J G, Wolfe L A, McGrath M J 1995a Exercise, posture, and back pain during pregnancy. 1: Exercise and posture. Clinical Biomechanics 10: 98–103

Dumas G, Reid J G, Wolfe L A, McGrath M J 1995b
  Exercise, posture, and back pain during pregnancy. 2:
  Exercise and back pain. Clinical Biomechanics 10:
  104–109

Endresen E 1995 Pelvic pain and low back pain in pregnant
  women. An epidemiological study. Scandinavian Journal of
  Rheumatology 24: 135–141

Farbrot E 1952 The relationship of the effect and pain of
  pregnancy to the anatomy of the pelvis. Acta Radiologica
  38: 403–417

Fast A, Shapiro D, Ducommun J, Friedmann L, Bouklas T,
  Floman Y 1987 Low back pain in pregnancy. Spine 12:
  368–371

Genell S 1949 Studies on insufficiencia pelvis (gravidarum et
  puerparum). Acta Obstetricia et Gynecologica
  Scandinavica 28: 1–33

Grünfeld B, Qvigstad E 1991 Disease during pregnancy [in
  Norwegian]. Tidsskrift för Norges Legeförening 111:
  1269–1272

Hauge-Lundby I, Stray-Pedersen B, Tellnes G 1991
  Common diagnoses for sick leave during pregnancy [in
  Norwegian]. Tidsskrift för Norges Legeförening 111:
  2833–2836

Heliovara M, Knekt P, Aromaa A 1987 Incidence and risk of
  herniated lumbar intervertebral disc or sciatica leading to
  hospitalization. Journal of Chronic Diseases 40: 251–258

Kristiansson P 1996 Back pain during pregnancy. Spine 21:
  702–709

Laslett M, Williams M 1994 The reliability of selected pain
  provocation tests for sacroiliac joint pathology. Spine 19:
  1243–1249

MacLennan A H, Nicolson R, Green R C, Bath M 1986
  Serum relaxin and pelvic pain in pregnancy. Lancet ii:
  243–245

Mantle M J, Greenwood R M, Curry H L F 1977 Backache in
  pregnancy. Rheumatology and Rehabilitation 16: 95–101

Östgaard H C, Andersson G B J 1991 Previous back pain and
  risk of developing back pain in a future pregnancy. Spine
  16: 432–436

Östgaard H C, Andersson G B J 1992 Low back pain post

partum. Spine 17: 53–55

Östgaard H C, Andersson G B J, Karlsson K 1991a
  Prevalence of back pain in pregnancy. Spine 16: 49–52

Östgaard H C, Wennergren M, Andersson G B J 1991b The
  impact of low back and pelvic pain on the pregnancy
  outcome. Acta Obstetricia et Gynecologica Scandinavica
  70: 21–24

Östgaard H C, Andersson G B J, Schultz A B, Miller J A A
  1993 Influence of some biomechanical factors on low back
  pain in pregnancy. Spine 18: 54–58

Östgaard H C, Zetherström G, Roos-Hansson E 1994a
  Reduction of back and posterior pelvic pain in relation to
  pregnancy. Spine 19: 894–900

Östgaard H C, Zetherström G, Roos-Hansson E 1994b The
  posterior pelvic pain provocation test in pregnant women.
  European Spine Journal 3: 258–260

Östgaard H C, Norén L, Östgaard S, Nielsen T F 1996a
  Reduction of sick leave for back or posterior pelvic pain in
  pregnancy. Acta Othopaedica Scandinavica Supplement
  270: 67: 45

Östgaard H C, Zetherström G, Roos-Hansson E 1996b
  Regression of back and posterior pelvic pain after
  pregnancy. Spine (in press)

Ransford A O, Douglas C, Mooney V 1975 The pain drawing
  as an aid to the psychologic evaluation of patients with low
  back pain. Spine 1: 127–134

Snijders C J, Seroo J M, Snijder J G N, Hoedt H T 1976
  Change in form of the spine as a consequence of
  pregnancy. Digest of the 11th international conference on
  medical and biological engineering, Ottawa, Ontario,
  pp 670–671

Sydsjö A, Sydsjö G, Wijma B 1989 High sick leave during
  pregnancy in an extensive compensation system [In
  Swedish]. Läkartidningen 86: 4141–4144

Walde J 1962 Obstetrical and gynecological pains, especially
  those contracted during pregnancy. Acta Obstetricia et
  Gynecologica Scandinavica (supplement) 2: 1–52

Young J 1940 Relaxation of the pelvic joints in pregnancy.
  Journal of Obstetrics and Gynaecology of the British
  Empire 47: 493–523

34. S-Relaxin and pelvic pain in pregnant women

P. Kristiansson

INTRODUCTION

Back pain during pregnancy is a frequent complaint, whose cause is unclear. Nine-month prevalence rates in the range of 48–90% have been reported, which is a remarkable increase of prevalence compared with the non-pregnant state (Biering-Sørensen 1982). In a prospective study (Kristiansson et al 1996a), it was shown that back pain started early in pregnancy, its incidence leveling off during the 24th week of gestation and returning to normal post partum. The increased prevalence rate and early onset indicate the importance of internal/hormonal factors as a cause of back pain during pregnancy.

Two studies of physical back status examination during pregnancy have shown that a pain provocation test aimed at verifying posterior pelvic pain has a high sensitivity and specificity (Kristiansson & Svärdsudd 1996, Östgaard et al 1994). This 'femoral compression test' was performed with the hip in 90° flexion, pain being provoked by an axial femoral pressure force of approximately 50–150 N applied to the knee. The results of the test were considered positive if pain was felt in the sacral area or in the buttock of the side tested. In the first study, the best discrimination between women who reported pain and women without back pain was achieved by combining tests (see Table 34.1). In addition, in order to see whether the test results were

Table 34.1 Sensitivity, specificity, and predictive value of pain-provoking tests aimed at the sacral region and symphysis among pregnant women who reported back or symphyseal pain at the test situation (number of test situations, $n = 155$) and among those who reported no back or symphyseal pain at the test situation (number of test situations, $n = 342$) Reproduced from Kristiansson & Svärdsudd 1996

Pain location and tests	Sensitivity	Specificity	Predictive value
Sacral spine			
pfc	69	90	76
tsl	64	89	77
tpsis	35	98	90
lt	24	96	74
plm	23	97	76
psig	23	98	81
pfc + tsl	72	88	74
pfc + tsl + tp	75	87	73
pfc + tsl + tp + lt	77	85	69
pfc + tsl + tp + lt + plm	81	84	69
pfc + tsl + tp + lt + plm + psig	83	83	68
Symphysis	87	85	51

pfc = painful femoral compression; tsl = tender sacrospinous ligament; tpsis = tender posterior superior iliac spine; lt = lumbar tenderness; plm = painful lumbar movement; psig = painful supine iliac gapping.

linked to the presence of pain or to other factors, i.e. whether the positivity of the test came and went with the reported pain, a longitudinal analysis was carried out in women who reported no pain at one visit followed by pain at the next visit, and freedom from pain at a third. For pain locations in the lower part of the back or in the pubic symphysis, there was a clear increase in the proportion of women with a positive test when the pain appeared and a clear decrease when it disappeared, indicating a causal relationship.

The outcome of the application of test combinations indicates that pain may be provoked from several structures, such as the sacrospinous/sacrotuberous ligament, the sacroiliac ligaments, the iliolumbar ligaments, and possibly others. These ligaments and surrounding structures are part of a functional system, and it seems reasonable to assume that the functional system, rather than individual ligaments, is affected and induces back pain during pregnancy (Kristiansson & Svärdsudd 1996).

The pregnant state affects the ligaments and bones in the pelvic region (Houghton 1975, Putschar 1976). As in other mammalian species, the reproductive hormones estrogen, progesterone, and relaxin may have a role in the connective tissue transformation of the pelvic joints in women (Wahl et al 1977).

Relaxin is a peptide hormone of the insulin-like growth factor family. Our knowledge of the role of relaxin in humans is still limited. The primary source of circulating relaxin is considered to be the ovary (Johnson et al 1991, Kristiansson et al 1996b). Circulating relaxin shows a marked increase in early pregnancy until a peak value at the 12th gestational week, followed by a decline until the 17th week, which is in turn followed by quite stable serum levels around 50% of peak value (Kristiansson et al 1996c). Three months after delivery, relaxin is not detectable in serum.

RELATIONSHIP BETWEEN RELAXIN AND PELVIC PAIN

MacLennan et al (1986a) found a significant association between severe incapacitating symphyseal pain and relaxin levels in late pregnancy, assessed by a heterologous radioimmunoassay

with antibodies raised against porcine relaxin. However, Petersen et al (1994) were unable to confirm the finding in a retrospective study comparing disabling pelvic pain with relaxin levels in the 30th gestational week analysed by a homologous enzyme-linked immunosorbent assay.

In a thorough analysis of the subject, Kristiansson et al (1996c) reported that relaxin might be involved in the development of pelvic pain in pregnant women. Their conclusion was based on serial measurements of back and pelvic symptoms, clinical back and pelvic status findings, and hormonal values in pregnant women who were sampled from the general population of pregnant women. There was a positive correlation between mean relaxin levels and pain with onset during pregnancy reported at the 36th gestational week that was located in the symphysis, the trochanteric region, or in combination in the sacral spine, symphysis, and lumbar spine. No correlation was found between relaxin levels and any pain location with the onset of pain before pregnancy. The proportion of women reporting pain in any of the above-mentioned locations or characterized by the combination of pain locations increased with increasing relaxin value (Table 34.2).

Among women with an onset of back pain during pregnancy, there was a positive significant correlation ($r = 0.27$, $p < 0.01$) between mean relaxin level and the outcome of the femoral compression test at the 36th gestational week: the more positive the test, the higher the mean relaxin levels. Women with a negative femoral compression test at the 36th week showed the lowest mean relaxin values (649 ± 25 ng/l), those with a unilaterally positive femoral compression test had slightly higher values (756 ± 76 ng/l), and those with a bilateral positive test had the highest values (945 ± 120 ng/l). There was no relationship between mean relaxin level and the result of the femoral compression test among women with onset of pain before pregnancy.

These observations suggest that relaxin might have a role in the changes in the pelvis during pregnancy, although not as profound as in several other mammalian species (Wahl et al 1977). In rodents and pigs, relaxin is needed to enlarge the birth canal to allow delivery. Infusion of estrogen

Table 34.2 Proportion of women ($n = 179$) with pelvic pain having an onset during pregnancy. According to relaxin levels the women are grouped into three groups

Pain location	Mean serum relaxin (ng/l)		
	< 420	$420 < = x < = 890$	>890
Trochanteric	0	1.9	8.1
Symphyseal	13.5	17.1	32.4
Sacral and symphyseal	18.9	36.2	46.0
Lumbar, sacral and symphyseal	21.6	44.8	54.1

leads to swelling of the symphyseal cartilage, and infusion of estrogen and relaxin transforms the cartilage into a flaccid ligament (Steinetz et al 1984). Relaxin alone has no profound effects in this respect (Crelin 1969).

In humans, the dependence of this relaxin effect seems to be a relic of a past stage in the evolution of the species (Johnson et al 1991), which is illustrated by the differences in secretion pattern among species. Rodents have their relaxin peak in late pregnancy just before delivery, whereas humans have their peak around the 12th gestational week (Kristiansson et al 1996c).

However, a residual effect in women might be remodeling of the connective tissue (MacLennan et al 1986b). A side-effect of this remodeling might be a predisposition to pain in the pelvic area. By employing pain-provoking tests, Kristiansson and Svärdsudd (1996) found that pain in the pelvic area was most likely to arise from the ligament system of the pelvis. The fact that the outcome of the most efficient of these pain-provoking tests, the femoral compression test, was closely related to mean relaxin levels is further support for the theory that relaxin is involved in the generation of pain.

These observations might have clinical relevance for the future. Today, pelvic pain is usually treated with belts or other mechanical support, or rest. If relaxin is a primary cause of pain, relaxin may be the target for treatment; those with a high relaxin level can be identified early during the pregnancy.

CONCLUSIONS

1. Back pain during pregnancy is a common complaint. The 30% of women with the highest pain score report great difficulties with normal activities. The back pain starts early in pregnancy and increases over time.

2. Pain provocation tests have a better discriminative power than do tests of configuration or mobility. The best discrimination between women who report pain in the lower back and women who do not is achieved by combining tests. This is an indication that several pain-releasing structures may be involved and that they form a functional unit.

3. Serum relaxin levels are significantly correlated with a history of pain located in the pelvic ring and with the outcome of a test provoking pain in this region. The observations support the view that relaxin is involved in the generation of pelvic pain in pregnant women.

REFERENCES

Biering-Sørensen F 1982 Low back trouble in a general population of 30-, 40-, 50-, and 60-year-old men and women. Study design, representativeness and basic results. Danish Medical Bulletin 29: 289–299

Crelin E S 1969 The development of the bony pelvis and its changes during pregnancy and parturition. Transactions of the New York Academy of Sciences 31: 1049–1058

Houghton P 1975 The bony imprint of pregnancy. Bulletin of the New York Academy of Medicine 51: 655–661

Johnson M R, Wren M E, Abdalla H, Kirkland A, Allman A C, Lightman S L 1991 Relaxin levels in ovum donation pregnancies. Fertility and Sterility 56: 59–61

Kristiansson P, Svärdsudd K 1996 Discriminatory power of tests applied in back pain during pregnancy. Spine 21: 2337–2344

Kristiansson P, Svärdsudd K, von Schoultz B 1996a Back pain during pregnancy. A prospective study. Spine 21: 702–709

Kristiansson P, Svärdsudd K, von Schoultz B, Wramsby H 1996b Supraphysiological serum relaxin concentration during pregnancy achieved by in-vitro fertilization is strongly correlated to the number of growing follicles in the treatment cycle. Human Reproduction 11: 2036–2040

Kristiansson P, Svärdsudd K, von Schoultz B 1996c Serum relaxin, symphyseal pain and back pain during pregnancy. American Journal of Obstetrics and Gynecology (in press)

MacLennan A H, Nicolson R, Green R C, Bath M 1986a Serum relaxin and pelvic pain of pregnancy. Lancet ii: 243–245

MacLennan A H, Green R C, Grant P, Nicolson R 1986b Ripening of the human cervix and induction of labor with intracervical purified porcine relaxin. Obstetrics and Gynecology 68: 598–601

Östgaard H C, Zetherström G, Roos-Hansson E, Svanberg B 1994 Reduction of back and posterior pelvic pain in pregnancy. Spine 19: 894–900

Petersen L K, Hvidman L, Uldbjerg N 1994 Normal serum relaxin in women with disabling pelvic pain during pregnancy. Gynecologic and Obstetric Investigation 38: 21–23

Putschar W G J 1976 The structure of the human symphysis pubis with special consideration of parturition and its sequelae. American Journal of Physical Anthropology 45: 589–594

Steinetz B G, O'Byrne E M, Butler M C, Hickman L B 1984 Hormonal regulation of the connective tissue of the symphysis pubis. In: Bigazzi M, Greenwood F C, Gasparri F (eds) Biology of relaxin and its role in the human. Excerpta Medica, Amsterdam, pp 71–92

Wahl L M, Blandau R J, Page R C 1977 Effect of hormones on collagen metabolism and collagenase activity in the pubic symphysis ligament of the guinea pig. Endocrinology 100: 571–579

35. Active straight leg raising test: a clinical approach to the load transfer function of the pelvic girdle

J. M. A. Mens   A. Vleeming   C. J. Snijders   H. J. Stam

INTRODUCTION

Pain in the lumbar spine and pelvic region frequently complicates pregnancy and delivery; the reported 9-month prevalence rate ranges between 48% and 56% (Berg et al 1988, Fast et al 1987, Mantle et al 1977, Östgaard et al 1991). In retrospective studies among young and middle-aged women with chronic low back pain, 10–28% state that their first episode of back pain occurred during a pregnancy (Biering-Sorensen 1983, Svensson et al 1990).

Hypotheses on pathogenesis focus on the changed load and the decreased stability of the pelvic girdle. Snijders et al (1993) describe the function of the pelvic girdle and lower spine in load transfer between trunk and leg. The idea that an increased lumbar lordosis is responsible for back pain during pregnancy is persistent (Fast et al 1987, 1990, Jacobson 1991, LaBan 1983), although lordosis during pregnancy is generally less than that post partum (Dumas et al 1993, Moore et al 1990, Snijders et al 1976).

It is obvious that weight gain from the fetus and uterus changes the load of the spine and pelvis. The increase in transverse and sagittal diameters of the abdomen (Östgaard et al 1993), the weight of the baby, and twin pregnancies (Mens et al 1996) are associated with the occurrence of pelvic girdle and low back pain. The weight gain of the mother during pregnancy seems not to be a risk factor (Fast et al 1987, Mantle et al 1977, Mens et al 1996, Saugstad 1991). Weakness of the oblique abdominal muscles and the changed direction in which they pull could interfere with their function as stabilizers of the pelvis (Snijders et al 1993).

Increase of movement of the sacroiliac joints

(SIJs) during pregnancy in an anatomic study (Brooke 1934), increased mobility and widening of the pubic symphysis (Abramson et al 1934, Heyman & Lundqvist 1932, Johanson & Järvinen 1957, Lynch 1920, Thoms 1936), and the gradual increase of pelvic pain during pregnancy (Kristiansson et al 1996, Mantle et al 1977, 1981, Mens et al 1996, Saugstad 1991) roughly parallel each other.

Increased mobility can be caused by hormones (Kristiansson 1995, MacLennan et al 1986), by weakening of the pelvic ligaments, as is the case in many animals (Sherwood 1988), or by increase of fluid in the SIJ (Lynch 1920, Sashin 1930).

Assessment of impairment of the pelvic joints frequently has been attempted in an objective way. Determination of mobility of the SIJ by palpation appears to be unreliable (Potter & Rothstein 1985). Tests based on the provocation of pain on mechanical stress have a high intertester reliability (Laslett & Williams 1994, Potter & Rothstein 1985), but the relationship of their outcome with instability is unclear (Dreyfuss et al 1994). In 1930 Chamberlain introduced a method to visualize radiographically the mobility of the SIJ (Chamberlain 1930). He described a higher position of the pubic symphysis at the weight-bearing side while standing on one leg. As far as we know, a correlation between this phenomenon and signs and symptoms has never been determined.

The existence of a Dutch 'Association for patients with pelvic complaints in relation to symphysiolysis' offered the opportunity to study a large number of patients with pelvic girdle pain. We noticed that in the supine position, active raising of one or both legs was weak in almost all of them. Many feel pain during active straight leg raising

(ASLR), but most patients feel as though they are paralysed. Because this sign was expected to be related to stress to the ligaments in the pelvis and/or lumbosacral junction, we investigated whether active raising could be influenced by approaches intended to change the position and/or mobility of the pelvic joints and lumbosacral junction. Jull et al (1993) use leg lifting as a standard load to investigate rotatory instability of the lumbar spine. As early as 1839, the Swedish gynecologist Cederschjöld reported 'an instantaneous relief in the pains and the ability to move the limbs when the hips are pressed hard together with the hands' (Genell 1949).

MATERIAL AND METHODS

Patients were selected from the outpatient clinic of the Institute of Rehabilitation Medicine of the University Hospital, Rotterdam. Included were non-pregnant women with pelvic girdle pain that started during pregnancy or within 3 weeks of delivery. Pelvic pain was defined as pain experienced between the plane through the four superior iliac spines and the transverse plane through the inferior border of the pubic symphysis. Pelvic girdle pain was defined as pelvic pain that was influenced by position and locomotion and localized to the posterior as well as at the anterior side of the pelvis.

The patients were asked what percentage of their pelvic girdle pain was felt at the worst side. Arbitrarily, 75% or more was classified as asymmetric pain.

The starting position for performing ASLR was a relaxed supine position with the legs straight passively in laterorotation and the feet 20 cm apart. The test was performed after the instruction 'Try to raise your legs, one after the other, above the couch for 5 cm without bending the knees'. Weakness was scored on a 4-point scale:

0 The patient feels no weakness and the examiner sees no abnormal pattern.
1 The patient feels weakness but the examiner sees no abnormal moving pattern.
2 The patient feels weakness and the examiner assesses that raising the leg causes difficulties.
3 There is inability to raise the leg.

Arbitrarily, a difference of 1 point or more between the left and right side was classified as asymmetric weakness.

Patients in our study were selected if pain and weakness were asymmetrically divided and both localized to the same side. We called this side the symptomatic side and the other the reference side.

Excluded from the study were patients with a fracture, neoplasm, inflammatory disease, or previous surgery of the lumbar spine or pelvis, and patients with signs indicating radiculopathy (asymmetric Achilles tendon reflex, hypesthesia in a radicular pattern, passive straight leg raising restricted by any pain before 45° or at any degree by pain in the lower leg).

The subject was asked whether the strength during ASLR changed (more, equal, or less) by the following modifications:

1. ASLR with the other hip passively flexed to 90°.
2. With the lower arm of the patient placed under the lumbar spine (the lower arm perpendicular to the trunk), with the intention of supporting lumbar lordosis.
3. ASLR with a pelvic belt just below the anterior superior iliac spines (ASISs) (high position).
4. ASLR with a pelvic belt at the level of the symphysis (low position).

A belt of non-elastic material was used (model 3221/3300 supplied by Rafys, Hengelo, The Netherlands) 5 cm wide at the anterior and 7 cm at the posterior side. The belt was fastened with Velcro so the tension could easily be adjusted. In a pilot study, we tested the minimum force needed. In most patients 50 N was sufficient to influence ASLR. Increased tension (up to 200 N) gave similar results to the 50 N tension. In loosening a tightly fixed belt, the effect generally disappeared suddenly between 20 and 50 N.

5. ASLR with the examiner's hand pushing on the ASIS of the symptomatic side in a medial as well as a cranial direction.
6. ASLR with the examiner's hand pushing on the contralateral ASIS. With a hand-held dynamometer (MicroFET, Hoggan Health Industries, Draper, Utah, USA), we measured the force applied. In most cases, 50 N was sufficient to influence ASLR.

7. With active rotation of the trunk in the direction of the raised leg in order to generate a contraction of the oblique abdominal muscles from cranial at the contralateral side to caudad at the ipsilateral side.

The instruction used was 'Try to reach with one hand in the direction of the knee at the other side as far as possible. Lift your shoulder and your head from the couch as far as possible, but take care that your other shoulder keeps in contact with the couch.

8. With active rotation of the trunk in the opposite direction by the same instruction at the other side.

X-rays in posteroanterior direction were made according to Chamberlain (1930). Tube film distance was 2 m. The patient was weight-bearing on one leg, alternately left and right, standing on a small bench, with the other leg hanging passively beside the bench. If the margins at the cranial side of the pubic bones were not in line with each other, the 'step' was measured in millimeters. A step with the reference side high was expressed as a positive value and with the symptomatic side high as negative. If both values were either positive or negative (see Table 35.2 below), or if the absolute value of the step was largest when the patient was standing on the symptomatic leg, an additional X-ray of the symphysis was taken in non-weight-bearing position (supine).

RESULTS

We report the results of the first 15 consecutive women who fulfilled the criteria. Their age ranged from 24 to 50 years, with a median of 32 years. Four women had one child, 11 had two or three children. The last delivery had occurred between 2.5 months and 25 years previously, with a median of 8 months. The percentage pain at the worst side was 75–100%, with a mean of 88.0%.

Eleven (73.3%) patients felt less strength during ASLR with the contralateral hip passively flexed (Table 35.1). Eight patients (53.3%) had more strength with a support of the lordosis by the lower arm (Table 35.1). With a belt, ASLR was more powerful in 12 patients (80.0%); half of them preferred the low position.

Table 35.1 Changes in strength during ASLR when performed with passive flexion of the contralateral hip (Hip flexion), with the lower arm placed under the lumbar spine (Lordosis), with a pelvic belt in the high position (Belt high) and in the low position (Belt low), with pressure of the examiner's hand on the ASIS at the ipsilateral side (Ipsilat pr), at the contralateral side (Contralat pr), with active trunk rotation in the direction of the leg that is raised (Ipsilat tr), and with active trunk rotation in the opposite direction (Contralat tr)

	Less strength (%)	Unchanged (%)	More strength (%)
Hip flexion	73.3	20.0	6.7
Lordosis	13.3	33.3	53.3
Belt high	0.0	40.0	60.0
Belt low	20.0	13.3	66.7
Ipsilat pr	0.0	6.7	93.3
Contralat pr	26.6	53.3	20.0
Ipsilat tr	20.0	20.0	60.0
Contralat tr	46.6	20.0	33.3

With pressure of the examiner's hand on the ipsilateral ASIS, ASLR was more powerful in all but one patient (Table 35.1). Pressure on the contralateral side did not influence the weakness in 8 patients, and resulted in an increase of weakness in 4. One patient had a preference for pressure of the examiner's hand on the reference side.

In 9 patients (60.0%), ASLR was less weak with contraction of the oblique abdominal muscles from cranial contralateral to caudad ipsilateral (Table 35.1). In 3 patients, this had no effect, and in 3 more weakness was noted. Three patients preferred ASLR with contraction of the abdominal muscles to caudad contralateral over contraction of the oblique abdominals to caudad ipsilateral.

Radiography

The measured malalignment of the upper margins of the pubic bones ranged between –6 and +7 mm (Table 35.2). The differences between the two X-rays at alternating one-leg standing ranged from 0 to 7 mm (mean 2.5 mm). The step standing on the leg at the reference side was on average +1.9 mm and at the symptomatic side –0.7 mm. In patients nos 5, 9, and 14, an additional X-ray was taken in the supine position without leg raising. In these patients, a step was seen in the non-weight-bearing situation (Table 35.2).

Table 35.2   Differences (in mm) between the heights of the upper margins of the pubic bones when standing on one leg, both at the reference side and at the symptomatic side

Patient	Step standing at reference side	Step standing at symptomatic side	Total shift	Step in supine position
1	+3	−1	4	
2	+2	0	2	
3	+3	−1	4	
4	+4	0	4	
5	0	−4	4	−3
6	+1	0	1	
7	+1	0	1	
8	+7	0	7	
9	+5	+2	3	+2
10	0	0	0	
11	0	0	0	
12	0	0	0	
13	0	0	0	
14	−1	−6	5	−6
15	+3	0	3	
Mean	+1.9	−0.7	2.5	

Positive value: step with the reference side high. Negative value: step with the reference side low.

DISCUSSION

It is not surprising that the approaches intended to change the position and/or mobility of the pelvic joints did not lead to identical results in each patient. Each approach has several effects, which might be contradictory on the strength of ASLR. For example, trunk rotation generates greater tension of the oblique abdominal muscles but goes together with flexion of the lumbar spine, and pressure at the ASIS fixes the pelvic bone at that side but is sometimes painful.

One of the most obvious reasons to explain weakness of ASLR is pathology of the hip flexor muscles. However, if this was the case in the patients described, the weakness should not have been influenced by, for example, pressure of the examiner's hand on the ASIS.

Neither is it a suitable explanation that weakness of ASLR is caused by increasing the lumbar lordosis: ASLR could be performed with the other leg with considerably less weakness; delordosing the lumbar spine by flexion of the other hip makes ASLR weaker in 73.3%, and lordosing the spine by a support strengthens ASLR in 53.3%. Several mechanisms may be responsible for the observation that increased lordosis goes together with increased strength in the majority of the patients. First, the mechanical relationship between lumbar spine and pelvis has to be explained.

During ASLR, the pelvic bone at the tested side has a tendency to rotate forward in relation to the rest of the pelvis and lumbar spine (DonTigny 1985). In the SIJ at the tested side, this causes (a tendency towards) counternutation. Subsequently, at the contralateral side, the sacrum has a tendency to rotate anteriorly in relation to the pelvic bone and generates (a tendency towards) nutation in the SIJ at that side. Moreover, owing to the weight of the lifted leg, the entire pelvis has a tendency to rotate during ASLR about a longitudinal axis in the direction of the lifted leg (Jull et al 1993). This causes a rotation at the lumbosacral junction in the opposite direction. The movements in the SIJ are linked by the iliolumbar ligaments to lumbosacral rotation in such a way that if lumbosacral rotation is restricted, the tendency to move in the SIJ is diminished, and vice versa. We propose calling this combination of movements 'lumbopelvic torsion'. It seems that stability of this system is necessary for an effective load transfer from spine to leg (Snijders et al 1993).

To consider unpleasant feelings during lumbopelvic torsion as being the cause of weakness during ASLR is compatible with the beneficial effect of the support of the lumbar lordosis, because of the influence of lordosis on axial rotation of the lumbar spine and on nutation–counternutation of the SIJ (Egund et al 1978,

Sturesson et al 1989, Weisl 1955). Passive flexion of the contralateral leg enhances lumbopelvic torsion by rotating the pelvic bone at that side backwards. Active trunk rotation in the direction of the leg that is raised stabilizes lumbopelvic torsion because the oblique abdominal muscular system pulls the pelvic bone into nutation and induces a rotation at the lumbosacral junction in the direction opposite to that during ASLR. Moreover, the tension in the oblique abdominal muscles enlarges intra-articular friction in the SIJ in the same way as a pelvic belt (Snijders et al 1993). A pelvic belt is a well-known stabilizer of the pelvic girdle (Abramson et al 1934, Berg et al 1988, Östgaard et al 1994, Thoms 1936, Vleeming et al 1992).

Table 35.2 shows that, in general, a step between the right and left pubic bones was larger standing on the leg of the reference side than of the symptomatic side. In some patients with a large displacement, X-rays were taken in the supine position during ASLR (Fig. 35.1). ASLR

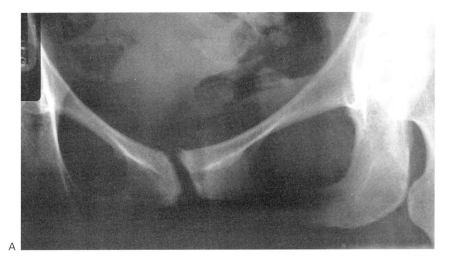

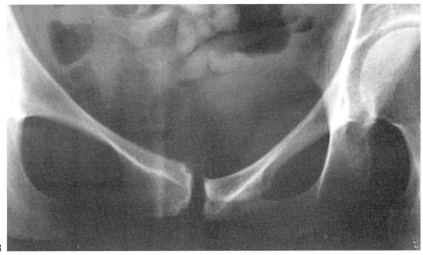

Fig. 35.1 X-rays during ASLR of a patient with a large displacement. (A) During ASLR of the right leg (reference side). (B) During ASLR of the left leg (symptomatic side). No malalignment of the pubic bones is seen during ASLR at the reference side. A step of about 5 mm is seen at the upper margins during ASLR on the symptomatic side. The projection of the left pubic bone is smaller than that of the right, indicating an anterior rotation of the left pelvic bone about an axis in the vicinity of the SIJ.

on the right side produced the same picture as standing at the left leg, and vice versa. Obviously, the pubic bone at the weight-bearing side is not displaced to cranial, as suggested by Chamberlain (1930), but the pubic bone at the non-weight-bearing side is forced inferiorly. Also the projection of the pubic bone at that side was smaller in a craniocaudad direction, so the pelvic bone was apparently rotated anteriorly. In patients nos 5, 9, and 14, an X-ray was taken in the supine position without ASLR. In each case, a step was seen. Little difference was seen between these X-rays and those standing on the symptomatic side. The step changed by 3–5 mm standing on the reference side. As a consequence, the step disappeared almost completely in patients 5 and 14. It seems that the value of the difference between the step in the non-weight-bearing situation and standing on one leg correlates better with the result of ASLR than do the size of the steps.

CONCLUSIONS

1. Decreased ability to perform ASLR correlates highly with the mobility of the pelvic joints as assessed by radiography.

2. In X-rays standing on one leg, symphyseal shear is not caused by a shift of the pubic bone at the weight-bearing side to cranial, but of the pubic bone at the non-weight-bearing side inferiorly.

3. ASLR seems to be a reliable test for the quality of the load transfer system between spine and leg. Weakness seems to be a key sign in patients with chronic pelvic girdle pain.

4. ASLR enables a better prediction of which measures will be helpful to treat chronic pelvic girdle pain. It is possible to test the usefulness of a pelvic belt, to evaluate what is the best position and the least needed tension. The results suggest that training of the oblique abdominals and enhancement of lordosis is beneficial in those patients.

5. In cases of weakness of the load transfer system between spine and leg, it is more logical to treat this weakness than just treat the resultant signs and symptoms by rest, medication, manipulation, etc.

6. Knowledge about understanding the mechanism of pelvic girdle pain is valuable for a better understanding of non-specific low back pain.

REFERENCES

Abramson D, Sumner M R, Wilson P D 1934 Relaxation of the pelvic joints in pregnancy. Surgery, Gynecology and Obstetrics 58: 595–613

Berg G, Hammar M, Möller-Nielsen J, Lindén U, Thorblad J 1988 Low back pain during pregnancy. Obstetrics and Gynecology 71: 71–75

Biering-Sorensen F A 1983 A prospective study of low back pain in a general population. I: Occurrence, recurrence and aetiology. Scandinavian Journal of Rehabilitation Medicine 15: 71–79

Brooke R 1934 Discussion on the physiology and pathology of the pelvic joints in relation to child-bearing. Proceedings of the Royal Society of Medicine 17: 1211–1217

Chamberlain W E 1930 The symphysis pubis in the roentgenexamination of the sacro-iliac joint. American Journal of Roentgenology and Radium Therapy 24: 621–625

DonTigny R L 1985 Function and pathomechanics of the sacroiliac joint. Physical Therapy 65: 35–44

Dreyfuss P, Dreyer S, Griffin J, Hoffman J, Walsh N 1994 Positive sacroiliac screening tests in asymptomatic adults. Spine 19: 1138–1143

Dumas G A, Reid J G, Wolfe L A 1993 Trunk posture and exercise during pregnancy. In: Eighth meeting of the European Society of Biomechanics, Rome, Italy, 1992. Abstracts. Journal of Biomechanics 26: 865

Egund N, Ollson T H, Schmid H, Selvic G 1978 Movements in the sacroiliac joints demonstrated with roentgen stereophotogrammetry. Acta Radiologica Diagnosis 19: 833–846

Fast A, Shapiro D, Ducommun E J, Friedmann L W, Bouklas T, Floman Y 1987 Low back pain in pregnancy. Spine 12: 368–371

Fast A, Weiss L, Ducommun E J, Medina E, Butler J G 1990 Low back pain in pregnancy. Abdominal muscles, sit-up performance, and back pain. Spine 15: 28–30

Genell S 1949 Studies on insufficientia pelvis (gravidarum et puerpartum). Acta Obstetricia et Gynecologica Scandinavica 28: 1–33

Heyman J, Lundqvist A 1932 The symphysis pubis in pregnancy and parturition. Acta Obstetricia et Gynecologica 12: 191–226

Jacobson H 1991 Protecting the back during pregnancy. American Association of Occupational Health Nursing Journal 39: 286–291

Johanson C E, Järvinen P A 1957 Factors affecting relaxation of the pelvis during normal pregnancy, delivery, and the puerperium. Acta Obstetricia et Gynecologica Scandinavica 36: 179–193

Jull G, Richardson C, Toppenberg R, Comerford M, Bui B 1993 Towards a measurement of active muscle control for lumbar stabilisation. Australian Journal of Physiotherapy 39: 187–193

Kristiansson P 1995 S-Relaxin – a marker for back pain during pregnancy. In: Vleeming A, Mooney V, Dorman T, Snijders C (eds) The integrated function of the lumbar spine and sacroiliac joint. ECO, Rotterdam

Kristiansson P, Svärdsudd K, von Schoultz B 1996 Back pain during pregnancy. A prospective study. Spine 21: 702–709

LaBan M M, Perrin J, Latimer F R 1983 Pregnancy and the herniated lumbar disc. Archives of Physical Medicine and Rehabilitation 64: 319–321

Laslett M, Williams M 1994 The reliability of selected pain provocation tests for sacroiliac joint pathology. Spine 19: 1243–1249

Lynch W F 1920 The pelvic articulations during pregnancy, labor, and the puerperium. Surgery, Gynecology and Obstetrics 30: 575–580

MacLennan A H, Nicolson R, Green R C, Bath M 1986 Serum relaxin and pelvic pain. Lancet 2: 243–245

Mantle M J, Greenwood R M, Currey H L F 1977 Backache in pregnancy. Rheumatology and Rehabilitation 16: 95–101

Mantle M J, Holmes J, Currey H L F 1981 Backache in pregnancy. II: Prophylactic influence of back care classes. Rheumatology and Rehabilitation 20: 227–232

Mens J M A, Vleeming A, Stoeckart R, Stam H J, Snijders C J 1996 Understanding peripartum pelvic pain implications of a patient survey. Spine 21: 1363–1370

Moore K, Dumas G A, Reid J G 1990 Postural changes associated with pregnancy and their relationship with low-back pain. Clinical Biomechanics 5: 169–174

Östgaard H C, Andersson G B J, Karlsson K 1991 Prevalence of back pain in pregnancy. Spine 16: 549–552

Östgaard H C, Andersson G B J, Schultz A B, Miller J A A 1993 Influence of some biomechanical factors on low-back pain in pregnancy. Spine 18: 61–65

Östgaard H C, Zetherström G, Roos-Hansson E, Svanberg B 1994 Reduction of back and posterior pelvic pain in pregnancy. Spine 19: 894–900

Potter N A, Rothstein J M 1985 Intertester reliability for selected clinical tests of the sacroiliac joint. Physical Therapy 65: 1671–1675

Sashin D 1930 A critical analysis of the anatomy and the pathological changes of the sacroiliac joints. Journal of Bone and Joint Surgery 12: 891–910

Saugstad L F 1991 Persistent pelvic pain and pelvic joint instability. European Journal of Obstetrics, Gynecology, and Reproductive Biology 41: 197–201

Sherwood O D 1988 Relaxin. In: Knobil E, Neill J, Ewing L L, Greenwald G S, Markert C L, Pfaff D W (eds) The physiology of reproduction. Raven Press, New York, pp 585–673

Snijders C J, Seroo J M, Snijder J G, Hoedt H T 1976 Change in form of the spine as a consequence of pregnancy. In: Digest of the 11th International Conference on Medical and Biological Engineering, Ottawa, 2–6 August, Abstract no 49.4

Snijders C J, Vleeming A, Stoeckart R 1993 Transfer of lumbo-sacral load to iliac bones and legs. I: Biomechanics of self-bracing of the sacro-iliac joints and its significance for treatment and exercise. Clinical Biomechanics 8: 285–294

Sturesson B, Selvic G, Uden A 1989 Movements of the sacroiliac joints. A roentgen stereophotogrammetric analysis. Spine 14: 162–165

Svensson H O, Andersson G B J, Hagstad A, Jansson P O 1990 The relationship of low-back pain to pregnancy and gynecologic factors. Spine 15: 371–375

Thoms H 1936 Relaxation of the symphysis pubis in pregnancy. Journal of the American Medical Association 106: 1364–1366

Vleeming A, Buyruk H M, Stoeckart R, Karamursel S, Snijders C J 1992 Towards an integrated therapy for peripartum pelvic instability: a study of the biomechanical effects of pelvic belts. American Journal of Obstetrics and Gynecology 166: 1243–1247

Weisl H 1995 The movements of the sacroiliac joints. Acta Anatomica 23: 80–91

Therapy

36. Behavioral analysis, fear of movement/(re)injury and behavioral rehabilitation in chronic low back pain

*J. W. S. Vlaeyen   A. M. J. Kole-Snijders   P. H. T. G. Heuts
H. van Eek*

INTRODUCTION

Chronic pain syndromes such as chronic low back pain are responsible for enormous costs for health care and society (Nachemson 1992). For these conditions, a pure biomedical approach often proves insufficient. Numerous studies have shown that there is little direct relationship between pain and disability (Waddell 1987) and suggest that the biopsychosocial approach offers the foundations of a better insight into how pain can become a persistent problem (Fordyce 1976, Turk et al 1983, Vlaeyen 1991). The main assumption is that pain and pain disability are not only influenced by organic pathology, if found, but also by biological, psychological, and social factors. As such, the distinction between somatogenic (real) and psychogenic (imaginary) pain is no longer considered relevant. In this chapter, the behavioral analysis of chronic pain will be discussed, special attention being paid to the role of fear in the development and maintenance of chronic pain disability, and the behavioral rehabilitation perspective of chronic pain management.

CHRONIC BACK PAIN AS A SOCIETAL PROBLEM

Many people suffer from low back pain in the course of their lives, of whom not all seek health care. In the majority of patients who seek care and refrain from work, the problem of pain resolves within a few weeks. Data presented by the Quebec Task Force on Spinal Disorders (Spitzer et al 1987) showed that 74% of the group of patients with acute back pain resumed work within 4 weeks of the onset of acute pain (Fig. 36.1). If a

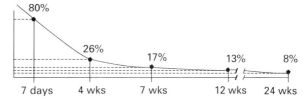

Fig. 36.1 The natural history of back pain. Percentage on sick leave in relation to pain duration since onset. (Based on Spitzer et al 1987; adapted with permission from Vlaeyen et al 1995b.)

person has not returned to work after 7 weeks, there is a 50% probability that he or she will still be off work at 6 months. About 8% of patients are still on sick leave 6 months after the onset of acute pain. Similar findings have been reported by Crook and Moldofsky (1994): if a worker has not returned to work by 3 months, there is a 50% probability that he or she will still be off work 15 months after onset.

The relatively small group of back pain patients who develop a chronic pain syndrome are responsible for 75–90% of the health-care and societal costs of back problems (Nachemson 1992). What are the reasons for this group becoming chronic pain sufferers? One possibility could be that these patients have more serious impairments than those who resume their daily activities earlier. However, no research supports this assumption. On the contrary, numerous studies have shown that there is no perfect relationship between impairment, pain and disability, and suggest that the behavioral or biopsychosocial approach offers the basis of a better insight into how pain can become a persistent problem (Fordyce 1976, Fordyce et al 1982, Turk et al 1983, Waddell 1987, Waddell et al 1984). The

435

main assumption is that pain and pain disability are influenced not only by organic pathology, if found, but also by psychological and social factors.

For example, from a biomedical view, a return to work should be encouraged only when the underlying pathology has healed, otherwise, the risks of reinjury and repeated failure would increase, subsequently leading to the enhancement of chronicity. From this biomedical perspective, staying off too long would be much safer than resuming work activities too early. Results reported by Crook and Moldofsky (1994), however, are in support of the conjecture that an early return to work contributes to a decrease (instead of an increase) in long-term work disability in musculoskeletal pain patients. Their arguments include the recognition that musculoskeletal incidents are increased by the immediate consequences, such as diminished pain, increased attention from others, avoidance of unpleasant and fearful situations, and the stabilization of the sick role. Moreover, longstanding avoidance leads to disuse of the musculature, which in turn augments the deficits in the necessary motor, social, and occupational skills. In other words, the pain disability is subject to a graded shift from structural/mechanical to cognitive/environmental control. Studies by Deyo et al (1986), Philips and Grant (1991), and Klenerman et al (1995) suggest that this shift occurs quite rapidly, probably within 4–8 weeks of the onset of acute pain.

BEHAVIORAL ANALYSIS

Today, pain is defined as not only a sensory experience, but also an emotional one. The International Association for the Study of Pain (1986) have proposed the following definition of pain: 'An unpleasant sensory and emotional experience associated with actual or potential tissue damage, or described in terms of such damage'. Within the behavioral sciences, the three-systems model of emotions has received considerable attention. According to this model, emotions are always subjective and never observable in themselves. They can only be inferred by their effects at some observable level (Öhman 1987). Likewise, (chronic) pain can best be approached as a hypothetical construct, but one which can be inferred

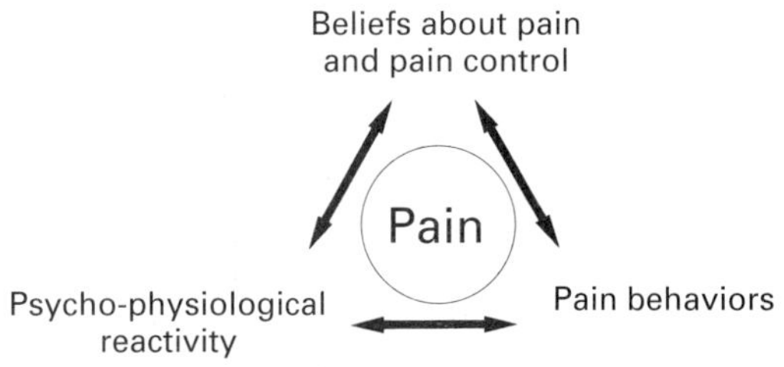

Fig. 36.2   Pain as a hypothetical construct that can only be inferred by observable psychophysiological reactivity, pain cognitions and pain behaviors. (Based on Öhman 1987 and Vlaeyen 1991.)

by at least three partially independent response systems: psychophysiological reactivity, beliefs about pain and pain control, and overt pain behaviors (Vlaeyen et al 1989) (Fig. 36.2).

Psychophysiological reactivity

When confronted with a stressor, an individual will respond automatically with an increase in sympathetic arousal. Evidence exists that patients with low back pain display elevations in paraspinal electromyographic activity and a delayed return to baseline following exposure to personally relevant and not just general stressors (Flor et al 1990). Increased sympathetic arousal to pain or psychosocial stressors may contribute to a reduced ability to tolerate pain, and subsequently to functional limitations and pain disability (Feuerstein 1991).

Beliefs about pain and pain control

Cognitive responses refer to the way in which the patient perceives and interprets his or her environment, and the extent to which he or she thinks that control can be exerted over the situation. One of the possible attributions is that pain is a sign of a serious health problem; this has been referred to as 'illness (or disease) conviction' (Pilowski 1994). Such an appraisal may be based on a misinterpretation of proprioceptive signals (Cioffi 1991). Moreover, there are reasons to believe that in chronic low back pain patients, a selective attention exists towards these proprioceptive signals, as a result of which they are more easily noticed and interpreted as 'dangerous' or 'signalling (re)injury'. An important consequence of this selective attention is somatic amplification and an increase in experienced pain intensity (Arntz et al 1991). In some chronic low back pain patients, the selective attention may extend towards an exaggeration of negative aspects of their situation in general. This more general appraisal process is referred to as 'catastrophizing' and is known to be associated with increasing distress. Distress symptoms can, in turn, increase pain by reducing pain tolerance levels and by triggering unnecessary sympathetic arousal (Ciccone & Grzesiak 1984).

Overt pain behaviors

Observable gross motor behaviors exhibited by pain patients are referred to in the literature as 'pain behaviors' (Fordyce 1976). Common examples of pain behaviors are verbal and non-verbal expressions, such as grimacing, lying down, using supportive devices, and complaining about pain, which communicate suffering to the social environment. Fordyce not only introduced the concept of pain behaviors, but also applied the operant conditioning principle to pain. When pain behavior is expressed by a patient, desirable things can happen (*positive reinforcement*) and unpleasant situations can be avoided (*avoidance learning*). By means of these environmental influences, pain disability can be maintained long after healing has occurred. The terms 'secondary gain' and 'tertiary gain' are sometimes used in this context. Secondary gain refers to the positive consequences that the patient experiences when pain is communicated through these pain behaviors. Tertiary gain refers to the positive consequences that the spouse or other family members experience because of the pain problem.

AVOIDANCE LEARNING AND FEAR

In 1982 Fordyce et al described how pain behavior may also result from avoidance learning, which has been classified under operant conditioning. Avoidance refers to 'the performance of a behaviour which postpones or averts the presentation of an aversive event' (Kazdin 1980). Avoidance learning has long been considered to underlie the formation of many so-called 'neurotic' symptoms (Kanfer & Philips 1970). In the case of pain, a patient may no longer perform certain activities because he or she anticipates that these activities increase pain and suffering. In the acute phase, avoidance behaviors such as resting, limping or the use of supportive equipment are effective in reducing suffering from nociception. Later on, these protective pain and illness behaviors may persist in anticipation of pain, instead of as a response to it. Longlasting avoidance of motor activities can have detrimental consequences, both physically (loss of mobility, muscle strength, and fitness, possibly resulting in the 'disuse syndrome'; Bortz 1984) and psychologically (loss of self-esteem, deprivation of reinforcers, depression, and somatic preoccupation). Philips and Jahanshahi (1986) found that, in a group of headache sufferers, avoidance was the most prominent behavior reported by these individuals. In their study, avoidance was not limited to avoidance of movement, but also withdrawal from social situations.

Philips (1987) argues in favor of a cognitive theory of avoidance behavior, rather than the operant theory. She takes the view that avoidance is influenced by the expectancy that further exposure to certain stimuli will promote pain and suffering. This expectancy is assumed to be based on previous aversive experiences in the same or similar situations. Philips also points to the similarities between the avoidance behavior displayed by pain patients and that by patients with phobias, and suggests that 'chronic pain and chronic fear – both aversive experiences which result in avoidance behavior – may share important characteristics' (Philips 1987, p 277). Recent studies have focused on the relationship between fear/anxiety and chronic pain, of which the object of fear has been fear of pain (Lethem et al 1983, McCracken et al 1992, 1993), fear of work-related activities (Waddell et al 1993) and fear of movement that is assumed to cause (re)injury (Crombez 1994, Kole-Snijders et al 1993, Kori et al 1990).

Fear of pain

In an attempt to explain how and why some individuals develop a chronic pain syndrome, Lethem et al (1983) introduced their 'fear-avoidance' model. The central concept of this model is fear of pain. 'Confrontation' and 'avoidance' are postulated as the two extreme responses to this fear, the former leading to the reduction of fear over time. The latter, however, leads to the maintenance or exacerbation of fear, possibly leading to a phobic-like state. The avoidance results in the reduction of both social and physical activities, which in turn leads to a number of physical and psychological consequences augmenting the disability.

In 1992 the Pain Anxiety Symptoms Scale (PASS; McCracken et al 1992) was developed to measure cognitive, physiologic, and motor aspects of fear of pain. The authors found correlations with measures of anxiety, cognitive errors, depression, and disability. In a second study (McCracken et al 1993), the authors showed that, in a group of CLBP patients, greater pain-related anxiety was associated with higher predictions of pain and less range of motion during a procedure involving a passive but painful straight leg raising test.

Fear of work-related activities

Chronic low back pain patients may fear not only pain, but also activities that are expected to cause pain. In this case, fear is hypothesized to generalize to other situations that are closely linked to the feared stimulus. Vlaeyen (1991) found that a group of 50 chronic low back pain patients had mean elevated scores that were clinically significant on the 'social phobia' and 'agoraphobia' scales of the Fear Survey Schedule (FSS-III; Arrindell et al 1990; Wolpe & Lang 1964).

More specifically, Waddell et al (1993) developed the Fear-Avoidance Beliefs Questionnaire (FABQ), focusing on the patient's beliefs about how work and physical activity affect his or her low back pain. The FABQ consists of two scales – fear-avoidance beliefs of physical activity and fear-avoidance beliefs of work – of which the latter was consistently the stronger. The authors found that fear-avoidance beliefs about work were strongly related to disability of daily living and work lost in the past year, more so than were biomedical variables such as the anatomic pattern of pain, its time pattern, and the severity of the pain.

Fear of movement/(re)injury

A more specific fear is fear of movement and physical activity that is (wrongfully) assumed to cause reinjury. In the above-mentioned study of Vlaeyen (1991), the same group of chronic low back pain patients scored clinically significant on the scale 'fear of bodily injury, death and illness' of the FSS-III (Wolpe & Lang 1964). Kori et al (1990) introduced the term 'kinesiophobia' (kinesis = movement) for the condition in which a patient has 'an excessive, irrational, and debilitating fear of physical movement and activity resulting from a feeling of vulnerability to painful injury or reinjury'. In accordance with Lethem et al (1983), Crombez (1994) empirically derived subgroups of 'avoiders' and 'confronters' from a sample of chronic low back pain patients. Although there were no differences found in gender, age, number of occasions of back surgery, use of medication, and reported pain intensity, 'avoiders' reported significantly more fear of pain and fear of injury than did confronters. When exposed to a maximal performance test (flexion and extension of the knee), confronters showed a significantly better performance than did avoiders.

Although fear of movement/(re)injury might well be an important predictor of pain disability in people with chronic low back pain, almost no empirical data confirming this hypothesis are currently available. In a recent study, Vlaeyen et al (1995a) took motor, psychophysiologic and self-report measures of fear from 33 chronic low back pain patients who were exposed to a single and relatively simple movement (to lift a 5.5 kg bag and hold it as long as possible). They demonstrated that the fear of movement/(re)injury was more prominent in males and in patients who received disability compensation. Fear of movement/(re)injury appeared to be closely related to measures of catastrophizing and depression, and, to a much lesser degree, to pain coping and pain intensity. Furthermore, subjects who reported a high degree of fear of movement/(re)injury showed more fear and stopped lifting the bag significantly sooner. In a subsequent study, using hierarchical regression analyses, the same researchers demonstrated that pain disability, as measured with the Roland Disability Questionnaire (Roland & Morris 1983), was best predicted by fear of movement/(re)injury, which was in turn best predicted by the level of catastrophizing. Socio-demographics, pain intensity levels, and biomedical status were also entered into the analyses but failed to appear in the regression equation (Vlaeyen et al 1995b).

These studies, as do the studies by Rose et al (1992) and Waddell et al (1993), provide support for the validity of the fear-avoidance concept. It should be noted, however, that these are cross-sectional in nature, leaving the question of whether fear of movement/(re)injury is secondary to the experience of low back pain or whether it is one of the determinants of becoming a chronic pain patient. The recent prospective study by Klenerman et al (1995) provides support for the latter. They collected both psychologic and biomedical measures from a sample of 300 acute low back pain patients within 1 week of presentation, and at 2 months, in order to predict 12 month outcome. The data showed that subjects who had not recovered by 2 months (7.3%) became chronic low back pain patients. Moreover, fear of pain turned out to be one of the most powerful predictors of chronicity.

Fear of movement/(re)injury is likely to influence patterns of performance of workers with low back pain in an occupational setting. Clinicians are often requested to make judgements about the present and future functional capacity of patients on the basis of dynamometry. The assumption hereby is that lumbar (isokinetic) dynamometry provides objective and unbiased measures, and that it can quantify maximal functional capacity. Menard et al (1994), for example, found a difference in the pattern of dynamometry in two groups of low back pain patients who differed only in the propensity of abnormal illness behavior (as indicated by the Waddell score), and proposed that fear of pain of movement might be one of the possible explanations. The plausability of this explanation is corroborated by earlier studies (Crombez 1994, Vlaeyen et al 1995a) in which a relationship between fear of movement/(re)injury and behavioral performance is demonstrated. This means that a valid assessment of functional capacity cannot be carried out without controlling for fear-avoidance beliefs.

Based on the findings of recent studies, a biopsychosocial model is tentatively suggested (Fig. 36.3) that represents how fear of movement/(re)injury possibly contributes to the maintenance of chronic pain disability, starting with the injury occurring during the acute phase. The painful experiences, which are intensified during movement, will elicit catastrophizing cognitions in some individuals and more adaptive cognitions in others. Patients who catastrophize are more likely to be fearful. Fear of movement/(re)injury subsequently leads to increased avoidance and, in the long term, to disuse, depression, and increased disability (Council et al 1988, Philips 1987). Both depression and disuse are known to be associated with decreasing pain tolerance levels (McQuade et al 1988, Romano & Turner 1985), hence promoting the painful experience. In addition to the avoidance

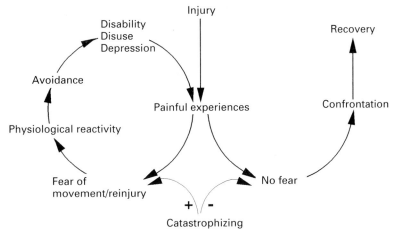

Fig. 36.3 Fear of movement/(re)injury as a determinant of chronic pain disability. (Adapted with permission from Vlaeyen et al 1995b.)

of fearful activities, pain disability may also persist because of the immediate consequences to which it leads, such as diminished pain, increased attention from others, and the avoidance of social conflicts or responsibilities. In patients likely to adapt, confrontation rather than avoidance is likely to occur, promoting health behaviors and early recovery. Future studies are needed to test the causality assumed in this model.

BEHAVIORAL REHABILITATION

The model outlined in Fig. 36.3 suggests that pain disability is subject to a graded shift from structural/mechanical to cognitive/environmental control. Consequently, the treatment of chronic low back pain is primarily focused not on removing an underlying organic pathology, but on the reduction of disability through the modification of environmental contingencies and cognitive processes. Behavioral rehabilitation is based on the biobehavioral model and integrates behavioral science and rehabilitation medicine. It deals with the application of cognitive–behavioral treatment programs in a rehabilitation center setting. Patients are given the opportunity to learn skills through graded training adapted to their physical status.

According to the three-systems model of emotions, a distinction can be made between treatment modalities that aim at the modification of the individual response system. Operant treatments are aimed at diminishing pain behaviors and augmenting activity levels through operant conditioning principles. Cognitive treatments have as their point of application beliefs about pain and pain control, while during respondent treatments patients learn relaxation skills and how to apply them in personally relevant stressful situations.

Operant treatments

Operant treatment is aimed at modifying the motor response system. The general goal of the treatment is to increase healthy behaviors and activity levels, and to decrease pain behaviors and excess disability. Variants of the programs are described by Fordyce (1976) and Roberts (1986). An operant treatment is not primarily aimed at

reducing self-reported pain intensity levels. Essential for this kind of intervention is the graded exposure to physical activities or work as treatment, in spite of pain. Also important is the reinforcement of healthy behaviors to prevent adaptation to the sick role. Variants of the operant treatment are called 'work hardening' (Matheson 1991) or 'graded activity programs' (Lindström et al 1992).

The program always starts with a number of baseline trials in which the patient exercises to the limit of tolerance. The therapist then sets a quota of exercises to be performed each session. Initial quota are lower than baseline levels, but they are increased systematically towards a preset goal. In situations where patients are not able actually to perform certain activities, shaping procedures can be applied during which the activities are relearned. For example, Vlaeyen et al (1990) developed a behavioral shaping program for a low back pain patient with sitting and standing intolerance. In contrast with the traditional medical approach, the patient exercises to the schedule (the patient rests after a certain amount of exercise has been performed) and not to tolerance level (the patient rests when the pain increases). This approach is different from that of the 'back schools' in that the latter rely primarily on providing information, while the operant approach provides the opportunity for the patient to experience that it is safe to move even when increasing his or her activity level. It is far more convincing for patients, especially fearful ones, actually to see themselves behaving differently than it is to be told that they are *capable of* behaving differently (Bandura 1977). An important component is the partner group instruction, during which partners are taught to recognize the difference between pain behavior and healthy behavior, to be more aware of their own responses towards these behaviors, and to attend more to healthy behaviors than to pain behaviors. Partner involvement facilitates generalization of change towards the home setting.

Cognitive treatment

Although there is no one cognitive therapy, common to all cognitive therapies is the modification of thoughts, feelings, and beliefs (Holzman & Turk 1986). In the cognitive group treatment described by Vlaeyen (1991), three phases can be distinguished: a reconceptualization phase, a skills acquisition phase, and a generalization phase.

The goal of the reconceptualization phase is to recast the pain experience in terms that imply self-control and resourcefulness.

In the skills acquisition phase, the patient exercises two types of imagery: imaginative transformation of the pain sensation and pain-incompatible sensory imagery. These techniques have been drawn from Diamond (1977) and Fernandez (1986). At the end of each session, patients are supplied with texts to read or a tape to listen to at least once a day.

During the generalization phase, the patients are asked to evaluate the different exercises. This information is then used to design an individually tailored audiotape, which the patient can use after discharge. Throughout the program, patients are given homework assignments after each session. These consist of brief, relevant reading assignments and audiotaped practice exercises based on the techniques taught during the sessions.

Respondent treatment

Respondent treatments are aimed at directly modifying psychophysiological reactivity and at teaching patients the skills necessary to respond with a relaxation response rather than with increased arousal when confronted by a personally relevant stressor. A convenient way to achieve this goal is by using the applied relaxation technique (APR; Öst 1988), possibly supported by electromyograph (EMG) biofeedback. The EMG feedback is basically employed to help patients recognize muscle tension and relaxation.

Here too, three phases can be distinguished. In the reconceptualization phase, the role of muscle tension in the maintenance of the pain problem is highlighted. By means of EMG-biofeedback, the patient is encouraged to identify tension-eliciting stimuli and to differentiate between muscle tension and relaxation. During the skills acquisition phase, the patient is taught the relaxation response according to the APR. During the generalization phase, the patient is gradually exposed to tension-eliciting stimuli and concomitantly encouraged to use the relaxation skills. As in the cognitive treat-

ment, patients attending the respondent treatment are also given homework assignments each session.

Extensive reviews on the effectiveness of these behavioral approaches to chronic low back pain include those reported by Turner and Chapman (1982), Linton (1986), Cohen et al (1989), and Vlaeyen et al (1995c). The overall conclusion is that operant treatment programs appear to increase physical activity levels and decrease pain behaviors, including medication intake. Initially, operant treatment programs were offered in the controlled environment of the hospital. Most of the recent studies have selected mildly disabled patients, for whom outpatient treatments appear suitable. Nicholas et al (1991, 1992) have demonstrated that an outpatient behavioral treatment can also be provided to moderately disabled people. Integration of the cognitive and operant treatments has been found to result in greater gains than when patients are offered operant treatments alone.

CONCLUSIONS

1. As other emotional experiences, pain is never directly observable in itself but can only be inferred through three observable response systems: psychophysiological reactivity, overt pain behaviors, and pain cognitions. Typical of emotional experiences, these response systems are loosely coupled and partially independent. This means that the everyday practice of considering pain to be identical to what is verbally reported must be rejected in a scientific analysis. Pain disability is a form of pain behavior, which, we must realize, is constantly being influenced by environmental consequences. Behavioral analysis specifies the causes of pain behaviors in terms of explicit environmental events that can be objectively identified and are potentially manipulable.

2. From a biopsychosocial perspective, the factors maintaining the pain problem can be quite different from those that initiated it. Pain disability is subject to a graded shift from structural/mechanical to cognitive/environmental control. This shift occurs quite rapidly, probably within 4–8 weeks. Similarly, the presence of demonstrable biomedical findings does not guarantee that psychological or social factors do not contribute to the level of pain disability.

3. Avoidance behavior is postulated to be one of the mechanisms in sustaining chronic pain disability. In the acute pain situation, avoidance of daily activities that increase pain is a spontaneous and adaptive reaction of the individual (Wall 1979); it usually allows the healing process to occur. In chronic pain patients, however, avoidance behavior appears to persist beyond the expected healing time and may subsequently lead to the 'disuse' syndrome (Bortz 1984). This is a detrimental condition, associated with physical deconditioning, in which performance of physical activities leads more easily to pain and physical discomfort, which in turn makes avoidance more likely. Avoidance may also lead to adaptation to a non-working status and a lack of work identity, making it more difficult for the patient to return to work or domestic activities. One of the reasons that avoidance behaviors persist is not the short-term effects of reduced suffering but the influence of certain beliefs and expectations (Philips 1987). If the individual believes that further exposure to certain stimuli will increase pain, harm, and suffering, avoidance or escape will probably occur.

4. Behavioral rehabilitation approaches are not set up to remove pain, nor to teach patients how to be more stoic or let them believe that it is all in their mind. The aim is to decrease pain disability levels and to provide patients with the opportunity to learn and practice skills to cope better with pain. For this, behavioral and biomedical sciences are integrated in a transdisciplinary working model, characterized by active patient participation. These approaches are promising and merit outcome research, including cost-effectiveness analyses.

5. Early identification of cognitive factors such as catastrophizing and fear of movement/(re)injury appears to be important in preventing chronic back disability. For this subgroup, a specific treatment might be applied. We know that for individuals suffering from phobias, graded exposure to the feared stimulus has proved to be a most effective treatment (e.g. Butler 1989). Consequently, for this chronic low back pain subgroup, a more systematic application of graded exposure to movement, such as described by Fordyce et al (1982) and Lindström et al (1992), is warranted. The movements that are chosen for such an exposure can best be matched with the work-related activities needed to resume the patient's job responsibilities. Randomized prospective research studies, including cost-effectiveness analyses, demonstrating the impact of such a customized approach are likely to be promising and are badly needed.

6. The available knowledge gained, both in the prediction of disability and in developing behavioral rehabilitation programs, should be applied to the field of secondary prevention (Linton 1987). Waiting until pain problems have fully developed into chronic and almost irreversible situations is ethically and economically unjustifiable.

REFERENCES

Arntz A R, Dreesen L, Merckelbach H 1991 Attention, not anxiety, influences pain. Behaviour Research Therapy 29: 41–50
Arrindell W A, Solyom C, Ledwidge B et al 1990 Cross-national validity of the five-components model of self-assessed fears: Canadian psychiatric outpatients data vs Dutch target ratings on the Fear Survey Schedule-III. Advances in Behaviour Research and Therapy 12: 101–122
Bandura A 1977 Self-efficacy: toward a unifying theory of behavioral change. Psychological Review 84: 191–215
Bortz W M 1984 The disuse syndrome. Western Journal of Medicine 141: 691–694
Butler G 1989 Phobic disorders. In: Hawton K, Salkovskis P M, Kirk J (eds) Cognitive behaviour therapy for psychiatric problems. A practical guide. Oxford Medical Publications, Oxford, pp 97–128
Ciccone D S, Grzesiak R C 1984 Cognitive dimensions of chronic pain. Social Sciences in Medicine 12: 1339–1345
Cioffi D 1991 Beyond attentional strategies: a cognitive–perceptual model of somatic interpretation. Psychological Bulletin 109: 25–41
Cohen M J, Naliboff B D, McArthur D L 1989 Implications of medical and biopsychosocial models for understanding and treating chronic pain. Critical reviews in Physical and Rehabilitation Medicine 3: 135–160
Council J R, Ahern D K, Follick M J, Kline C L 1988 Expectancies and functional impairment in chronic low back pain. Pain 33: 323–331
Crombez G 1994 Pijnmodulatie door anticipatie [Pain modulation through anticipation]. Doctoral dissertation, University of Leuven, Belgium
Crook J, Moldofsky H 1994 The probability of recovery and return to work from work disability as a function of time. Quality of Life Research 3 (supplement 1): 97–109
Deyo R, Diehl A, Rosenthal M 1986 How many days of bed rest for acute low back pain? New England Journal of Medicine 315: 1064–1070
Diamond M J 1977 Hypnotizability is modifiable: an alternative approach. International Journal of Clinical and Experimental Hypnosis 25: 147–166
Fernandez E 1986 A classification system of cognitive coping strategies for pain. Pain 26: 141–152

Feuerstein M 1991 A multidisciplinary approach to the prevention, evaluation, and management of work disability. Journal of Occupational Rehabilitation 1: 5–12

Flor H, Birbaumer N, Turk D C 1990 The psychobiology of chronic pain. Advances in Behaviour Research and Therapy 121: 47–84

Fordyce W E 1976 Behavioural methods for chronic pain and illness. CV Mosby, St Louis

Fordyce W E, Shelton J L, Dundore D E 1982 The modification of avoidance learning in pain behaviours. Journal of Behavioural Medicine 5: 405–414

Holzman A D, Turk D C 1986 Pain management, a handbook of psychological treatment approaches. Pergamon Press, New York

International Association for the Study of Pain, Subcommittee on Taxonomy 1986 Classification of chronic pain, descriptions, descriptions of pain syndromes and definitions of pain terms. Pain (supplement) 3: 1–225

Kanfer F H, Phillips J S 1970 Learning foundations of behavior therapy. John Wiley & Sons, New York

Kazdin A E 1980 Behaviour modification in applied settings, (revd edn). Dorsey Press, Homewood, IL

Klenerman L, Slade P D, Stanley I M et al 1995 The prediction of chronicity in patients with an acute attack of low back pain in a general practice setting. Spine 4: 478–484

Kole-Snijders A M J, Vlaeyen J W S, Boeren R G B, Schuerman J A, van Eek H 1993 Validity of the Tampa Scale for kinesiophobia – Dutch version (TSK-DV) for chronic low back pain patients. Paper presented at the 7th World Congress on Pain, Paris

Kori S H, Miller R P, Todd D D 1990 Kinisophobia: a new view of chronic pain behaviour. Pain Management Jan/Feb: 35–43

Lethem J, Slade P D, Troup J D G, Bentley G 1983 Outline of a fear-avoidance model of exaggerated pain perceptions. Behaviour Research and Therapy 21: 401–408

Lindström I, Öhlund C, Eek C et al 1992 The effect of graded activity on patients with sub-acute low back pain: a randomized prospective clinical study with an operant conditioning behavioural approach. Physical Therapy 72: 279–290

Linton S J 1986 Behavioural remediation of chronic pain: a status report. Pain 24: 125–141

Linton S J 1987 Chronic pain: the case for prevention. Behaviour Research and Therapy 4: 313–317

McCracken L M, Gross R T, Sorg P J, Edmands T A 1993 Prediction of pain in patients with chronic low back pain: effects of inaccurate prediction and pain-related anxiety. Behaviour Research and Therapy 31: 647–652

McCracken L M, Zayfert C, Gross R T 1992 The Pain Anxiety Symptoms Scale: development and validation of a scale to measure fear of pain. Pain 50: 67–73

McCracken L M, Gross R T 1993 Does anxiety affect coping with pain? Clinical Journal of Pain 9: 253–259

McQuade K J, Turner J A, Buchner D M 1988 Physical fitness and chronic low back pain. Clinical Orthopaedics and Related Reseach 233: 198–204

Matheson L N 1991 Integrated work hardening. In: Mayer T G, Mooney V, Gatchel R J (eds) Contemporary conservative care for painful spinal disorders. Lea & Febiger, Philadelphia, pp 346–363

Menard M R, Cooke C, Locke S R, Beach G N, Butler T B 1994 Pattern of performance in workers with low back pain during a comprehensive motor performance evaluation. Spine 2: 1359–1366

Nachemson A L 1992 Newest knowledge of low back pain. Clinical Orthopaedics 279: 8–20

Nicholas M K, Wilson, P H, Goyen J 1991 Comparison of cognitive–behavioural group treatment and an alternative non-psychological treatment for chronic low back pain. Pain 48: 339–347

Nicholas M K, Wilson, P H, Goyen J 1992 Operant–behavioural and cognitive–behavioural treatment for chronic low back pain. Behaviour Research and Therapy 29: 225–238

Öhman A 1987 The psychophysiology of emotion: an evolutionary-cognitive perspective. Advances in Psychophysiology 2: 79–127

Öst L G 1988 Applied relaxation: description of an effective coping technique. Scandinavian Journal of Behaviour Therapy 17: 83–96

Philips H C 1987 Avoidance behaviour and its role in sustaining chronic pain. Behaviour Research and Therapy 25: 273–279

Philips H C, Grant L 1991 The prevention of chronic pain and disability: a preliminary investigation. Behaviour Research and Therapy 29: 443–450

Philips H C, Jahanshahi M 1986 The components of pain behaviour report. Behaviour Research and Therapy 24: 117–125

Pilowsky I 1994 Pain and illness behaviour: assessment and management. In: Wall P D, Melzack R (eds) Textbook of pain. Churchill Livingstone, Edinburgh, pp 1309–1320

Roberts A H 1986 The operant approach to the management of pain and excess disability. In: Holzman A D, Turk D C (eds) Pain management. A handbook of psychological treatment approaches. Pergamon Press, New York, pp 10–30

Roland M, Morris R 1983 A study of the natural history of back pain. I: Development of a reliable and sensitive measure of disability in low back pain. Spine 8: 141–144

Romano J M, Turner J A 1985 Chronic pain and depression. Does the evidence support a relationship? Psychological Bulletin 97: 18–34

Rose M, Klenerman L, Atchinson L, Slade P D 1992 An application of the fear-avoidance model to three chronic pain problems. Behaviour Research and Therapy 30: 359–365

Spitzer W O, LeBlanc F E, Dupuis M et al 1987 Scientific approach to the assessment and management of activity-related spinal disorders: report of the Quebec task Force on Spinal Disorders. Spine 12 (supplement 7): S1–S59

Turk D C, Meichenbaum D, Genest M 1983 Pain and behavioural medicine. A cognitive–behavioural perspective. Guilford Press, New York

Turner J A, Chapman, C R 1982 Psychological interventions for chronic pain: a critical review. II: operant conditioning, hypnosis, and cognitive–behavioural therapy. Pain 12: 23–46

Vlaeyen J W S 1991 Chronic low back pain. Assessment and treatment from a behavioural rehabilitation perspective. Doctoral dissertation, University of Limburg, Maastricht, The Netherlands

Vlaeyen J W S, Snijders A M J, Schuerman J A, van Eek H, Groenman N H, Bremer J J C B 1989 Chronic pain and the three-systems model of emotions. A critical examination. Critical Reviews in Physical and Rehabilitation Medicine 2: 67–76

Vlaeyen J W S, Groenman N H, Thomassen J et al 1990 A behavioural treatment for sitting and standing intolerance in a patient with chronic low back pain. Clinical Journal of Pain 5: 233–237

Vlaeyen J W S, Kole-Snijders A M J, Boeren R G B, van Eek H 1995a Fear of movement/(re)injury in chronic low back pain and its relation to behavioural performance. Pain 62: 363–372

Vlaeyen J W S, Kole-Snijders A M J, Rotteveel A R, Ruesink R, Heuts P H T G 1995b The role of fear of movement/(re)injury in pain disability. Journal of Occupational Rehabilitation 5: 235–252

Vlaeyen J W S, Haazen I W C J, Kole-Snijders A M J, van Eek H, Schuerman J A 1995c Behavioural rehabilitation of chronic low back pain: comparison of an operant, an operant–cognitive and an operant–respondent treatment.

British Journal of Clinical Psychology 34: 95–118

Waddell G 1987 A new clinical model for the treatment of low back pain. Spine 12: 632–644

Waddell G, Main C J, Morris E W, DiPaola M P, Gray I C M 1984 Chronic low back pain, psychologic distress and illness behaviour. Spine 9: 209–213

Waddell G, Newton M, Henderson I, Somerville D, Main C 1993 A Fear-Avoidance Beliefs Questionnaire (FABQ) and the role of fear-avoidance beliefs in chronic low back pain and disability. Pain 52: 157–168

Wall P D 1979 On the relation of injury to pain. Pain 6: 253–264

Wolpe J, Lang P J 1964 A fear schedule for use in behaviour therapy. Behaviour Research and Therapy 2: 27–30

37. Treatment of pelvic instability

D. Lee

INTRODUCTION

Instability of the lumbar spine and pelvic girdle is recognized as a significant contributor to low back pain (Panjabi 1992, Richardson & Jull 1995, Schneider 1995, Vleeming et al 1995a). Instability can be defined as a loss of the functional integrity of a system that provides stability. In the pelvic girdle, there are two systems that contribute to stability: the osteoarticularligamentous and the myofascial. Vleeming and Snijders (Snijders et al 1992, Vleeming et al 1990a, 1990b, 1995a) refer to these two systems as 'form closure' and 'force closure'. Together they provide a self-locking mechanism that is extremely useful in rehabilitation.

'Form closure refers to a stable situation with closely fitting joint surfaces, where no extra forces are needed to maintain the state of the system' (Snijders et al 1992, Vleeming et al 1990b, 1995a). The degree of inherent form closure of any joint is dependent on its anatomy. There are three factors that contribute to form closure: the shape of the joint surface, the friction coefficient of the articular cartilage, and the integrity of the ligaments that approximate the joint.

The shape of the sacroiliac joint (SIJ) is highly variable both between and within individuals. In the skeletally mature, S1, S2, and S3 contribute to the formation of the sacral surface, and each part can be oriented in a different vertical plane. In addition, the sacrum is wedged anteroposteriorly. These factors provide resistance to both vertical and horizontal translation. In the young, the wedging is incomplete such that the SIJ is planar at all three levels and is vulnerable to shear forces until ossification is complete (the third decade of life).

The articular cartilage lining the SIJ is unusual. The sacral surface is lined with smooth hyaline cartilage whereas the iliac surface is lined with a rough type of fibrocartilage. Vleeming et al (1990a, 1990b) studied the friction coefficient of the SIJ and found that the coarse cartilage texture contributed to the ability of the joint to resist translation. The coarseness of the iliac cartilage increases with age (Bowen & Cassidy 1981). The complementary ridges and grooves in the mature SIJ (Solonen 1957, Vleeming et al 1990a, 1990b) also increase friction and thus contribute to form closure.

The SIJ is surrounded by some of the strongest ligaments in the body. The long dorsal sacroiliac (SI) ligament tightens during sacral counternutation or anterior rotation of the innominate and will limit this motion (Vleeming et al 1995b). The sacrotuberous and interosseus ligaments tighten during sacral nutation or posterior rotation of the innominate and limit this motion (Vleeming et al 1989a, 1989b, 1995a). The ventral SI ligaments are the weakest of the group and are supported anteriorly by the integrity of the pubic symphysis. These ligaments contribute to both form and force closure.

Panjabi has proposed a conceptual model that describes the interaction between the components of the spinal stabilizing system (Panjabi 1992). In this model, he describes the neutral zone, which is a small range of displacement near the joint's neutral position in which minimal resistance is given by the osteoligamentous structures. The neutral zone is easily palpated; the barriers to the zone are called R1 (first resistance) in manual therapy terms (Maitland 1986). The range of the neutral zone may increase with injury, articular degeneration (loss of form closure), and/or weakness of the stabilizing musculature (loss of force closure). When the SIJ is unstable, the neutral zone is increased.

The clinical tests that are used to detect this increase in neutral zone, or loss of form closure, evaluate the ability of the joint to resist pure vertical and horizontal plane translation. An unstable SIJ has a softer end-feel of motion, an increased quantity of translation, and a variable symptom response. If the joint is irritable, the test may provoke pain. If the instability is long-standing and asymptomatic, the tests are often not provocative.

'In the case of force closure, extra forces are needed to keep the object in place. Here friction must be present' (Snijders et al 1992). Joints with predominantly flat surfaces are well suited to transfer large moments of force but are vulnerable to shear. Factors that increase intra-articular compression will increase the friction coefficient and the ability of the joint to resist translation.

The muscles that contribute to force closure of the SIJ posteriorly include the erector spinae, multifidus, gluteus maximus, latissimus dorsi, and biceps femoris. The fibers of the gluteus maximus muscle run perpendicular to the plane of the SIJ and blend with the thoracodorsal fascia and the contralateral latissimus dorsi (Vleeming et al 1995a). Compression of the SIJ occurs when the gluteus maximus and the contralateral latissimus dorsi contract. This oblique system crosses the midline and is a significant contributor to load transference through the pelvic girdle during rotational activities and during gait (Vleeming et al 1995a).

The thoracodorsal fascia is tensed by contraction of both the gluteus maximus and latissimus dorsi as well as the erector spinae muscle. The fascia and the erector spinae muscle increase compression posteriorly through the SIJ by approximating the posterior aspect of the innominates (Snijders et al 1995, Vleeming et al 1995a). This system counteracts sacral nutation and is supported by the sacrotuberous ligament, which is in turn reinforced by the biceps femoris muscle.

Underlying all of these muscles and critical to their function is the transversus abdominis. Recent research has shown that the transversus abdominis muscle is a primary stabilizing muscle for the lumbar spine (Hodges & Richardson 1995a). It has a large attachment to the deep layers of the thoracodorsal fascia and is recruited *prior* to the initiation of any movement of the upper or lower extremity. In a study of patients with chronic low back pain, it was found that there was a timing delay during which the transversus abdominis muscle failed to contract prior to the initiation of arm and/or leg motion (Hodges & Richardson 1995b). Hodges concludes that 'a significant motor control deficit is present in people with chronic low back pain which is primarily associated with the control of contraction of transversus abdominis. The failure of the stabilization mechanism with subjects in the LBP [low back pain] group indicates that the normal strategy used by the body to control intervertebral motion and stiffness is inefficient.' This is extremely significant research with respect to rehabilitation of the unstable lumbopelvic region and is the point at which muscle re-education begins.

In a separate study, Hides et al (1994) found wasting and local inhibition at a segmental level of the lumbar multifidus muscle in all patients with a first episode of acute/subacute low back pain. In a follow-up study (Hides et al 1995), they found that, without therapeutic intervention, multifidus did not regain its original size or function and the recurrence rate of low back pain over an 8-month period was very high. They also found that the deficit could be reversed with an appropriate exercise program.

Anteriorly, the muscles that contribute to force closure of the pelvic girdle are the oblique abdominal and the contralateral adductor muscles (Snijders et al 1995). These muscles are activated in standing and unsupported sitting, and become quiet when the legs are crossed. The oblique abdominals are thought (Richardson & Jull 1995) to be prime movers and initiators of movement and depend on the prior contraction of the transversus abdominis for stabilization of the trunk (Hodges & Richardson 1995a).

In standing and walking, the pelvic girdle is stabilized on the femur by the coordinated action of the gluteus medius and minimus and contralateral adductor muscles. Although these muscles are not directly involved in force closure of the

SIJ, they are a significant factor in pelvic girdle function and are reflexly inhibited when the SIJ is unstable.

The muscles of the pelvic floor appear to play a vital role in the function of the other muscle groups. These muscles anchor the apex of the sacrum and control sacral nutation. Hodges found that some patients with chronic low back pain were unable to recruit the transversus abdominis without prior contraction of the pelvic floor.

Weakness, or insufficient recruitment and/or timing, of these muscle groups reduces the force closure mechanism through the SIJ. The patient then adopts compensatory movement strategies to accommodate the weakness. This can lead to decompensation of the lower back, hip, and knee.

Instability of the pelvic girdle can be due to articular and/or myofascial factors. Loss of the ligamentous support will lead to articular instability. When the joint is unstable, the quantity of translation will be increased and the end-feel of motion will be soft on stability testing. When unstable, the SIJ is vulnerable to locking with one articular surface translated, or sheared, relative to the other. The sacrum may shear unilaterally in an anterior or posterior direction (Fig. 37.1). This is not the same motion as sacral nutation or counternutation. These motions are physiologic angular motions that occur during normal move-

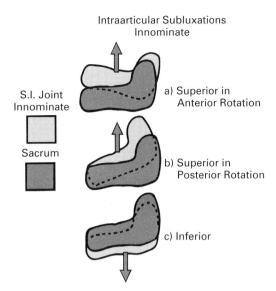

Fig. 37.2   The innominate may shear unilaterally in a superior or inferior direction and is commonly associated with anterior or posterior rotation. The degree of translation is magnified in this figure for ease of illustration.

ments of the trunk and lower extremity. Sacral shear lesions commonly occur during lifting and twisting. The innominate may shear superiorly or inferiorly with an element of anterior or posterior rotation (Fig. 37.2). These shear lesions commonly occur when unanticipated vertical loads occur through the leg. There will always be a loss of muscle function when the SIJ is unstable and/or locked. Clinically, the posterior fibers of gluteus medius as well as the gluteus maximus muscle are significantly affected when the SIJ is unstable.

Even when the SIJ is stable, loss of muscle strength and timing can lead to myofascial instability of the lumbopelvic region. In this instance, stability testing of the SIJ will reveal a normal quantity of translation as well as a normal end-feel of motion. The stability tests are key differential diagnostic tests in the clinical evaluation of SIJ mobility and stability. Muscle weakness can be detected with specific manual methods (Kendall et al 1993). Careful observation of how the synergists are recruited to assist the weak muscle during these tests is required to detect any substitution strategies (Richardson & Jull 1995). The loss of muscle support (force closure) can lead to secondary articular instability.

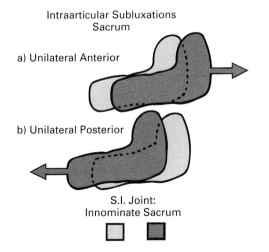

Fig. 37.1   The sacrum may shear unilaterally in an anterior or posterior direction. The degree of translation is magnified in this figure for ease of illustration.

METHOD OF DIAGNOSIS

Articular stability – form closure

The following tests examine the ability of the SIJ to resist vertical and horizontal translation forces (shear) that are applied passively to the non-weight-bearing joint (Lee 1992, 1995) (Fig. 37.3). With the patient supine and the knees and hips flexed, the sacral sulcus just medial to the posterior superior iliac spine (PSIS) is palpated with the long and ring fingers while the index finger of this hand palpates the lumbosacral junction (Fig. 37.4). The long and ring fingers monitor translation between the innominate and the sacrum while the index finger notes any movement between the pelvic girdle and the L5 vertebra.

To test anteroposterior translation, a posterior pressure is applied to the innominate through the iliac crest and the anterior superior iliac spine (ASIS). The relative mobility is noted posteriorly (Fig. 37.5). The end of the range of motion is reached when the pelvic girdle rotates as a unit beneath the L5 vertebra. The motion is compared with that of the opposite SIJ. The quality of the end-feel, the quantity of translation, and the reproduction of any symptoms are noted.

To test superoinferior translation, a superior/inferior pressure is applied to the innominate through the distal end of the femur or through the ischial tuberosity. The relative mobility is noted posteriorly. The end of the range of motion is reached when the pelvic girdle is felt to bend laterally beneath the L5 vertebra. The motion is compared with that of the opposite SIJ. The quality of the end-feel, the quantity of translation, and the reproduction of any symptoms are noted.

An unstable SIJ has a softer end-feel of motion, an increase in the quantity of translation, and a variable symptom response. If the joint is irritable, the test may provoke pain. If the instability is long-standing and asymptomatic, the tests are often not provocative. A study is currently underway to assess the intertester reliability and validity of these tests.

Myofascial stability – force closure

The aim of the following tests is to evaluate the stability of the lumbar spine and pelvic girdle under increasing loads. In addition, motor control patterns are evaluated. In patients with chronic low back pain, it has been shown (Richardson & Jull 1994) that, at low load levels, endurance rather than strength is the main deficit. The tests therefore involve an isometric contraction for a set period of time. When in dysfunction, a muscle may display an inability to sustain a hold or

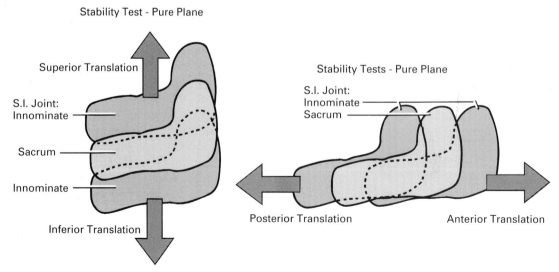

Fig. 37.3   The stability tests evaluate the ability of the SIJ to resist pure planar forces in the superoinferior and anteroposterior planes.

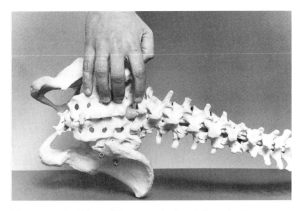

Fig. 37.4 Position of the posterior hand for palpation during stability testing of the SIJ.

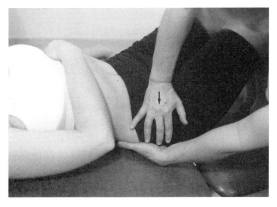

Fig. 37.5 A posterior pressure is applied through the innominate to test anteroposterior translation stability of the SIJ.

produce a more phasic, jerky pattern of contraction when the hold is sustained. Since the emphasis of this chapter is on treatment of instability, the reader is referred to Kendall et al (1993) and Richardson and Jull (1994, 1995) for elaboration on the details of these tests. Only the principles will be described here.

Transversus abdominis/multifidus

The patient lies prone and a pressure biofeedback unit (Hodges 1995b, Richardson & Jull 1994, 1995) is placed underneath the abdomen to monitor the patient's ability to sustain a neutral lumbar spine position during the test. The cuff is inflated to a base level of 70 mmHg. The patient is instructed to draw the stomach up and in towards the chest (abdominal hollowing). The lower abdomen is palpated to ensure contraction of the transversus abdominis. The multifidus muscle is palpated to ensure its co-contraction with the transversus abdominis. Any substitution strategies by rectus abdominis and the oblique abdominals are observed, and the pressure change in the biofeedback cuff is noted. Ideally, the pressure should drop by 6–8 mmHg. Large pressure decreases indicate that the patient is using the rectus abdominis to flex the lumbar spine. Pressure increases indicate that the lumbar lordosis is increasing and that the neutral spinal position has been lost.

If the patient is able to recruit the transversus abdominis appropriately, the test is progressed through increasing degrees of difficulty in the supine position. With the patient supine, the hips and knees are flexed and the pressure biofeedback unit is placed beneath the lumbar spine. The cuff is inflated to a base level of 40 mmHg and the patient is asked to 'hollow the abdomen'. The ability to do so is noted as in the prone test. The pressure should increase by no more than 10–15 mmHg. Loads are increased through the upper and lower extremity in a progressive manner, increasing both the weight and the lever arm (Fig. 37.6). A static holding test is advocated by Richardson and Jull (1994, 1995) because these muscles are required to contract for prolonged periods of time during stabilization of the spine. The patient should be able to sustain a 10 s hold repeated 10 times.

Gluteus medius

The function of this muscle is observed during gait and one-legged standing. There should be very little adduction of the pelvic girdle on the weight-bearing leg. The test described by Kendall et al (1993) is used specifically to test the posterior fibers of gluteus medius. The patient lies on his or her side with the leg to be tested uppermost. With the knee extended, the leg is positioned in slight extension, abduction, and external rotation. The patient is requested to hold the trunk and the leg still as support is released. The response is then observed. The patient with a poorly functioning gluteus medius

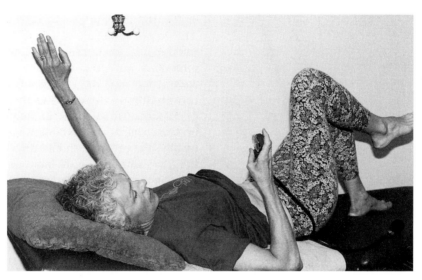

Fig. 37.6   The ability to maintain a neutral lumbar spine under increasing loads is evaluated with a pressure biofeedback unit (Richardson & Jull 1994, 1995).

will tend to rotate the pelvis backwards to facilitate the use of the tensor fascia lata. Alternately, he or she may side-flex the spine in an attempt to hold the leg. In both cases, stabilization of the lumbar spine has been lost in an attempt to achieve the task demanded. If the patient can hold the proper trunk and leg position for 10 s, resistance is applied to the leg into flexion, adduction, and internal rotation. When the posterior fibers of gluteus medius are weak, the leg gives easily. In addition, atrophy of the upper lateral quadrant of the buttock can be seen and felt.

Gluteus maximus

The function of this muscle is also observed during gait. It should contract just after heel strike (Inman et al 1981). When the gluteus maximus is weak, the buttock appears flattened. The muscle is specifically tested in the prone position (Kendall et al 1993). The patient is asked to squeeze the buttocks together and the ability to do so is palpated. If the patient is able to generate an effective contraction isometrically, he or she is then asked to perform a concentric contraction by extending the femur with the knee flexed. Resistance is then applied to the extended femur. Careful observation of the effects of this

contraction on the position of the lumbar spine gives the examiner further information on the ability of the patient to stabilize effectively.

Anterior oblique system – oblique abdominal/contralateral adductors

In chronic low back/pelvic girdle pain, the patient often loses the ability to dissociate movement between the trunk and the femur at the hip joint. When the hip joint becomes 'functionally rigid', more stress is placed on the SIJ and the joints of the low back. To specifically test the anterior oblique system, the patient lies supine with the hips and knees flexed. He or she is asked to lift the buttocks off the table (bridge). From this position, the patient is asked to keep the knees still and to rotate (not side-bend) the trunk to the left and right. When he or she is unable to dissociate the trunk from the legs, the knees will move from side to side and most of the movement will occur in the lumbar spine. When the patient is able to dissociate this motion, the trunk will rotate as a unit at the hip joints, and the knees will remain stationary.

These are a few examples of how the functional biomechanics can be incorporated into assessment in the clinical setting. The list is not exhaustive and the reader is referred to Kendall et al (1993) for further tests of specific muscle length and strength.

TREATMENT

It is extremely important to treat the entire functional complex, i.e. the lumbar spine, the pelvic girdle, the hip joint, and the lower extremity. If the ascending and descending influences are ignored, the outcome will not be satisfactory. The following treatment program is not meant to be exclusive of others but is merely intended to present the principles required for an effective program. Initially, each system is treated specifically. This is followed by a global approach through functional exercises.

The osseous system

All fractures or bone pathology must be treated first. The system is the responsibility of the orthopedic surgeon and is dealt with elsewhere in this text.

The articular system

Once the osseous system is stable, attention is directed to articular function. Any restrictions of the hip, knee, and/or foot that could increase stress on the SIJ are mobilized. In addition, any locking of the SIJ (shear lesion) is treated.

Sacral shear lesion

The mode of onset is traumatic, usually a lifting injury associated with a twist. The patient often reports hearing and feeling a pop and a sharp pain localized to the locked SIJ at the time of the injury.

Rotation of the sacrum between the two innominates is noted on both forward and backward bending during both standing and sitting. The ability to laterally translate the pelvic girdle in the coronal plane during lateral flexion of the trunk is unilaterally restricted, and the ipsilateral kinetic tests (Gillet's test) into extension and flexion are limited.

The sacrum is rotated (i.e. a deep sacral sulcus together with an anterior sacral base and a posterior inferior lateral angle on the *opposite side*) in all positions of the trunk – hyperflexion, neutral, and hyperextension. The intra-articular joint glides are restricted (particularly in the anteroposterior plane) on the locked side.

Anterior shear lesion of the sacrum at the right SIJ. An anterior shear lesion of the sacrum at the right SIJ is diagnosed when the joint is restricted on the right and the sacrum is rotated to the left. The manipulative reduction is illustrated in Fig. 37.7. With the patient in the right side-lying position, the lower leg extended, and the upper hip and knee flexed, the thoracolumbar spine is rotated until L5–S1 is felt to be fully rotated to the left. The lateral aspect of the spinous process of the L5 vertebra is firmly stabilized with one thumb to maintain the rotation at the lumbosacral junction. With the other hand, the left innominate and the lumbosacral unit are rotated to the right *about a pure vertical axis through the pelvic girdle* to the motion barrier, allowing the table to stabilize the right innominate. From this position, a high-velocity, low-amplitude thrust is applied through the left innominate and the sacrum to produce posterior translation of the right sacral base relative to the right innominate. Following reduction of the shear lesion, the stability tests for the SIJ are repeated. In this instance, an increase in anteroposterior glide will be palpated on the right.

Posterior shear lesion of the sacrum at the right SIJ. A posterior shear lesion of the sacrum at the right SIJ is diagnosed when the joint is restricted on the right and the sacrum is rotated to the right. The manipulative reduction is illustrated in Fig. 37.8. With the patient prone and the right hip and knee flexed over the side of the table, the right sacral base is palpated with the heel of the left hand. With the other hand, the right iliac crest and ASIS are palpated. A posterior glide is applied to the innominate against the fixed sacrum. When the motion barrier has been reached, a high-velocity, low-amplitude thrust is applied to the sacrum in an anterior direction. Following reduction of the shear lesion, the stability tests for the SIJ are repeated. In this instance, an increase in anteroposterior glide will be palpated on the right.

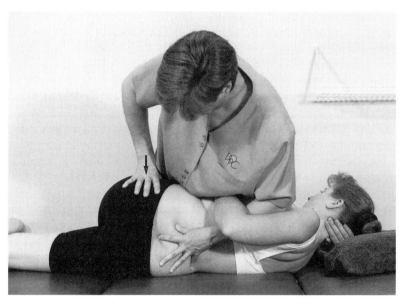

Fig. 37.7   The manipulative reduction technique for an anterior shear lesion of the sacrum at the right SIJ.

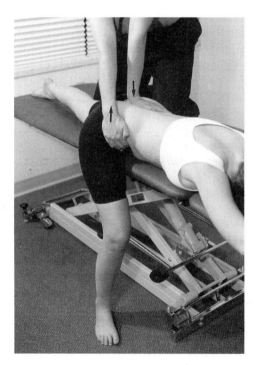

Fig. 37.8   The manipulative reduction technique for a posterior shear lesion of the sacrum at the right SIJ.

Innominate shear lesion

The mode of onset is traumatic, a fall on the buttocks being a common cause. If the vertical force occurs posterior to the axis of rotation, the superior shear lesion will be associated with anterior rotation of the innominate. If the vertical force is anterior to this axis, the shear lesion will be associated with posterior rotation.

The pain may be acute or chronic, localized to the SIJ, and/or distally referred to the knee, depending upon the stage of pathology. Secondary problems at the lumbosacral junction frequently occur. Coccygodynia secondary to the altered pull of the sacrospinous ligament is a common complaint. Unilateral weight-bearing, walking, and sitting on the effected side aggravate the symptoms.

Marked intrapelvic torsion is noted in both forward/backward bending of the trunk in standing and sitting. The ability to laterally translate the pelvic girdle in the coronal plane during lateral flexion of the trunk is unilaterally blocked, and the ipsilateral kinetic (Gillet) tests into both flexion and extension are limited.

The innominate is positioned superiorly and is either posteriorly or anteriorly rotated relative to the innominate of the opposite side. The L5 vertebra and the sacrum are rotated towards the side of the posteriorly rotated innominate. When the superior shear lesion occurs in anterior rotation, the tension of the sacrotuberous ligament is markedly reduced. However, posterior rotation of the innominate increases the tension of the sacrotuberous ligament, and when the superior shear lesion occurs in posterior rotation, the tension of the sacrotuberous ligament can feel normal. The lesion is always intra-articular, so the joint glides are restricted. Following reduction, repeated testing of stability (pure planar glides) reveals the underlying instability, which must exist for the shear lesion to occur.

Unilateral shear lesion of the innominate – superior with anterior rotation/posterior rotation. The patient is prone if the shear lesion is associated with anterior rotation, and supine if associated with posterior rotation. The therapist stands at the end of the table facing the patient. With both hands, the patient's lower leg, proximal to the talocrural joint, on the side being treated is grasped. The motion barrier is reached by applying a longitudinal pull through the leg. A high-velocity, low-amplitude tug is applied through the leg to the SIJ. A second therapist may assist by stabilizing the inferolateral aspect of the sacrum with the heel of one hand. Following reduction, the stability tests for the SIJ are repeated. In this instance, an increase in superoinferior glide will be palpated on the side of the shear lesion.

The myofascial system

There are no manual therapy techniques to tighten lax ligaments, so form closure cannot be improved through physiotherapy. Articular dysfunction with or without pain rapidly leads to inhibition of slow-twitch muscle fibers (Richardson & Jull 1994). The impact on function is a reduced ability to sustain a muscle contraction. Functionally, this means that one cannot sustain postures or appropriately stabilize a joint for prolonged periods of time. Loss of muscle strength and patterning will lead to myofascial instability. This lack of tonic control or static stabilization is reflected in the subjective complaints of patients suffering from instability in the pelvic girdle. Frequently, they complain of an inability to sit, stand, forward bend, lie supine, or walk for prolonged periods of time. They report that they must periodically change positions to keep the pain within tolerable limits. The goal of rehabilitation in the presence of articular and/or myofascial instability within the pelvic girdle is to improve force closure and thus facilitate the self-locking mechanism of the pelvic girdle through appropriate exercise and re-education of movement patterns. It is important to remember that the articular, neural, and myofascial systems are interdependent, and although they have been divided for discussion, rehabilitation must address all components simultaneously.

The temporary application of an external support can be very helpful during the early stages of rehabilitation. The support should be worn at all times when weight-bearing. Sclerosing injections into the dorsal SI ligaments have shown some promise in affording relief for patients with permanent instability (Dorman et al 1995).

In rehabilitation, both strengthening and endurance of the weakened muscles must be addressed. The aim of this program is to reactivate the stabilizing muscles, retrain their holding capacity, and retrain their ability to automatically contract appropriately with other synergists to support and protect the spine/pelvic girdle under various functional loads. Richardson and Jull (1994) have devised a four-stage program that can be applied to the posterior oblique, anterior oblique, and longitudinal systems as described by Vleeming et al (1995a). This integrated program is useful in the rehabilitation of instability of the pelvic girdle, although no outcome studies have been carried out to validate the approach.

The first stage of the program (stage 1) requires isolation and facilitation of the key muscles involved in stabilization of the trunk and pelvic girdle. Once the patient can effectively recruit and sustain a holding contraction, the exercise is made more challenging by introducing limb movement, reducing the base of support and then increasing the load (stage 2). Stage 3 involves stabilization during controlled movement through the lumbar spine and pelvic girdle, and stage 4 requires stabilization during high-speed motions. Very few people require stage 4 stabilization. In fact, high-speed exercise has been shown (Richardson & Jull 1995) to reduce the ability to stabilize the trunk. Slow, controlled movements with increasing loads is what most people need to function.

The thoracodorsal fascia, and the ability to render it taut, is paramount to the function of the posterior oblique system. When the fascia is taut, loads can be transferred from the trunk to the lower extremity. This is facilitated by the co-contraction of the prime movers, including the oblique abdominals, the latissimus dorsi, and the gluteus maximus muscles. However, underlying this is the preactivation of the transversus abdominis, which must contract first to stabilize the spine through the thoracodorsal fascia (Hodges & Richardson 1995b). This is where the rehabilitation program begins for everyone.

The patient lies either supine or prone with the pressure biofeedback unit placed beneath the lumbar spine/lower abdomen. The patient is instructed first to draw the coccyx towards the pubic symphysis (recruit the pelvic floor) and then to draw the belly button backwards and up towards the spine (abdominal hollowing; Richardson & Jull 1994, 1995). The principles and explanation of this exercise have been described above. The holding capacity is retrained by asking patients to perform their maximum number of 10 s hold repetitions. This number may vary between exercise sessions depending on their level of fatigue. The goal is to reach 10 repetitions of 10 s holds. If the patient cannot recruit the transversus abdominis in this position, the four-point kneeling position is an effective place to start (Richardson & Jull 1995).

The exercise is progressed to stage 2 by introducing lower or upper extremity motion, first in supine or prone and then in sitting. In the supine position with the hips and knees flexed, the patient is required to maintain the lumbar neutral position and then slowly to let the knee fall to one side, or the leg move towards extension. The load and the lever arm may be progressed in this same position by asking the patient to lift the foot up off the table while maintaining the hip and knee flexed. A progression from this would be to extend this leg slowly out to 45°. This is performed unilaterally and can be progressed to alternate leg extensions. If possible, it is important to ensure that the transversus abdominis is contracting prior to the initiation of any limb movement. The same exercises may be performed sitting on a gym ball or lying supine on a long roll (Fig. 37.9). By making the base unstable, the exercise and the ability to stabilize become more difficult without moving into the next stage. Rolls and gym balls facilitate the rehabilitation of automatic reactions that are necessary for function.

In the prone and sitting positions, multifidus may be facilitated (Richardson & Jull 1994, 1995) by applying a local stretch and asking the patient to 'swell' the back simultaneously. This muscle should co-contract with transversus abdominis to assist in lumbopelvic stability. This contraction may be monitored manually during the other exercises.

Once the patient is able to recruit the deeper abdominals and multifidus, attention can be focused on the prime movers, the oblique abdominals, gluteus medius, maximus, and latissimus dorsi. At all times during these exercises, stabilization of the trunk is maintained.

If the gluteus maximus is poorly recruited, or if it is weak, it should be isolated and facilitated at this time. This is done in the prone position by asking the patient to squeeze the buttocks together and sustain the contraction for 10 s. A surface electromyography (EMG) unit can provide a useful biofeedback system for this muscle. The exercise is progressed by having the patient lie prone over a gym ball and asking him or her to stabilize the trunk and then lift the extended thigh.

A further progression would be to have the patient lie supine with the hips and knees flexed. The patient is asked to stabilize the trunk and then to lift the buttocks so that the thighs and trunk are parallel. From this position, a rotation force is applied to the pelvic girdle through the left and right ASISs. The patient resists this force, not allowing any motion to occur. This isometric contraction requires recruitment of the oblique abdominals (part of the anterior and posterior oblique system). A further challenge is to place the patient's calves over a gym ball and perform the same exercise (Fig. 37.10). It is the application of the principles that is important, the

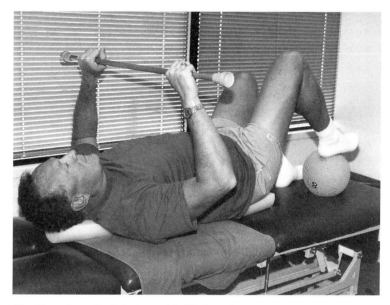

Fig. 37.9 Stage 2 – isolation and facilitation of the stabilizers of the trunk with an unstable base (1/2 roll), unilateral leg motion (supported), and bilateral upper extremity motion.

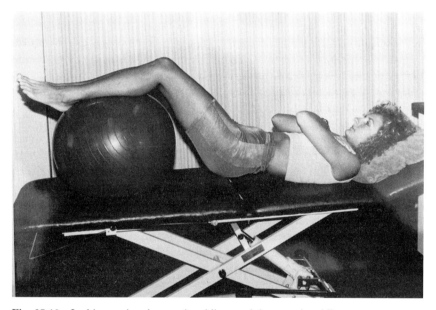

Fig. 37.10 In this exercise, the anterior oblique and the posterior oblique systems are facilitated.

specific exercise being left to the imagination of both the patient and the therapist. Stabilize the trunk, initiate a motion with the extremity, and then challenge the balance.

A functional way to train the gluteus maximus is to have the patient practice going from sitting to standing with a stabilized trunk using primarily the gluteus maximus. To be done properly, this exercise requires control of the lumbar spine and pelvic girdle through the deep abdominals/multifidus and the pelvic floor, and a very strong buttock. Leg extension machines (Apex Leg Press;

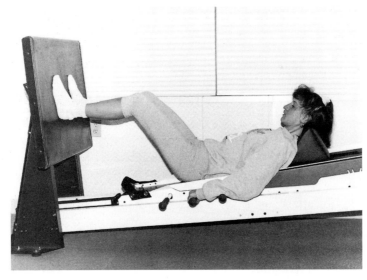

Fig. 37.11   The Shuttle MVP is useful for progressing trunk stabilization by increasing loads through either the lower or the upper extremity. Exercises can be carried out in side-lying or four-point kneeling to decrease the base of support and increase the challenge.

Medical Exercise Thigh Trainer; Shuttle MVP or 2000–1) can help to strengthen the gluteal group. On the Shuttle, patients can initially exercise in the supine position with either one or two feet on the foot plate. With the trunk stabilized, they push against a variable resistance, which can be increased as tolerated (Fig. 37.11). They are progressed from this position to four-point kneeling (a more unstable base). Superb control has been achieved when, in a four-point kneeling position with the hands on the foot plate, they are able to control the trunk position and press the body away with the hands and shoulders. This is still a stage 2 exercise.

The posterior fibers of gluteus medius weaken when the SIJ is unstable. This has profound effects on walking and load transference through the hip joint. The secondary consequences of a Trendelenberg gait on the SIJ and the lumbar spine can be significant. Rehabilitation of the gluteus medius begins in the side-lying position with a pillow between the knees. The patient is shown where to palpate the muscle posteriorly and taught which compensatory movement strategies to avoid (posterior rotation of the trunk and side-flexion of the trunk). Initially, with or without a surface EMG unit, the patient is asked

to lift the medial aspect of the knee off the pillow. Careful observation of substitution strategies is required at this stage. The exercise is progressed by asking the patient to lift the knee off the pillow and to extend it while maintaining the correct position of the trunk and hip. The knee is then flexed and lowered onto the pillow. This exercise may be performed at a later time (still in stage 2) on the Shuttle in the side-lying position. In addition, the Fitter board (sideways slider unit) is extremely useful in rehabilitating the gluteus medius and the contralateral hip adductors while maintaining a stabilized trunk (Fig. 37.12).

A progression of exercises for the anterior oblique system begins with transversus abdominis and the pelvic floor. Once the patient can stabilize the trunk, the exercises that differentiate the trunk from the femur can begin. Alana Parker, a Feldenkrais physiotherapist from San Francisco, has incorporated the use of styrofoam rolls into her Feldenkrais exercises. They are extremely effective in the rehabilitation of the anterior oblique system and also in teaching patients to differentiate motion. To begin with, the patient is supine with the hips and knees flexed. A styrofoam roll, one foot in length, six inches in diameter and cut in half lengthwise, is placed horizontally beneath the

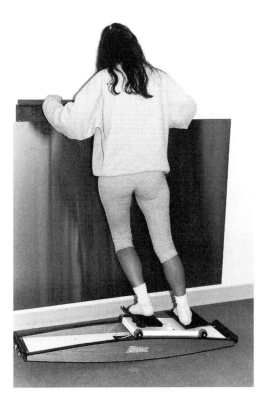

Fig. 37.12 The Fitter board requires stabilization of the trunk, activation of gluteus medius and the contralateral adductors, coordination, and balance.

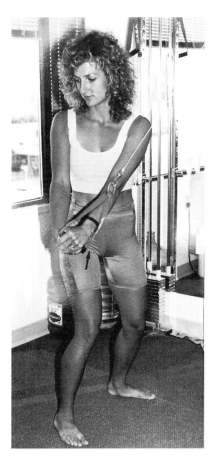

Fig. 37.13 Using pulleys, the patient is taught to stabilize the trunk and to dissociate motion between the trunk and the lower extremity by rotating through the hip joint (arrow).

low back. The patient is asked to stabilize the trunk and then to flex and extend the trunk, not in the lumbar spine or pelvis but at the hip joints, keeping the knees still. When the patient has mastered sagittal plane motion, the roll is placed longitudinally along the spine and pelvis, and the patient is asked to stabilize the trunk and then to rotate, not side-bend, the trunk relative to the fixed femurs at the hip joint. This exercise is progressed by removing the roll, having the patient bridge (recruit the gluteus maximus) and then rotate the trunk at the hip joints in the unsupported position. This motion recruits the oblique abdominals and the contralateral adductors very effectively.

To make this exercise functional, pulleys are used. In a standing position, the patient is required to pull the weight either up or down using a rotary motion, not through the trunk but through the hip joint (Fig. 37.13). This exercise requires effective stabilization of the trunk via the transversus abdominis, multifidus and pelvic floor, and active recruitment of the latissimus dorsi, gluteus maximus, gluteus medius, contralateral adductors and oblique abdominals. All of these muscles are important in stabilization of the pelvic girdle through the posterior, anterior, and oblique systems. The load is increased as tolerated and the speed is maintained at a low level.

At this time, wobble boards or long rollers can be used to challenge balance in standing. Patients, must stabilize the trunk and shift their weight from side to side, forward and back, or do full squats or upper extremity work.

All exercise equipment can be adapted to fit into the principles of stabilization therapy. Only imagination limits the exercise program once the principles are understood. Thus exercises can be adapted to meet the demands of the patient's work and recreation. This program is less 'muscle specific' and more functionally oriented. It is important not to progress faster than motion can be controlled. The early stages are the most difficult to teach and often take the longest time to master. Diligence is rewarded with fewer setbacks. If limb motion is added, or the load is increased, beyond that which can be controlled centrally, the pain will increase.

According to the protocol advocated by Richardson and Jull (1994), stage 3 exercises involve controlled motion of the *unstable region*. This stage is much more advanced and is only given when required by an individual's work or sport. Programs include concentric and eccentric work with variable resistance in all three planes: sagittal, coronal, and transverse. At this stage, the various isokinetic machines (Medex: Medical exercise rotation trainer) as well as any pulley apparatus can be useful. Rotation is often not well tolerated by those with a true articular instability of the SIJ when the pelvis is fixed either in an apparatus or in sitting. Before this exercise can be effective, a stabilization program is needed.

CONCLUSIONS

1. Patients presenting with instability of the pelvic girdle can be very challenging to treat.

2. If the joint has become locked, exercises alone will not bring a successful resolution.

3. Without exercises, manipulation of the SIJ leaves the patient vulnerable to shearing or locking again.

4. Together, manual therapy and exercises based on sound scientific principles help to restore the force closure mechanism which the patient requires for a return to function.

REFERENCES

Bowen V, Cassidy J D 1981 Macroscopic and microscopic anatomy of the sacroiliac joint from embryonic life until the eighth decade. Spine 6(6): 620–628

Dorman T A, Cohen R E, Dasig D, Jeng S, Fischer N, DeJong A 1995 Energy efficiency during human walking before and after prolotherapy. In: Vleeming A, Mooney V, Dorman T, Snijders C J (eds) Second interdisciplinary world congress on low back pain. San Diego, CA, 9–11 November, pp 645–649

Hides J A, Stokes M J, Saide M, Jull G A, Cooper D H 1994 Evidence of lumbar multifidus muscle wasting ipsilateral to symptoms in patients with acute/subacute low back pain. Spine 19(2): 165–172

Hides J A, Richardson C A, Jull G A 1995 Multifidus inhibition in acute low back pain: recovery is not spontaneous. Proceedings of the 9th biennial conference of the Manipulative Physiotherapists Association of Australia. Gold Coast, Queensland, pp 57–60

Hodges P W, Richardson C A 1995a Neuromotor dysfunction of the trunk musculature in low back pain patients. Proceedings of the World Confederation of Physical Therapists congress, Washington, USA

Hodges P W, Richardson C A 1995b Dysfunction of transversus abdominis associated with chronic low back pain. Proceedings of the 9th biennial conference of the Manipulative Physiotherapists Association of Australia. Gold Coast, Queensland, pp 61–62

Inman V T, Ralston H J, Todd F 1981 Human walking. Williams & Wilkins, Baltimore

Kendall F P, Kendall McCreary E, Provance P G 1993 Muscles: testing and function, 4th edn. Williams & Wilkins, Baltimore

Lee D G 1992 Intra articular versus extra articular dysfunction of the sacroiliac joint – a method of differentiation. IFOMT Proceedings, 5th international conference. Vail, Colorado, 1–5 June, pp 69–71

Lee D G 1995 Contemporary positions of the sacroiliac joint. Key note address. Proceedings of the 9th biennial conference of the Manipulative Physiotherapists Association of Australia. Gold Coast, Queensland, pp 74–83

Maitland G D 1986 Vertebral manipulation, 5th edn. Butterworths, London

Panjabi M M 1992 The stabilizing system of the spine. I: Function, dysfunction, adaptation, and enhancement. Journal of Spinal Disorders 5(4): 383–389

Richardson C A, Jull G A 1994 Concepts of assessment and rehabilitation for active lumbar stability. In: Boyling J D, Palastanga N (eds) Grieve's modern manual therapy of the vertebral column, 2nd edn. Churchill Livingstone, Edinburgh, pp 705–720

Richardson C A, Jull G A 1995 Muscle control – pain control. What exercises would you prescribe? Manual Therapy 1(1): 2–10

Schneider G 1995 The reliability of an exercise regime to limit episodes of lumbar instability. Proceedings of the 9th biennial conference of the Manipulative Physiotherapists Association of Australia. Gold Coast, Queensland, pp 140–144

Snijders C J, Vleeming A, Stoeckart R 1992 Transfer of lumbosacral load to iliac bones and legs. 1: Biomechanics of self-bracing of the sacroiliac joints and its significance for treatment and exercise. In: Vleeming A, Mooney V, Snijders C J, Dorman T (eds) First interdisciplinary world congress on low back pain and its relation to the sacroiliac joint. San Diego, CA, 5–6 November, pp 233–254

Snijders C J, Vleeming A, Stoeckart R, Kleinrensink G J, Mens J M A 1995 Biomechanics of sacroiliac joint stability: validation experiments on the concept of self-locking. In: Vleeming A, Mooney V, Dorman T, Snijders C J (eds)

Second interdisciplinary world congress on low back pain. San Diego, CA, 9–11 November, pp 77–91

Solonen K A 1957 The sacroiliac joint in the light of anatomical roentgenological and clinical studies. Acta Orthopaedica Scandinavica Supplement 27: 1–127

Vleeming A, Wingerden J P, Snijders C J, Stoeckart R, Stijnen T 1989a Load application to the sacrotuberous ligament: influences on sacroiliac joint mechanics. Clinical Biomechanics 4: 204–209

Vleeming A, Stoeckart R, Snijders C J 1989b The sacrotuberous ligament: a conceptual approach to its dynamic role in stabilizing the sacroiliac joint. Clinical Biomechanics 4: 201–203

Vleeming A, Stoeckart R, Volkers A C W, Snijders C J 1990a Relation between form and function in the sacroiliac joint. 1: Clinical anatomical aspects. Spine 15(2): 130–132

Vleeming A, Volkers A C W, Snijders C J, Stoeckart R 1990b Relation between form and function in the sacroiliac joint. 2: Biomechanical aspects. Spine 15(2): 133–135

Vleeming A, Snijders C J, Stoeckart R, Mens J M A 1995a A new light on low back pain. In: Vleeming A, Mooney V, Dorman T, Snijders C J (eds) Second interdisciplinary world congress on low back pain. San Diego, CA, 9–11 November, pp 149–168

Vleeming A, Pool-Goudzwaard A L, Hammudoghlu D, Stoeckart R, Snijders C J, Mens J M A 1995b The function of the long dorsal sacroiliac ligament: its implication for understanding low back pain. In: Vleeming A, Mooney V, Dorman T, Snijders C J (eds) Second interdisciplinary world congress on low back pain. San Diego, CA, 9–11 November, pp 123–137

38. Mechanics and treatment of the sacroiliac joint

R. L. DonTigny

The purposes of this chapter are threefold. The first is to describe the functions of the sacroiliac joints (SIJs) in terms of movement, structure, ligamentous influence, and principles of mechanics. The second is to describe the pathomechanics and their various clinical manifestations. The third is to offer various principles of treatment to restore normal function and prevent dysfunction.

In order to gain some appreciation of the motion that occurs in the SIJ, palpate your own posterior superior iliac spines (PSISs) while seated. Translate your left knee anteriorly and your right knee posteriorly and notice the movement that takes place (Fig. 38.1). Reverse the translations a few times. Hold the right leg in posterior translation and rotate your trunk to the right and then to the left. Note how rotation to the right is enhanced and rotation to the left is inhibited. Now repeat this exercise with a belt tightened snugly around the pelvis, below the iliac crests. Note how pelvic motion is restricted.

This teaches us that motion in the SIJs may facilitate trunk rotation and dysfunction may inhibit it. Note also that this movement of the innominate bones occurs on an axis at the ischial tuberosities.

MOVEMENT AND STRUCTURE

Movements of the innominate bones and the sacrum are only somewhat interdependent. With flexion of the lumbar spine, there is a tendency toward a movement of the sacrum on the stabilized innominate bones, termed ventral inclination or nutation, and with extension, dorsal or

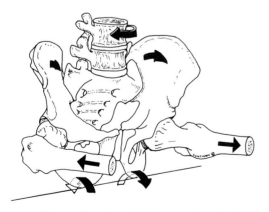

Fig. 38.1 Translation of the thighs in opposite directions when seated causes the innominate bones to rotate on an axis just beneath the ischial tuberosities and can facilitate or inhibit trunk rotation.

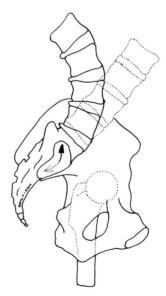

Fig. 38.2 Expected movement of the sacrum with flexion and extension on the stabilized innominate bones.

461

contranutation occurs, probably on a transverse axis (Fig. 38.2).

Weisl (1953) found that the sacrum descends between the innominate bones with superincumbent weight-loading when moving from a supine to an erect posture, putting a tensile stress on the posterior interosseous ligaments (Fig. 38.3A). For the innominate bones to achieve a similar movement, they would have to move on a transverse axis through the SIJ (Fig. 38.3B).

The innominate bones do not normally move on the sacrum on such a transverse sacroiliac (SI) axis, but rotate anteriorly and posteriorly on an acetabular axis (Fig. 38.4). Although this may raise or lower the sacrum, it does not necessarily cause any movement in the SIJs when the innominates move together, as it is diametrically opposed to the probable SI axis. Note the increase in lumbosacral shear with anterior rotation.

The variation in configuration of the joint surfaces is such that if movement of the sacrum were unrestricted by ligaments, the superincumbent weight would cause the S1 segment of the sacral surface of the SIJ to move downwards and separate from the S1 segment of the ilial surface of the SIJ, with a corresponding decrease in joint friction. Similarly, caudally, the S3 segment of the sacral surface would tend to rise and separate from the S3 segment of the ilial surface (Fig. 38.5) (DonTigny 1994).

LIGAMENTOUS INFLUENCE AND FUNCTIONAL MECHANICS

Structurally, the sacrum is suspended from the ilia by the dense posterior interosseous ligaments and functions as the reverse of a keystone by hanging more deeply between the ilia with increased

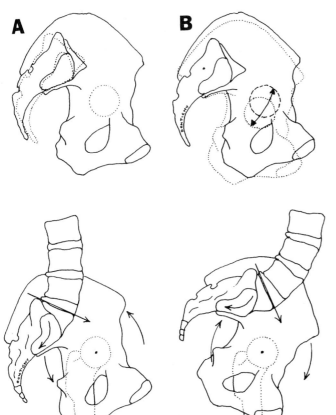

Fig. 38.3 (A) Unloaded sacrum (dotted line) moves deeper between the ilia when loaded with the superincumbent weight. (B) Relative position of the innominate bones to the sacrum before (dotted line) and after (solid line) loading. Note the change in position of the acetabula relative to the SIJ when the innominate bone moves on an axis through the sacrum.

Fig. 38.4 (A) With pelvic flexion, the SIJ is more posterior to the acetabula, making the legs appear to be relatively shorter when standing and longer when sitting. The body of the sacrum is more horizontal, decreasing shear. (B) With anterior rotation of the innominate bones on an acetabular axis, the SIJ moves anteriorly and superiorly to the acetabula, increasing apparent leg length when standing and making the legs appear shorter when sitting. Shear is increased on the body of the sacrum.

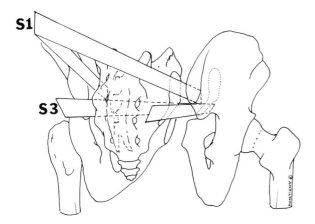

Fig. 38.5 Angulation of the S1 and S3 surfaces of the SIJs. Unrestricted loading of the body of the sacrum would tend to decrease friction at both S1 and S3.

loading. The PSISs converge slightly with increased weight-loading on the sacrum. Vukicevic et al (1991) found that the joints do not approximate with weight-loading as long as the posterior interosseous ligaments are intact. This indicates that loading of the posterior interosseous liga-

ments could decrease friction on the surfaces of the SIJ. If the sacrum functioned as a keystone, the joint surfaces would approximate and the PSISs would diverge. The superincumbent weight is transferred from the sacrum through the posterior interosseous ligaments to the innominate bones and not through the SIJs, which are, in my opinion, essentially non-weight-bearing.

Superincumbent weight-loading on the sacrum causes it to incline ventrally (nutate), increasing tensile stress on the posterior interosseous ligaments. This causes the caudal end of the sacrum to move posteriorly, creating a counterbalancing tensile stress on the sacrotuberous and sacrospinous ligaments. These balanced tensile forces result in a force couple and a tendency to rotate around a transverse axis created by and perpendicular to the force couple (Fig. 38.6) (DonTigny 1994).

If these forces are balanced bilaterally on the sacrum, a transverse axis is established through the sacrum but not necessarily through the joints. As these tensile forces vary with applied force, so will the transverse axis tend to vary. This trans-

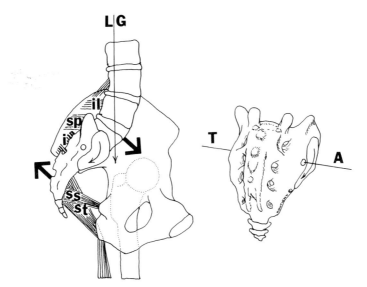

Fig. 38.6 The sacrum and its superincumbent weight, through the line of gravity (LG), is supported by and exerts a tensile stress on the iliolumbar ligaments (il), the short posterior SI ligaments (sp) and the posterior interosseous ligaments (i). A secondary tensile stress is exerted on the sacrotuberous (st) and sacrospinous (ss) ligaments, creating a force couple (large arrows). The moment of force created by the couple serves as a transverse axis (TA) of rotation. The location of this axis may vary depending upon the direction of the applied forces.

verse axis would be force dependent but not anatomically dependent, and would explain the difficulty in locating a precise anatomically dependent transverse axis.

Vukicevic et al (1991) found that removal of the posterior interosseous ligaments causes the SIJs to become profoundly unstable. They also found that the posterior interosseous ligaments can sustain a wide range of loading without pelvic or sacral deformation even after the elimination of the sacrotuberous and sacrospinous ligaments. Proper function is dependent upon a balance of tensile stress on these ligaments. This balance of forces is assisted by the biceps femoris acting, in many people, through the sacro-tuberous ligament, the piriformis, and the lower fibers of the gluteus maximus, acting to prevent further posterior movement of the distal sacrum, and (among others) the abdominal muscles and the latissimus dorsi.

To further ensure the stability of the SIJs, the orientation of the posterior ligaments (Fig. 38.7) and of the sacrotuberous and sacrospinous ligaments (Fig. 38.8) causes a movement of the ilia toward the sacrum on the axis created by the moment of the force couple. The opposing surfaces of the SIJs are drawn tightly together, increasing friction and protecting the joints from shearing with increased weight-loading (DonTigny 1994). Posterior rotation of the innominate bones around the acetabular axis further tenses these ligaments and increases friction and load-transmitting capabilities (Vleeming et al 1989a, 1989b), but would not be expected to cause the innominates to move further posteriorly on the sacrum. As this mechanism appears to be very strong and effectively limits further motion posteriorly of the innominates on the sacrum, we may probably conclude that the SIJ is not susceptible to injury through minor trauma with posterior asymmetric rotation of the innominate bones on the sacrum.

Dorsal inclination of the sacrum (contranuta-tion) with extension of the spine is blocked anatomically by the broad sacral surfaces of the S1 segments moving posteriorly against the ilial surfaces, and the angular change of the S3 segments blocks the distal sacrum as it moves ventrally (see Fig. 38.5 above).

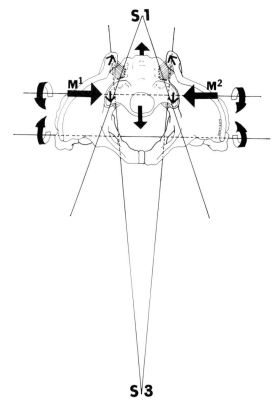

Fig. 38.7 Top view of the pelvis. As the body of the sacrum tends to move anteriorly and downwards with superincumbent tensile stress, and is not restricted anatomically by the S1 or the S3 ilial surface, the joint surfaces tend to separate. The joint surfaces only approximate through the action of the moments of force (M^1 and M^2) created by the force couples established by the secondary tensile stress on the sacrotuberous ligaments.

Extension of the spine would appear to be accompanied by and increased with an anterior rotation of the innominate bones on the sacrum; however, in the standing position, Russek (1976) demonstrated that extension of the spine caused the line of gravity to shift posteriorly to the ground reaction force vector through the acetabula. The superincumbent weight posterior to the acetabula increased pelvic flexion (nutation) and decreased the lumbosacral angle.

Mechanics during ambulation

After initial impact of the foot while ambulating, the quadriceps functions to decelerate knee flexion and then the hamstrings work with the quadri-

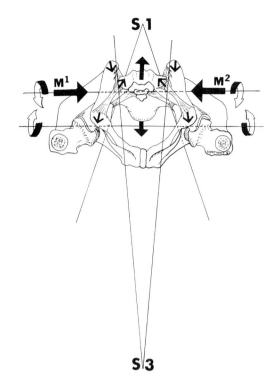

Fig. 38.8 Bottom view of the pelvis. Note the direction of tensile stress and compare it with the variation in the angulation of structure of the surfaces of the SIJs.

ceps to pull the knee posteriorly into terminal extension. The lateral insertions of the hamstrings provide lateral stability for the knee and limit anterior shearing of the distal femur on the tibial condyles, which protects the anterior cruciate ligament. Simultaneously, the hamstrings stabilize the ipsilateral innominate bone to maintain self-bracing in that SIJ, and the sacrotuberous ligament serves as an extension of the tendon of the biceps femoris to stabilize the sacrum, which all serves to anchor the anterior inclination and rotation of the trunk on the contralateral side through the oblique posterior fascia.

This pelvic deceleration and stabilization momentarily arrests and then reverses the anterior inclination of the trunk at two-point support. The trunk is never actually tilted posteriorly, but moves anteriorly and posteriorly with rotation and counter-rotation in relation to the mean forward inclination once each step and twice each stride. This rhythmic oscillation begins with pelvic deceleration, which causes each vertebra to de-

celerate sequentially, probably causing a flattening and recovery of the spinal curves with loading and unloading of the discs. Thorstensson et al (1984) found the excursion of this oscillation to be about 2.0–2.5 cm at L3 and about 1.0–1.5 cm at C7. This indicates that the spinal curves may act as a decreasing waveform and function to dampen this rhythmic sacrocranial vertebral oscillation, as the movement at C7 was less than that at L3. Not only do the spinal ligaments store and release energy with this oscillation, but the discs also appear to undergo an intermittent compression. This may also serve to store and release energy, may have a pumping action to circulate spinal fluid, and may assist in nutrition of the discs.

This oscillation serves to control the anterior inclination of the trunk and facilitates ambulation through these brief reversals. The SIJ on the side of initial impact self-braces unilaterally to provide stabilization to the lumbosacroiliac complex during this oscillation. Also, during this brief interval at initial impact and two-point support, maximum anterior trunk inclination coincides with the position of maximum counter-rotation of the upper trunk. The gluteus maximus on the side of initial impact functions with the contralateral latissimus dorsi across the bearing SIJ to enhance self-bracing (Gracovetsky 1995, Vleeming et al 1995a). Any pathology that may exist in the SIJ that interferes with normal function in the joint or prevents self-bracing could cause loss of control of this rhythmic sacrocranial vertebral oscillation. This might increase shear forces on the lower lumbar discs, increase a spondylolisthesis, or cause an unstable segment.

Counter-rotation is basic to and serves to enhance the efficiency of bipedal ambulation as certain lines of fascia serve to facilitate certain muscle groups. Energy is stored by stretching the muscles and fascia of the trailing arm and shoulder, the abdominal external oblique with the contralateral internal oblique, and when the hip flexors and quadriceps of the trailing leg are on stretch. With the derotation and posterior recovery of the trunk at two-point support, the hip flexors raise the trailing leg slightly, releasing the energy stored in the tightened fascia and propelling the leg forward for the next step.

After initial impact, to facilitate the forward swing of the trailing leg and to lengthen the step, the pelvis swings anteriorly in the horizontal plane in response to previously tightened fascia. The gluteus maximus undergoes an eccentric contraction to control and decelerate the pelvic swing, to decrease the impact loading of the next step as it continues to maintain ipsilateral self-bracing.

I speculate that counter-rotation tends to open the posterior aspect of the S1 segment of the SIJ on the side of self-bracing just as the extension of the trailing leg releases tension on the sacrotuberous ligament (Figs 38.9 and 38.10). This tensile release is directed diagonally across the sacrum toward the short posterior SI ligament on the side of self-bracing and creates a force-dependent oblique axis. Although the moment of the force couple on the side of self-bracing draws the innominate into the sacrum, the moment of the force couple on the contralateral side is away from the sacrum and causes a release of self-bracing, with a tendency for the contralateral innominate to move away from the sacrum. Note how the angulation of the S1 segment of the SIJ on the side of impact loading and self-bracing lines up with the direction of the deceleration force. The sacrum appears to skew slightly and undergo a slight oscillatory movement. All of these forces are probably damped by the high coefficient of friction of these joints.

Levin (1995) described the sacrum as being tethered in three-dimensional space and restrained by 12 tension vectors in such a way that any change in tension in one part of the structure would alter tension in all parts of the structure. He proposed that this structure functions in a similar way to a tension icosahedron. This concept is vital to understanding the nature of the function of the lumbosacroiliac complex as a self-compensating force couple with a variable, force-dependent transverse axis. This tension structure as a force couple accommodates, mitigates, balances, stores, and redirects various forces such as linear velocity, linear acceleration and deceleration, linear momentum, angular acceleration

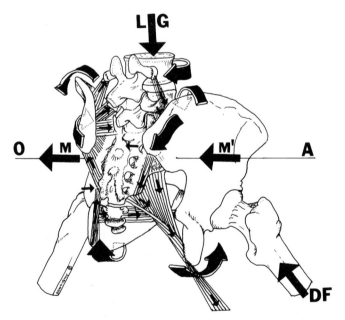

Fig. 38.9 On the side of initial impact the deceleration force (DF) and the pull of the hamstrings and sacrotuberous ligament create a force couple with a moment (M') that maintains self-bracing and stabilizes contralateral counter-rotation of the trunk. On the side of extension, the force couple is reversed creating a moment (M) that decreases self-bracing and releases stored energy. These two different moments result in an oblique axis of sacral movement (OA).

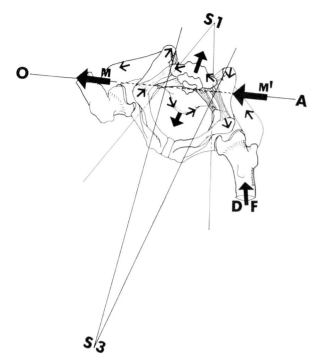

Fig. 38.10 Bottom view of the pelvis, comparing pelvic motion with ligamentous stress, angulation of joint surfaces, and a probable oblique axis.

and deceleration, angular momentum, and the rate of change of momentum, which affect the pelvis and its principle ligaments (DonTigny 1994).

DYSFUNCTION AS A PATHOLOGICAL RELEASE OF SELF-BRACING

Low back pain most frequently occurs during a transition from an erect posture to a trunk-forward posture (or reverse) while lifting, bending, or lowering. The superincumbent weight moves anteriorly to the acetabula, creating a force in anterior rotation of the innominate bones around the acetabular axis and away from the position of self-bracing. The movement loosens the sacrotuberous ligaments, decreasing friction and self-bracing principally at the S3 segments of the SIJs, and leaving the superincumbent weight somewhat suspended from the posterior interosseous ligaments. The helical structure of the sacrotuberous ligaments allows a greater storage

of energy with self-bracing. The pathological release of self-bracing can be expected to cause a relative uncoiling of their helix.

Probably the most critical support necessary to maintain self-bracing when leaning forward is a strong voluntary contraction by the abdominal muscles to lift and stabilize the anterior pelvis. As the abdominal muscles are relaxed when standing and do not automatically contract when leaning forward, they frequently fail to provide adequate anterior pelvic support in the transition to and from the trunk-forward position (DonTigny 1979). Failure voluntarily to contract a strong muscle group or inability to contract a weak muscle group predisposes the SIJs to dysfunction (SIJD) and injury from an anterior rotation of the innominate bones on the sacrum, even from minor trauma. This may occur when leaning forward if the innominate bones lack support and rotate upwards posteriorly and downwards anteriorly around an acetabular axis immediately prior to the trunk moving forward, or when lifting, if the trunk extends on the anteriorly rotated innominate bones. SIJD may also occur during coughing or straining if the increased intra-abdominal pressure spreads the innominate bones and anteriorly rotates them on the sacrum (DonTigny 1985). The rapid release of balanced forces in this complex may cause sudden stress on the hamstrings, the gluteus maximus, the paravertebral extensors, and the piriformis.

As the posterior interosseous ligaments and the iliolumbar ligaments are prestressed with the superincumbent weight in the trunk-forward position, there is a continuing tendency for the distal aspect of the sacrum to swing posteriorly on the transverse axis of the SIJs, tensing the sacrotuberous and sacrospinous ligaments to maintain self-bracing. However, when the innominate bones begin to rotate upwards posteriorly and downwards anteriorly, they move on an acetabular axis and decrease self-bracing. This allows the innominate bone to rotate cephalad and laterally at the S3 segment of the sacral surface of the SIJ and, anteriorly, caudad, and laterally on the S1 segment of the sacral surface of the SIJ on the acetabular axis. Fixation probably occurs near or at the S3 segment at the posterior inferior iliac spine (PIIS) (Fig. 38.11) (DonTigny 1994).

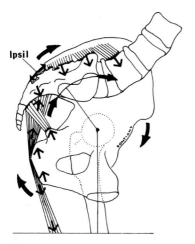

Fig. 38.11 Pathological release of self-bracing with failure of the force couple and resultant movement of the innominate bones on the sacrum on an acetabular axis. This stretches the superficial long posterior SI ligament (lpsil) and the sacrospinous ligament. An imbalance of tensile forces may cause a shearing stress of the ligamentous and tendinous attachments to the ischial tuberosity.

The movement of the PSISs cephalad and laterally on the sacrum with SIJD (DonTigny

1979) stretches the superficial long posterior SI ligament (DonTigny 1993, Vleeming et al 1995b) and is measurable (DonTigny 1990a). This may cause pain at its insertion into the caudal margin of the PSIS and along the lateral border of the sacrum. Prolonged stretch may weaken the attachment and cause local decalcification (Hackett & Huang 1961).

Although tensile stress is decreased on the sacrotuberous ligaments with SIJD, it is increased on the sacrospinous ligaments (Fig. 38.12). The sacrotuberous ligament attaches more cephalad on the sacrum and more caudad on the innominate than does the sacrospinous ligament. These ligaments work together with normal self-bracing, but are stressed quite differently with the pathological release of self-bracing with SIJD. Levin (1996, personal communication) reported commonly finding exquisite pain and tension in the sacrospinous ligament while palpating vaginally and an immediate release of tension with mobilization to the self-bracing position.

Point tenderness due to this fixation is common at the PIIS, but not obvious as it is frequently

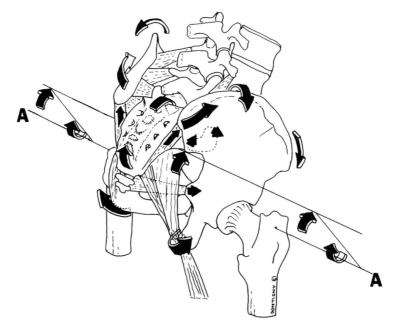

Fig. 38.12 Oblique view of some of the forces involved with the pathological release of self-bracing on an acetabular axis (AA) and initial application of force at the PIIS. Spinous extension is increased and thus stress on the iliolumbar ligaments may be decreased with a lack of support of the anterior pelvis. Ligamentous tethering by the superficial long posterior SI ligament and by the sacrospinous ligament limits dysfunction.

obscured by local edema that must be removed with deep massage prior to being able to identify the tenderness with deep palpation. The sacral origin of the piriformis muscle may be separated from its secondary origin at the upper margin of the greater sciatic notch of the ilium and may also cause pain in this immediate area, although the body of the piriformis is more caudal to the PIIS and deeper.

The movement of the innominate bone cephalad and laterally on the sacrum tends to separate the sacral origin of the gluteus maximus from its ilial origin. If extensive, the fibers of this muscle may be separated on a line from the PSIS diagonally downward to its insertion at the greater trochanter and iliotibial tract. This may precipitate a trochanteric bursitis, impair extensor stability, and cause pain down the iliotibial tract into the lateral aspect of the knee capsule.

As the PSIS rotates anteriorly with SIJD the tension on the iliolumbar ligaments may be decreased, decreasing lumbosacral stability, further increasing the anterior inclination of the sacral plateau, and resulting in increased shear forces on the discs, increased stress on a spondylolisthesis, or the appearance of an unstable lumbosacral segment. Damping of local oscillation or vibration could be impaired, thus allowing vibrational tissue creep to increase instability and shear.

As the innominate bones move anteriorly, downward, and laterally on the S1 segment of the sacral surface, the joint space is opened centrally, the anterior joint capsule is stretched and may be torn, and synovial fluid may leak from the joint. On arthrography of the SIJ, Fortin (1995) reported finding contrast medium surrounding the L5 nerve root and within the substance of the psoas muscle. He suggested that leakage of inflammatory mediators from a rent in the anterior capsule of a dysfunctional SIJ may explain the leg pain some of these patients experience. The same mechanism may separate the ilial origin of the iliacus muscle from its sacral origin and also be a cause of pain in this immediate area.

As a tear or injury to the capsule of the knee joint may inhibit the function of the quadriceps muscle, it seems possible that a tear of the capsule of the SIJ could cause a similar muscle inhibition. Dorman et al (1995) found that when the innominates are held in anterior rotation, the gluteus medius is inhibited. Other muscles may be similarly affected. This should be determined before concluding that the disc is at fault.

With SIJD, the ischial tuberosities may approximate to the coccyx, decreasing tension on the sacrotuberous ligaments and probably also distorting the muscles and fascia of the pelvic diaphragm. The ramifications of this have yet to be determined.

The patient may acquire a tendinitis of the biceps femoris at the ischial tuberosity because of an imbalance of forces across the ischial tuberosity (see Fig. 38.11 above). Abnormal stress on the biceps femoris may strain the ligaments of the head of the fibula and continue distally causing pain in the peroneus longus. Vleeming et al (1995a) found that the peroneus longus may provide up to 18% of the stability of the sacrotuberous ligament through the kinetic chain.

Pain on sitting

In the standing posture, the line of gravity is posterior to the acetabula, causing the innominates to rotate downwards posteriorly on an acetabular axis and enhance self-bracing. This movement is reinforced by buttressing of the femoral heads. In the sitting posture, the weightbearing on the ischial tuberosities tends to force the ilia apart. With SIJD, the ischial tuberosities are posterior to their normal position and weightbearing on them in sitting increases the anterior rotation strain on the capsule and other structures.

Pain on an increase of intra-abdominal pressure

The increase of intra-abdominal pressure associated with coughing or straining can be expected to spread the innominate bones on the sacrum and may precipitate or exacerbate SIJD. Stabilization of the SIJs by manual compression of the iliac crests will usually allow the patient to cough in comfort and implicates the SIJs, rather than an associated increase in intradiscal pressure, as the painful source (DonTigny 1985, 1990b).

Abdominal pain

Pain may be experienced in the abdomen at Baer's SI point and varies with stress on the SIJ. This point has been described as being on a line from the umbilicus to the anterior superior iliac spine (ASIS) 5 cm from the umbilicus (Mennell 1952) and may be misdiagnosed as appendicitis or ovarian pain. Norman (1968) reported injecting the SIJs to relieve lower abdominal pain. Wilson (1967) warned that painful radiation from the lower lumbar joint has led to unnecessary removal of pelvic organs.

SIJD with pregnancy

SIJD is a common uncomfortable complication of pregnancy. As weight increases on the anterior pelvis and pelvic support weakens, an anterior rotation strain occurs at the SIJs and may result in dysfunction (DonTigny 1979). Another factor is the hormonal influences of relaxin during the final stages of pregnancy. This softens and relaxes the SI ligaments and the symphysis pubis, which makes these areas less stable and more prone to injury (Abramson et al 1934, Thorp & Fray 1938). Kristiansson (1995) found that back pain during pregnancy was clearly associated with serum levels of relaxin.

Changes in apparent leg length

In the normal standing posture, the SIJs are positioned slightly posterior to the acetabula. With SIJD, the SIJs are positioned more cephalad and anteriorly, as in Fig. 38.4 above. This change in relationship results in a higher iliac crest when the patient is standing, an apparently longer leg length when the patient is supine, and an apparently shorter leg when the patient is sitting.

Common varieties of SIJD

Bilateral dysfunction

Bilateral SIJD is the most common type of dysfunction (DonTigny 1973, Swart 1923). It is most frequently overlooked because it is symmetric and most tests look for asymmetry as a sign of pathology. With this dysfunction, the iliac crests and PSISs are equally high on both sides when standing. The legs appear to be of equal length when supine, and, with the standing flexion test, both PSISs will appear to rise with trunk flexion at the same rate, although neither will actually move on the sacrum. The pelvis will be inclined anteriorly (although not necessarily increasing the lordosis), giving the impression of tight hip flexors. Bilateral SIJD also tends to flare the iliac crests, which then approximate with manual correction.

Unilateral dysfunction

If the dysfunction is unilateral, the crest on the affected side will be higher when standing and the leg on that side will appear to be longer when the patient is supine. The PSIS will be higher on the painful side when standing and the sacral plateau will tilt away from the side of pain. Any resultant lateral shift will be away from the side of pain, and a compensatory scoliosis may occur toward the painful side when standing. Even though the PSIS will be higher on the side of dysfunction, the level of the iliac crests may appear to be nearly the same. Because the acetabulum on the painful side moves downwards and posteriorly with reference to the SIJ, that leg will appear to get shorter when the patient moves from supine to the long sitting position. The decrease in tension on the sacrotuberous ligament may allow some sacral torsion. A bilateral anterior oblique SIJD may also occur that is similar to the unilateral SIJD, but both sides are involved (DonTigny 1993).

A complication of bilateral SIJD

A complication of bilateral SIJD may exist in the form of a secondary vertical shifting of the SI segment (DonTigny 1979, 1993). The anterior rotation fixation, which appears to occur at the PIISs, causes a movement of the PSISs cephalad and lateral on the sacrum. This opens the SIJs slightly, decreasing friction in the S1 segment of the joint, which may then allow the S1 ilial surface of the SIJ to slip cephalad on the S1 sacral surface of the SIJ. The initial point of binding seems to act as a pathological axis of rotation to allow this secondary shifting.

This secondary shift may occur suddenly with initial impact while walking, causing the patient to collapse without warning. Dorman (1995) described this as 'the slipping clutch syndrome'. This is frequently referred to as an up-slip or a posterior innominate lesion, and may be mistaken for an anterior dysfunction on one side and a posterior dysfunction on the other. The iliac crest on the more painful side will be slightly lower than the other when standing and the leg on that side will appear to be shorter when the patient is supine. The PSIS will be lower on the more painful side when standing and the sacral body will tilt toward the side of pain. Any resultant lateral shift will be toward the more painful side and a compensatory scoliosis may develop away from the side of pain. The pubis on the painful side may shift cephalad at the symphysis. I find no true posterior dysfunction of the SIJs, probably because the self-bracing mechanism prevents dysfunction posteriorly and because all of these described dysfunctions can be corrected and self-bracing restored with the same basic mobilization.

Recognition and diagnosis

Depending upon the degree and the severity of the dysfunction and the many and varied congenital anatomic aberrations in this region, nearly all of the described manifestations may occur some of the time and one should be aware of the various relationships. Recognition and diagnosis of SIJD can be made with the identification of a few of the manifestations that occur most frequently. These are the change in apparent leg length, pain deep in the area of the PIIS, and pain at the PSIS at the attachment of the superficial long posterior SI ligament. Slightly less frequently, pain should be sought at the attachment of the short posterior SI ligament on the medial aspect of the PSIS, a painful separation of the fibers of the gluteus maximus from the PSIS to the posterior trochanter, and pain in the sacrospinous ligament.

EVALUATION AND CORRECTION OF SIJD

To be valid, a test must be an appropriate, purposeful procedure to determine how and to what degree a lesion or dysfunction varies from normal function. SIJD is seldom included in procedures for evaluation of low back pain, and the majority of tests presently used do not reveal the dysfunction when it exists, so must be considered inappropriate (or misinterpreted).

The passive straight leg raising test

The passive straight leg raising (PSLR) test can be very helpful in the differential evaluation of SIJD. This test is generally interpreted rather narrowly relative to suspected nerve root pain and possible disc involvement, even though false positive and false negative results are common. The signs themselves are not false, but the hypothesis relative to their interpretation may be in error. Grieve (1981) has stated that a disc lesion is not a prerequisite of pain with PSLR and, even if present, need not necessarily have anything to do with causing pain, other than possibly making it worse.

Bohannon et al (1985) found a constant relationship between PSLR, pelvic rotation, and the pelvic angle. Pelvic rotation occurred in every subject by 9° of PSLR and usually before 4°. Every 2.7° of PSLR to the horizontal is accompanied by 1.7° of PSLR to the pelvic angle and 1° of pelvic rotation to the horizontal. Any restriction in pelvic rotation can affect the PSLR test. Cibulka et al (1986) found that SIJD can cause a hamstring strain, and Hiltz (1976) found that SIJD could cause sciatic pain.

The PSLR test cannot be considered negative if it does not cause pain. The pull of the hamstrings on the ischial tuberosity with PSLR causes a force in posterior rotation that may ease the pain of SIJD. As the examiner lowers the leg at the conclusion of the PSLR test, ipsilateral pain in the low back may be increased if the patient attempts to assist the examiner and actively holds back or lowers his or her own leg with the hip flexors. Mens et al (1995) found an apparent weakness of active straight leg raising with chronic back pain. Leg raising was made more powerful when the examiner stabilized the ipsilateral innominate bone at the ASIS. The contraction of the iliacus tends to pull the ipsilateral innominate anteriorly on the sacrum, increasing the pain of SIJD.

Two tests help to confirm the SIJs as the most likely location of this pain:

1. The fault is in the SIJ and not in the iliopsoas muscle if the patient stabilizes the anterior pelvis with the abdominal muscles by raising the head and shoulders, or if the examiner stabilizes the ASIS with his hand and the patient is then able to raise or lower the leg without discomfort.

2. If the abdominal muscles are weak and unable to support the anterior pelvis, the patient should actively lower the leg with the hip extensors against resistance applied by the examiner. The resultant force in posterior rotation will ease the pain of SIJD.

Mennell (1952) noted that as the ipsilateral innominate bone moves posteriorly with PSLR, the sacrum is carried posteriorly on the contralateral innominate: contralateral pain in the low back is indicative of SIJD on the contralateral side. Self-bracing is increased on the ipsilateral side with PSLR and released on the contralateral side. An increase of ipsilateral pain in the low back with PSLR is indicative of the complication of bilateral SIJD previously described.

Thus, when performing the PSLR, one must enquire whether the test increases pain or eases pain in the ipsilateral low back, or causes pain in the back on the contralateral side, or both. Does it cause or increase leg pain? Is the pain deep between the hamstrings along the course of the sciatic nerve or is the pain in the biceps femoris and peroneus longus – or is it just a tight hamstring?

CONFIRMATION AND CORRECTION

As SIJD occurs with a pathological release from the self-bracing position, all that is necessary to restore function is to return the joint to the self-bracing position (DonTigny 1993, 1994). As the legs appear to become longer with SIJD, they can be expected to shorten with correction. The key is to move the PSIS caudad and medially on the sacrum where the fixation occurs. The apparent shortening of the leg that occurs with correction is a measurable, objective, positive, and predictable sign that relieves pain and restores function to the SIJ.

An apparent shortening will occur with correction no matter whether the leg appears to be longer or shorter on the more painful side or whether the legs appear to be of equal length. This apparent shortening is accompanied by a measurable movement of the PSISs caudad and medially on the sacrum (DonTigny 1990a).

It is not a difference in leg length that causes dysfunction in the SIJs but rather the dysfunction that causes the changes in leg length. As leg length changes quickly and easily with mobilization, heel lifts are unnecessary.

The procedure to correct and confirm SIJD is performed with the patient supine on a plinth. The examiner stands at the foot of the plinth, grasps each ankle with a saddle grip, approximates the malleoli in the midline, and notes the comparative length of each leg. The relative position of each medial malleolus is an extension of the position of each ipsilateral acetabulum and indicative of the relative position of that acetabulum to the sacrum.

As the fixation is posteriorly and may act as a pathological axis of rotation, it is possible to mobilize the anterior pelvis cephalad or caudad, causing the legs to appear to shorten or lengthen without effecting a correction to the self-bracing position. One must mobilize the posterior aspect of the innominate caudally.

A very simple and safe method of mobilization to the self-bracing position is to stand to one side of the patient, grasp an ankle with both hands, gently raise the leg to about 40–50° of PSLR and put a strong, sustained pull on that leg in the long axis for about 5 s. No jerking, popping or twisting is necessary. Put that leg down and again examine the relative length at the malleoli. That leg will now appear to be shorter than it was previously. Repeat this procedure with the other leg, and that leg will also appear to shorten. Repeat this with the first leg again and it will appear to shorten even more. Keep repeating this procedure while alternating sides until no more apparent shortening occurs. The SIJs are high-friction joints and must be wobbled back into self-bracing a little bit at a time, rather like a stuck drawer. This takes a little patience, but is painless and well tolerated by the patient. The legs should appear to be of equal length after correction.

Any of several methods may be used to rotate the innominate bones posteriorly on the sacrum. The leg can be used as a lever, the innominate may be grasped directly and rotated posteriorly, or muscle energy techniques may be used (Fig. 38.13). Always examine the apparent leg length at the malleoli before and after each procedure. The dysfunction may occasionally be so tight that it may not release with the initial attempt at correction. Simply go to the other side and correct that and then come back to the first side; it will release much more easily and the leg will get shorter. It is very interesting and enlightening to mobilize or pull on a long leg or a short leg and watch it become shorter.

The patient must begin self-mobilization exercises as soon as possible after onset to correct the dysfunction and to maintain the correction. Once the basic principle is understood, a wide variety of exercises can be employed to accomplish a correction (DonTigny 1993). Either a direct stretch (Fig. 38.14) or a strong isometric hip extension (Fig. 38.15) may be used. Any of these exercises may be used depending upon convenience, ability, and individual efficacy of response. The selected exercises should be done alternately on each side at least three times (right, left, right, left, right,

left). If pain is severe, the exercises should be repeated every few hours throughout the day for 4 or 5 days, then 3–4 times daily for a week, and then as needed. Self-correction at bedtime allows the joints to stay unstressed during the hours of sleep.

PREVENTION OF ONSET OR RECURRENCE

SIJD may be effectively prevented by actively supporting the anterior pelvis to maintain the self-bracing mechanism when standing and especially prior to leaning forward to perform any task. A concurrent contraction of the gluteus maximus muscles serves to reinforce self-bracing. Muscles that are weak must be strengthened. To maintain self-bracing, it is more effective to actively contract a weak abdominal muscle group than to have a strong muscle group and not actively contract it.

Support

A good lumbosacral support or belt can be helpful to stabilize the unstable joint. It should be put on when the patient is supine and after a correction has been made. If the support is put on without

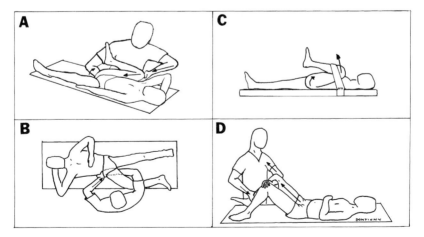

Fig. 38.13 Various methods of manual correction of dysfunction to restore self-bracing. (A) Using the leg as a lever. (B) Direct mobilization to cause the PSISs to move caudally and medially on the sacrum. (C) Isometric hip extension against a strap (Swart 1923). (D) Using the contralateral knee as a fulcrum while distracting the thigh and pelvis with the forearm. Just enough pressure is put on the lower leg with the other hand to keep the knee from extending. This is a very effective method of correction, simple and painless.

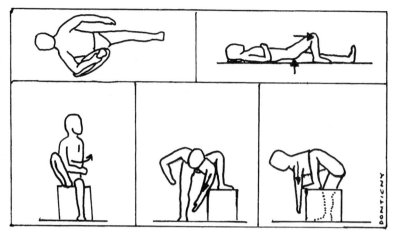

Fig. 38.14   Restoration of the self-bracing position using a direct stretch can be carried out while sitting, standing or lying.

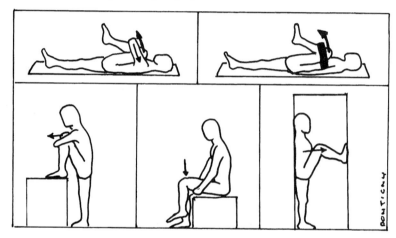

Fig. 38.15   Muscle energy techniques can be used in a variety of positions.

correcting the dysfunction, it may increase pain by increasing pressure on the uncorrected joints.

Frequency of occurrence

An outcome audit of 145 patients with low back pain in 1969 found 80% to have SIJD. Physical therapy treatments averaged 5.9 per patient (DonTigny 1973). In 1971 a similar audit of 54 consecutive outpatients with low back pain revealed that 83.3% had SIJD. Treatments averaged 2.9 per patient, and relief was frequently dramatic (DonTigny 1973). Shaw (1992) carried out a study of 1000 consecutive cases and found 98% to have SIJD. This is in agreement with the present observations.

CONCLUSIONS

1. The lumbosacroiliac complex appears to function as a self-compensating force couple with a moment of force that serves as a variable, force-dependent transverse axis, usually through the posterior aspect of the SIJ. This force couple increases joint stability through a principle of self-bracing, which allows greater ligamentous tension for the storage and release of energy and serves to balance forces of gravity, weight-loading, inertia, rotation, and acceleration and deceleration.

2. A pathological release of self-bracing may occur if the abdominal muscles fail to support the anterior pelvis when the line of gravity moves anteriorly. The innominate bones then move on

the SIJs on an acetabular axis, with fixation that may be extra-articular. The resulting lesion may mimic disc dysfunction or may give the impression of a multifactorial etiology and prevents normal function of the force couple.

3. Treatment of SIJD is the restoration of the self-bracing position through the manual correction of the innominate bones caudad and medially on the sacrum. The legs always appear to shorten with this correction. Prevention of SIJD is by

stabilizing the anterior pelvis with an active contraction of the abdominal muscles to maintain self-bracing, especially when leaning forward.

4. The most likely underlying cause of idiopathic low back pain is this subtle, measurable, reversible, biomechanical lesion. It is a commonly overlooked variation from normal, is easily corrected, and can be prevented with proper exercise. A thorough examination of the SIJs must always be included in the evaluation of low back pain.

REFERENCES

Abramson D, Roberts S M, Wilson P D 1934 Relaxation of the pelvic joints in pregnancy. Journal of Surgery, Gynecology and Obstetrics 58: 595–613

Bohannon R W, Gajdosik R, LeVeau B F 1985 Contribution of pelvic and lower limb motion to increases in the angle of passive straight leg raising. Physical Therapy 65: 474–476

Cibulka M T, Rose S J, Delitto A, Sinacore D R 1986 Hamstring muscle strain treated by mobilizing the sacroiliac joint. Physical Therapy 66: 1220–1223

DonTigny R L 1973 Evaluation, manipulation and management of anterior dysfunction of the sacroiliac joint. The DO 14: 215–216

DonTigny R L 1979 Dysfunction of the sacroiliac joint and its treatment. Journal of Orthopaedic and Sports Physical Therapy 1: 23–35

DonTigny R L 1985 Function and pathomechanics of the sacroiliac joint: a review. Physical Therapy 65: 35–44

DonTigny R L 1990a Measuring PSIS movement. Clinical Management 10: 43–44

DonTigny R L 1990b Anterior dysfunction of the sacroiliac joint as a major factor in the etiology of idiopathic low back pain syndrome. Physical Therapy 70: 250–265

DonTigny R L 1993 Mechanics and treatment of the sacroiliac joint. Journal of Manual and Manipulative Therapy 1: 3–12

DonTigny R L 1994 Function of the lumbosacroiliac complex as a self-compensating force couple with a variable, force-dependent transverse axis: a theoretical analysis. Journal of Manual and Manipulative Therapy 2: 87–93

Dorman T A 1995 Failure of self-bracing at the sacroiliac joints: the slipping clutch syndrome. In: Vleeming A, Mooney V, Dorman T, Snijders C J (eds) Second interdisciplinary world congress on low back pain. San Diego, CA, 9–11 November, pp 653–656

Dorman T A, Brierly S, Fray J, Pappani K 1995 Muscles and pelvic clutch: hip abductor inhibition in anterior rotation of the ilium. Journal of Manual and Manipulative Therapy 3: 85–90

Fortin J D 1995 Sacroiliac joint injection and arthrography with imaging correlation. In: Lennard T A (ed.) Physiatric procedures. Hanley & Belfus, Philadelphia. Reprinted in Vleeming A, Mooney V, Dorman T, Snijders C J (eds) Second interdisciplinary world congress on low back pain. San Diego, CA, 9–11 November, pp 533–544

Gracovetsky 1995 Locomotion. Linking the spinal engine with the legs. In: Vleeming A, Mooney V, Dorman T, Snijders C J (eds) Second interdisciplinary world congress on low back pain. San Diego, CA, 9–11 November, pp 171–173

Grieve G P 1981 Common vertebral joint problems. Churchill Livingstone, New York

Hackett G S, Huang T C 1961 Prolotherapy for sciatica from weak pelvic ligaments and bone dystrophy. Clinical Medicine 8(12): 2301–2316

Hiltz D L 1976 The sacroiliac joint as a source of sciatica: a case report. Physical Therapy 56: 1373

Kristiansson P 1995 S-Relaxin. A marker for back pain during pregnancy. In: Vleeming A, Mooney V, Dorman T, Snijders C J (eds) Second interdisciplinary world congress on low back pain. San Diego, CA, 9–11 November, p 204

Levin S M 1995 The sacrum in three-dimensional space. In: Vleeming A, Mooney V, Dorman T, Snijders C J (eds) Second interdisciplinary world congress on low back pain. San Diego, CA, 9–11 November, pp 625–633

Mennell J B 1952 The science and art of joint manipulation: the spinal column. J & A Churchill, London

Mens J M A, Vleeming A, Snijders C J, Stam H J 1995 Active straight leg raising. A clinical approach to the load transfer function of the pelvic girdle. In: Vleeming A, Mooney V, Dorman T, Snijders C J (eds) Second interdisciplinary world congress on low back pain. San Diego, CA, 9–11 November, pp 207–220

Norman G F 1968 Sacroiliac disease and its relationship to lower abdominal pain. American Journal of Surgery 116: 54–56

Russek A S 1976 Biomechanical and physiological basis for ambulatory treatment of low back pain. Orthopaedic Review 5(4): 21–31

Shaw J T 1992 The role of the sacroiliac joint as a cause of low back pain and dysfunction. In: Vleeming A, Mooney V, Snijders C J, Dorman T (eds) First interdisciplinary world congress on low back pain and its relation to the sacroiliac joint. San Diego, CA, 5–6 November, pp 67–80

Swart J 1926 Osteopathic strap technique. Joseph Swart, Kansas City

Thorp D J, Fray W E 1938 The pelvis joints during pregnancy and labor. Journal of the American Medical Association 111: 1162–1166

Thorstensson A, Nilsson J, Carlson H, Zomlefer M R 1984 Trunk movements in human locomotion. Acta Physiologica Scandinavica 121: 9–12

Vleeming A, Stoeckart R, Snijders C J 1989a The sacrotuberous ligament: a conceptual approach to its dynamic role in stabilizing the sacroiliac joint. Clinical Biomechanics 4: 201–203

Vleeming A, Wingerden J P van, Snijders C J, Stoeckart R, Stijnen T 1989b Load application to the sacrotuberous ligament: influences on sacroiliac joint mechanics. Clinical Biomechanics 4: 204–209

Vleeming A, Snijders C J, Stoeckart R, Mens J M A 1995a A new light on low back pain. The selflocking mechanism of the sacroiliac joints and its implications for sitting, standing and walking. In: Vleeming A, Mooney V, Dorman T, Snijders C J (eds) Second interdisciplinary world congress on low back pain. San Diego, CA, 9–11 November, pp 149–168

Vleeming A, Pool-Goudzwaard A L, Hammudoghlu D, Stoeckart R, Snijders C J, Mens J M A 1995b The function of the long dorsal sacroiliac ligament: its implication for understanding low back pain. In: Vleeming A, Mooney V, Dorman T, Snijders C J (eds) Second interdisciplinary world congress on low back pain. San Diego, CA, 9–11 November, pp 125–137

Vukicevic S, Marusic A, Stavljenic A, Vujicic G, Skavic J, Vukicevic D 1991 Holographic analysis of the human pelvis. Spine 16: 209–214

Weisl H 1953 The relation of movement to structure in the sacroiliac joint. PhD Thesis, University of Manchester, UK

Wilson J C Jr 1967 Low back pain and sciatica: a plea for better care of the patient. Journal of the American Medical Association 200: 705–712

39. Treatment of gravitational strain pathophysiology

M. L. Kuchera

INTRODUCTION

Gravitational force is constant and a greatly underestimated systemic stressor. Of the many signature manifestations of gravitational strain pathophysiology (Kuchera 1995a), the most prominent are *altered postural alignment* and *recurrent somatic dysfunction*. Signs and symptoms of low back pain, pain referred to the extremities, headache, fatigue, and weakness often become apparent only after key host compensatory mechanisms are activated or overwhelmed. These symptoms, as well as several visceral complaints, are frequently secondary to the underlying somatic pathophysiology but are rarely considered as such. Examination of patients' pathophysiology due to gravitational strain is likely to reveal postural decompensation, chronic or recurrent strains and sprains, pseudoparesis, recurrent articular dysfunction, recurrent myofascial trigger points, and ligamentous laxity, often in combination. The key to efficient diagnosis and therefore effective treatment is the realization that these seemingly diverse signs and symptoms are manifestations of pathophysiologic change resulting from a common musculoligamentous strain pattern caused by the stress of gravity.

Recognizing gravitational strain pathophysiology facilitates the selection of new and different therapeutic approaches for familiar problems. The precise approach selected for each patient and its predicted outcome are strongly influenced by the ratio of *functional disturbance* to *structural change* specific to that individual. Successful treatment protocols must establish attainable structural and functional goals. These are based upon modifying underlying pathophysiology and bio-mechanical stressors. Thus treatment incorporates therapeutic methods directed at local tissue biodynamics, but when gravitational strain contributes to the underlying pathophysiology, strategies for systemic integration of postural alignment must also be integrated.

Major goals for treating patients with gravitational strain pathophysiology include restoring local tissue function while simultaneously promoting central integration to obtain optimal biomechanical alignment for the individual. Treatment components may include, but are not limited to, orthotics, manipulation, prolotherapy, exercise protocols, muscle re-education initiatives, physical therapy modalities, and patient education (Table 39.1). Not all of these modalities will be required in every patient. Neither will every patient respond as expected, even when the optimum combinations are applied. Nonetheless, the incorporation of strategies for limiting gravity-induced dysfunction frequently salvages previously unsuccessful but seemingly well-designed protocols for low back pain treatment. Failure to reduce gravitational strain results in continued biomechanical stress and strain on an already compromised structure. This produces a predictable alteration of the tissue biodynamics and a return of somatic dysfunction.

This chapter discusses clinical ramifications of gravitational strain pathophysiology (GSP) and outlines practical and effective local and systemic management strategies.

DIAGNOSIS AND TREATMENT APPROACHES

GSP: local underlying tissue biodynamics

Numerous authors (Beal 1987, Denslow & Chase

Table 39.1   Suggested treatment of the components of GSP

*Local treatment**

Finding	Treatment approach(es)
Myofascial trigger points	Manipulation (local and reflex) (esp. muscle energy/counterstrain) Stripping masage Myofascial spray and stretch Procaine injections Physical therapy adjuncts (Ultrasound – pulsed, iontophoresis, vapocoolant then warm packs)
Muscle spasm	Manipulation (local and reflex) (esp. soft tissue/counterstrain) Stretching exercises Myofascial spray and stretch Therapy adjuncts (interferential, ultrasound)
Pseudoparesis	Stretching of antagonists Strengthening exercises Manipulation (local & reflex) Physical therapy adjuncts (Russian stimulation, tapotement)
Ligamentous laxity Functional hypermobility	Manipulation to adjacent hypermobility Protective short-term bracing Regional muscle strengthening exercises (see above)
Structural hypermobility	All of above for functional can be applied Prolotherapy
Somatic dysfunction	Manipulation (local and reflex) Range of motion exercises

*Systemic integration treatment**

Finding	Treatment approach(es)
Patterns of trigger points, muscle spasm, pseudoparesis	Muscle re-education Janda's protocol Proprioceptive retraining Manipulation (regional, local, reflex) Nutritional/metabolic care Postural alignment
Patterns of recurrent somatic dysfunction	Manipulation (regional, local, reflex) Postural alignment

*Postural alignment treatment**

Primary plane of involvement	Treatment approach(es)
Sagittal plane	Levitor orthotic Pelvic coil exercises Regional manipulation Bilateral alteration of heel-to-anterior-sole height Patient education

Table 39.1   *(Contd)*

Coronal plane	Unilateral heel or sole lift Foot orthotics Konstancin exercises Regional manipulation
Horizontal plane	Unilateral alteration of heel-to-anterior-sole height Regional manipulation

*Requires elements in other two categories for lasting success.

1962, Freeman 1957, Jungmann & McClure 1963, Kendall et al 1993) have researched posture and the adaptive response of somatic structures to gravitational strain. Resultant pathophysiologic changes in these stressed somatic tissues are the source of many patient complaints, including local and referred pain syndromes (Kuchera 1995a). Positive modification of underlying tissue biodynamics is the desired end result of each element of the treatment protocol, and the extent to which this is possible determines the prognosis. This section will concentrate on the local tissue characteristics of chronic, recurrent somatic dysfunction and subsequent anatomic change in posturally related muscles and ligaments.

The term 'somatic dysfunction' was originally coined by the osteopathic profession to describe the asymmetry, restricted motion, and tissue texture changes palpable in certain dysfunctional physiologic states. The term has been generally adopted and is listed in the International Classification of Disease (ICD-9-CM) as a codable diagnosis, listed by regions of the body (739.0–739.9). Somatic dysfunction is specifically defined as 'impaired or altered function of somatic tissues – skeletal, arthrodial, and/or myofascial – and its related neural, vascular and lymphatic elements'. Early in the process of biomechanical strain, somatic dysfunction often exists alone and is reversible. As structural change is introduced, somatic dysfunction becomes more common, but its treatment in isolation restores only a portion of the patient's regional and total function.

Treatment of skeletal/arthrodial somatic dysfunction is most specifically addressed with manipulation. While symmetry is often restored with manipulation, it is most important to maximize stable, physiologic motion in the area and improve tissue level health. Considerable variability exists

Table 39.2   Choice of manipulative technique

Technique	Tissues responding best	Tissues responding poorly
Direct method of treatment		
High-velocity, low-amplitude (HVLA)	Fibrotic, structurally shortened tissues	Acutely painful or spastic, abundant edema, patient guarding, osteoporosis
Muscle energy	Functionally or structurally shortened, myofascial trigger points, mild-to-moderate muscle spasm	Acute spasm, non-cooperative patient
Inhibition	Acute spasm, myofascial trigger points	Chronic, structurally shortened, fibrosis
Stretching	Functionally or structurally shortened muscle, myofascial trigger points, mild muscle spasm, myofascial trigger points	Acute muscle spasm
Fulford (percussion hammer)	Chronic viscous change, traumatic fascial patterns	Fracture, bruising at site
Indirect method of treatment		
Counterstrain	Acute spasm, myofascial trigger points, edema, pain	Chronic, structural shortening
Myofascial release	Edema, traumatic fascial patterns	Chronic, structural shortening
Ligamentous balancing	Most situations	—

in the choice of manipulative technique (Table 39.2); however, the choice of technique is less important than accomplishing certain goals. These goals are:

1. to provide restitution of lost normal motion
2. to modify protective, compensatory, or dysfunctional physiologic mechanisms in the regional tissues affected
3. to remove central physiologic mechanisms perpetuating somatic dysfunction
4. to modify physical and physiologic impediments to the above goals.

Later in this chapter, specific considerations for reaching these goals in the lumbosacroiliac region will be presented.

Treatment of gravity-induced myofascial dysfunction

Gravitational strain predictably initiates dysfunction in postural muscles and their antagonists. Postural muscles, structurally adapted to resist prolonged gravitational stress, generally resist fatigue. When overly stressed, however, these same postural muscles become irritable, tight, and shortened (Janda 1986). The antagonists to these postural

muscles demonstrate inhibitory characteristics described as 'pseudoparesis' (a functional, non-organic weakness) or 'myofascial trigger points with weakness' when they are stressed (Janda 1986, Kendall et al 1993). A neurologic examination, including functional muscle testing, is essential in evaluating patients with suspected GSP because muscular weakness or cramping is present in isolated or apparently neurologically related areas.

The pattern of hyperactive and inhibited muscles seen in gravitational strain patients is presented in Table 39.3. Travell myofascial trigger points arise independently in both overworked postural muscles and their dysfunctional antagonists (Travell & Simons 1983). Clinicians will recognize from their own experience with chronic low back patients that many of the muscles listed in this section are repeatedly treated, often in isolation, with good but transient results. Recognition that gravity is a stressor capable of initiating recurrent patterns of local and systemic dysfunction significantly expands a physician's diagnostic and therapeutic perspectives. If part of the pattern is recognized, seeking dysfunction in other parts of the pattern not previously considered is warranted.

Table 39.3   Muscle response to gravitational strain

Region	Postural muscle response (spasm)	Phasic muscle response (pseudoparesis)
Cervical/upper thoracic	Upper trapezius Levator scapulae Pectoralis major (upper part) Pectoralis minor Cervical erector spinae Scalenus muscles Sternocleidomastoid	Latissimus dorsi Mid/lower trapezius Rhomboids Anterior cervical muscles
Lumbar/lumbopelvic	Tensor fasciae latae Hamstrings Hip adductors (short adductors) Gastrocnemius/soleus Piriformis Iliopsoas	Quadriceps Abdominals Gluteus maximus

Myofascial dysfunction, including the presence of myofascial trigger points, is a specific form of somatic dysfunction with subjective pain, recordable weakness, and autonomic and vascular–lymphatic characteristics (Kuchera 1997). In prolonged myofascial strain, both structural (anatomic) and functional (physiologic and biochemical) changes occur, leading to sustained changes in myofascial length. In response to gravitational strain, postural muscles are typically shortened. Significantly, studies (Gossman et al 1982) suggest that

deleterious change is most pronounced in shortened, as opposed to lengthened, muscles. Numerous patient complaints can be directly attributed to gravity-induced muscle dysfunction, both spastic and inhibited muscles (Table 39.4).

Even though the dysfunction induced by gravitational stress and strain is muscle-specific, general patterns are documented to be characteristic and predictable (Institute for Gravitational Strain Pathology 1992, Janda 1986, Jungmann & McClure 1963, Kuchera 1995a, Travell & Simons

Table 39.4   Common muscle symptoms arising from gravitational strain

Structure	Spastic muscle symptom
Iliopsoas	Inability to stand straight (psoas posturing); knees flexed; recurrent L1–2 somatic dysfunction; pain referral to back and anterior groin; positive Thomas test
Quadratus lumborum	Low back pain referred to the groin and hip; exhalation 12th rib somatic dysfunction; diaphragm restriction
Hamstrings	Pain sitting or walking; pain disturbs sleep; pain referral to posterior thighs; straight leg raising limited mechanically
Piriformis	Pain down posterior thigh; may entrap peroneal portion of sciatic nerve; perpetuated by SI dysfunction; associated with pelvic floor dysfunction, dyspareunia, and prostatodynia
Thigh adductors (short)	Pain referral to inguinal ligament, inner thigh, and upper medial knee
Gastrocnemius–soleus complex	Nocturnal leg cramps; pain referral to upper posterior calf, instep, and heel

Structure	Inhibited muscle symptom
Gluteus minimus	Pain characteristic when arising from chair; pain referral to buttock, lateral, and posterior thigh; 'pseudosciatica'; antalgic gate; positive Trendelenburg test
Gluteus medius	Pain aggravated by walking; pain referral to posterior iliac crest and SIJ; positive Trendelenburg test
Gluteus maximus	Restlessness; pain sitting or walking up hill; antalgic gait; SI instability
Vastus muscles	Buckling knee; weakness going up stairs; thigh and knee pain; chondromalacia patellae
Rectus abdominis	Increased lordosis; constipation
Tibialis anterior	Pain referred to great toe and anteromedial ankle; may drag foot or trip when tired

1983, 1992). Travell and Simons (1983, 1992) definitively describe and map individual myofascial trigger points but also consistently report associated trigger point patterns in myotatic units. The myotatic unit, composed of muscles sharing the same functional responsibilities or stress, is at increased risk of myofascial dysfunction. Failure to look and treat beyond the individual pain generator increases the risk of its recurrence.

Travell and Simons' local treatment techniques for myofascial trigger points are described in detail in several texts (Simons & Travell 1989,

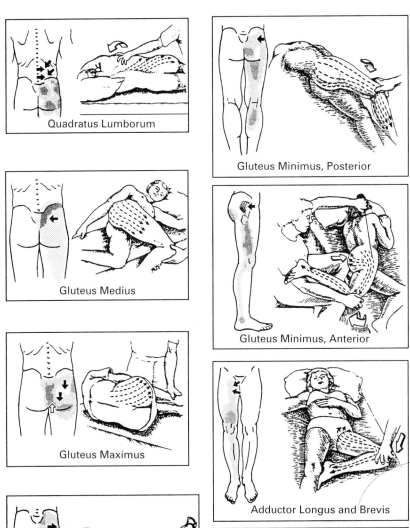

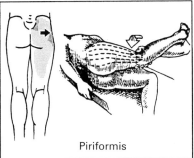

 Pain Pattern 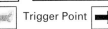 Trigger Point

Fig. 39.1 Travell trigger point pain patterns common in patients with GSP. Local treatment with vapocoolant spray and stretch technique requires postural alignment and systemic integrating techniques to avoid recurrence. (Adapted with permission from Simons 1987.)

Travell & Simons 1983, 1992). Figure 39.1 summarizes the pain referral patterns and positions used in applying vapocoolant myofascial spray and stretch to the muscles most commonly involved in gravitational strain. Figures such as this, however, fail to incorporate Travell and Simons' advocacy of treating underlying precipitating and perpetuating causes, including gravity-induced postural stress. Specific techniques for the treatment of local tissue change are only a part of the successful treatment protocol for myofascial dysfunction.

According to Jungmann (1961), 'the ilio-psoas muscle is in the forefront of the structures which oppose the thrust of gravity on the spine and pelvis'. Thus it is liable foremost to be affected by gravitational strain. Correction of iliopsoas muscle shortening, with or without trigger points, is therefore pivotal in achieving postural realignment (Kuchera 1995a). During acute spasm, 'counterstrain' manipulation is much more effective than the spray and stretch technique. Treatment begins by locating the exquisitely tender iliacus point

described by Jones (1993). In the supine position, the patient's legs and hips are flexed to approximately 90°, with the foot of the involved side crossed over the opposite ankle. The hips are allowed to externally rotate by letting the knees separate. This general position is then modified by careful and precise positioning to relax the iliopsoas muscle. The appropriate position is ascertained by an immediate 70% (or more) reduction in tenderness/pain to direct palpation of Jones' iliacus point. Once located, the position is maintained for 90 s. This 'position of ease' (Fig. 39.2) reduces noxious afferent stimuli conveyed to the spinal cord and positioning of antagonist muscles reflexly relaxes the shortened spastic iliopsoas. The extremities are then slowly and passively extended back onto the treatment table. Associated L1 or L2 arthrodial dysfunction is almost always found with a shortened spastic iliopsoas muscle and should also be specifically addressed. Manipulative treatment to remove this somatic dysfunction is essential for achieving and then maintaining normal iliopsoas muscle function.

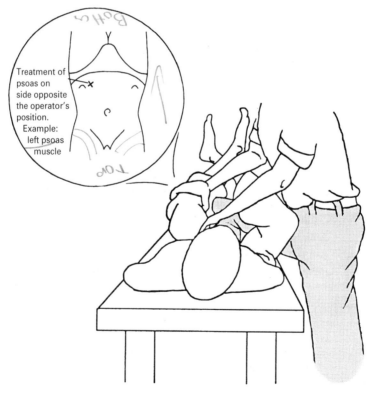

Fig. 39.2 'Position of ease' in iliopsoas counterstrain technique.

The treatment of local myofascial trigger points is not limited to the use of procaine injections or vapocoolant technique. According to Travell and Simons (1983, 1992), many other techniques, including manipulation, are effective in removing this and other myofascial dysfunction. All are easily integrated in treatment protocols that address systemic neuromusculoskeletal dysfunction (Kuchera 1997).

Myofascial dysfunction is capable of initiating and maintaining pain syndromes, systemic dysfunction, and instability. Therefore, appropriate local treatment remains a vital component in protocols in which this dysfunction is identified. It must, however, be integrated with systemic strategies designed to reduce perpetuating biomechanical strain and to coordinate peripheral and central mechanisms associated with muscular function.

Muscular re-education

Gravitational strain initially precipitates and perpetuates dysfunctional patterns (Janda 1986, Travell & Simons 1983, 1992) in the postural muscles and their antagonists by creating systemic imbalance. Beyond the local changes described in the preceding section, resulting afferent proprioceptive imbalance affects systemic neuromuscular reflex mechanisms associated with the maintenance of posture.

The central nervous system functions by coordinating systemic *patterns of movement* rather than by producing isolated muscle activation. Movement precedes postural control and is necessary to alter it (Knott & Voss 1968). Thus postural realignment cannot occur without local manipulation or systemic muscular re-education. Conversely, re-establishment of normal muscle function and central nervous system regulation of movement patterns are dependent on postural realignment. Therefore, coordinated, functional movement patterns and postural realignment are interdependent.

Jungmann recognized gravity's propensity to create both local and systemic patterns of dysfunction. Treatment of gravitational strain pathophysiology was therefore directed to include the integration of body systems (Institute for Gravi-

tational Strain Pathology 1992, Kuchera 1995a). His treatment protocol was designed to re-educate and repattern systemic functions such as walking and breathing while reducing systemic stress through postural realignment.

Jungmann's observations have been more recently complemented by those of Janda (Kuchera 1995b). With regard to integrated muscular dysfunction, Janda (1986) notes:

development of tightness and/or weakness in certain muscles may be considered as a systemic and characteristic deviation in the functional quality of these muscles. The final result of this deviation is then a general imbalance within the whole muscular system.

Janda's approach to treatment also combines local treatments with functionally oriented, systemically integrated activities.

Ultimately, the clinical goal is to return the patient who has GSP to optimal function. To address the interdependence of postural stability, consistent proprioceptive input, and coordinated movement patterns, a carefully constructed program, including patient education, is required. The range of therapeutic protocols designed to normalize movement patterns within the gravitational field is beyond the scope of this chapter; nonetheless certain principles can be enunciated for reaching this goal:

1. *Seek biomechanical stability.* This provides a balanced platform from which to operate. If orthotics are required, they should be worn consistently while in the upright position. This is especially important early in the 're-education' period while the central nervous system is integrating the evolving postural alignment.

2. *Stretch tight postural muscles or other shortened muscles.* Tight muscles should be stretched before attempting to strengthen inhibited, weakened muscles. Attempts to reverse this order are typically frustrating because inhibition from the shortened antagonist interferes with programs designed to strengthen the weakened phasic muscles.

3. *Keep functional units in careful balance with one another through proprioceptive retraining.* This will greatly facilitate treatment and forestall the recurrence of dysfunction. This can be accomplished with the use of a tilt board or other

adjunctive devices, or through a combination of specific exercises (Janda 1986).

4. *Re-educate the CNS to respond to rapid change.* Janda describes methods of increasing the speed of muscular contraction to help protect the musculoligamentous system from rapidly changing stresses.

Lewit (1985) argues that somatic dysfunction is most frequently the cause of faulty movement patterns potentiated by muscle imbalance and postural overstrain. If this is even partially true, muscular re-education and postural balancing must be considered in the design of a successful and lasting treatment protocol.

Prolotherapy for hypermobile regions

Gravitational force is constant; specific stress vectors and inherent host factors resisting the imposed forces will, however, vary between individuals. Anatomic and biomechanical factors interacting with congenital and acquired susceptibilities will modify an individual's response to physical stressors. Transitional (junctional) areas have an anatomic predisposition to develop histological, physiological, dysfunctional and structural changes in response to stress. These cross-over areas and their protective/supportive structures are particularly susceptible to gravitational strain, somatic dysfunction, postural decompensation, and injury. Congenital ligamentous susceptibility to GSP exists in those with connective tissues disorders such as Ehlers–Danlos syndrome or Ollier's disease. Acquired susceptibility is found in individuals with ligamentous laxity from direct macrotrauma or sustained biomechanically induced microtrauma.

The histologic junctional zones created by connective tissue attachments of ligaments, tendons, and joint capsules are also vulnerable to the biomechanical stress of postural decompensation (Cantu & Grodin 1992, Hackett 1958). This is especially true for the fibro-osseous junctional attachments of restraining ligaments. The viscous components of chronically stressed ligaments undergo progressive change (Kuchera 1995c). The change begins with edema in the region of their fibro-osseous junction, which is tender to palpation.

New collagen, with a half-life of 10–12 months, realigns the connective tissues in response to stress vectors, perpetuates the resultant posture and maintains biomechanical amplification of gravitational stress. Chronic stress, thus amplified, modifies connective tissue structure and reduces its ability to compensate for gravitational stress. Eventually, ligamentous laxity and hypermobility occur.

Not all hypermobile areas are 'structural'. Functional or compensatory hypermobility occurs early in response to adjacent areas of hypomobile somatic dysfunction. Compensatory hypermobility disappears when the somatic dysfunction is removed. If left long enough, however, compensatory hypermobility will structurally adapt to the constant functional demand. This results in a permanent viscous change in the musculoligamentous structures. Differentiation between functional and structural hypermobility is needed because treatment for the two types is quite different. Figure 39.3 depicts specific tests of sacroiliac (SI) instability.

Continuous gravitational stress initiates ligamentous strain, responsible for continued chronic and recurrent pain, especially affecting the neck and low back (Hackett 1959). Common ligamentous pain patterns arising from the lumbosacroiliac region are shown in Fig. 39.4. Further postural stress on these hypermobile structures increases discomfort. These patients are unable to sit or stand in the gravitational field for any period of time because they are unable to find a position of comfort. Their condition is sometimes referred to as the 'cocktail party syndrome' (Dorman & Ravin 1991). When these patients lie down and remove the longitudinal effect of gravity, they experience bilateral low back pain, which often takes more than 30 min to subside. Vleeming et al (1995) attributes this symptom to pain referral to the long dorsal SI ligament. Ligamentous strain also affects tensegrity (Levin 1995), thereby influencing structures that may be quite distant from the locally hypermobile site.

In a homeostatic attempt to stabilize hypermobility and protect joint structures, the body responds by deposition of calcium along lines of stress (Wolff's Law). This produces exostoses at attachments of postural muscles and ligaments.

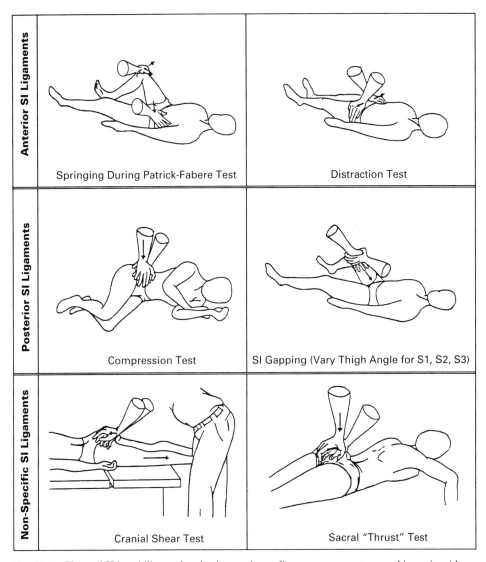

Fig. 39.3 Tests of SI instability apply selective tension to ligamentous structures seeking pain with local hypermobility. This permits isolation of the involved ligament.

Often, calcification of the entire ligament takes place. Bony exostoses and ligamentous calcification provide radiographic evidence of chronic stress on these structures. This process occurs relatively early to the iliolumbar ligament, whose purpose is to stabilize the lumbar spine with respect to the pelvis and to permit postural function in the gravitational field. Subjective or subclinical pain elicited by palpation over iliolumbar ligament attachments may be the first sign of postural decompensation of the lumbopelvic junction.

Signs and symptoms of structural hypermobility indicate stress surpassing homeostatic capabilities, and a need for stabilization. Conservative protocols that strengthen muscle to supplement the function of weakened ligaments may be considered. Proliferant therapy, or prolotherapy, is also capable of eliminating structural hypermobility and is the treatment of choice for other patients with ligamentous laxity. Prolotherapy is described in Chapter 40 in this volume, but two points need to be re-emphasized here.

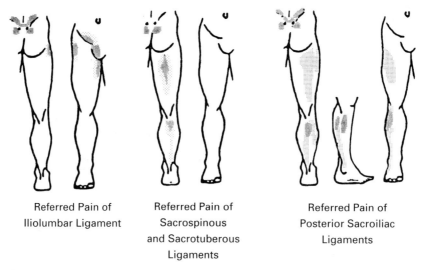

Referred Pain of
Iliolumbar Ligament

Referred Pain of
Sacrospinous
and Sacrotuberous
Ligaments

Referred Pain of
Posterior Sacroiliac
Ligaments

Fig. 39.4   Common ligamentous pain patterns arising from gravitational strain and postural malalignment. (Adapted from Hackett 1958.)

1. Prolotherapy should be reserved for structural (as opposed to functional) hypermobility.

2. If prolotherapy is improperly applied by failing to address the alignment and motion aspects of the underlying gravitational stress problem, the clinical results will be unsatisfactory or, at best, transient.

In GSP, soft tissue structures are affected early and then progress through dysfunction towards anatomic structural change. Examination should assess the status of the underlying tissues in the spinal transition areas and the support structures involved in the maintenance of postural alignment. Historical, palpatory, and radiologic analyses provide clues to the location and status of involved ligaments. Functional and stress testing of the underlying tissues is a practical way of assessing the extent of their involvement in the process. Palpation evaluates tissue texture changes, including edema at fibro-osseous junctions and signs of ligamentous laxity. Differentiation of structural and functional laxity may involve evaluation of a conservative therapeutic trial. Special attention is paid to dysfunction or instability in the lumbosacroiliac complex. This is discussed below.

Treatment of SI and pelvic dysfunction with manipulation

Diagnosis and management of recurrent somatic

dysfunction in the lumbosacroiliac region is particularly relevant in reducing myofascial dysfunction (Travell & Simons 1992) and low back pain (Kuchera & Kuchera 1994a). Shaw (1992) confirms the ubiquity (98%) of sacroiliac somatic dysfunction in 2000 consecutive cases of low back pain. It is also ubiquitous in patients with GSP (Kuchera 1995b) and is therefore an integral part of the treatment of postural decompensation (Kuchera 1995a).

SI function and dysfunction are best assessed by applying a consistent palpatory examination and adopting the criteria and nomenclature of one of several postulated models. The lumbosacroiliac region is, unfortunately, the site of the greatest number of congenital spinal anomalies, including facet asymmetry. This complicates the interpretation of palpatory findings. For this reason, appropriate diagnosis of somatic function and low back dysfunction should not be based solely on static anatomic landmarks; asymmetric landmark interpretation should always be coupled with motion testing in the region. Figure 39.5 shows the static and dynamic palpatory findings associated with a variety of pelvic somatic dysfunctions (Kuchera & Kuchera 1994a).

DonTigny (1995a) describes the lumbosacroiliac complex as a 'self-compensating force couple that accommodates, mitigates, balances, stores and redirects various forces affecting the pelvis and its

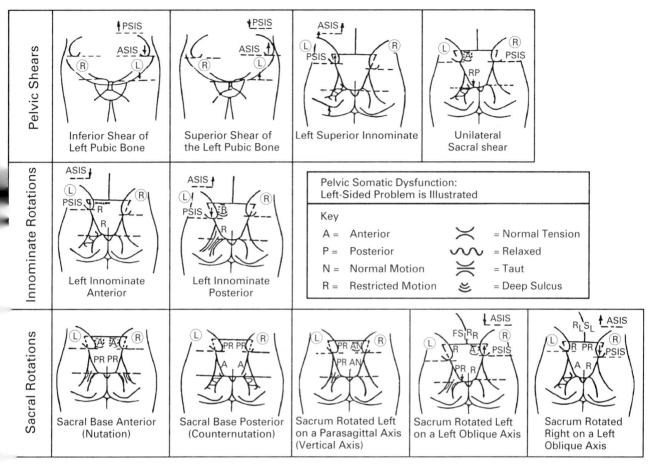

Fig. 39.5 Palpatory diagnostic characteristics associated with specific pelvic somatic dysfunctions. (Adapted from Kuchera & Kuchera 1994b.)

principle ligaments'. This complex is dependent upon stable yet unimpeded motion of somatic structure. Transfer of weight-bearing force through the lumbosacroiliac complex during posture and gait is largely responsible for the dynamic physiologic motions described around various axes (Kuchera & Kuchera 1994a). It is also consistent with the description (DonTigny 1995a) of balanced ligamentous and gravitational tensile stresses in determining a location for a transverse sacral axis that is force dependent rather than anatomy dependent.

Stability of the SI joint (SIJ) (Fig. 39.6) is dependent upon 'force-closure' and 'self-bracing' mechanisms (Vleeming et al 1995). GSP is capable of disturbing both these mechanisms, leading to instability. Postural stress in the sagittal plane activates the systemic patterns of muscle dysfunction

described by Janda (1986) and by Travell & Simons (1983, 1992), as previously outlined in Table 39.3 and Fig. 39.1 respectively. This posturally induced stress disturbs stability by causing imbalance in the four major muscles involved in force closure: the erector spinae, gluteus maximus, latissimus dorsi, and biceps femoris. Additionally, anterior displacement of the gravitational line decreases anterior pelvic support, thus disturbing self-bracing (DonTigny 1995b). Structural loss of tensegrity can also result in instability (Levin 1995).

Posturally induced sacral instability predisposes to recurrent SI somatic dysfunction. Reduction of force closure and self-bracing protective mechanisms during periods of sacral loading significantly increase the potential for non-physiologic unilateral sacral and innominate shear somatic

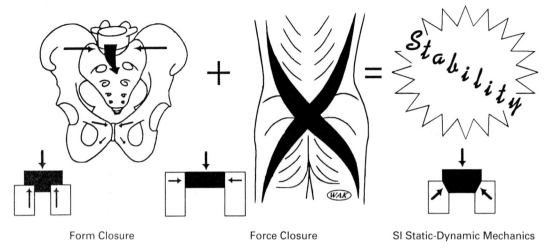

Form Closure   Force Closure   SI Static-Dynamic Mechanics

Fig. 39.6 Stability in the SIJ arises from combination of self-bracing and force closure mechanisms responsive to gravitational stress. (Adapted with permission from Vleeming 1995.)

dysfunctions. They are called 'non-physiologic' because they do not occur about an axis and are not motions normal to the SIJ. These dysfunctions are easy to diagnose if looked for, easy to fix if found, but will perpetuate patient problems and prevent the success of otherwise effective treatment regimes unless addressed (Kuchera & Kuchera 1994a). These dysfunctions are often misdiagnosed as discogenic disease or other multifactorial etiologies of low back pain.

These non-physiologic pelvic shear somatic dysfunctions must be diagnosed and treated if postural realignment and reduction of musculo-ligamentous strain are to occur. One or more traumatically induced pelvic shear somatic dysfunctions – sacral shear, innominate shear, and pubic shear – occur when patients, for example, unexpectedly step into a pothole or off a step or curb that they did not anticipate. Force is transferred up the lower extremity or into the ischial tuberosity with this and similar mechanisms of injury. This upward force is met by the body's weight and body momentum moving in a downward direction. The result is a shearing force along the SI articulation. The shape of the SI articulation influences the movement of the SIJ during the shear and results in fairly predictable static palpatory landmarks accompanied by restricted SI function. Pubic shears also possess distinctive palpatory characteristics.

Pubic shear somatic dysfunction responds well to direct-method, muscle-energy manipulative techniques. The somatic dysfunction 'barrier' is engaged by rotating one half of the pelvis against the restriction (Fig. 39.7). The patient is then asked actively to attempt to rotate the pelvis away from that impediment as the physician applies resistance isometrically. In each of these positions, the physician positions the patient and holds the knee so that either activation will pull the origin of those muscles in the appropriate direction to correct the somatic dysfunction present. Upon patient relaxation, the physician rotates the pelvis further, through the dysfunctional barrier to a new barrier. This is repeated approximately three times. Prior to muscle-energy activation, sufficient thigh adduction to gap SI dysfunction or abduction to gap pubic somatic dysfunction will help to localize these techniques for optimum effect.

While a number of manipulative techniques are described in the osteopathic literature (e.g. Greenman 1989, Kimberly 1980), a straight longitudinal high-velocity, low-amplitude (HVLA) 'tug' through the same lower extremity is often successful in addressing sacral or innominate shear diagnoses. The soft tissue 'slack' of the knee and hip is first eliminated with steady traction and encouragement of the patient to relax his or her muscles. An HVLA tug is then

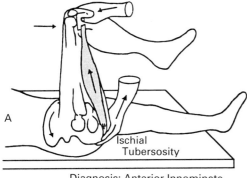

Diagnosis: Anterior Innominate
Treatment: Muscle energy activation
using the hamstring muscles

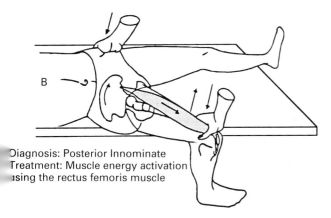

Diagnosis: Posterior Innominate
Treatment: Muscle energy activation
using the rectus femoris muscle

Fig. 39.7   Muscle energy manipulation (A) Treating anterior innominate rotation or inferior pubic shear somatic dysfunctions with muscle energy direct technique employs the hamstrings to 'pull' one half of the pelvis through the somatic dysfunction barrier. (B) Activation of the rectus femoris muscle against resistance rotates half of the pelvis anteriorly to correct either posterior innominate rotation or superior pubic shear somatic dysfunction. (Reprinted with permission from Kuchera 1995c.)

Right Sacral Shear

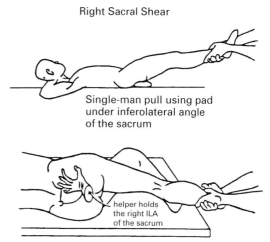

Single-man pull using pad
under inferolateral angle
of the sacrum

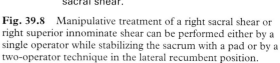

helper holds
the right ILA
of the sacrum

Two-man pull using an assistant
to stabilize the inferolateral angle
of the sacrum on the side of the
sacral shear.

Fig. 39.8   Manipulative treatment of a right sacral shear or right superior innominate shear can be performed either by a single operator while stabilizing the sacrum with a pad or by a two-operator technique in the lateral recumbent position. (Reprinted with permission from Kuchera 1995c.)

applied against resistance applied to the sacrum at the inferolateral angle (Fig. 39.8). This is often effective in re-establishing both static alignment and dynamic motion characteristics in the SIJ.

Not all somatic dysfunctions affecting the pelvis are traumatically induced as are the shears. Most other somatic dysfunctions occur during execution of daily activities. Simply walking engages a number of physiologic axes, and momentary disruption of coordination during the walking cycle can result in a number of somatic dysfunction diagnoses involving the sacrum and/or the innominates. Prolonged shifting of weight onto a potential axis of motion engages it and predisposes to somatic dysfunction around that axis. Right-handed golfers, for example, have a propensity (Kuchera 1995a) towards the development of right rotation about a right oblique sacral axis. This has been postulated to result from shifting weight onto the right upper pole of the sacrum during the golf swing. In the general population, the most common compensatory (non-traumatic) pattern of somatic dysfunction in the pelvis includes a left rotation about a left sacral oblique axis and an anteriorly rotated right innominate. Manipulation effectively and immediately corrects these pelvic somatic dysfunctions, although they may spontaneously resolve over time and during repeated routine patient movements (Kimberly 1980).

Unless normal motion within the lumbosacroiliac complex is re-established, postural alignment and systemic integrating techniques are destined to fail. Conversely, patterns of somatic dysfunction will recur in gravitational strain patients treated with manipulation only.

Treatment of spinal somatic dysfunction with manipulation

Correction of spinal somatic dysfunction is also essential to accomplish local, postural, and systemic treatment goals in patients with GSP. Prerequisite segmental and regional palpatory methods delineate characteristics used in classifying somatic dysfunction and strongly influence the choice of manipulative technique (see Table 39.2 above).

Segmental testing (Fig. 39.9) can be active or passive (Kuchera 1995a). Passive motion testing assesses the quality of the 'barrier' or 'end-feel' in the minor and involuntary range of a synovial joint's physiologic range of motion. A somatic dysfunction barrier will characteristically have an abrupt and resistant end-feel, whereas the physiologic barrier in the opposite direction will be resilient. In contradistinction, one form of active segmental motion testing involves requesting the patient to provide backward and forward bending as the physician monitors the effect by palpation near the articular facets. Regardless of the type of motion testing selected, if the same diagnostic procedures are first well defined, interexaminer reliability for determining segmental somatic dysfunction is high.

Segmental somatic dysfunction can interfere with treatment of GSP even when otherwise appropriate treatment protocols are offered. While the precise mechanisms have not been isolated, the role that somatic dysfunction plays in

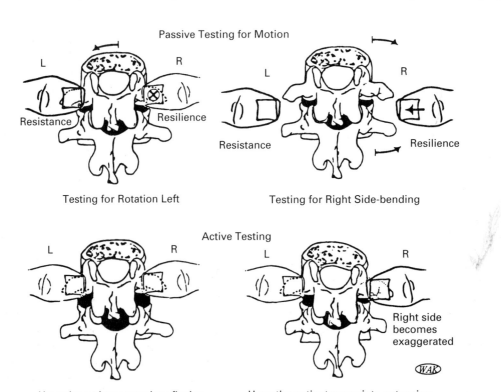

Fig. 39.9 Motion testing. *Passive motion testing* (top) involves the physician pressing alternately over each transverse process and translating between spinal segments to assess the quality of the barrier at the end of motion. In the diagram, the left thumb meets sudden resistance in both side-bending and rotation while the end-feel for both is springy under motion initiated by the right thumb. The somatic dysfunction diagnosis is a spinal segment that is side-bent right and rotated left (NS$_R$R$_L$). In *active motion testing* (bottom), the patient flexes and extends while the physician palpates the motion near the articular pillars. In the diagram, both thumbs move forward equally with flexion. With extension, the right facet closes but the left does not. At the end of extension, the right transverse process is more posterior than the left. Here the dysfunction is flexed, rotated and side-bent right (FR$_R$S$_R$). (Reprinted with permission from Kuchera 1995c.)

influencing the central integration of pro-prioceptive and nociceptive input has been implicated by many clinicians. Others view somatic dysfunction as a mechanical deterrent to postural realignment. Regardless of the mechanism, correction of segmental somatic dysfunction plays an important role in the restoration of joint motion and the ability of the patient to respond positively to postural treatment protocols.

Spinal somatic dysfunction is especially common at craniocervical, cervicothoracic, thoracolumbar, lumbopelvic, and SI junctions (Dunnington 1964, Heilig 1983, Zink & Lawson 1979). In regional testing, the fascia associated with these transition zones is carried in a variety of directions and is named by the direction in which the tissues move most freely. Compensatory fascial preference patterns (Zink & Lawson 1979) successively alternate direction at each transition zone. A side-bending curve to the right, for example, is balanced by a side-bending curve to the left in the adjacent structural region. Each region that prefers to rotate better to the right alternates with an adjacent region preferring to rotate to the left. Compensatory fascial patterns are, in this way, balanced and alternating. Traumatically induced fascial patterns do not alternate and tend to be unbalanced. Skeletal, arthrodial, and myofascial structures in transition areas also tend to move in the direction of fascial freedom. In this manner, a fascial preference pattern determined by regional testing provides insight into the direction and amount of compensation permitted in a patient who is biomechanically stressed. Correction of regional somatic dysfunction is also considered important in permitting postural realignment and preventing the recurrence of dysfunctional posture.

Postural alignment in the gravitational field influences both somatic and visceral functions. Facilitated segments, established by afferent stimuli originating at the cross-over and apical spinal segments along these curves (Kuchera & Kuchera 1994a), have lower thresholds to somatic, visceral, and psychoemotional stressors, and mediate somatosomatic, somatovisceral, viscerosomatic, and some viscerovisceral reflexes (Fig. 39.10). Organs and other structures obtaining their primary innervation from these facilitated segments will

often exhibit dysfunctional pathology related to hypersympathetic activity (Kuchera & Kuchera 1994b). Travell and Simons (1992) present similar explanations for myofascial trigger point characteristics.

Without therapeutic intervention, studies reveal that individuals with posturally induced strain patterns will have somatic dysfunctional patterns that can be mapped like fingerprints and are roughly recognizable years after initial documentation (Denslow & Chace 1962). Likewise, if postural imbalance is experimentally introduced with a single non-therapeutic heel lift, specific patterns of somatic dysfunction and segmental facilitation are induced.

Regardless of the technique selected, both the peripheral input and the central response components must be accommodated. Therefore, manipulation of afferent musculoskeletal input from articular and myofascial somatic dysfunction remains an essential element in all treatment protocols described in this chapter. Likewise, the more systemic elements described in Table 39.1 above must be integrated, or else manipulation alone will provide only transient relief. When manipulation is used alone in these patients, somatic dysfunction often recurs in predictable patterns and creates a patient who is dependent on these manipulative procedures for temporary relief.

Treatment of static–dynamic postural alignment

The most obvious effect of gravitational strain can be evaluated by careful assessment of an individual's posture in each of the cardinal planes. 'Ideal' *static* postural alignment transfers gravitational force along structures adapted for weight-bearing. This minimizes energy expenditure by postural muscles and limits biomechanical strain on postural ligaments. *Dynamic* postural alignment is constantly adjusted by mechanical neuromuscular coordination as the individual maintains or changes position. Musculoligamentous function significantly influences and is affected by dynamic postural alignment. A thorough palpatory examination of somatic structures and an analysis of weight-bearing motions including gait, along with

Precipitation, Perpetuation, and Facilitation

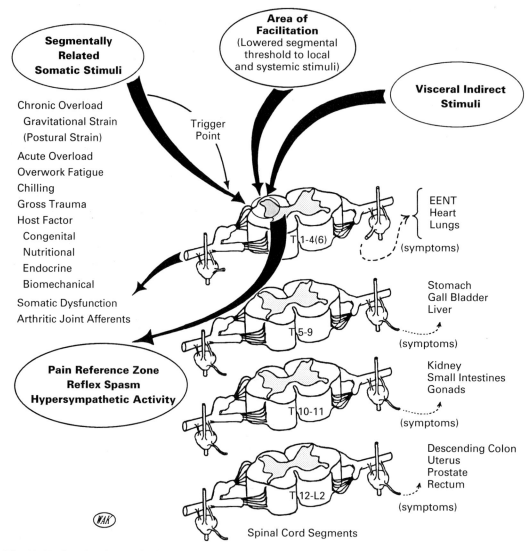

Fig. 39.10 Local and systemic stimuli from somatic and visceral sources can be magnified or perpetuated through central processes such as facilitation. Facilitated segments lower thresholds to a wide range of stressors and behave like 'neurologic lenses' (Korr 1947) focusing that stress to create predictable pain patterns, autonomic disturbances, and other dysfunction. Gravitational strain acts on local tissues to create a somatic stressor while influencing the location of facilitated segments at areas of postural change.

routine neurologic and somatic testing, provide clinical clues to the inherent capability of the neuromusculoskeletal system to balance and maintain biomechanical alignment.

Any deviation from an ideal postural alignment will biomechanically amplify gravitational stress on individual structures (Kapandji 1974). When the viscoelastic deformation properties of postural muscles, restraining ligaments, and other connective tissues are unable to resist the stress imposed, neuromuscular reflex activity is automatically and subconsciously initiated to maintain postural equilibrium. Continuous gravitational stress on these structures results in various combinations of predictable pathophysiologic change, as outlined above. All of the cardinal planes of motion are affected. The pattern of structures involved is dependent on which of the cardinal postural planes is most stressed. Strain is accentuated and perpetuated by inadequate host compensatory mechanisms. Individual postural alignment conforms to inherent connective tissue structure in addition to the cumulative functional demand placed upon it by static and dynamic postural conditions. Using this information constructively necessitates the evaluation of both dynamic and static factors. Analysis of dynamic attributes suggests which exercise prescription and other rehabilitative elements might be integrated into the complete treatment protocol. Analysis of static posture provides insight into the use of orthotic devices to modify gravitational stress caused by

biomechanical risk factors associated with alignment.

Standing radiographic studies provide specific quantitative data used in designing treatment to counteract the biomechanical consequences associated with *static* postural alignment variations. Many radiographic postural measurements have been statistically associated with low back pain and other gravitational stress-induced clinical findings (Kuchera 1995a). Using a standardized radiographic protocol (Willman 1977), objective and reproducible measurements are easily and accurately obtained (Kuchera et al 1990). Anteroposterior (AP) X-rays are measured to assess static posture in the coronal and horizontal planes. Lateral films provide sagittal plane measurements.

Radiographic measurements outside normative ranges (Fig. 39.11) help to delineate the biomechanical disadvantage placing increased func-

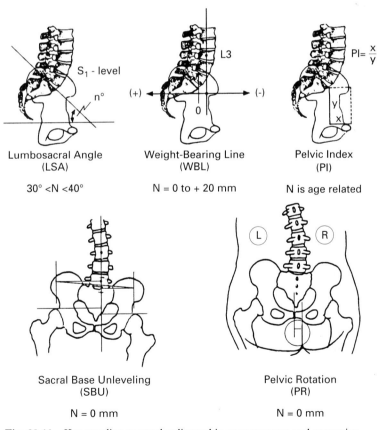

Fig. 39.11 Key standing postural radiographic measurements and normative ranges. (Reprinted with permission from Kuchera & Kuchera 1994b.)

tional demand upon low back structures. The greater the biomechanical deviation from normative postural ranges, the more likely it is that postural homeostatic mechanisms will fail. Resultant somatic dysfunction and musculoligamentous strain are common in postural decompensation affecting all planes. Furthermore, chronicity and severity of gravitational strain can combine to create gross structural change as well. For example, sagittal plane postural decompensation has been strongly implicated in L5–S1 spondylolysis and/or isthmic spondylolisthesis (Kuchera 1987, Kuchera & Kuchera 1994a).

One static radiographic measurement, Jungmann's (Institute for Gravitational Strain Pathology 1992) Pelvic Index (PI), is an infrequently reported but extremely valuable measurement for objectively evaluating chronic intrapelvic gravitational strain. This measurement (Fig. 39.11) represents the relative position of the sacrum with respect to the innominate (pelvic) bones. An understanding of the biomechanics involved (Fig. 39.12) readily suggests that the PI objectively quantifies the

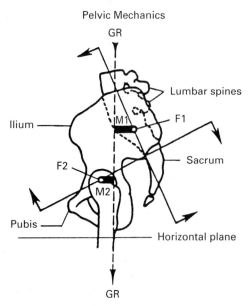

Fig. 39.12 Intrapelvic rotations occur biomechanically about their axes (F1 and F2) in relation to the gravitational line (GR). The sacrum rotates anteriorly (nutates) because weight-bearing falls anterior to its S_2 axis. The innominates rotate posteriorly because weight-bearing is posterior to the femoral axis. (Reprinted with permission from Institute for Gravitational Strain Pathology 1992.)

accumulated pelvic effect of the battle between gravity and homeostatic mechanisms that help the body's posture to resist it. This and other static postural measurements may be followed over time to provide objective, graphical documentation of the patient's progress.

Postural strain in the sagittal plane is suspected in individuals with thoracic kyphosis and/or hyperlordosis in the lumbar or cervical regions. It is almost invariably present in those with L5–S1 isthmic spondylolisthesis. Patients with sagittal plane decompensation are frequently observed to have slightly flexed knees owing to psoas involvement. Postural stress reflexly weakening the vastus medialis and lateralis muscles manifests as buckling knees and patellofemoral tracking problems. The abdomen protrudes, even if the individual is not overweight.

Chronic stress placed on those ligaments that are resisting the accentuation of sagittal postural curves results in sclerotomal/ligamentous pain patterns. Bilateral iliolumbar ligament involvement is common and easily palpated. Figures 39.1 and 39.4 above summarized pain patterns commonly referred from the musculoligamentous structures of the low back, pelvic girdle, and lower extremities that are strained by gravitational stress. Thus observational, palpatory, and historical clues are readily available to the clinician who entertains a diagnosis of GSP.

Most pelvic braces are static, designed only for acute situations. These are therefore inadequately designed to treat chronic postural change. Their continued use subverts inherent function and will weaken postural muscles. Only one pelvic orthotic device currently marketed, the Levitor (Progressive Appliance Corp., Rangeley, Maine, USA), is both dynamic and designed to be worn for prolonged periods of time in direct biomechanical opposition to the decompensating effect of gravitational strain in the sagittal plane (Fig. 39.13). It does not replace muscular action and its prolonged use therefore does not create the muscle weakening side-effect seen with static braces. The combination of a Levitor orthosis with other conservative postural treatment components – manipulation, physical therapy, exercise, and patient education – is more effective than using those components alone in the care of

Pelvic Lever Action

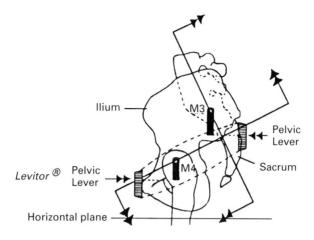

Cross Section of the Levitor ®

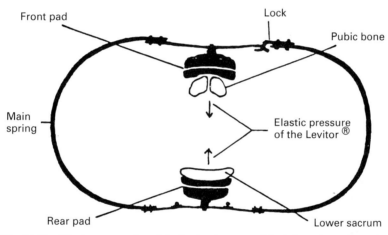

Fig. 39.13   The leverage action of the Levitor is accomplished through precise pad placement to resist gravitationally induced counter-rotation between the sacrum and innominates (see Fig. 39.12). The anterior pad is placed on the anterosuperior aspect of the pubes; the sacral pad is placed below the S_2 axis. (Reprinted with permission from Institute for Gravitational Strain Pathology 1992.)

patients with chronic low back pain (Kuchera & Jungmann 1986).

The Levitor pelvic orthotic device weighs 150–200 g. It is constructed of a special aluminum alloy with a high tensile strength. It is designed to transfer approximately 3.2 kg pressure to the pubic rami and the sacrum below its S2 pivot. This pressure application induces counter-rotation of the sacrum with respect to the innominates, reversing gravitationally induced musculoliga-

mentous strain. In a patient population carefully selected to meet Levitor inclusion criteria (Institute for Gravitational Strain Pathology 1992), 86% responded with reduction of pain. In another study (Kuchera & Jungmann 1986), 76% of difficult-to-manage low back pain patients demonstrated objective improvement of sagittal plane postural radiographic measurements, compared with 33% of those treated with physical therapy, manipulation, exercise, and patient education alone.

496 THERAPY

Pansystemic manipulation of somatic dysfunction is also vital in creating a successful postural treatment protocol in the sagittal plane. Hypomobility, in the presence of adapting postural homeostatic mechanisms, disrupts the realignment process and creates the potential for new or aggravated pain from musculoligamentous strain.

Postural stress in the coronal plane also contributes to the development of low back pain. Low back pain in these patients is typically accompanied by unilateral iliolumbar ligament strain and quadratus lumborum tightness. Acquired postural patterns in the coronal plane commonly include a single 'C-curve' or the double 'S-type' curve. Regardless of the number of curves,

musculoligamentous structures on the concave side of a curve are shortened while those on the convex side are stretched. Biomechanically, postural stress in the horizontal plane accompanies that in the coronal plane.

Treatment approaches for postural alignment in the coronal and horizontal planes parallel those discussed above for modifying posture in the sagittal plane, varying only in the specifics of type of exercise or orthotic. Konstancin exercises (Kuchera & Kuchera 1994b) replace the pelvic coil; orthotics, if selected, are typically placed inside or built into the shoe (Fig. 39.14). Unilateral heel or sole lifts to affect primarily posture in the coronal plane, and/or unilateral alteration

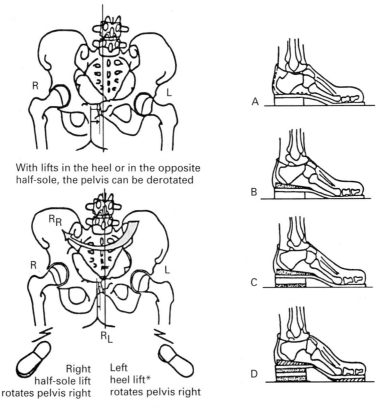

With lifts in the heel or in the opposite half-sole, the pelvis can be derotated

Right half-sole lift rotates pelvis right   Left heel lift* rotates pelvis right

Fig. 39.14 Lift therapy to heel and/or anterior sole requires gradual implementation to permit somatic and central mechanisms an opportunity to adjust to change. The heel lift is usually used for levelling the sacral base, and the half-sole is used for derotation if needed. Typically, lifts are started at 2–4 mm (B) and increased by that amount every 2–4 weeks. To prevent foot dysfunction, not more than 12 mm should be placed under a heel without modifying the entire sole (D). Lifts can be added inside the shoe (B) built onto the outside of the shoe, or a combination of both (C–D). Accurate lift measurements are made at the midcalcaneal line. (Reprinted with permission from Kuchera 1995c.)

of heel-to-anterior-sole height to affect primarily the horizontal plane, are common in these treatment protocols (Irvin 1991, 1995, Kuchera 1995a, Kuchera & Kuchera 1994a, Peterson 1983). See Chapter 9 in this volume for further information.

Although typically named for the plane of maximal asymmetry, synchronous postural changes in the three cardinal planes are linked biomechanically (Kuchera & Irvin 1987). Recognition of this potential for triplanar decompensation and a more thorough understanding of the pathophysiologic changes resulting in the stressed somatic tissues provides a unified approach into the treatment of an otherwise disparate range of pain and dysfunctional syndromes.

SUMMARY

Postural stress due to gravity presents with several signs and symptoms. These are elucidated by careful history, observation of posture, radiographic postural measurements, palpable diagnosis of recurrent arthrodial and myofascial dysfunctions, and localization of ligamentous strain. Patients with high functional demand in the sagittal plane are more likely to develop significant low back pain, hyperlordosis, spondylolysis, and isthmic L5–S1 spondylolisthesis (Kuchera 1995a). These patients typically complain of easy fatiguability. Many have been inappropriately diagnosed as having primary fibromyalgia syndrome (Kuchera & Kuchera 1994b). Most significantly, however, these patients typically present with a history of treatment failure for their chronic, recurrent low back pain and dysfunction.

Spinal somatic dysfunction occurring at postural cross-overs and other transition zones as a result of gravitational strain creates facilitated segments. These facilitated segments function as a 'neurologic lens' (Korr 1947), focusing stress on associated visceral and somatic structures alike. Thus, patients with GSP also have a higher incidence of somatovisceral activation of functional disorders such as irritable bowel syndrome or dysmenorrhea (Kuchera 1995a). Treatment of postural disorders to promote better weight-bearing alignment not only decreases musculoligamentous signs and symptoms, but also provides a wide range of welcomed and sometimes unexpected systemic benefits for the patient.

Prevention is the best solution for ligamentous laxity and other structural decompensations that complicate the prognosis for conservative care. The possibility of successfully applying this approach is enhanced by early identification of patients with biomechanical risk factors and recognition of symptoms associated with strain. The goal in prevention is reduction of these risk factors and strengthening of host factors before structural changes in the ligaments are permanent.

Integrated treatment protocols, combining a number of elegant somatic treatment techniques, including manipulation, somatic stabilization, and orthotics, have been proven to be clinically effective in the treatment of patients with GSP. During the course of postural alignment and local treatment, afferent information conveyed to the CNS from peripheral receptors in tendons, ligaments, muscle, and other somatic tissue results in a modification of the central response. Muscle re-education and other systemic integrating treatment schemes are prescribed to promote coordinated sequencing of muscle firing, important in rehabilitating the patient and maintaining local therapeutic benefits. Local, postural, and systemic integrating techniques are combined to provide a lasting clinical outcome greater than that achieved by the sum of the individual components.

The integration of treatment goals and modalities as recommended in this chapter will benefit those individuals with demonstrable pathophysiology due to gravitational strain. These benefits:

- significantly reduce patient symptoms
- potentially prevent permanent or structural change
- often arrest further decompensation when there has been structural change from the pathophysiologic process
- occasionally reverse a portion of the structural change.

Most importantly, this approach is capable of salvaging well-planned and faithfully executed protocols that have previously failed to accomplish their desired clinical goals.

CONCLUSIONS

1. Patients with gravitational strain pathophysiology (GSP) present with recurrent pain, patterns of somatic dysfunction including trigger points and reflex somatovisceral symptoms.

2. The diagnosis of GSP is based on clinical history, observation with radiographic evaluation of posture, and palpatory diagnosis of the functional characteristics of skeletal, arthrodial and myofascial structures.

3. Treatment of GSP prevents musculoligamentous strain, improves posture, enhances somatic healing, decreases musculoligamentous symptoms and alleviates recurrent dysfunction.

4. A treatment protocol for GSP appropriately employs manipulation, somatic stabilization or orthotics, as well as muscular and proprioceptive re-education. It represents an integrative biomechanical and neurophysiological approach to maximizing homeostasis and structure-function interrelationships in the body unit.

REFERENCES

Beal M C 1987 Biomechanics: a foundation for osteopathic theory and practice. In: Northup G W (ed.) Osteopathic research: growth and development. American Osteopathic Association Press, Chicago, pp 37–57

Cantu R I, Grodin A J 1992 Myofascial manipulation: theory and clinical application. Aspen Publishers, Gaithersburg, Maryland

Denslow J S, Chace J A 1962 Mechanical stresses in the human lumbar spine and pelvis. In: Beal M (ed.) 1993 American Academy of Osteopathy yearbook: selected papers of John Stedman Denslow, DO. American Academy of Osteopathy, Indianapolis, pp 99–108

DonTigny R L 1995a Function of the lumbosacroiliac complex as a self compensating force couple with a variable, force-dependent transverse axis: a theoretical analysis. In: Vleeming A, Mooney V, Dorman T J, Snijders C J (eds) Second interdisciplinary world congress on low back pain. San Diego, CA, 9–11 November, pp 501–512

DonTigny R L 1995b Mechanics and treatment of the sacroiliac joint. In: Vleeming A, Mooney V, Dorman T, Snijders C J (eds) Second interdisciplinary world congress on low back pain. San Diego, CA, 9–11 November, pp 515–529

Dorman T A, Ravin T H 1991 Diagnosis and injection techniques in orthopedic medicine. Williams & Wilkins, Baltimore

Dunnington W P 1964 A musculoskeletal stress pattern: observations from over 50 years' clinical experience. Journal of the American Osteopathic Association 64: 366–371

Educational Council on Osteopathic Principles (ed.) 1995 Glossary of osteopathic terminology. In: AOA yearbook and directory of osteopathic physicians, 86th edn. American Osteopathic Association Press, Chicago, p 701

Freeman J T 1957 Posture in the aging body. Journal of the American Medical Association 165(7): 843–846

Gossman M R, Sahrmann S A, Rose S J 1982 Review of length-associated changes in muscle. Physical Therapy 62(12): 1799–1807

Greenman P E 1989 Principles of manual medicine. Williams & Wilkins, Baltimore

Hackett G 1958 Ligament and tendon relaxation treated by prolotherapy, 3rd edn. Charles C Thomas, Springfield IL, pp 4, 27–34

Hackett G 1959 Low back pain. Industrial Medicine and Surgery 28: 416–419

Heilig D 1983 Principles of lift therapy. In: Peterson B (ed.) Postural balance and imbalance. American Academy of Osteopathy, Newark, CT, pp 113–118

Institute for Gravitational Strain Pathology 1992 The Jungmann concept and technique of antigravity leverage, 2nd edn, revised. Maine Printing Exchange, Rangeley

Irvin R E 1991 Reduction of lumbar lordosis by use of a heel lift to level the sacral base. Journal of the American Osteopathic Association 91(1): 34–44

Irvin R E 1995 Is normal posture a correctable origin of common, chronic, and otherwise idiopathic discomfort of the musculoskeletal system? In: Vleeming A, Mooney V, Dorman T, Snijders C J (eds) Second interdisciplinary world congress on low back pain. San Diego, CA, 9–11 November, pp 425–460

Janda V 1986 Muscle weakness and inhibition (pseudoparesis) in back pain syndromes. In: Grieve G P (ed.) Modern manual therapy of the vertebral column. Churchill Livingstone, Edinburgh, pp 197–200

Jones L (1993) Strain and counterstrain. American Academy of Osteopathy, Indianapolis

Jungmann M 1961 Abdomino-pelvic pain caused by gravitational strain. Southwestern Medicine 42(11): 501–508

Jungmann M, McClure C W 1963 Backaches, postural decline, aging and gravity-strain. Proceedings of the New York Academy of General Practice, New York City, October 17

Kapandji I A 1974 Physiology of the joints, vol. III. Churchill Livingstone, New York

Kendall F P, McCreary E K, Provance P G 1993 Muscles: testing and function, with posture and pain, 4th edn. Williams & Wilkins, Baltimore

Kimberly P (ed.) 1980 Outline of osteopathic manipulative procedure, 3rd edn. KCOM Press, Kirksville

Knott M, Voss D E 1968 Proprioceptive neuromuscular facilitation: patterns and techniques, 2nd edn. Harper & Row, New York

Korr I M 1947 The neural basis of the osteopathic lesion. Journal of the American Osteopathic Association 47: 191–198

Kuchera M L 1987 Postural decompensation in isthmic L5–S1 spondylolisthesis. Journal of the American Osteopathic Association 87(11): 781

Kuchera M L 1995a Gravitational strain pathophysiology,

parts I and II. In: Vleeming A, Mooney V, Dorman T, Snijders C J, (eds) Second interdisciplinary world congress on low back pain. San Diego, CA, 9–11 November, pp 659–693

Kuchera M L 1995b Gravitational strain pathophysiology and 'Unterkreuz' syndrome. Manuelle Medizin 33(2): 56

Kuchera M L 1995c Gravitational stress, musculoskeletal strain, and postural alignment. Spine, State of the Art Reviews 9(2): 463–490

Kuchera M L 1997 Travell myofascial trigger points. In: Ward R (ed.) Foundations for osteopathic medicine. Williams & Wilkins, Baltimore

Kuchera M L, Irvin R E 1987 Biomechanical considerations in postural realignment. Journal of the American Osteopathic Association 87(11): 781–782

Kuchera M L, Jungmann M 1986 Inclusion of Levitor orthotic device in the management of refractive low back pain patients. Journal of the American Osteopathic Association 86(10): 673

Kuchera W A, Kuchera M L 1994a Osteopathic principles in practice, 2nd edn, revised. Greyden Press, Columbus, OH

Kuchera M L, Kuchera W A 1994b. Osteopathic considerations in systemic dysfunction, 2nd edn, revised. Greyden Press, Columbus, OH

Kuchera M L, Bemben M G, Kuchera W A, Willman M 1990 Comparison of manual and computerized methods of assessing postural radiographs. Journal of the American Osteopathic Association 90(8): 714–715

Levin S M 1995 The sacrum in three-dimensional space. Spine, State of the Art Reviews 9(2): 381–388

Lewit K 1985 Manipulative therapy in rehabilitation of the motor system. Butterworths, London

Peterson B (ed.) 1983 Postural balance and imbalance. 1983 yearbook of the American Academy of Osteopathy. American Academy of Osteopathy, Newark, CT

Shaw J T 1992 The role of the sacroiliac joint as a cause of low back pain and dysfunction. In: Vleeming A, Mooney V, Dorman T, Snijders C J (eds) First interdisciplinary world congress on low back pain and its relation to the sacroiliac joint. San Diego, CA, 5–6 November, pp 67–80

Simons D G 1987 Myofascial pain syndrome due to trigger points. In: Goodgold J (ed.) Rehabilitation medicine. CV Mosby, St Louis, pp 686–723

Simons D G, Travell J G 1989 Myofascial pain syndromes. In: Wall P D, Melzack R (eds) Textbook of pain, 2nd edn. Churchill Livingstone, Edinburgh, pp 368–385

Travell J G, Simons D G 1983 Myofascial pain and dysfunction: the trigger point manual, vol. I. Williams & Wilkins, Baltimore

Travell J G, Simons D G 1992 Myofascial pain and dysfunction: the trigger point manual, vol. II. Williams & Wilkins, Baltimore

Vleeming A, Snijders C J, Stoeckart R, Mens J M A 1995 A new light on low back pain: the selflocking mechanism of the sacroiliac joints and its implications for sitting, standing and walking. In: Vleeming A, Mooney V, Dorman T, Snijders C J (eds) Second interdisciplinary world congress on low back pain. San Diego, CA, 9–11 November, pp 149–168

Willman M K 1977 Radiographic technical aspects of the postural study. In: Peterson B (ed.) 1983 Postural balance and imbalance. American Academy of Osteopathy, Newark, CT, pp 140–143

Zink J G, Lawson W B 1979 An osteopathic structural examination and functional interpretation of the soma. Osteopathic Annals 7: 12–19

40. Pelvic mechanics and prolotherapy

T. Dorman

INTRODUCTION

Back pain has been the starting point for the recent surge in our interest in the function and dysfunction of the human pelvis. The old model of disc disease has been insufficient to account for the size of the problem, the poor correlation between anatomic abnormalities in the discs as seen on modern imaging (Jensen 1994), and the persistence of pain and dysfunction in the face of anatomically corrective surgery. A group of persistent clinicians have found that manipulation and certain injection techniques, including prolotherapy, have yielded positive clinical results. This has led to an odyssey consisting of some clinical research and a fresh look at some basics regarding form and function. A wonderful interaction has developed between these clinicians and the research department of Erasmus University in Rotterdam under the leadership of Andry Vleeming. A new understanding of the function of ligaments is leading to an appreciation of their role in disease. In fact, a new category of disease is emerging – that of 'mechanical disease'. Orthopedic medicine is the branch of medicine that deals with these problems.

ORTHOPEDIC MEDICINE AS A DISCIPLINE

James Cyriax of London first coined the term 'orthopedic medicine' in 1929, separating the management of soft tissues by non-surgical techniques from orthopedic surgery. He later became the father of orthopedic medicine. He made many contributions, but above all he brought a Renaissance approach to this evanescent subspecialty. His pristine paradigm applies today just as much as previously. The rest of so-called traditional medicine has drifted somewhat in the last decades of the twentieth century into an operational mode of standards of care and set routines, which have developed a slight tendency to degenerate into a stoichiometric relationship between standardized diagnostic groups on the one hand and therapeutic interventions on the other. The orthopedic medical tradition has maintained a dynamic relationship between the patients' symptoms and signs on the one hand and intervention on the other. Each evaluative step is a challenge to the current diagnostic hypothesis; each therapeutic intervention is in the nature of an experiment. The outcome of the experiment denies or confirms (in that order) the hypothesis that was the clinical point of departure. Accordingly, the management of cases by this approach is one of a dynamic interaction predicated on the intellectual agility of the operator.

The physician (operator) bases his work on a continual assessment of the patient and his responses. Each experiment or therapeutic intervention is based on the clinician's understanding of orthopedic medicine, the essentials of which are an appreciation of the behavior of the fascial ligamentous system of the body, and an understanding of secondary phenomena related to the associated organ systems, particularly the central nervous and the muscular systems. The initial clinical findings raise a diagnosis with perhaps a short list of differential diagnoses; from this an initial experiment is constructed. The experiment might consist of the evaluation of a range of movement, pain provocation by a contracting muscle, or a test question.

In orthopedic medicine, laboratory and imaging investigations are, by and large, useless. They are, of course, useful in the broader context of a medical evaluation in searching for (and in the context of orthopedic medicine ruling out) more serious disease, such as pathological fractures. In the life of the human, the degenerative process, as it is called, takes it toll. This degenerative process has counterparts in the external appearance of the organism as well as the internal appearance – i.e. the findings on images. So, from an orthopedic physician's perspective (and only after the appropriate ruling out process has been undertaken), an overinterpretation of images can at times be confusing as it might divert an unwary clinician's attention to an organ that is anatomically abnormal, degenerate, etc. but not the cause of the presenting problem, usually a pain.

Accordingly, a guiding rule in clinical orthopedic medicine is to base one's empiric approach on the *clinical manifestations*. Success in this branch of medicine is based on the clinician's ability to imbibe this philosophical approach. The details of the clinical approach are outlined best in Cyriax's texts (1982, 1984) and secondarily in the writings of the present author (Dorman 1991). In a broader context, the philosophical paradigm is that of Karl Popper (1959), an acknowledged guide to the scientific method that has been the engine for the periodic success of our civilization since Grecian times and during the Renaissance. Orthopedic medicine has not taken hold of the imagination of the medical profession during this century in spite of its fantastic effectiveness. Why? The blame lies in the failure of philosophy, as pointed out by Ayn Rand (Peikoff 1991).

CONCEPTS IN ORTHOPEDIC MEDICINE

Pain patterns

On the basis of clinical experience, a number of rules have been defined regarding pain. First, we should dwell briefly on this word 'rules'. In the English language, this word serves double duty. Here, we are discussing observed patterns in nature, rather than the dictates of morals or governments. These patterns within nature are based on observation and, for the clinician, on *clinical* observation. Advances in science are based on observation, even when these observations contradict expectations.

Accordingly, the orthopedic physician evaluates pain patterns based entirely on the accumulated experience of the *empiric* approach.

In the 1930s, J J Kellgren, a teacher and researcher in America, used a noxious stimulus (6% saline injection) instilled in various somatic locations in volunteer subjects (his medical students) and asked them to draw pain patterns. This research served the basis for a subsequent understanding of the observed phenomena of referred pain from the fascial ligamentous (musculoskeletal) system. The obvious next step was to identify similar pain patterns in injured individuals and to attempt to relieve their pain (at least temporarily) with local anesthesia injected at the same sites. This was performed by George Hackett, an industrial surgeon active in the Midwest of the USA in the 1940s and 1950s. Resistance to acceptance of these patterns arose early. Anatomic knowledge of the distribution of the nerves, a knowledge of embryological development and patterns, as well as the concept of pain distribution in the anatomic counterpart of nerve roots, divisions of the brachial or lumbar plexus, and peripheral nerves, prevailed from anatomic knowledge. Kellgren's and Hackett's patterns did not correspond with this expectation, and the term 'unscientific' was applied. In fact, these observations were the quintessence of the empiric method: they were based on clinical observations.

An attempt at treatment followed. With the recognition that fascial layers can be strained and ligaments relaxed from the mechanical 'wear and tear' of the moving parts of the body, attempts at refurbishing these structures with prolotherapy were made. It was found – again, empirically – that it was possible to abolish a large portion of the painful syndromes with which the patients presented. In addition to confirming the effectiveness of proliferant injections in experimental animal models (Hackett & Henderson 1955), Hackett also reported a 90% clinical improvement in the patients whom he managed in his capacity as an industrial surgeon (Hackett 1958, 1959, Hackett et al 1961). It was during this period that a collation between the clinical recognition of pain patterns on the one hand and the empiric use of proliferant injections on the other was brought together, with the initial salutary results, marking the second landmark in the evolution of the specialty of orthopedic medicine.

History-taking

The orthopedic physician takes a history with an inquiring mind. On the one hand, he has ready in his subconscious a portmanteau of familiar pain diagrams, recurrent patterns with which the body responds when injured, an understanding of the mechanics of the fascial ligamentous (tensegrity) system, a knowledge of secondary manifestations from the response to chronic pain, the neurological, muscular and psychological secondary phenomena, which are often dominant historically, an understanding of the mechanisms of injury from falls, thrusts and so on, and, finally, a familiarity with the response of soft tissue to injury, which, in certain areas of the body, is peculiar. With this array of keys, the patient is approached in an attempt to unlock the puzzle.

Every clinical presentation in orthopedic medicine is such a puzzle. The skill of history-taking is, on the one hand, simple, but, on the other, represents the highest degree of clinical sophistication. The most difficult instruction to trainees is not to jump to conclusions but to maintain a neutral position towards the diagnostic keys that come to mind first from the history. The quintessence of the empiric method is one of *disproving* a hypothesis, and only when the disproof fails can a diagnosis be accepted. Accordingly, the tests of the diagnosis include further probing questions and, finally, intervention. A diagnosis is not established until *after* the cure is achieved and an adequate follow-up time of observation has passed. Accordingly, a section on 'history-taking' (anamnesis) in orthopedic medicine is impossible to write. No two cases are identical, and there is no ritual, catechism, or litany to follow. The golden rule is never to ask direct questions when indirect questions are possible. Questions should be phrased so as to *deny* a hypothesis, if possible, because the outcome of the empiric approach, in the clinical setting in orthopedic medicine, is always the response of the subject, an alteration in pain being the most common.

History-taking should, however, include a detailed account of the mechanics of an injury. In the situation where machinery or automobiles are involved, it is advantageous to learn about, for example, the speed of impact, the amount of damage to the vehicles, the site of damage to the vehicles, and the presence or absence of restraints. When pain arises, the time of arrival of pain in relation to the time of injury should be noted. (It is a characteristic of ligament injuries that there is a delay between the injury and the onset of the resultant pain.)

Tensegrity

The one-eyed man is blessed in the land of the blind. On the other hand, not every seer is truthful. Modern scientific research has shown us that some paradigms are confirmed objectively, yet are counterintuitive. Examples of this from physics are the notion that matter and energy are interchangeable, and that wave forms and particles both represent the same thing. Skepticism in the face of counterintuitive new concepts is healthy. In contrast, rejecting them merely *because* they are counterintuitive denies us great benefit. Into this category of counterintuitive yet valuable concepts we need to place *tensegrity*.

The term was introduced in 1929 by the famous architect, Buckminster Fuller (1975), composed from the words 'tension' and 'integrity'. There are instances in our daily lives where we have come to accept the transfer of mechanical forces diffusely. Instances of this are the transfer of the weight of an automobile via air and rubber (we call it the inner tube and tire sitting on the rim of the wheel of the car) to the ground, or the observation that a truss is stronger in supporting weights than the sum of its parts. Structural engineers will confirm that tension-reinforced concrete supports cantilevered weight and changing stress better than does the amorphous material. Biological structures are uniformly found to be tensegrity models. Forces are dispersed through the system diffusely, tension and compression acting in an integrated way. The familiar example is the geodesic dome seen in exhibitions, in which the center of gravity is right in the middle where nothing exists at all. The fascial ligamentous skeletal system, which is the framework of our bodies, is such a tensegrity model. For a discussion of the physics and the anatomy, the reader is referred to Chapters 1 and 10 in this volume.

The importance of this concept to the orthopedic physician is that it helps to explain commonly observed associations. Forces are transferred diffusely through a system; they tend to concentrate or accumulate at sites of increased mobility or where the direction of mobility changes. Examples of this are at the sites of the axial skeleton where the mechanics change: both ends and the thoracolumbar junction. Strains accumulate at the sites where the fascial layers are firmly attached to the periosteum, i.e. the compression members. Examples of this are the lateral epicondyle of the humerus, the tips of the transverse processes of the vertebrae, the posterior superior iliac spine, the whole of the iliac crest and its three lips on both sides, and the shin bone. (The astute reader will note a correlation between these areas of attachment and the 18 sites defined as tender spots in fibromyalgia.)

Fault propagation

Another concept with which one needs to be familiar is that of *fault propagation* or crack propagation. It is a common experience that when fabric begins to fray, for example in front of the knee in a pair of trousers, with worsening decay of the fabric, the one hole enlarges indefinitely while the rest of the fabric remains relatively well preserved. Once a weakness occurs and passes a certain threshold of enlargement, further progression of the weakness at the site is rapid. This is a phenomenon characteristic of many materials. It is also true for the fascial ligamentous envelopes of the body. In contrast to the fabric on trousers, the natural healing process of the body combats our internal fault propagation. However, when the balance of destructive forces exceeds the reparative capability, this concept becomes applicable. This, together with the torque arising from asymlocation (see below) of the sacrum, characteristically causes ligamentous and fascial strains at remote sites after an interval. These sites are usually the neck and the thoracolumbar junction, in that order. Repeated strain eventually passes the threshold whereby fault propagation occurs. Accordingly, it is usual to find that a person with a low back injury develops neck pain after an interval, typically 3 months. The several faults in the fabric of the fascial ligamentous diffuse organ may become fixed. The body eventually heals the injury in the newly displaced forms, hence, the change in body contour with aging. When this phenomenon occurs irregularly, prolonged periods of fascial strain at the 'weak points' occur, which is responsible for the persistent and recurrent exacerbation of pain.

Posain

It is a common experience of patients with ligamentous and fascial injuries that they are unable to maintain one position or another for a long time. Typically, an individual with low back pain will state that he is unable to sit more than half an hour without being compelled by his pain to get up and move around. On occasion, other positions provoke this pain (Ongley et al 1987).

What, one might ask, is the reason? When any ligament is placed under stress, even a mild stress, it becomes after a while a source of pain that gradually becomes intolerable; the individual is compelled to move. How is it, then, that adopting what would normally be an acceptable comfortable position provokes this positional pain, i.e. 'posain', in injured people? The cause is that in these individuals torque is transferred through the system. This is somatic dysfunction, an internal derangement of the symmetry and correct alignment of the axial skeleton. It is the *exaggerated asymmetry* that provokes the unusual strain. These patients usually report a pain in one side of the back, for example over one sacroiliac (SI) articulation posteriorly. The pain may radiate via the buttock down the leg. The term 'posain' was introduced by this writer in the 1980s as a convenient 'language handle' for this phenomenon.

Nulliness

Another common experience – a law of nature, if you like – is that individuals with posain also suffer from 'numbness', by which they mean a sense of numbness, but when examination is performed no anesthesia is identified, however careful the neurological testing. This might even include nerve conduction studies or evoked potential studies. This false sense of numbness is, however, real to the patients, and, when asked to draw diagrams of the distribution of this phenomenon, it is found to match the patterns discussed earlier and first identified clearly by Hackett. This phenomenon has been defined by this writer as 'nulliness', in an attempt to coin a word that would imply a numb-like sensation without an objective counterpart. Since this author proposed the term 'nulliness' in the 1980s, it has gained wide acceptance as a distinct characteristic of strained ligaments.

These patterns of nulliness are referred. Each ligament has a characteristic pattern or patterns of its own; each ligament has a limited repertoire of patterns. When the sensory input from the ligament is reduced, as for example with the application of local anesthesia at the site of strain, this symptom disappears. A characteristic of nulliness is that the patient reports that stroking the affected area (the site to which the symptom is referred) is either pleasant or neutral. It is not unpleasant. In contrast, when stroking an area of the body where numbness is present following neurotmesis, the patient reports showers of pins and needles and an unpleasant sensation from the stroking. This is a strikingly useful clinical differentiating point.

Form and force closure

The importance of friction in the function of the SI joints (SIJs) has been conveyed through the introduction of the contrasting concepts of form closure and force closure (see also Chapter 3 in this volume).

Form closure refers to a stable situation with closely fitting joint surfaces. In an idealized model of form closure, weight-bearing (and the transfer of other forces) would be achieved through snugly fitting geometrical forms alone. Functional analysis of living joints shows that various mechanical refinements are usually present in each. In the case of the SIJ, the additional factors are distinct. On first inspection, the sacrum appears to be wedged between the ilia. It has, however, been shown that, on standing, the closed kinematic chain is based on lateral pressures through the

rough surfaces of these joints. This has been termed force closure (see Chapter 3). In the SIJ, both a compressive lateral force and friction are needed to withstand vertical loads. Shear at the SIJ is prevented by a combination of the specific anatomic features (form closure) and the compression generated by ligaments and muscles acting across the high friction surfaces (force closure). These concepts are considered in Chapters 3 and 6 in this volume.

Movement and governance of the SI articulation

In the first century BC, Hippocrates recognized some movement of the SIJ in parturition but regarded it as otherwise immobile (Lynch 1920). Diemerbroch (1689) raised the suggestion that the articulation has some movement even in the non-pregnant individual. The joint was categorized as a diarthrosis in 1864 by Von Luschka. The first supposition of a fixed axis of rotation came from research at the start of the twentieth century. A recognition that buttock and leg pain may arise from hypermobility of the joint was raised by Goldthwait and Osgood in 1905 (Goldthwait 1945). Movement of these joints has been accepted since then. However, in a surprising stampede, the causes of pain in the buttock and leg were, since 1934, ascribed exclusively to the then newly described complications of disc injuries (Mixter & Barr 1934). Interest in the movement of the SIJ has subsequently waned in spite of a number of specific studies.

Since 1954, and based on Weisl's (1953) work, the normal presence of some movement in the joint has become received opinion. That this movement is tangible we have only recently come to appreciate (see Chapter 13 in this volume). Nonetheless, unsubstantiated statements by some individuals expressing the view that mobility is absent in the SIJ in adults (apart from the pregnant state), or that if movement occurs it is so slight as to be immaterial, can still be heard. Movement in living humans has been demonstrated stereophotogrammetically (Sturesson et al 1989), with radiology by the placement of Kirschner wires in sacrum and ilium (Colachis et al 1963, Kissling 1995) and observing the external movement, and through actual measurements of iliac positions with calipers (LaCourse et al 1990, Pitkin & Pheasant 1936). Motion at the SIJs is maintained even in advanced age (Vleeming et al 1992). Movement of these joints has been recognized in manual medical circles through methods of palpation throughout the history of osteopathy (Goldthwait 1945) and also well established in physiotherapy circles (DonTigny 1993, Hesch 1994).

Governance of the joint is seemingly very little by way of the joint capsule itself, but mainly through the tightening of the several periarticular ligaments (see below). The capsule of the SIJ has been shown radiologically to be frequently incomplete (Aprill 1992). An analysis of movement at either SI articulation calls into question movement at the other two joints of the pelvic ring. Although interconnected through the soft tissues, the relative movement of each of the bones versus the others in the three directions of space, let alone the interaction with the fascial tube of the whole organism, creates a three-dimensional puzzle of great complexity.

The osteopathic profession has labored with the classification of the dysfunctions of the axial skeleton for over a hundred years. A recent classification (Greenman 1989) has brought some order into a subject that was previously marred with terminological turmoil. A reproducible, practical, and uniformly applicable form of measurement of the relative movements of the four elements – (1) fascia; (2) sacrum; (3) left ilium; and (4) right ilium – has not been found. The art of manual palpation has not, so far, yielded satisfactory interobserver consistency in measurements to be acceptable for modern statistical analysis. It remains, therefore, an impression, a *Gestalt*, of the admittedly growing cadre of manual medical therapists that these movements can be palpated and treated. That manual treatment can be beneficial is now official (Schekelle et al 1991), although the *modus operandi* of the various therapies remains empirical.

What can be said regarding the attendant ligaments and other soft tissue structures surrounding this joint? What role do any of them have in the governance of function? Interestingly, recent research has shown that the large ligamentous bands, recognized of old in the pelvis, play a substantial role in the governance of the sacrum. Finally, to the extent that there is a modal, i.e. a most typical, pattern of movement round an hypothetical 'axis', it turns out that the deep posterior interosseous ligaments of the SIJ play that role (Egund et al 1978, Sturesson et al 1989).

Asymlocation

From the foregoing, it might be appreciated that the sacrum can become trapped asymmetrically between the ilia. The adducting forces active in the pelvis are apt to maintain this position even indefinitely. This asymmetry is physiologic. With ligament relaxation, it is apt to become exaggerated. The demarcation between the normal or physiologic asymmetry and an abnormal one, which in turn leads to somatic dysfunction, is not one that can be defined anatomically or physiologically with any precision. It is a clinical (osteopathic) observation, however, that with a partial or complete correction of asymmetry, pain and dysfunction diminish or disappear. Conceptually, therefore, 'asymlocation' is a term this writer has coined for referring to this asymmetry. It is intended to be a neutral term that does *not* define dysfunction *per se*.

Function of specific ligaments

Nutation winds up the dense interosseous ligaments of the SIJ, tightening and approximating the auricular surfaces, and inducing the phenomenon of force closure. The very important, and hitherto neglected, long dorsal SI ligament is, however, relaxed in nutation and tensed in counternutation (see Chapter 3 in this volume). Clinicians need to keep in mind that pain localized within the boundaries of the long dorsal SI ligament might represent a spinal condition of sustained counternutation of the sacrum. In contrast, the sacrotuberous ligament is tightened in nutation (see Chapter 3). It functions as an extension of biceps femoris, assisting in the control of self-locking of the pelvis. Thus contraction of the biceps femoris pulls on the soft tissues at the sacral side of the SIJ, thereby governing nutation. The gluteus maximus, with its broad origin from the posterior and lateral aspect of the sacrum and sacrotuberous ligament below, as well as the fasciae above, is inserted predominantly into the greater trochanter of the femur. Its fascial origin is partly contiguous with the thoracolumbar fascia. The thoracolumbar fascia is now known to transfer force across the midline in concert with the contralateral latissimus dorsi (see Chapter 3). Increased tension of the sacrotuberous ligament will preclude normal nutation of the SIJ. It can be seen, therefore, that all these large flat muscles and their fascial components work in conformity.

Muscles

Judging by their attachments, various muscles are probably involved, directly or indirectly, in force closure of the SIJ. The indirect effect is by modulation of the tension of ligaments and fascia. Each of these muscles has been shown to have a somewhat variable 'function' depending on the position of the two SIJs. It should be remembered that these articulations are braced in nutation on stance, a situation that alternates between the sides in optimal healthy functioning. The SI articulations tend to manifest some degree of bracing at most times. This is inherent to the tensegrity model. The degree of nutation/counternutation, interacting with the tension of the soft tissues around them, is variable. It affects, and is altered by, muscle action. The demarcation between normal and pathologic (positioning) is inconstant and has led to some confusion of terminology. The common tendency for the articulation to drift into the suboptimal chronic position of an 'anterior ilium' (i.e. a counternutated position) on one or both sides has been classified clinically (DonTigny 1993) as pathologic, although an objective confirmation for this is still unavailable (see Chapter 38 in this volume).

An analysis of 100 healthy individuals has shown that the abductors of the hip, predominantly the gluteus medius, come into action when the ilium is rotated posteriorly, presumably at the moment of heel strike during walking (Dorman et al 1995a). Additionally, four muscles will be analysed as examples of modulators of fascial tension.

First, the *erector spinae*, through its extending effect on the spine and its substantial sacral attach-

ments, might be expected to promote nutation. As the muscle is a summation of many intersegmental units (catalogued under one name), it is likely that facilitation of select subsegments of this group of motorneurons might fire independently in certain situations. Here is one of the many instances in which it is difficult to ascribe a prime movement to a trunk muscle because of the integrated function of the whole trunk.

Second, the *gluteus maximus* muscle is also of interest. One might note its large size in the biped upright human stance in contrast to its diminutive mass in monkeys, which are essentially quadruped (Lovejoy 1983). Some of the horizontal fibers of the gluteus maximus might be expected, on contraction, to have a direct compressive effect on the SI articulations. The fibers attached to the sacrotuberous ligament are more interesting. (The terms 'origin' and 'insertion' are more confusing than helpful here.) When these fibers contract and raise the tension of the sacrotuberous ligament, self-locking is promoted and nutation governed. This is another example in which, besides the 'prime function' of the muscle, one must recognize its role in modulating the tension of ligaments and fasciae. The effect on the sacrum of increasing the tension in the sacrotuberous ligament is variable; it depends on posture and the existing degree of nutation.

Third, the *latissimus dorsi* muscle is linked across the midline through the thoracolumbar fascia to the contralateral gluteus maximus. These seem to function in concert in trunk rotation. The thoracolumbar fascia can itself be tensed by the erector spinae muscle (Vleeming et al 1995). A correlation between the developmental mass of the erector spinae and the tension in the thoracolumbar fascia has been demonstrated. An image of some of the interactions can be gleaned from Figs 3.8 and 3.9.

Last, *biceps femoris* serves as an example of a limb muscle acting on what has traditionally been called its origin, also as a tensor of a ligament. The biceps femoris muscle has been shown in the experimental situation to alter the tension of the sacrotuberous ligament. In some specimens, the attachment to the ischium is minimal, demonstrating again that the main function is one of integrated tension modulation of the soft tissues, thereby controlling the main clutch of the trunk, the SI articulations (Wingerden et al 1993), with incidental contact via a 'toggle', the ischium. Not surprisingly, the measured tension in the ligament has been shown to be affected by the degree of nutation of the sacrum and position of the rest of the body, which is by inference thought to affect the resting tension of the fascial ligamentous 'tube' of the trunk.

Do any muscles maintain a state of continuous contraction to maintain the state of force closure – bracing – of the SI articulations? From a biomechanical perspective, something akin to a spring is 'needed' to maintain the loaded closure pressure. It seemed, therefore, paradoxical that in unconstrained sitting and standing electromyograph (EMG) testing showed the gluteus maximus and biceps femoris to be silent (Snijders et al 1995a). In this form of standing, it turns out that the internal oblique abdominal muscles are under continuous tension. It is an observation that voluntary muscles tend to relax cyclically (when they do not relax, fatigue, spasm, and trigger points develop). Nature's solution emerged from an experiment designed to falsify the hypothesis of muscle contributions to self-bracing. It turns out that when the legs are crossed, the internal oblique abdominal muscles relax (see Fig. 3.10). It appears that the trunk is rotated slightly, placing the fascial tube of the body under slight tension. It is this tension which maintains compression of the pelvis. One ischium is subject to increased weight-bearing, and the tension measured in the latissimus dorsi of one side and the gluteus maximus of the other is increased. This balance can be maintained for some time, but creep in the soft tissue is apt to give enough slack after an interval, which will reflexly 'wake up' the 'guardian' internal oblique muscles. It is now that the sitting subject instinctively reverses, changes over to crossing the other leg, an experience we have all noticed subjectively (Snijders et al 1995a). It would be surprising if force closure were dependent on muscle action at rest, for example in sitting. Therefore, the observation that adequate tension is generated in the fascia and ligaments to ensure force closure of the SI articulations by passive stretching, i.e. by crossing the legs, is a reassuring and subtle instance of energy conservation.

Walking

We see, therefore, that the ligamentous and fascial surrounding structures (augmented by the large, flat musculature on *both sides* of the body) are importantly responsible for ipsilateral force closure of the SI articulation. The posterior layer of the thoracolumbar fascia acts as a large transmission belt. It is almost certain that, in walking, integrated action occurs between these several separately named anatomic entities. Additionally, if, for one reason or another, the functioning of one component of this conglomerate is less than optimal, the role is taken over by the remaining functionally intact elements. The compression members (bones) of the pelvis might be said to toggle with each step. There is alternating locking and release of the SIJs in stance and swing. If one of these functions remains locked, or is otherwise impaired, walking can still take place because of the independent reserve function of the peripheral joints and muscles. It is proposed here that there is a complex interaction between all these elements in stance and swing, including:

1. storage and release of elastic antigravitational energy (Dorman 1992, Dorman et al 1995)
2. interactive complex motion of the compression and tension members of the pelvis, and the surrounding ligaments and fasciae.

The momentum in walking is a uniquely human physiologic process based on the peculiar anatomy of the SI articulations. The joint can be thought of as a multidirectional force transducer integrating the several functions of the pelvis discussed herein. The transducer involves an induction of energy and forces (Snijders et al 1992). This integrated function calls for a new concept. Accordingly, it has been proposed in a recent article that a new term be coined for this purpose, which would facilitate further discussion on the subject. The term offered was 'transduction' (Dorman & Vleeming 1995). Transduction is the process of the transfer of forces, both elastic and gravitational, between the pelvic components in kinetic motion.

Recapitulation

The pelvis is central, both anatomically and functionally, in the human frame, which from a functional point of view can be analysed as a walking machine. This article has brought together evidence for a new understanding of the role of the SIJ as the key element in the pelvis. It allows the 'walking machine' to transfer forces back and forth between the components of this 'machine'. Stance is afforded through force closure, which ensures stability. The joint allows the transfer and modulation of forces on the swing side. The integrated function of the whole pelvis facilitates efficient alternation of self-locking and energy transfer between the sides with each step. In order to comprehend this article, a number of new concepts are required.

1. Force closure is a new concept defining the clutch-like bracing of a link in the closed kinematic chain of stance through friction, a function peculiar to the human SIJ. It differs from form closure.

2. Effective self-locking of the SI articulation is achieved through both form and force closure. Nutation winds up most of the ligaments in the area. Without nutation, effective self-locking would not occur. Note that a 'flexed' (or non-loaded) spine increases counternutation, tending to destabilize the pelvis.

3. Locomotion transfers antigravitational and elastic energy back and forth between the moving parts. This is an essential function in walking because of the need to step, in contrast to the even movement of rolling stock.

4. The ligaments around the joint play an essential role in its function.

5. These roles include that of storage and release of elastic energy.

6. An additional role is participation in the *diffuse* transfer of tension forces through the thoracolumbar fascia and, by analogy, through other fascial layers.

7. The role of all the muscles in the trunk and lower limb is contributory, mostly as a modulator of tension in the ligaments and fascia.

8. The integrated function of these elements and forces is a characteristic of the human pelvis, ideally adapted to walking. It is proposed here that this integrated function be called 'transduction'.

SYNDROME RECOGNITION

Orthopedic physicians recognize a large inventory of syndromes: clusters of symptoms and signs, usually matching distinct pain diagrams, which characterize specific mechanical dysfunctions. Some of these syndromes are dominated by symptoms that are secondary to the underlying mechanical cause. Many of these have been outlined by Cyriax (1982) and Dorman (1990) and could not be detailed comprehensively in this chapter. A few illustrative examples will suffice.

'My back goes out'

In this syndrome, patients report episodes in which, unexpectedly and suddenly following a slight movement, most characteristically rising from a stooped position with a slight degree of rotation in a casual manner and without a great weight, a severe, sudden onset, asymmetric back pain occurs, usually with radiating pain via one buttock down the leg. The patient is unable to stand straight. When examined acutely, these individuals are unable to form the normal lumbosacral lordosis, are able to flex forward, have marked asymmetry in side-bending and rotation at the lumbopelvic level, frequently suffer from marked straight leg raising limitation on the painful side, may have secondary weakness due to pain, but do not suffer reflex suppression or sensory deficits. These individuals are frequently responsive to manipulative therapy. In its absence, the episodes typically recover in between 2 weeks and 2 months, but individuals with this phenomenon are prone to recurrences.

When examined by osteopathic methods, marked dysfunctions in the pelvis are always identifiable in the acute condition. It is the thesis of this chapter that the phenomenon is one whereby the sacrum becomes asymmetrically entrapped. Forces acting in the soft tissues, particularly in the upright human, are adducting. (This becomes obvious from viewing the sacrum as being suspended between the ilia.) The pelvis, being a tensegrity ring, functions as a whole. When pain occurs, secondary muscle spasm disallows relaxation and restoration of symmetry of the sacrum between the ilia. The natural resolution of such an episode typically occurs in about 2 weeks. It is proposed here that the mechanism(s) of this resolution include one or more of the following factors:

1. either bone and ligament molding occurring within 2 weeks
2. natural slippage of the displaced parts
3. the parts returning to normal through relaxation of the soft tissues or through manipulation
4. a combination of all of these.

Further discussion on the mechanics of the pelvis can be found later in this chapter, as well as in Chapter 3 in this volume.

Toggling pain

It is this writer's clinical observation over 20 years that a characteristic of low back pain associated with a dysfunction of the pelvic ring is its asymmetry. The pain may be sensed over the midline in the low back, but in these cases invariably also over one SI articulation in the buttock. When it is referred, the pain is referred down the lower limb and is on the same side. Another characteristic is that, if the pain abates, recurrences sometimes occur on the other side, although most individuals with these episodes of pain suffer from it predominantly on one side. Most frequently, the other side is also occasionally affected. This is because an unstable sacrum between the ilia can get entrapped in more than one way, putting strain on the ligaments of the other side, which become the source of posain and nulliness.

Sacrotuberous ligament

This ligament, or distal 'stay' of the pelvis, is often strained in SIJ dysfunction because it is further out in the radius of the pelvis (Fig. 40.1). It should be remembered that more than one pattern of pain occurs and that individuals may vary in how it affects them. Nonetheless, the repertoire of patterns is small.

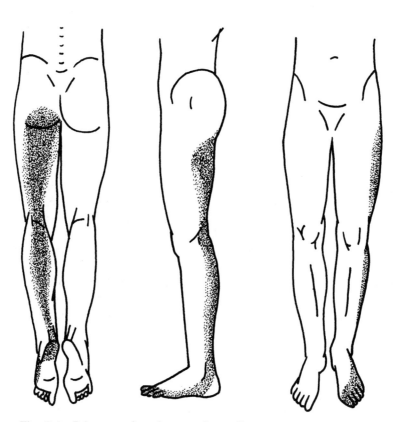

Fig. 40.1 Pain pattern from the sacrotuberous ligament.

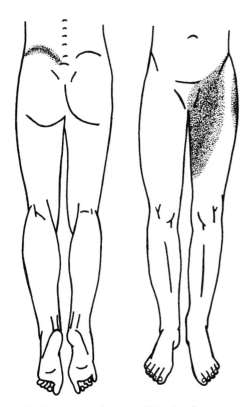

Fig. 40.2 Pain pattern from the iliolumbar ligament.

Iliolumbar ligament sprain

This ligament, being the major stay of the relationship of the pelvis to the lower lumbar vertebrae, is also frequently involved as a source of pain in pelvic dysfunctions (Fig. 40.2). Of interest is that an asymmetry in physical findings is usual on examination when the subject is tested standing. It will be found that side-bending to one side provokes the pain, while rotation to the other also does so. (Note that one has not specified in which direction it is provoked. The ligament is a twisted three-dimensional structure, and the only consistent finding is that side-bending and rotation are painful in opposite directions).

Sciatica

This term implies pain in the low back with radiation down the lower limb posteriorly via the buttock. It is well recognized that radiculopathy, usually due to pressure on the dural sleeve of one of the lumbar nerve roots, can be responsible for this pain. On the other hand, 'sciatica' is more often due to referred pain from the sacrotuberous ligament. In this case, the pain may 'skip' the popliteal space, but the patterns of pain are often indistinguishable on pain diagrams. Straight leg raising is also not a useful discriminant, through stretching the sciatic nerve in the popliteal fossa or through dorsiflexing the foot at a strategic position of straight leg raising is less poor a differentiator. (Both maneuvers stretch the fascial sleeve of the leg and the branches of the sciatic nerve.) The association of neurologic signs, the presence of tenderness at the attachment of the sacrotuberous ligament at the inferolateral angle of the sacrum, as well as historical clues, such as posain and nulliness, are more useful.

Gluteus medius syndrome

As the gluteus medius has a specific role in locking the SI articulation on the stance side, it is subject to reflex inhibition when the ilium on the affected side is in a forward position (DonTigny 1985). This can be manifested clinically by an alteration in its contraction visible over the buttocks as an individual bends forward, and also identifiable on examination in the side-lying position (Dorman 1994). Tenderness is also found on deep palpation just under the rim of the iliac crest.

Piriformis syndrome

As the piriformis muscle plays a major role in stabilizing the pelvis and is an important muscle traversing the SIJ, it is not surprising that it is strained at times when the pelvis is dysfunctional. The patient reports pain in the middle of the buttock, down the middle aspect of the thigh to the level of the popliteal fossa, affected by certain movements. Testing the muscle when maximally stretched provokes severe pain and yields the diagnosis.

Slipping clutch syndrome

This newly recognized syndrome is characteristic of about 15% of subjects suffering from back pain due to SI ligamentous dysfunction (Dorman

1994). The patients report episodes of giving way of one leg. The phenomenon of giving way is painless, although occasionally they are injured after a fall. Not all the patients, in fact, fall down, as they often catch themselves. The phenomenon of the limb giving way invariably occurs as the affected side enters into stance and is thought to represent slight slippage due to failure of the force closure of the joint, which should occur normally at this moment. As force closure is dependent on, amongst other things, the normal elastic function of the posterior SI ligaments, it is not surprising that relaxation of these structures can be responsible for mechanical dysfunction, as well as being a source of pain. These individuals respond to therapy with prolotherapy. In fact, it is through the healing effect of therapy that this syndrome recently came to light by serendipity.

SIJ pain

Pain over the joint, at times with radiation posteriorly via the inferior aspect of the buttock and the posterior part of the thigh, is a characteristic feature of a sprain of the posterior SIJ ligament and occurs not infrequently in isolation. It has the characteristic of posain, is aggravated at the end of the day after an individual has been physically active, and also responds to injection therapy.

The response to manipulation

Most of the syndromes surrounding the pelvis, as well as those created remotely through the axial skeleton through the tensegrity and fault propagation phenomena discussed earlier, are due to a single cause. This is relaxation of the ligaments controlling the tensegrity unit we call the pelvis. This is the source of most mechanical dysfunctions. The dysfunctions themselves lead to, or aggravate, strains of fascia and ligaments. A vicious cycle develops. Muscle spasm is secondary. Its manifestations are very well recognized in pain management circles.

Patients with these dysfunctions frequently report that manipulation in the hands of a manual therapist allows them temporary, intermittent relief from pain. Not infrequently, the situation worsens gradually over the years, so that patients seen after one or two decades of recurrent episodes of pain

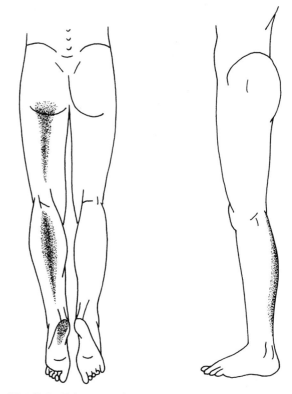

Fig. 40.3   Pain pattern from the sacrospinous ligament.

report that the pain has become continuous. Nonetheless, the hallmark of this syndrome is that the pain was intermittently, temporarily relieved early in the history. The improvement from manual therapy is due to a realignment of the pelvic bones. The recurrences are due to ligament relaxation, which allows recurrent dysfunctions. The specific characteristic of the dysfunction at one time might vary. It is proposed here, however, that the episodic improvement with manipulation is the hallmark of the ligament dysfunction in the axial skeleton, usually in the pelvic ring.

Common factors in these syndromes

The thrust of the discussion so far is that all of the above clinical phenomena arise from *one* underlying phenomenon, that of ligament relaxation and asymlocation in the pelvis. This is the term used to convey the concept that in the tensegrity model that we call the human pelvis, the sacrum is held or trapped between the ilia. It is prone to being held in a somewhat asymmetric position between them. This tends to place an asymmetric stain on the soft tissues, fasciae and ligaments. With a certain degree of relaxation of the ligaments, there develops a tendency for this asymmetry to advance to a point of exaggeration akin to the phenomenon of fault propagation in mechanics. When this threshold is passed, recurrent entrapment of the sacrum asymmetrically amounts to a mechanical dysfunction, i.e. to, in osteopathic terminology, *somatic dysfunction*.

This is in turn apt to provoke secondary phenomena, which have been listed here as the 'mini' syndromes characteristic of the human pelvis. Some of these show themselves with ligament symptoms alone, some muscle dysfunction or spasm, and some, through the phenomenon of transfer of torque through the axial skeleton, are manifested in the neck or the thoracolumbar junction. The underlying fault is in the soft tissues of the pelvis.

An understanding of the role of the pelvis in locomotion and the attendant dysfunctions is, in this writer's opinion, the third great landmark in orthopedic medicine, the first being the introduction of testing soft tissues by altered tension (Cyriax), and the second, the recognition of pain patterns in scleratomes and the introduction of prolotherapy (Hackett).

ONGLEY'S TECHNIQUE

From the discussion in this chapter so far, the reader will have drawn the logical conclusion that the optimal management should be one of restoration of symmetry followed by some measure or other to maintain the improved position. This is, indeed, exactly what is achieved with Ongley's technique.

It goes without saying that this routine starts with diagnosis. The diagnosis has to be based on a *clinical assessment* of the cause of the back pain, followed by a manipulation that should be so vigorous as to restore the pelvis to full symmetry and abolish any tendency for recurrence, which might be due to adhesions. Accordingly, it is an advantage if the patient can be maximally relaxed. A manipulation by the more popular and more gentle techniques of muscle energy, or even of

gentle thrust, might be quite sufficient to restore a patient to *temporary* comfort but not to restore the joint to optimal alignment nor completely release any adhesions that might be formed from prolonged malalignment. With this technique, therefore, the manipulation is *vigorous*.

In order to facilitate this manipulation (and it is intended to be performed once only), there is an advantage if dilute lidocaine (local anesthesia) is injected into the soft tissues guarding the pelvis, particularly the posterior SI articulation, and also the ligaments around the lumbosacral junction, the iliolumbar ligaments, and the capsules of the zygoapophyseal joints at the two lowest levels of the spine. The details of the injection routine are detailed elsewhere (Dorman 1991). At times, individuals suffer from marked pain from a peripheral fascial strain, such as along the iliac crest from the fascia overlying the gluteus medius muscle. This can be relieved on this occasion with a local anesthetic injection, usually including small amounts of triamcinolone (an injectable steroid). It is important, however, not to place steroid injections into mechanically essential ligaments, for instance the posterior SI ligaments.

A manipulation that is a modification of an osteopathic technique is used next, restoring the pelvis to as much symmetry as possible. This is in turn followed with proliferant therapy injections to the stabilizing ligaments of the pelvis, in particular the three layers of the posterior SI ligaments, paying particular attention to the deepest and central part. Droplet infiltrations of proliferant injections are also placed along the iliolumbar ligaments, the zygoapophyseal joint capsules of the two lowest levels of the lumbar spine, along the transverse processes to make contact with the intertransverse ligaments at their periosteal attachments, into the supraspinous and interspinous ligaments of the lowest levels, and also treating the fascia over the erector spinae at the upper level of the sacrum. This can also be achieved through a single needle insertion point in the midline opposite L5. For details of the injection techniques, the reader is referred to Dorman (1991, 1993).

Finally, the patients are encouraged to perform the full range of movement 'exercises' to encourage healing in the natural lines of strain.

This concept is based on an understanding of Wolff's Law (Wolff 1870). This routine, as practiced by a number of doctors in California, was found to have a salutary effect, and, under the guidance of its author, M J Ongley, a double-blind clinical study was conducted. This study confirmed the experimenters' initial clinical impression of its benefit (Ongley et al 1987). A criticism (which in the view of this writer was inapplicable) was leveled at the study in that it measured four variables: manipulation, local anesthesia, select use of triamcinolone, and prolotherapy. It is this author's belief that the study evaluated a *method* and that a logical separation of the components is inappropriate. This criticism, however, was accepted by two of the co-authors, and a second double-blind study was conducted to evaluate the single variable of prolotherapy. Not surprisingly, the results were also meaningful in a statistical sense, but the disparity between the groups was much less than in the first study. These studies, however, represented a clinical landmark, tending to confirm the hypothetical framework that is outlined here. The theoretical basis for the study included a number of tenets:

1. The SI articulations move normally in life.
2. The SI articulations can become entrapped asymmetrically – asymlocation.
3. Management by Ongley's technique promotes or restores a return to symmetry (LaCourse et al 1990)
4. Injections of irritants into ligaments do in fact produce a proliferating effect.
5. The benefit of the proliferating effect exceeds any disadvantage, such as prolonged inflammation or scarring.
6. The benefit is apt to last for long periods, warranting the use of this invasive routine.

These individual issues have all been tested.

PROLOTHERAPY

To the histologist, the process of repair of connective tissue is simple. Therefore, it has not been a subject of recent publications. The inflammation that precedes and initiates the repair process of connective tissue was described first by Eli Mechnikoff (1893), and more detailed descriptions of the dynamic process were elaborated by Cohnheim (1889), who studied the process microscopically in the living capillaries of rabbit ears, which, owing to the thin nature of the tissue, lend itself to such a live study. Modern pathological preparations of (dead and fixed) histology allows us to study an imaged representation of a moment in time, and only through serial histological studies of parallel situations can we approximate an understanding of the dynamic process. Nonetheless, enough information is available from a combination of these methods to state unequivocally that healing in connective tissues is a dynamic process initiated by the injury. Through a combination of the humoral agents of inflammation liberated by the cells at the site of the injury and an interaction with the mesenchymal migrant cells, both from the hemopoietic system and of mesenchymal origin, such as fibroblasts, the cascade of healing is initiated.

What is the endpoint of healing? This differs depending on variables. These include:

- the extent and severity of the injury
- whether the damage to tissue was permanent or reparable
- the nature of the injured tissue (some tissues respond differently)
- the strength of the healing stimulus
- the duration of the stimulus.

An extraordinary observation of the healing process in almost all tissues is the phenomenon of cessation of healing. Experiments have shown that after resection of half a liver in experimental dogs, the remaining tissue grows appropriately to the right size, mass, and biochemical capacity. Regeneration then ceases. The servomechanism by which the intact organism regulates the termination of the healing process is unknown. This specific topic is a subcategory of the more general issue of morphogenetics. The whole process of maintenance of size and form appropriate to the age, size, and biochemical requirements of organs remains an enigma in contemporary biological sciences, one marked by the extraordinary absence of discussion of the problem in scientific circles. (In case the reader is in any doubt, the genome, the genetic information transmitted through the DNA, is inadequate in addressing this whole issue.)

The process of inflammation initiates repair following injury to the mesenchyme. Connective tissue, which is of interest in the context of this review article – i.e. collagenous tissue such as ligaments, fasciae, and tendons – is subject to repair through the same mechanism. There is no mystery in this subject. As discussed elsewhere in this review, it is a clinical observation that the repair process of these ligamentous fascial structures is at times deficient or incomplete. The terms 'deficient' and 'incomplete' are relative in the sense that clinical experience has shown that enhancement of the repair process yields superior clinical results. Accordingly, it is assumed in orthopedic medical circles that the natural healing process following certain injuries may be inadequate or abnormal. Be that as it may, the provocation of hypertrophy of collagenous ligamentous, fascial, and tendinous tissue is a confirmed observation.

In summary, prolotherapy is the provocation of the laying down of increased amounts of *normal* collagenous material in ligament, tendon, or fascia, which enhances the function of these tissues at the site concerned. The process is achieved by provoking inflammation at the site concerned.

Historical review

The first description of the intentional provocation of scar formation is found in Hippocrates' writing two and a half millenia ago (Lynch 1920). Hippocrates describes the insertion of searing needles into the anterior capsule of the shoulder in order to stabilize shoulders in javelin throwers, the warriors of Sparta. It is interesting that shoulder instability amongst contemporary sportsmen is still recognized and still responds to proliferant therapy. Since the advent of the hollow needle, the need for searing (a technique also used in racehorses, where it is called 'firing') is no longer necessary. The irritant can be introduced in a more sophisticated manner through a hollow needle by injection to the appropriate site.

The modern use of sclerotherapy dates back to the herniologists in the era before antiseptic surgery. In 1837 Valpeau of Paris described the use of scar formation in hernias for their repair. The genealogy of herniology, and later the management of hydroceles and a variety of vein sclerosis

techniques, was reviewed extensively earlier this century by Yeomans (1939), and the tradition of vein sclerosis persists into contemporary medical times. Earl Gedney, an osteopath from Philadelphia familiar with the sclerosing techniques of herniologists and venologists, was the first to introduce injection techniques for ligaments (Gedney 1937). Gedney injected a 'hypermobile SIJ' first with salutary results. The term 'sclerotherapy' continued to be used for about two decades until the mid-1950s, when the great organizer of prolotherapy, George Hackett, acquired the skills of injection techniques from the osteopathic profession, evaluated its benefit in an initial series of studies, and published a number of articles about his experiences. This culminated in a short textbook, the third edition of which was published in 1958, and the tradition of his textbook has been maintained into modern times (Hackett 1958).

Optimal healing

Scar tissue has a number of mechanical properties which differ from those of normal connective tissue and are considered to be disadvantageous. Scars can be recognized histologically as different from normal connective tissue. It was Hackett who realized that, in situations where ligaments are 'relaxed' (his term for ligament insufficiency), hypertrophy of the ligament represented an advantage, contrasting with scar formation, which would be a disadvantage. Was there any prospect of achieving ligamentous hypertrophy without scarring? In setting out a therapeutic 'road map', Hackett envisaged (as far as we know) that the injections should:

- be effective
- provoke as little pain as feasible
- be safe
- be easy to learn and perform
- require the minimal number of repetitions
- work generically, i.e. be effective in as many subjects as possible
- yield hypertrophy of normal tissue
- avoid scarring.

The therapeutic window

Following this 'road map', there evolved quite

rapidly in the 1940s and 50s a series of informal empiric trials, first in animals and later in patients with injured ligaments, of the use of a number of sclerosing agents, renamed 'proliferant agents' by Hackett. It transpired that a great deal of benefit could be achieved clinically by the use of a number of agents. As elsewhere in therapeutics, it has been found that synergy can be achieved with a modicum of polypharmacy. A number of agents used in the past include extracts from several plants, the least unfamiliar being psyllium seed extract or Sylnasol, a product no longer available, and an extract from fish oil, still available in the pharmacopeia – sodium morrhuate. The chief proliferant agents as judged by the frequency of usage are, however, (1) glucose, (2) glycerin, and (3) phenol. They are usually used in the following combination:

- phenol   1.25%
- glucose   12.5%
- glycerin   12.5%
- made up with 0.5% of lidocaine for local analgesia in water.

(This preparation is also called P25G or P2G.)

Klein (1995) and Banks (1991) have classified the injectable proliferating solutions that initiate the wound healing cascade into:

1. Irritants, which cause a direct chemical tissue injury that attracts granulocytes. Phenol, quinine and tannic acid are agents in this category.

2. Osmotic shock agents, which cause bursting of cell membranes, leading to local tissue damage. Hyperosmolar dextrose (12.5–15% maximum) and glycerin are examples of the most commonly used agents in this category.

3. Chemotactic agents, which activate the inflammatory cascade. Sodium morrhuate is a prototype of this group. These compounds are the direct biosynthetic precursors of the mediators of inflammation, i.e. prostaglandins, leukotrienes, and thromboxanes.

4. Particulates, such as pumice flour, which are small particles on the order of 1 μm that lead to longer-lasting irritation and the attraction of macrophages to the site.

Evidence of proliferant effect

An extensive literature exists documenting histo-logical scar formation in the mode of sclerotherapy (Yeomans 1939). This old research has not been subject to contemporary confirmation in a scientific mode, but every pathologist will report scar formation from time to time in biopsies obtained for a variety of purposes in routine surgical and medical practice. This is considered to be accepted general knowledge. Research in the context of the use of proliferant therapy needs therefore to be seen as an addition to the established body of knowledge regarding the healing of connective tissue.

Hackett reported in the 1950s on the histological changes of the Achilles tendon of rats treated with proliferant therapy. These were uncontrolled studies and were considered entirely satisfactory proof of the proliferant effect in the limited circles, the Sclerotherapy Society, that had adopted these techniques. They were ignored by the rest of the medical establishment.

The next landmark in the study of prolotherapy was a blinded animal study combining histology, electron microscopy, and mechanical evaluation of rabbit ligaments. King Liu (King Liu et al 1983) and his team used sodium morrhuate in the medial collateral ligaments of rabbit knees. The histological and mechanical beneficial effects of proliferant therapy in this experimental model were categorically established.

The remaining, and it seems to this writer, minor question of a parallel phenomenon on human tissue was established by taking biopsies (Klein et al 1989) of posterior SI ligaments before and after treatment in three patients with chronic low back pain. Treatment consisted of a series of six weekly injections into lumbar and SI ligaments, fascia, and facet capsular sites using a connective tissue proliferant (dextrose–glycerine–phenol) combined with mobilization and flexion/extension exercises. Post-treatment biopsies 3 months after completion of the injections demonstrated fibroblastic hyperplasia on light microscopy and increases in average ligament diameter on electron microscopy from a pre-treatment value of $0.055 \pm 0.26\,\mu m$ to $0.087 \pm 0.041\,\mu m$ post-treatment ($p < 0.001$). Range of motion significantly improved post-treatment in rotation ($p < 0.001$), flexion ($p < 0.015$), and side flexion ($p < 0.001$), as did visual analog pain ($p < 0.001$) and disability ($p < 0.001$) scores.

Figure 40.4 illustrates the histology of human ligaments before and after prolotherapy. Figure 40.5 shows electronmicrographs of the same samples.

Mechanics and ligament proliferation

Accepting, then, that prolotherapy provokes hyperplasia of ligament tissue, an increased amount of collagen, and the absence of damage, as far as can be judged histologically, an assessment was needed regarding the mechanical effect of prolotherapy in human ligaments to match the mechanical observations made by King Liu mentioned above.

This issue was addressed through the treatment of the joint capsule and injured ligaments of the knees of athletes who had suffered injuries from

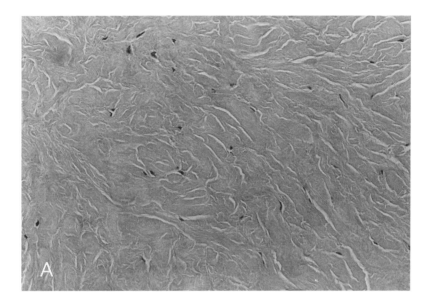

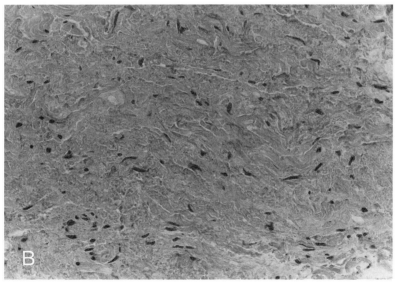

Fig. 40.4 Black and white reproduction of H&E representative slides of ligament histology (A) before and (B) after prolotherapy. Note the increased waviness representing collagen and the increased number of fibroblast nuclei. Of significance is the *absence* of features of inflammation or disease.

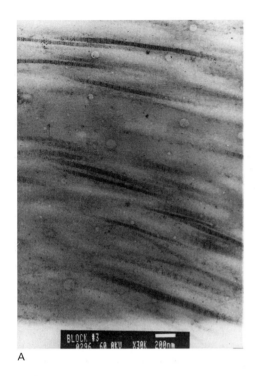

A

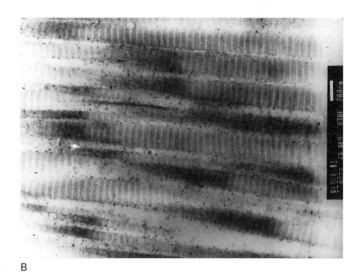

B

Fig. 40.5 Electron microscopy longitudinal cuts of ligament tissue (A) before and (B) after prolotherapy. Note the increase in size of the collagen fibers as well as the increase in variation of the size of these fibers.

athletic misadventure. The study was conducted during a 9-month period in a private orthopedic office. Thirty patients with knee pain were seen during the enrolment period, but in the cases of only five knees (in four patients) was it possible to obtain measurements after treatment because the equipment was available only for 9 months and many of the athletes, after clinical improvement, failed to return for repeat measurements. All the selected subjects had substantial ligament instability. All measurements were taken by one researcher. The patients underwent multiple injections. They were followed routinely and repeat measurements were obtained within 9 months. Subjective symptoms were elicited at entry and exit from the study. Ligament stability was measured by a commercially available computerized instrument that measures ligament function objectively and reliably in a complete three-dimensional format (Oliver & Coughlin 1985, Selsnick et al 1986). It consists of a chair equipped with a six-component force platform and a six-degree of freedom electrogoniometer. With computer integrated force and motion measurements, a standardized series of clinical laxity tests can be performed and an objective

report obtained. Prior studies have compared clinical testing with objective tests (Daniel et al 1985) and have established reproducibility (Highgenboten 1986). The proliferant solution used in these cases was P25G. The proliferant injections were 'peppered' into the lax ligament(s), usually at 2-weekly intervals, each offending ligament being treated an average of four times. A total of between 30 and 40 cm^3 of the proliferant solution is injected into the appropriate portion of the joint ligaments. Details regarding the injection technique can be found in the original publication (Ongley et al 1988).

Wolff's Law

It has been established since the turn of the last century that the mechanical components of mammalian bodies, i.e. the musculoskeletal system, which, of course, includes ligaments, fasciae, and tendons, respond to the lines of force through reinforcement. This has been called Wolff's Law after the scientist who first described the lines of force in bony trabeculae (Wolff 1870).

This is a time to remind ourselves that the laws of nature are the observations that scientists and physicians make about patterns characteristic of nature. This observation of the nature of healing in mesenchymal tissues in the presence of forces and movement is, by and large, the basis on which modern theories of early mobilization after disease and the use of exercises and mobilization in rehabilitation and physiotherapy have gained a wide (and rightly deserved) reputation. The use of exercises and mobilization in orthopedic medicine is no exception. Although the observation that healing in the presence of movement is an advantage with the use of prolotherapy, it is but an empirical observation, this issue not (yet) having been subjected to experimental study. It is, however, a strong impression of this writer, based on 20 years of clinical experience, that it is true.

Summary

In summary, it can be stated that the 'road map' set out by Hackett has been achieved. The style and routine of the use of proliferant injections have been defined elsewhere (Dorman 1991). The safety of the proliferant injections has been confirmed (Dorman 1993), and the mechanical and clinical outcome also established (Ongley et al 1987). It can therefore be stated in summary that the technique of injection of irritant material into connective tissue – ligament, fascia, and tendon – is now known to provoke hyperplasia of normal connective tissue, which enhances the function of these tissues. These functions represent mechanical strength (binding) as well as the storage and release of elastic energy, enhancing the efficiency and also the normal range of movement.

ELASTICITY OF LIGAMENTS – A NEW UNDERSTANDING

Conventional wisdom has it that ligaments serve as bindings between bones, and that their function is merely that of holding the structures together. It was a clinical observation of this writer, however, that individuals whose backs were treated with proliferant therapy improved in their agility, their range of movement, and the facility with which they functioned after treatment, raising the possibility that the efficiency of movement had

been restored (quite independently of the fact that they had become pain-free). This, together with the recognition by podiatrists (see also Chapter 21 in this volume) that elasticity is stored and released in the lower limbs with walking, and the recognition of the role of ligaments as stores of elastic energy in running and galloping animals (Alexander 1988), seemed to point quite obviously to the role of elastic recoil in the ligaments of the pelvis as contributors to the efficiency of human locomotion and walking.

A theoretical construct was thus developed postulating that the human frame is an integrated mechanism for efficient walking and that energy is stored, released and transferred back and forth within this mechanism in a manner somewhat analogous to that of the restoration of anti-gravitational energy by a descending pendulum in a long case clock. The additional horological analogy of release of elastic energy in a spring seemed to apply to the torque of the torso and almost certainly to the torque of the ligaments controlling the pelvis as it became recognized that, with each step, the iliac bones move on a diagonal axis. Even though the movements are of low amplitude, the cumulative mass of the ligaments concerned seemed to store a substantial amount of energy.

This hypothetical model led to experiments aimed at measuring the contribution of the movements of these various parts to the efficiency of walking. This was in turn measured by assessing the oxygen consumption at the maximal speed of walking of 10 experimental subjects (Dorman et al 1993), and these experiments confirmed this hypothetical construct. Finally, a similar experiment with oxygen consumption was undertaken with patients before and after treatment with Ongley's technique. This showed an average increase in efficiency of walking after treatment of 38% as measured by oxygen consumption at a maximum walking speed (Dorman et al 1995b). This experiment closed the circle, so to speak, bringing together the clinical management of patients and the theoretical concepts regarding the function of ligaments and the role of the pelvis in the physiology of walking. From these combined observations, the following conclusions can be drawn:

1. Internal movement occurs in the human pelvis with every step. The SI articulation closes (force closure) on the stance side and opens on the swing side.

2. With this movement, energy is stored elastically in the soft tissues, predominantly the posterior SI ligaments. This energy is released in the swing phase and contributes to the efficiency of walking.

3. The role of the pelvis is to transfer the energy of locomotion, both the antigravitational swing of the pendulums (the four limbs) and the torque from the soft tissues including the trunk. The term 'transduction' has been coined to convey this concept (Dorman & Vleeming 1995).

4. Ligament relaxation can be responsible for asymlocation, at times progressing to dysfunction in the pelvis, which in turn can lead to:
   a. a series of painful syndromes in and around the human pelvis
   b. the transfer of torque through the tensegrity mechanism to other sites in the axial skeleton, particularly the cervical spine and the thoracolumbar junction.

5. Restoration of normal mechanics through manipulation is effective.

6. When ligament relaxation alone or associated with fault propagation at a proximal or remote site has led to permanent changes in ligaments or fasciae, treatment with prolotherapy is restorative.

7. The management of these conditions is dependent on the clinician's understanding of concepts in orthopedic medicine.

CONCLUSIONS

1. Clinicians dealing with pain and dysfunction in the musculoskeletal system will benefit from acquiring an understanding of this organ system as a ligamentous fascial system. The fasciae are continuous, and mechanical factors regulate this system. Disorders in the mechanics lead to clinical counterparts that are recognizable through traditional medical approaches, i.e. syndromes and diseases. The clinician's tools for management are:
   a. history-taking
   b. an understanding of the mechanics of injury
   c. recognition of pain patterns, anatomically and temporally
   d. an understanding of the physiological role of the human pelvis and disordered mechanics.

On this basis, clinical diagnoses should be made in all cases, leading to rational therapy.

2. Mechanical considerations include recognition of asymlocation, of abnormal entrapment within the tensegrity adductor mechanism of the pelvis, and of normal, and at times abnormal, position, leading to the secondary phenomena of pelvic somatic dysfunction.

3. Ligament attenuation, weakness, or 'relaxation' is a contributory underlying mechanical cause, which is in turn aggravated by the increased tension on the dysfunctional ligaments.

4. Ligaments can be refurbished with prolotherapy.

5. Dysfunctional pelvises lead to a number of distinct clinical syndromes, all of which have a mechanical cause, often aggravated by secondary muscular and neurological phenomena. Definitive treatment is based on the recognition and correction of the mechanical causes, using secondary measures for the associated muscular and neurologic phenomena if they are maintained through a vicious cycle.

6. The predominant tools for the management of orthopedic medical problems are manipulation and prolotherapy.

REFERENCES

Aprill C N 1992 The role of anatomically specific injections into the sacroiliac joint in low back pain and its relation to the sacroiliac joint. In: Vleeming A, Mooney V, Snijders C J, Dorman T (eds) First interdisciplinary world congress on low back pain and its relation to the sacroiliac joint. San Diego, CA, 5–6 November pp 373–380

Banks A 1991 A rationale for prolotherapy. Journal of Orthopaedic Medicine 13(3): 54–59

Cohnheim J 1889 Lectures on general pathology (English translation). London

Colachis S C, Worden R E, Bechtol C O et al 1963 Movement of the sacro-iliac joint in the adult male: a preliminary report. Archives of Physical Medicine and Rehabilitation 44: 490–498

Cyriax J 1982 Textbook of orthopaedic medicine, vols 1 and 2, 8th edn. Baillière Tindall, London

Cyriax J 1984 The illustrated manual of orthopaedic medicine, 2nd edn. Butterworths, London

Daniel D M, Malcolm L L, Losse G, Stone M L, Sachs R, Burks R 1985 Instrument measurement of anterior laxity of the knee. Journal of Bone and Joint Surgery (US) 67: 720–725

Diemerbroch I 1689 The anatomy of human bodies (trans. W. Salmon). Brewster, London

DonTigny R L 1985 Function and pathomechanics of the sacroiliac joint: a review. Journal of the American Physical Therapy Association 65(1): 35–44

DonTigny R L 1993 Mechanics and treatment of the sacroiliac joint. Journal of Manual and Manipulative Therapy 1(1): 3–12

Dorman T 1991 Treatment for spinal pain arising in ligaments – using prolotherapy: a restrospective survey. Journal of Orthopaedic Medicine 13(1): 13–19

Dorman T 1991 Diagnosis and injection techniques in orthopedic medicine. Williams & Wilkins, Baltimore

Dorman T 1992 Storage and release of elastic energy in the pelvis: dysfunction, diagnosis, and treatment. Journal of Orthopaedic Medicine 14: 54–62

Dorman T A 1993 Prolotherapy: a survey. Journal of Orthopaedic Medicine 15: 2

Dorman T 1994 Failure of self bracing at the sacroiliac joint: the slipping clutch syndrome. Journal of Orthopaedic Medicine 16: 49–51

Dorman T, Vleeming A 1995 Self-locking of the sacroiliac articulation. Spine, State of the Art Reviews: Prolotherapy in the lumbar spine and pelvis 9: 407–418

Dorman T A, Buchmiller J C, Cohen R E et al 1993 Energy efficiency during human walking. Journal of Orthopaedic Medicine 15(3): 64–67

Dorman T, Brierly S, Fray J, Pappani K 1995a Muscles and pelvic gears: hip abductor inhibition in anterior rotation of the ilium. Journal of Orthopaedic Medicine 17(3): 96–100

Dorman T A, Cohen R E, Dasig D et al 1995b Energy efficiency during human walking: before and after prolotherapy. Journal of Orthopaedic Medicine 17: 1

Egund N, Olson T H, Schmid H, Selvik G 1978 Movement in the sacroiliac joints demonstrated with roentgen stereophotogrammetry. Acta Radiologica Diagnosis 19: 833–846

Fuller R B 1975 World game lecture series. University of Pennsylvania Museum, Philadelphia

Gedney E H 1937 Hypermobile joint. Osteopathic Profession 4: 30–31

Goldthwait J E 1945 Essentials of body mechanics in health and disease, 4th edn. J B Lippincott, Philadephia

Greenman P E 1989 Principles of manual medicine. Williams & Wilkins, Baltimore

Hackett G S 1958 Ligament and tendon relaxation treated by prolotherapy, 3rd edn. Available from Hemwall G. Institute in Basic Life Principles. Box One, Oak Brook, IL 60522–3001

Hackett G S 1959 Low back pain. Industri Med Surgery Sept: 416–419

Hackett G S, Henderson D G 1955 Joint stabilization: an experimental, histologic study with comments on the clinical application in ligament proliferation. American Journal of Surgery 89: 968–973

Hackett G S, Huang T C, Raftery A et al 1961 Back pain following trauma and disease – prolotherapy. Military Medicine 49: 517–525

Hesch J 1994 The Hesch method of treating sacroiliac joint dysfunction. Available from 14117 Grand Ave, NE, Albuquerque, NM 87123–1802

Highgenboten C L 1986 The reliability of the Genucom knee analysis system. The second European congress of knee surgery and arthroscopy, Basel, Switzerland

Hippocrates. The genuine works of Hippocrates 1946 (trans. F Adams). Williams & Wilkins, Baltimore

Jensen M C 1994 Magnetic resonance imaging of the lumbar spine in people without back pain. New England Journal of Medicine 331: 69–73

King Liu Y, Tipton C, Matthews R D et al 1983 An in situ study of the influence of a sclerosing solution in rabbit medial collateral ligaments and its junction strength. Connective Tissue Research 11: 95–102

Kissling R O 1995 The mobility of the sacro-iliac joint in healthy subjects. In: Vleeming A, Mooney V, Dorman T, Snijders C J (eds) Second interdisciplinary world congress on low back pain. San Diego, CA, 9–11 November, pp 409–422

Klein R 1995 The theory and practice of prolotherapy, 12th Annual AAOM Meeting, Palm Springs, CA

Klein R, Dorman T, Johnson C 1989 Prolotherapy in back pain. Journal of Neurology, Orthopedic Medicine and Surgery 10: 123–126

LaCourse M, Moore K, Davis K, Fune M, Dorman T 1990 A report on the asymmetry of iliac inclination: a study comparing normal, laterality and change in a patient population with painful sacro-iliac dysfunction treated with prolotherapy. Journal of Orthopaedic Medicine 12: 3

Lovejoy C O 1988 Evolution of human walking. Scientific American 259(5): 118–125

Lynch F W 1920 The pelvic articulations during pregnancy, labour and puerperium: an X-ray study. Surgery, Gynecology and Obstetrics 300: 357–580

McNeil Alexander R 1988 Elastic mechanism in animal movement. Cambridge University Press, New York

Metchnikoff E 1893, republished 1968 Lectures on the comparative pathology of inflammation. Dover Publications, New York

Mixter W J, Bar J S 1934 Rupture of intervertebral disc with involvement of spinal canal. New England Journal of Medicine 211

Oliver J H, Coughlin L P 1985 An analysis of knee evaluation using clinical techniques and the Genucom knee analysis system. Accepted for presentation at the scientific program, American Orthopedic Society for sports medicine interim meeting. Las Vegas, Nevada

Ongley M J, Klein R G, Dorman T A et al 1987 A new approach to the treatment of chronic back pain. Lancet 2: 143–146

Ongley M J, Dorman T A, Eek B C et al 1988 Ligament instability of knees: a new approach to treatment. Manual Medicine 3: 151–154

Peikoff L 1991 Objectivism: the philosophy of Ayn Rand. Dutton, New York

Pitkin H C, Pheasant H 1936 Sacrarthrogenic telalgia. A study of sacral mobility. Journal of Bone and Joint Surgery (US) 18

Popper K R 1959 The logic of scientific discovery. Basic Books, New York

Schekelle P G, Adams A H, Chassin M R, Hurwitz E L, Phillips R B, Brook R H 1991 The appropriateness of spinal manipulation for low-back pain. Available from Rand, 1700 Main Street, PO Box 2138, Santa Monica, CA 90407–2138

Selsnick H, Oliver J, Virgin C 1986 Analysis of knee ligament testing – Genucom and clinical exams. Presented at the AOSSM. Annual meeting, Sun Valley, Idaho

Snijders C J, Vleeming A, Stoeckart R 1992 Transfer of lumbosacral load to iliac bones and legs. 1: Biomechanics of self bracing of the sacroiliac joints and its significance for treatment and exercise. In: Vleeming A, Mooney V, Snijders C J, Dorman T (eds) First interdisciplinary world congress on low back pain and its relation to the sacroiliac joint. San Diego, CA, 5–6 November, pp 233–254

Snijders C J, Bakker M P, Vleeming A, Stoeckart R, Stam H J 1995a Oblique abdominal muscle activity in standing and in sitting on hard and soft seats. Clinical Biomechanics 10(2): 73–78

Snijders C J, Slagter A H E, van Strik R, Vleeming A, Stoeckart R, Stam H J 1995b Why leg crossing? The influence of common postures on abdominal muscle activity. Spine 20: 1989–1993

Sturesson B, Selvik G, Udén A 1989 Movement of the sacroiliac joints: a roentgen stereophotogrammetic analysis. Spine 14(2): 162–165

Vleeming A, van Wingerden J P, Dijkstra P F, Stoeckart R, Snijders C J, Stijnen T 1992 Mobility in the sacroiliac joints in the elderly: a kinematic and radiologic study. Clinical Biomechanics 7: 170–176

Vleeming A, Pool-Goudzwaard A L, Stoeckart R, van Wingerden J P, Snijders C J 1995 The posterior layer of the thoracolumbar fascia: its function in load transfer from spine to legs. Spine 20: 753–758

van Wingerden J P, Vleeming A, Snijders C J, Stoeckart R 1993 A functional–anatomical approach to the spine–pelvis mechanism: interaction between the biceps femoris muscle and the sacrotuberous ligament. European Spine Journal I(2): 140–144

Weisl H 1953 The relation of movement to structure in the sacro-iliac joint. PhD thesis, University of Manchester, UK

Wolff J 1870 Die innere Architektur der Knochen. Arch Anat Phys 50

Yeomans F C (ed.) 1939 Sclerosing therapy: the injection treatment of hernia, hydrocele, varicose veins and hemorrhoids. Williams & Wilkins, Baltimore

41. Assessment and treatment of sacroiliac joint dysfunction utilizing isolated resistance training and manual mobilization in a chronic worker's compensation population

M. D. Avillar   J. G. Keating   V. Sims

INTRODUCTION

Incidences of lower back pain continue to escalate, both in number and in total cost to health-care systems (Kelsey & White 1980). This trend of increased injury and cost continues in spite of large increases in research and funding that is directed at all areas of spine care. Low back pain is a 50 billion dollar a year growth industry in our society (Graves et al 1990a).

Waddell (1980) states that there has been an epidemic of low back pain in the Western world since 1956. The reason behind this phenomenon is unclear; however, it is believed that the increase can be attributed to increasingly sedentary lifestyles and the sedentary work roles that are developed in a society based on information.

Treatment plans that deal with chronic low back pain have not changed in their basic make-up for the past 40 years. The most common method of treatment for any form of low back pain is bedrest and analgesics. However, there is no documentation that this is an effective treatment regime (Twomey & Taylor 1995).

Exercise has been proposed to remedy low back pain since Samuel Gowers (1904) advocated an active rehabilitation program for his patients. Exercise as a form of treatment is only now gaining widespread acceptance as an effective method of dealing with low back pain. A number of differing types of exercise have been prescribed to deal with chronic low back pain. The different forms of exercise training vary widely from the rarely used heavy resistance training, general conditioning, cardiovascular endurance training, and training with light weights at high repetitions, to any number of various combinations (Foster & Fulton

1991). Clinical settings have generally utilized a basic general conditioning approach teamed with lower body stretches, Williams flexion stretches, McKenzie extension stretches, and physical therapy modalities (Polatin 1990).

Increasing the strength of the low back musculature has been postulated to prevent low back pain (Foster & Fulton 1991, Graves et al 1990a, Kelsey & White 1980, Waddell 1980). The specifics of how actually to increase the strength of the lower back is an issue of debate among clinicians (Rissanen et al 1995). Resistance exercises that are effective in strengthening extensors of the low back region are hotly debated (Pollock et al 1989). The erector spinae that dominate the low back region present a unique problem of how to isolate the muscle group for strengthening. In common everyday activity, the hip flexors and gluteals overpower the lumbar extensors and shield them from exercise (Graves et al 1994). The shielded lumbar extensors may predispose the low back to injury and the development of a chronic pain cycle. Machine-driven lumbar rehabilitation designed to isolate the lumbar extensors has begun to show strong results in decreasing subjective patient pain reports and restoring subject functional status (Carpenter et al 1991, Nelson et al 1995, Risch et al 1992).

An area relevant for low back pain that has attracted increased scrutiny in the past 10 years is the sacroiliac joint (SIJ). This new-found interest in the SIJ deals with the possible relationship that the SIJ has with chronic low back pain. The SIJ as an area of pain generation has been overlooked since Mixter and Barr introduced the herniated nucleus pulposus (HNP) to the medical world (Mixter & Barr 1934). Prior to Mixter and Barr's

HNP observations, the SIJ was frequently cited as a possible etiology for pain in the low back (Vleeming et al 1993). Fifty years after the initial realization that the lumbar disc is involved in low back pain, the idea of the herniated lumbar disc mediating all forms of low back pain syndromes has been discounted. It seems quite obvious that there are a variety of structures associated with low back pain; these can be commonly damaged in vigorous or in repetitive daily activities.

A number of problems arise in dealing with the accurate diagnosis of SIJ dysfunction (SIJD). One problem occurs in that the pain patterns are similar to those of other common low back pain disorders. A diagnostic conundrum presents owing to the fact there are no concrete uniform criteria dealing with SIJD (van Duersen et al 1990). Practitioners have in the past dumped a number of undiscernible low back pain problems into the SIJD category. This practice has led, historically, to a lack of credibility being given to the diagnosis of SIJD. Another problem involved with the diagnosis of SIJD is the nature of the activity that causes the injury. Activities that can commonly cause SIJD (Box 41.1) are very similar to activities that are found to cause more commonly accepted low back pain disorders. Owing to these diagnostic and historical problems, a common practice of overlooking SIJD as a possible pain source has evolved in most mainstream orthopedic practices (Shaw 1993). In most circles, the diagnosis is completely overlooked or cast off as one of quackery.

Box 41.1   Common causes of SIJD

Trauma to buttocks	Repetitive end of range flexion/extension movements
Overall joint laxity	Automobile accident with one leg fully extended
Postpartum	Lifting injury in an awkward position
Twisting movements with weight	Shearing type movements
Repetitive lifting movements	

Theories relating to a possible pain mechanism associated with SIJD come from a number of areas: muscle imbalance, regionalized muscle or ligamentous sprain/strain, sacral and/or ilial misalignment, and SIJ capsule tears. Sacroiliitis is considered to be the most common form of SIJ pain (Bernard & Cassidy 1993). The exact mechanism causing the inflammation at or near the SIJ is frequently unclear. Muscle imbalance has also been cited as a possible cause of pain. The muscle imbalance theory maintains that the joint itself is unaffected, but that the musculature surrounding the SIJ is in some form of dysfunction (Kermond 1995). This dysfunction could limit the flexibility of the dynamic muscles of the low back and ultimately begin a syndrome of chronic disuse, culminating in decreased function and pain. SIJ capsule tearing could occur from an intense trauma to the SIJ or from a shearing type movement and/or blow to the SIJ. This overall degeneration of the connective sheath surrounding the SIJ has provoked growing interest in radiologists and orthopedic surgeons. SIJ capsule ruptures are observed by injecting into the joint capsule contrast materials that can provide radiographic evidence of abnormality (Schwarzer et al 1994).

The treatment protocol described in this article utilizes an extensive evaluation of the SIJ. If SIJD is diagnosed, a manual correction technique is employed; this technique is aimed at producing symmetric bony landmark alignment for the SIJ and the surrounding structures. After the manual therapy is completed, an aggressive specific lumbar extensor resistance exercise program is undertaken. The evaluation of program success involves the change in subjective complaints of pain, objective changes in subject lumbar extensor strength, and objective change in subject work status prior to and following the protocol. This project is part of a resurgence among conventional mainstream caregivers (medical doctors, orthopedic surgeons, exercise therapists, and physical therapists) who have become interested in SIJD as a possible cause for chronic low back pain.

METHODS

Worker's compensation subjects presented to an orthopedic surgeon's practice because of low back pain. The low back pain had to be of a chronic nature (4 weeks or longer) to be considered for this project. All subjects presented with specific complaints of pain in the SIJ area. The specific low back pain complaints were documented by use of pain diagrams (Schwarzer et al 1994). Subjects were examined for low back pain and showed no neurological signs of lumbar disc abnormality.

The diagnosis of SIJ dysfunction was determined by the anatomic location of patient pain, response to SIJ provocation testing, and manual testing abnormalities seen during movements that are combined with bilateral symmetry abnormalities. If one or more of the tests in each category was positive, and a specific region of pain was present at the SIJ, the patient was diagnosed as having SIJD. The series of tests that are used to diagnose SIJD are seen in Boxes 41.2–41.4.

Box 41.2 SIJ provocation tests

Distraction	Thigh thrust
Compression	Pelvic torsion right
Iliac shear	Pelvic torsion left
Yeoman's	Figure 4/Patrick's
Posterior	Gaenslen's

Box 41.3 Manual dynamic SIJD tests

Sitting flexion test (long sit test)	Standing flexion test
	Supine long sit test
March/stork test	

Box 41.4 Static bilateral alignment testing for SIJD

Symmetrical alignment (supine) of the ASIS
Symmetrical alignment (supine) of the iliac crests
Symmetrical alignment (supine) of the PSIS
Palpation for sacral obliquity (prone)
Symmetric alignment (supine) of the symphysis pubis
Sacral border and PSIS tender to pressure

Manual dynamic testing

The supine long sitting test is performed with patient supine on an examining table. The examiner begins by placing his thumbs under the inferior border of each medial malleolus. The two medial malleoli are brought together for comparison, the knees being fully extended and all musculature relaxed. The patient then flexes into the seated position with knees extended, while looking at the ceiling. Again the lower body musculature should be relaxed. Great care is taken to make sure the subject is in a symmetric position at all times; if not, a false positive can occur due to patient positioning. The test is positive if the positioning of the malleoli, comparing pre-long sit and post-long sit, has created a discrepancy. The discrepancies between the malleoli during the long sit test are assessed for non-symmetric interaction. A positive test results when observable change occurred in relative leg length differences between the two positions.

The standing flexion test is performed with patient standing, knees straight, and feet pointing straight ahead. The examiner's thumbs are placed on the inferior aspect of the left and the right posterior superior iliac spine (PSIS). The patient bends slowly forward as far as possible. A positive test occurs when one PSIS has moved more cranially than the opposite PSIS.

The sitting flexion test is performed when the patient is in a seated position on the table. The examiner's thumbs are placed on PSISs, and the patient is than asked to bend forward slowly from the neutral position. The gluteals should not be allowed to lift off the examining table. A positive test occurs if one PSIS moves to a superior position with respect to the other. The superior PSIS is considered to be the dysfunctional side. The standing flexion test is the same design as the sitting flexion test except that the subject is standing and may not bend his knees.

The march/stork test is performed as the patient is standing in the neutral position. One of the examiner's thumbs is placed on the right PSIS while the other thumb is placed on the dorsal surface of the sacrum, placing the thumbs into a position of alignment. The patient then flexes at the hip on the side being examined. The PSIS should travel in a downward direction in comparison to the thumb acting as sacral marker. If there is no downward motion of the PSIS that is being examined, the test is considered to be positive.

Static symmetry tests

Assessment of bilateral ASIS symmetry occurs with the subject in the supine position. Anterior superior iliac spine (ASIS) positioning is carried out by placing the volar surface of the distal thumb on the underside of each ASIS. The height of each spine is compared in a horizontal plane. A positive ASIS test results when the height of one of the ASISs is greater than that of the opposite ASIS.

Assessment of the iliac crests occurs as follows. The apexes of the iliac crests are found with the subject in the supine position. Iliac crest positioning is carried out by placing the volar surface of the proximal index finger on the crest of the ilia. The height of each ilium is compared, utilizing the finger positioning, in a vertical plane. Great care should be taken to ensure that the subject is in a symmetric position when being assessed. A positive iliac crest test results when the height of one of the iliac crests is superior to that of the opposite one.

Assessment of bilateral PSIS symmetry occurs with the subject in the prone position. PSIS positioning is done by placing the volar surface of the distal thumb on the dorsal surface of each PSIS. The height of each PSIS is compared with that of the other in a horizontal plane. A positive PSIS test results when the height of one of the PSISs is greater than that of the opposite one. This test is difficult to assess when subjects are obese.

Assessment of sacral obliquity occurs with the subject in the prone position. The dorsal surface of the coccyx is bilaterally palpated using the volar surface of the distal thumbs. In this part of the assessment, the thumb should act as an outliner and not as a pressure point on the landmarks (pressure in this test can be used to detect whether the sacrum is tender to touch at the sacral borders and the PSIS). The examiner should move his thumbs cranially up the sacral border to each fused segment of the sacrum. At each fused segment of the sacrum, the heights of the bony landmarks, should be compared with each other in the horizontal plane. If one thumb is more posterior than the other, a positive test has occurred. It is a common occurrence in SIJD to elicit pain with pressure at different sacral segment levels. This production of pain can be used as a diagnostic tool for SIJD.

The pubic symphysis is located on the subject in the supine position. Both thumbs are placed on the anterior portion of the pubis. If one thumb is more posterior than the other, the test is positive. Another sign that the pubic symphysis is mediating pain is a sharp pain in the groin when the manual correction technique is being performed. This is most notable during the setting of the pubes (see below).

Diagnostic assessment

The assessment procedure for SIJD takes into account a number of signs and symptoms. In order to diagnose SIJD, the evaluator should have a combination of results: positive pain pattern for SIJD (Fortin et al 1994a, 1994b), an objective result in SIJ testing, and abnormal static SIJ landmarks (Shaw 1993). Pain generation upon provocation testing is a positive indicator of SIJD, as is having a common SIJD injury mechanism in the history. The SIJD provocative testing and common injury mechanisms are not, however, an absolute necessity for making the diagnosis. The different SIJD tests and signs are described in Boxes 41.2–41.4 (descriptions of the static and dynamic tests are given in the previous section).

If there is no pain over the SIJ region, or pain cannot be alleviated by manual mobilization, the subject should not be considered to have SIJD. No particular set of diagnostic criteria is generally used for the diagnosis of SIJD. The lack of a 'gold standard' in the diagnosis of SIJD is in part due to great differences in the literature about which SIJ test can be used as a valid predictor of SIJD (Cibulka et al 1993, Laslett & Williams 1994, Potter & Rothstein 1985).

Patients who are acutely injured (4 weeks or less) are not suitable for discussion of this SIJ treatment protocol. The majority of low back pain cases will naturally resolve in a 4–6 week period (Andersson 1981).

It should be noted that if the only objective measure for low back pain is asymmetric alignment of the ilial and sacral landmarks, this asymmetry alone is not enough evidence for the diagnosis of SIJD. Landmarks that are asymmetric are very common in asymptomatic subjects, as well as in low back pain sufferers and subjects with SIJD. Visualized abnormality on static or dynamic testing can be expected in asymptomatic patients, and painless SIJ asymmetry may not mediate low back pain. If the proper symptoms and pain patterns are not present, other diagnoses should be explored. The overzealous application of these SIJ correction techniques can only water down the overall understanding of the effectiveness of manual correction in a chronic low back pain population.

The series of steps behind the overall diagnosis for SIJD is as follows: low back pain assessment utilizing extension, flexion, or lateral side-bending movements to alleviate pain and/or numbness in lower limbs or low back (Donelson 1980). If these treatment measures do not resolve the situation, the subject's history should be checked to see whether SIJD is indicated. It should be elicited that pain patterns are physiologic for SIJ injury (Fortin et al 1994a, Waddell 1980, Keating et al 1995). Patient ilial and sacral landmarks (Box 41.4) should be evaluated for possible asymmetry, and SIJ dynamic and provocation testing (see Boxes 41.2 and 41.3 above) conducted. Manual correction techniques are utilized to produce symmetry in pertinent landmarks (see below). It should be observed whether manual corrections increase the pain-free end of range flexion/extension movements and/or decrease subjective pain ratings in the low back.

Treatment

The rehabilitation process consisted of the symmetric alignment of the SIJ's bony landmarks utilizing manual mobilizations. Following the manual corrections, an extensive dynamic resistance training program (MedX, Ocala, FL, USA) specific to the lower back was performed, in conjunction with the introduction of a general conditioning program. The general conditioning program consists of machine progressive resistance exercises (PREs) for the legs, upper torso, and abdominal muscle groups. In addition, a common program of lower body and lumbar extension stretching was given for home use.

On the first visit to the rehabilitation area, the subjects were manually mobilized into symmetric sacral and ilial positions and given a home exercise program that had basic pelvic stabilization and flexibility stretches, and McKenzie extension exercises. On the second visit to the rehabilitation unit, the SIJ was re-evaluated. Following the manual correction, the patient was then assessed for initial isolated lumbar strength. The assessment of patient back strength was determined by the utilization of an isometric strength testing device. The testing device used was a MedX lumbar extension unit as described by Avillar (1995) (see also Chapter 46 in this volume).

After the initial strength test (visit 2), the subjects began dynamic training on the lumbar extension machine. The dynamic training consisted of a concentric and an eccentric movement phase, the eccentric phase being emphasized. The training was performed until the subject reached volitional muscle failure, i.e. he lifted the weight until he could no longer exercise. The goal of this training is an exercise session of 1 set, 12–20 repetitions, in a 75–120 s period. The volitional failure method (Pollock et al 1989) utilizes a progressively heavier weight at exercise, the weight being slowly lifted each time until it cannot be lifted correctly (no preset number of repetitions). If 15–20 repetitions were successfully completed in 110+ s, the training weight for the next session would be raised by 10%. The training regimen continued twice per week until the patient was discharged. Isometric tests were administered once a month.

Manual mobilization of SIJD

The sacroiliac (SI) manual corrections that were performed on the SIJD population were always in the order of correcting iliac non-symmetry, then ASIS discrepancy, and finally sacral obliquity. Iliac positioning was considered to be of greater importance than possible non-symmetric sacral positioning. Hence, iliac asymmetry was treated before any sacral rotation. It is important to note that many different iliac and sacral alignment procedures have appeared in the literature (e.g. Cibulka 1993, Keating et al 1995).

The following methods were used for manual mobilization, these being selected because of the therapists' familiarity with the systematic procedure. This familiarity had been developed by over 10 years of experimentation with different SI mobilization techniques.

After the diagnosis of SIJ involvement is made, the following manual corrections should be performed. If a subject presents with one ilium superior to the other, the term 'upslip' is applied to the superior side. This iliac upslip in the supine position (observed with the long sit, iliac crest, and ASIS tests; see Box 41.3 above) is treated with the subject supine, the leg on the superior side being externally rotated and fully extended. The leg is then held in a fully extended, relaxed position at 30–45° from the table. A gentle but forceful sustained traction is applied to the leg in a series of three pulling motions. If the traction maneuver does not produce symmetric ilial positioning, reproduce the mobilization. If the subject presents with an iliac upslip in the prone position (observed with the long sit, PSIS, and iliac crest tests; Box 41.4), treatment follows the aforementioned steps for an upslip, but the subject is in the prone position. The traction force should not cause any pain to the subject.

If the right ilium is rotated into a posterior position, the right ASIS will be depressed and/or more cranial than the left ASIS. If the ASISs are not in symmetric positions, the following corrections (the 'push–pull' technique) are used. The technique activates the hip flexors on the right and the hip extensors on the left. As the subject is supine with the hips flexed at 90° and the knees bent, the examiner has the subject pull the right knee toward the chest while the examiner provides resistance above the knee in the anterior thigh. The left knee is simultaneously driven in a downward direction in which the examiner also resists the movement in the posterior thigh. These movements are isometric contractions performed 3–5 times per session, with a resistance applied for 3–5 s. The patient movement force is at an exertion level of 80–100%. If the left ilium is

rotated into a posterior position, the aforementioned corrections are used with the actions of the hip extensors and hip flexors being reversed.

If the right ilium is rotated in an anterior position, the right ASIS will be elevated and/or posterior to the left ASIS. The aforementioned 'push–pull' method will be used again, this time activating the hips extensors on the right and hip flexors on the left. If the left ilium is rotated in an anterior position, the same mobilization is used in accordance with the right ilium anterior rotation technique, the only difference being the use of the opposite limbs from those in the description above.

If the sacrum is rotated in a posterior position on the right side, the following technique is used for correction. The subject lies on his right side with the hips flexed at an angle of approximately 70–80° (almost a fetal position). The right knee is flexed at a 90° angle, and the left leg is fully extended and relaxed over the right thigh. The examiner places one hand under the subject's right knee and the other hand on the medial side of the right ankle. The subject holds the right leg up at approximately 30–50° while the examiner pushes the leg down using the hand positioned on the ankle (dynamic contraction). This movement is repeated in a series 3–5 times.

If SIJD is present, and the mobilization is done correctly, the patient will feel a pulling sensation in both the PSISs. The more notable sensation is in the opposite PSIS when the subject is lying on one side. It is of great importance that the quadriceps and/or the hamstrings are not activated when this 'piriformis' exercise is performed. If these muscles are active in the contraction, the resistance to the examiner's movement will be much greater and the pressure to the movement will be felt in the patient's quadriceps or hamstrings instead of the PSISs.

If the sacrum is rotated posteriorly on the left side, the same technique is used as described above for the right rotated sacrum. The only differences is that the subject will lie on his left side and the movements are carried out on the left leg.

If the right symphysis pubis is superior to the opposite pubis, the following mobilization will produce symmetry and decrease pain when adducting the knees at the end of the mobilizations (setting the pubes). The subject will activate the left rectus abdominis and the right hip adductors. While the subject is supine, he is instructed to push his left shoulder off the table (in a sit-up style contraction) while the examiner provides resistance to the movement at the shoulder. When the subject's torso has lifted 5–10 cm off of the table, the movement is blocked by the examiner. The right hip is flexed at 45–55° and will simultaneously adduct, the examiner providing resistance to the movement above the knee. These movements last 3–5 s and are performed in a series of three.

The same mobilization as described in the paragraph above is performed if the left symphysis pubis is superior to the right and if a sharp pain is present in the groins when setting the pubes. The only difference is that the opposite movements are conducted for a left- as opposed to a right-sided problem.

After all of the necessary manual mobilizations have been completed, and symmetric alignment has been achieved, mobilization of the pubes will be last (this is referred to as setting the pubes or 'shot-gunning' the pubes). In this technique, the subject is supine with the hips flexed at 45° and the feet positioned almost side by side (in a 'butterfly position'). The examiner's elbow is placed at one side of the inner knee, the other hand locking down on the opposite inner knee. The subject is instructed to adduct his knees together at 80–100% of maximal force for 3–5 s. This is done three times. It is common for an audible click to be present, which should not be painful. After setting the pubes, the sacral and ilial landmarks are checked for symmetry, objective dynamic testing is performed, and the subject can describe pain changes.

The observation of the bony landmarks and the dynamic tests will not always go to a perfect degree of symmetry. If the unsymmetric bony landmarks occur after mobilization, and pain has not been alleviated, the SIJD subject should be re-evaluated and the maneuvers performed again. If symmetry is never gained, it may not be a plausible goal. This may be due to intrinsic asymmetric landmarks, lack of clinician expertise, or lack of pain generation from the SIJD complex.

It has been this team's observation that these cases are in a large minority of SIJD sufferers.

Pain scores. Subjects were asked to score their pain level prior to each rehabilitation session. The pain rating was the average level of pain that the subject felt before entering the building for rehabilitation. The visual analog scale for pain rating that was used is as follows:

0 No pain
1–2 Occasional pain
3–4 Mild constant pain
5–6 Moderate constant pain
7–8 Unable to carry out daily activities
9–10 Emergency: need to see a doctor.

Work status. Subject work status was taken at the initial visit and on discharge from the program. The following rating system accompanied the subject's level of work:

0 No work
1 Sedentary duty
2 Light duty
3 Moderate duty
4 Fully duty

Sedentary duty consisted of lifting a maximum 5 kg and occasionally lifting and carrying such articles as dockets, ledgers, and small tools. Light duty consisted of lifting a maximum of 10 kg. with frequent lifting and/or carrying of objects weighing up to 5 kg. Moderate duty consisted of lifting up to 25 kg and frequent lifting and/or carrying of objects weighing up to 10 kg. Full duty consisted of the normal 40 hour-a-week job that was done prior to injury.

Discharge from the program. Subjects were given a 1-month prescription for (twice a week) physical therapy. At the 1 month mark, subjects were reviewed for the following criteria: strength improvement, compliance to program, and pain status. Criteria for discharge from the program included: goals being achieved, non-physiologic strength decreases at isometric (IM) testing, and continued non-physiologic pain patterns or complaints (Waddell 1980). Consideration of surgery for the SIJ occurred if patients went through the rehabilitation program, did not receive relief after 8 weeks of treatment, and continued to report physiologic pain patterns (Schwarzer et al 1994).

RESULTS

Forty-two females qualified for SIJ mobilization and isolated lumbar strength analysis in a 6-month period from March to September 1994. For gender population characteristics, see Table 41.1. Analysis of variance (ANOVA) reveals that the average pain score on the visual analog scale significantly decreased ($p < 0.001$), from an initial 6.2 to final average of 2.9. ANOVA reveals that work status increased significantly ($p < 0.001$) from an initial average work level of 2.6 to a discharge work level of 3.7. The average IM torque increased significantly ($p < 0.01$) from an initial IM average of 123.9 Nm to a final IM average of 153.5 Nm (+23.8%). ANOVA showed that IM torque increased significantly ($p \leqslant 0.01$) at all standardized test points throughout the pain-free range of motion (ROM) during IM testing (Fig. 41.1). The pain-free ROM did not change during the program. The average number of rehabilitation visits for the female population was 15.4 sessions.

Thirty-seven males qualified for this analysis from March to September 1994. ANOVA revealed the following results. The average pain score on the visual analog scale significantly ($p < 0.001$) decreased from an initial visit average of 5.5 to a discharge average of 2.1 (scale above). Work status increased significantly ($p < 0.001$) from an initial visit work level of 3.2 to a work level of 3.7 on discharge from the program. The average IM torque scores increased significantly ($p < 0.01$) from an initial IM average of 217.1 Nm to a final IM average of 276.1 Nm (+27.2%). IM torque increased significantly ($p \leqslant 0.01$) at all standardized test points throughout the pain-free ROM during IM testing (Fig. 41.2). The pain-free ROM increased significantly ($p \leqslant 0.01$) from initial ROM (0–46°) to final ROM (0–50°). The average number of male rehabilitation visits was 14.3 sessions.

In comparing male and female populations, ANOVA reveals no significant difference ($p > 0.05$) in initial pain rating, final pain rating, final work status level, length of low back pain previous to SIJ protocol entry, average lumbar IM strength

Table 41.1 SIJD population characteristics

Gender	n	Age (Years)	Height (cm)	Weight (kg)	Low back pain prior to program (months)	Pre-pain (0–10)*	Post-pain (0–10)*
Male	37	40.1	180.3	90.4	5.5	5.5	2.1
Female	42	38.1	164.1	66.6	5.9	6.2	2.9

*See 'Pain score' section for description.

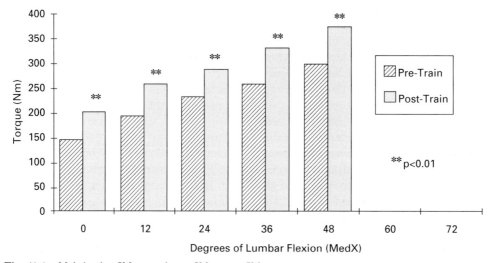

Fig. 41.1 Male lumbar IM strength: pre-IM to post-IM.

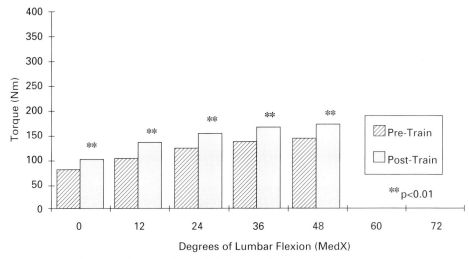

Fig. 41.2 Female lumbar IM strength: pre-IM to post-IM.

DISCUSSION

change, number of rehabilitation sessions, and group age. Significant differences ($p \leq 0.05$) occur in total IM torque produced, group height, and group weight, the male group having greater values for these three aspects.

DISCUSSION

These data indicate that the SIJ mobilization and isolated lumbar strengthening protocol is effective in reducing subject self-reported pain levels and increasing the subject functional working status. Objective measurements of improvement are witnessed by the increasing strength values seen on lumbar extension strength testing (lumbar IM torque) and in the increasing levels of subject work status. These objective changes occur with subjective decreases in self-reported pain levels in a chronic workers' compensation low back pain population.

Comparing the male and female group characteristics, ANOVA reveals that the populations are homogenous in nature, barring gender-based differences. The areas in which there are no significant differences are numerous. The gender-based differences occur in group height, weight, and the overall total lumbar IM torque produced, differences that are to be expected when comparing male and female groups.

The study of the effects of manual mobilization on the SIJ, and low back pain in general, have yet

to be examined. The effects of machine-driven isolated lumbar resistance training on low back pain sufferers, let alone those people who may suffer with SIJD, have yet to be fully investigated. To our knowledge, this is the only study that has had a well-defined SIJD group that was manually mobilized into symmetric SIJ position and then trained in an isolated lumbar extension device. This is also one of the few studies dealing with the SIJ that has objective evidence (increased strength gain, increased work status level) along with subjective reports of decreased pain when utilizing a specific treatment protocol.

This information shows an objective functional restoration of subject strength and work status in a chronic low back pain population within a workers' compensation population. This protocol warrants scrutiny due to: overall effectiveness, method of SIJD assessment and diagnosis, and the combination of manual treatment and aggressive isolated lumbar machine-driven exercise.

CONCLUSIONS

1. This study reveals very positive results in the areas of self-reported subjective decrease in low back pain, as well as objective increases in lumbar strength and increased functional status (work level).

2. This unique combination of manual therapy and aggressive resistance training in a chronic

low back pain population requires further enthusiastic investigation due to its effectiveness and the efficient treatment period for a traditionally difficult population.

3. An obvious question arises of what the individual effects of the isolated strength training versus the effects of the SIJ mobilization techniques were.

4. The issues behind the causative nature of these results requires that this project be investigated at greater length.

5. Two main points involving this population bear mentioning: subjects were utilizing the worker's compensation system, and they had chronic complaints of low back pain lasting for longer than 5 months prior to entry into this program.

Considering these two important issues in dealing with this study population, the results are remarkable. This evaluation and treatment method for the SIJD is an attempt to treat a subcategory of low back pain that has not in the past been well defined nor treated in a consistent manner.

ACKNOWLEDGMENTS

I would like to thank the entire staff at the Keating Group for their help in assembling this chapter. I especially want to thank the amazing interns (Jennifer, Chris, Chrissy, Mark, and Molly) from the University of Florida who spent countless hours at bizarre and tedious tasks to prepare this information.

REFERENCES

Andersson G 1981 Epidemiological aspects of low back pain in industry. Spine 6: 53–60

Avillar M, Sims V, Keating J, Stinchcomb P, Herrberg J 1995 The effect of a seven week sacroiliac joint mobilization and stabilization program on a low back pain population. In: Vleeming A, Mooney V, Dorman T, Snijders C (eds) Second interdisciplinary world congress on low back pain. San Diego, CA, 9–11 November, pp 305–321

Bernard T, Cassidy D 1993 The sacroiliac joint syndrome: pathophysiology, diagnosis, and management. In: Vleeming A, Mooney V, Snijders C, Dorman T (eds) First interdisciplinary world congress on low back pain and its relation to the sacroiliac joint. San Diego, CA, 5–6 November, pp 120–143

Carpenter D M, Graves J E, Pollock M L et al 1991 Effect of 12 and 20 weeks of resistance training on lumbar extension torque production. Physical Therapy 71: 580–588

Cibulka M, Delitto A, Erhard R E 1993 Pain patterns in patients with and without sacroiliac joint dysfunction. In: Vleeming A, Mooney V, Snijders C, Dorman T (eds) First interdisciplinary world congress on low back pain and its relation to the sacroiliac joint. San Diego, CA, 5–6 November, pp 363–370

Donelson R 1980 The McKenzie Approach to evaluating and treating low back pain. Orthopaedic Review 19(8): 681–686

Fortin A, Dwyer S, West J, Pier J 1994a Sacroiliac joint: pain referral maps upon applying a new injection/arthrography technique. I: Asymptomatic volunteers. Spine 19(13): 1475–1482

Fortin A, Aprill C, Ponthieux B, Pier J 1994b Sacroiliac joint: pain referral maps upon applying a new injection/arthrography technique. 2: Clinical evaluation. Spine 19(13): 1483–1489

Foster D, Fulton M 1991 Back pain and the exercise prescription. Clinics in Sports Medicine 10(1): 197–209

Gowers S 1904 Lumbago: its lessons and analogues. British Medical Journal 1: 117–121

Graves J E, Pollock M L, Carpenter D M et al 1990 Quantitative assessment of full range-of-motion isometric lumbar extension strength. Spine 15(4): 289–294

Graves J, Webb D, Pollock M et al 1994 Pelvic stabilization during resistance training: its effect on the development of lumbar extension strength. Archives of Physical Medical Rehabilitation 75: 210–215

Keating J G, Sims V, Avillar M D 1995 Sacroiliac joint fusion in a chronic low back pain population. In: Vleeming A, Mooney V, Dorman T, Snijders C (eds) Second interdisciplinary world congress on low back pain. San Diego, CA, 9–11 November, pp 361–365

Kelsey J L, White A A 1980 Epidemiology and impact of low-back pain. Spine 5(2): 133–140

Kermond W 1995 Early intervention low intensity exercise therapy in work related acute lumbar sprain injuries. Presented at Exercise rehabilitation of the spine: update '95, Orlando, FL, 6–8 April

Laslett M, Williams M 1994 The reliability of selected pain provocation tests for sacroiliac joint pathology. Spine 19(1): 1243–1249

Mixter W J, Barr J S 1934 Rupture of the intervertebral disc with involvement of the spinal canal. New England Journal of Medicine 211: 210–215

Nelson B, O'Reilly E, Miller M, Hogan M, Wegner J, Kelly C 1995 The clinical effects of intensive, specific exercise on chronic low back pain: a controlled study of 895 consecutive patients with 1-year follow-up. Orthopedics 18(10): 971–981

Polatin P 1990 The functional restoration approach to chronic low back pain. Journal of Musculoskeletal Medicine 7(1): 17–30

Pollock M, Leggett S, Graves J, Jones A, Fulton M, Cirulli J 1989 Effect of resistance training on lumbar extension strength. American Journal of Sports Medicine 17(5): 624–629

Potter N, Rothstein J 1985 Intertester reliability for selected clinical tests of the sacroiliac joint. Physical Therapy 65: 1671–1675

Risch S, Norvell N, Pollock M et al 1992 Lumbar strengthening in chronic low back pain patients. Spine 18(2): 232–238

Rissanen A, Kalimo H, Alaranta H 1995 Effect of intensive training on the isokinetic strength and structure of lumbar muscles in patients with chronic low back pain. Spine 20: 333–340

Schwarzer A, Aprill C, Bogduk N 1994 The sacroiliac joint in chronic low back pain. Spine 20(1): 31–37

Shaw J L 1993 The role of the sacroiliac joint as a cause of low back pain and dysfunction. In: Vleeming A, Mooney V, Snijders C, Dorman T (eds) First interdisciplinary world congress on low back pain and its relation to the sacroiliac joint. San Diego, CA, 5–6 November, pp 67–80

Twomey L, Taylor J 1995 Exercise and spinal manipulation in the treatment of low back pain. Spine 20(5): 615–619

van Deursen L, Patijn J, Ockhuysen A, Vortman B 1990 The value of some clinical tests of the sacroiliac joint. Journal of Manual Medicine 5: 96–99

Vleeming A, Stoeckart R, Snijders C 1993 A short history of sacro-iliac research. In: Vleeming A, Mooney V, Snijders C J, Dorman T (eds) First interdisciplinary world congress on low back pain and its relation to the sacroiliac joint. San Diego, CA, 5–6 November, pp 5–11

Waddell G 1980 Nonorganic physical signs in low back pain. Spine 5(2): 117–125

42. Evaluation and treatment of the most common patterns of sacroiliac joint dysfunction

J. Hesch

INTRODUCTION

The sacroiliac joint (SIJ) has been implicated as a source of low back pain by many clinicians and researchers, including Lee (1989, 1992) and Vleeming and Mooney (1992). There is an inter-disciplinary interest in the role of the SIJ and low back pain and its functional relation to the musculoskeletal system (Vleeming et al 1992, 1995). The SIJ may cause pain due to disease, inflammation, or movement dysfunction. Move-ment dysfunction may exist as hypermobility or hypomobility. According to Porterfield and DeRosa (1991), the normal SIJ functions as a triplane shock absorber and transfers upper body weight into the pelvis and lower extremities, and participates in the absorption of the force of heel strike. If the SIJ is hypomobile, it cannot effectively absorb stress from activities of daily living, and other structures may be overstressed, thus contributing to muscu-loskeletal pain and dysfunction. Examples are low back pain and hip pain. Ligamentous and capsular pain may be present if one or more of the pelvic bones has moved beyond the normal range of motion and became stuck, thus perpetuating soft tissue pain. Treatment can often produce dramatic results in a short period of time by passively restoring normal motion. In this example, the hypomobility is transient and is appropriately referred to as apparent hypomobility. True hypo-mobility or status hypomobility is much more resistant to treatment and at times non-responsive. Often, degenerative changes or disease has occurred over time, and thus normal mobility cannot be restored. Mild forms of true hypermobility can be managed readily, whereas moderate and severe forms are quite challenging. Other authors have addressed true hypermobility and instability within this book.

Apparent hypermobility and apparent hypo-mobility often coexist. Mobility testing of the pelvis reveals one direction of decreased mobility, whereas testing in the opposite direction reveals increased mobility. This is quite common, and treatment directed at restoring normal movement in the direction of hypomobility usually also restores normal movement in the direction of the apparent hypermobility. This chapter addresses common patterns of apparent hypomobility and apparent hypermobility.

It is an established fact that the SIJ has a small amount of functional motion, as does the symphysis pubis (Vleeming et al 1992). There may be a greater than normal amount of motion due to trauma, repetitive overload, inflammation, hormonal laxity, or heredity. Bernard (1992) has demonstrated through fluoroscopy that the SIJ does move with manually applied loads such as those utilized in evaluation and treatment. What has not been established is whether or not manual clinical tests and treatments specifically affect *only* the SIJ. It may be that mobility is evaluated and treated manually as part of the integrated system of the spine, pelvis, and hip. The SIJ is part of this system, and it does not function in an isolated fashion. Mobility tests that attempt to isolate actual joint play may yield useful information about the system; however, we cannot say with certainty that mobility tests exclusively isolate *only* the SIJ.

For several reasons, specific joint mobility tests (also called spring tests) may yield information about perceived movement that may be greater than the actual movement that occurs. The bony landmarks used are at a distance to the joint and may thus amplify perceived motion. The spring test may be applied in one plane and yet may produce triplane motion in the joint, and the kinesthetic information may therefore seem amplified. A spring test may induce simultaneous motion at both SIJs and the symphysis pubis. A small degree of cartilage and bone deformation may also occur. Last, in spite of our best efforts to isolate the joint, the test might actually incorporate the lumbopelvic–hip region. These reasons do not detract from the clinical utility of the spring tests, as they evaluate an important and often overlooked aspect of joint function, which is joint play. This will be addressed later.

PALPATION OF LUMBOPELVIC LANDMARKS

Even though it is part of a standard lumbopelvic evaluation, accurate palpation of lumbopelvic landmarks in standing and sitting can at times be difficult owing to muscular response to gravity. In standing, the pelvic posture can be influenced by biomechanical dysfunction above and below the pelvis. Palpation of the landmarks in supine and prone lying may yield more accurate information about the isolated lumbopelvic structure as the influence of the upper and lower body is reduced. A higher inter- and intrarater agreement has been observed with supine and prone palpation as part of an evaluation protocol (Ellis et al 1989). An abbreviated evaluation that addresses bony palpation is presented in Fig. 42.1. Evaluation should also include palpation of all soft tissues, especially muscles and ligaments. A distinction needs to be made between *positional dysfunction* and *movement dysfunction*. Positional dysfunction describes how it is positioned; movement dysfunction describes how it cannot move. Evaluation and treatment that rely on position alone are at best speculative. Movement testing is presented below.

The client should lie in a symmetric posture. Record findings on only one side of the body and check the appropriate side. When findings are symmetrical place an = sign in front of the first box.

Side of body:	☐ Right	☐ Left

Supine palpation

Leg length	☐ Long	☐ Short
ASISs	☐ Anterior	☐ Posterior
ASISs	☐ Superior	☐ Inferior
ASISs	☐ Medial	☐ Lateral
Anterior iliac shelves (The anterior iliac shelf is the 5 cm portion of the ilium above the ASIS)	☐ Superior	☐ Inferior
Pubic bones (entire length)	☐ Anterior	☐ Posterior

Prone palpation

PSISs	☐ Anterior	☐ Posterior
Posterior iliac shelf (The posterior iliac shelf is the superior portion of the ilium that is midway between the midline of the spine and the most lateral pelvis)	☐ Superior	☐ Inferior
Ischial tuberosity	☐ Superior	☐ Inferior
Sacral palpation bilaterally at S1, S2, S3, S4 and S5	☐ Anterior	☐ Posterior
Sacral inferior lateral angles	☐ Superior	☐ Inferior
L5 position	☐ Rotates left	☐ Rotates right
L5 response to prone press-up	☐ Rotates left	☐ Rotates right

Sitting palpation

L5 in flexion	☐ Rotates left	☐ Rotates right
L5 in extension	☐ Rotates left	☐ Rotates right
L5 in neutral	☐ Rotates left	☐ Rotates right

Fig. 42.1 Bony position palpation of the pelvis and L5.

PELVIC MOBILITY AND JOINT SPRING TESTS

Mobility tests can be general or specific. For example, an anteriorly directed force on the left of the sacrum at the level of the joint (S1, S2, and S3) induces a right rotational force and is a joint spring test. In contrast, right active lumbar and pelvic rotation is a general mobility test. Both types of test are important in evaluating clients with suspected SIJ dysfunction. The specific joint spring tests give more information about joint and ligament function. The general mobility tests will give more information about whole patterns of motion influenced by several joints and several muscle groups. The following gross motion tests are presented in the literature and are in fairly common use: the standing trunk flexion test, standing hip flexion (Gillet's) test, sitting flexion test, and long sit test (Potter & Rothstein 1985). These gross motion tests implicate faulty motion of the pelvis as a unit but are not very specific; however, they are often utilized to evaluate purported faulty 'sacroiliac joint motion'. The SIJ is within the pelvis, and a more appropriate description might be 'faulty lumbopelvic–hip' motion. These tests are useful screening tests but cannot provide the same information as the spring tests.

It is nearly impossible to perform a joint spring test in standing. It is much easier to perform isolated joint spring tests with the client supine and prone. As the SIJ functions as a shock absorber, the spring tests might be able qualitatively to assess that function. The use of the term 'spring' seems very appropriate when testing the quality of pelvic joint play as there is a very discernable elastic feel in loading the pelvic joints, in imparting the actual spring test, and in the quality of recoil.

Walker (1992) asks a relevant question with regards to motion testing:

Is the motion present adequate in total range to be detected by observation and manual palpation, as extensively described by several clinicians? The minimal range of motion present in probably most of the population casts doubt on whether therapists can detect 1 to 3 degrees or 1 to 3 mm of motion occurring specifically at the SIJ. Perhaps the term *play* (joint play) should be used when referring to the SIJ, as *motion* implies quantity of motion similar to other synovial joints, which does not appear to be the case.

The SIJ does not exist in isolation with regard to anatomy and function. Perhaps more important than the fact that motion occurs within the SIJ is the concept that it occurs *through* the SIJ. Proper function of pelvic articulations requires the ability to translate forces through these articulations and to dissipate forces via viscoelastic properties. Articular spring tests are useful in evaluating these important properties of pelvic joint function.

Specific pelvic joint spring tests

All tests are carried out first on one side and then the other. Spring tests are always used even if the pelvis is symmetric as movement dysfunction may still be present. Firm and increasing pressure is applied to the part being tested until motion no longer occurs. At this point the soft tissue and joint slack is taken up and maintained before imparting the spring test. The actual spring test is then performed when an additional force is imparted. The spring test should therefore test primarily joint play (qualitatively) in the joint, and to a lesser extent a response in the surrounding soft tissue. When performing the spring test, take note of the quality of the initial load, the end feel of the spring test, and the feel of recoil, as well as the subjective response. Retest several times if unsure. When evaluating the recoil, it is important to return to the point at which the slack is taken up, rather than abruptly letting go. The quality of the perceived joint play is rated as normal, hypomobile, or hypermobile. A 0–6 scale can also be utilized (Paris 1991):

0 = ankylosis or no detectable movement
1 = considerable limitation in movement
2 = slight limitation in movement
3 = normal (that is, for the individual)
4 = slight increase in motion
5 = considerable increase in motion
6 = unstable.

Of course, there is a degree of subjectivity in rating joint play. Skill in joint spring testing comes with practice and training. Spring tests are not used to determine whether pain is present when one is evaluating biomechanical function of the pelvic girdle. It is not uncommon for clients to have biomechanical dysfunction that is sub-threshold, so pain is not present. Additionally, the forces imparted with clinical tests applied to the knee do not replicate physiological forces (Noyes 1977), and this might also be true for the pelvis. However, if pain is encountered, it is acknowledged, the test is modified or deferred, and an interpretation of the pain is attempted.

Spring tests can be measured with force transducers, for example MicroFET™ muscle testing device (Hoggan Health Industries, Draper, UT, USA). This is a hand-held instrument that measures the amount of force applied by the clinician. After taking up the slack in the joint, the clinician can then apply an additional force and determine how much force is applied when joint play is perceived. Both sides are compared. The clinician can measure pre- and post-treatment force. Most force transducers used in the clinic describe force in pounds, or kilograms, although force described in Newtons (N) accounts for the influence of gravity. For the benefit of the inter-disciplinary audience, all three measures will be presented. The spring tests average 88 N (20 lb, 9 kg) for taking up the slack and up to 176 N (40 lb, 18 kg) to apply the spring test. The force needed may vary from person to person. The above averages serve as a guideline with which to develop the skill of applying the spring tests. The appropriate amount of force is the least amount that yields useful information without increasing pain. The initial load takes from 2–3 s and performing the spring test takes 1–2 s, as does assessing the recoil.

A study was performed to determine whether therapists could learn accurately to produce specific forces to the lumbar spine (Keating et al 1993). The authors concluded that therapists can learn to quantify applied forces, which has implications for evaluation and communication of joint behavior. This study is encouraging and a similar study with forces applied to the pelvis is needed.

The basic sacroiliac joint spring tests

1. Prone sacral rotation (Fig. 42.2). With the client prone, apply the ulnar border or the heel of your hand on the left side of the sacrum at

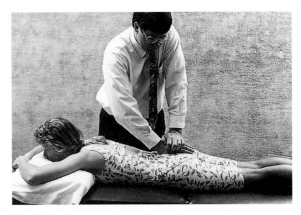

Fig. 42.2   Prone sacral rotation spring test.

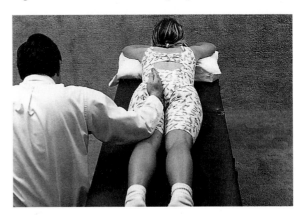

Fig. 42.3   Prone sacral side-bending spring test.

the joint level (S1, S2, and S3). You must be medial to the posterior superior iliac spine (PSIS) to assure that you do not have contact on the ilium. Apply an anteriorly directed force of up to 88 N (20 lb, 9 kg) to take up the slack in the joint, and then an additional force of up to 176 N (40 lb, 18 kg) to assess joint play. Repeat the test on the other side. Pressure on the left side induces right rotation; pressure on the right induces left rotation.

2. Prone sacral side-bending (Fig. 42.3). With the client prone, palpate the coccyx and locate the inferior lateral angles of the sacrum by pushing laterally and superiorly with your thumbs. You will have to depress the soft tissue to make bony contact. Then place the ulnar border of your hand on the left inferior lateral angle. Apply a superior force of up to 88 N (20 lb, 9 kg) to take up the slack. Only a minimal additional force of up to 49 N (11 lb, 5 kg) is required to assess joint play. Repeat the test on the right side.

3. Supine posterior rotation of the ilium (Fig. 42.4). With the client supine, place as much contact as possible with one hand on each ilium. The hand should mold to the anterior ilium to maximize comfort. Take up the slack on one side by applying up to 88 N (20 lb, 9 kg), directed at a 45° angle. The force applied is a posterior rotary force. After taking up the slack, apply an additional force up to 176 N (40 lb, 18 kg) to assess joint play. Repeat the test on the other side.

4. Prone anterior rotation of the ilium (Fig. 42.5). With the client prone, place the heel of your hand on the left superior ilium, just above and lateral to the PSIS. Apply a pure anterior force with up to 88 N (20 lb, 9 kg) of force to take up the slack. Then apply an additional force up to 176 N (40 lb, 18 kg) to assess joint play. Repeat the test on the right side.

5. Prone anterolateral glide of the ilium (Fig. 42.6). With the client prone, place the heel of your hand on the posterior ilium, including the medial portion of the PSIS and the portion of the ilium above and below the PSIS. Take care not to include the sacrum or the test will be invalid. Apply up to 88 N (20 lb, 9 kg) of force directed anterolaterally at a 45° angle. After taking up the slack in the joint, apply an additional force up to 18 kg to assess joint play. Repeat the test on the other side.

A convenient grading form for basic spring tests is available (Fig. 42.7).

EVALUATION AND TREATMENT CONSIDERATIONS

A diagnosis is established by a physician prior to using this approach to evaluation and treatment. Mechanical pain responds rather quickly to mechanical treatment, and thus care is not prolonged in the absence of progress. Whether or

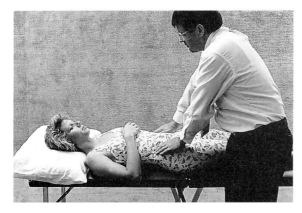

Fig. 42.4   Supine posterior rotation of the ilium spring test.

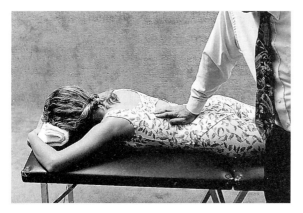

Fig. 42.5   Prone anterior rotation of the ilium spring test.

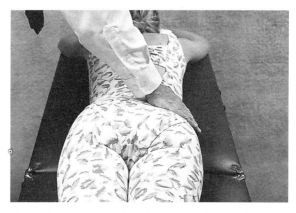

Fig. 42.6   Prone anterolateral glide of the ilium spring test.

	Hypomobile	Hypermobile
1. Sacral rotation (prone)	☐	☐
2. Sacral side-bending (prone)	☐	☐
3. Posterior rotation of the ilium (supine)	☐	☐
4. Anterior rotation of the ilium (prone)	☐	☐
5. Anterolateral ilium glide (prone)	☐	☐

Fig. 42.7   Basic pelvic spring test grading form.

not this approach is effective can usually be determined within 2–3 visits, up to a maximum of 6. Previous to utilizing this approach, a thorough evaluation is performed, including the lumbar spine, the hip joints, a review of medical tests, history-taking, neurological screening, and consultation as appropriate. This approach can easily be integrated or interfaced with other approaches to low back pain.

Caution is warranted and treatment may be contraindicated in the presence of poor rapport, severe protective muscle guarding, no direction of movement that eases pain, recent herniated nucleus pulposus with nerve root compromise, paresthesia or sensory loss below the knee, and undiagnosed pain. This list is not exhaustive, and sound clinical judgement always takes precedence.

Treatment should be tolerated with minimal, if any, discomfort. Treatment is usually perceived as relieving pain and is always discontinued if pain increases to a moderate degree during the procedure. If painful, reassessment is carried out to determine the appropriate course of action. This method of evaluation emphasizes the role of joint function and treats on the basis of faulty joint play. It acknowledges that there is a relationship between pain and function, and that treatment should address both. The rationale for this treatment approach has been presented elsewhere (Hesch et al 1992).

THE MOST COMMON PATTERN OF LUMBOPELVIC MOVEMENT DYSFUNCTION

The most common pattern of faulty lumbopelvic movement dysfunction is based on the evaluation of palpation and spring tests described earlier. In an outpatient physical therapy clinic, this pattern is encountered on a daily basis. In certain patients, this pattern appears to be the root cause of the lumbopelvic pain syndrome; in others, it is only a contributing factor. There are many other patterns of lumbopelvic movement dysfunction, which are described in detail elsewhere (Greenman 1996, Hesch 1996). Based on this method of evaluation, 90% of the patient population with SIJ dysfunction will also have joint dysfunction of the lumbar spine (Kraemer, unpublished data).

There are eight components of the most common pattern. Patients typically present with all eight, but occasionally may have fewer:

1. left posterior pubic bone
2. left sacral rotation
3. left sacral side-bending fixation
4. right anterior ilium
5. left posterior ilium
6. type I right inflare
7. type I left outflare
8. type II left lumbar flexion movement dysfunction.

Left posterior pubic bone

Positional dysfunction. The entire anterior surface of the left pubic bone is posterior in relation to the right.

Movement dysfunction. Spring tests at the symphysis pubis are rarely utilized as palpatory findings correlate very highly with the spring test findings, and clients are often quite tender even with mild pressure. If an anterior-to-posterior spring test is performed, it will reveal hypermobility on the left and hypomobility on the right.

Other findings. Tenderness of the soft tissue overlying the left pubic bone and at the left sacrospinous ligament may correlate with a posterior pubic bone. No doubt, changes in the dimension of the sciatic notch would accompany a pubic shift, and there may be adverse tension or compression of sciatic notch contents.

Treatment. See Fig. 42.8.

Left sacral rotation

Positional dysfunction. With the patient prone, the entire left side of the sacrum is prominent as the sacrum appears rotated left about a vertical axis.

Movement dysfunction. The prominent left side will have decreased anterior mobility; the deep right side will have increased anterior mobility (spring test 1).

Other findings. Sacral rotation has a direct effect on L5–S1 facet motion.

Treatment. See Fig. 42.9.

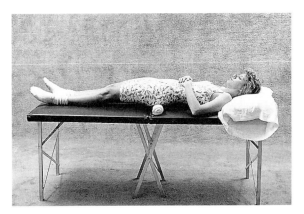

Fig. 42.8   Self-treatment for left posterior pubic bone. *Patient Position*: supine with hips and knees in neutral position. *Self-treatment*: place a rolled (7 cm diameter) towel horizontally under the left ischium and maintain for 2–5 min. Then retest via palpation.

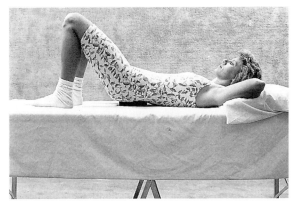

Fig. 42.9   Left sacral rotation treatment. *Patient position*: supine with hips and knees flexed. Padded dowel placed vertically on the left side of the sacrum to encompass L5–S1, and S1–3. Padded dowel is 2.5 cm × 10 cm wood dowel covered with pipe foam for comfort. *Treatment*: maintain this position for 2 min. After treatment, retest mobility.

Left sacral side-bending fixation

Positional dysfunction. The left inferior lateral angle will be inferior in relation to the right.

Movement dysfunction. There is a lack of superior glide when tested at the left inferior lateral angle (spring test 2).

Other findings. Sacral side-bending can perpetuate faulty lumbosacral motion coupling.

Treatment. See Fig. 42.10.

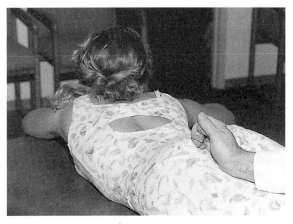

Fig. 42.10   Left sacral side-bending treatment. *Patient position*: prone with the trunk side-bent to the right. This is done to minimize left lumbosacral facet compression during mobilization, and to pull the sacrum into right side-bending. *Therapist position*: the ulnar border of the hand is on the undersurface of the inferior lateral angle of the sacrum on the left side. *Treatment*: gently take up any available slack and perform five gentle oscillations. The combined force to take up the slack and perform oscillations rarely exceeds 137 N (31 lb, 14 kg). After treatment, retest mobility with the spring test.

Right anterior ilium

Positional dysfunction. The anterior superior iliac spine (ASIS) anterior, medial, and inferior; anterior iliac shelf inferior; posterior superior iliac spine PSIS anterior; posterior iliac shelf superior; and ischial tuberosity superior.

Movement dysfunction. Reduced posterior rotation (spring test 3).

Other findings. Dysfunction of the anterior ilium is very common (DonTigny 1993), particularly on the right side, but rarely on the left. It is a common postural adaptation due to asymmetric sitting posture, getting in and out of the car in a hurried fashion thus twisting the spine on the pelvis, holding babies supported on one side of the pelvis, etc. It is present to some degree in most of the adult population and is often asymptomatic. In acute injuries, the client may have had an anterior ilium for quite some time, then overloaded the joint and soft tissues, enhancing a pattern that was previously quiescent. Anterior ilium is a contributor to faulty biomechanics of the spine and lower extremity, and is therefore often addressed in clients who do not appear to have sacroiliac joint pain. Anterior ilium

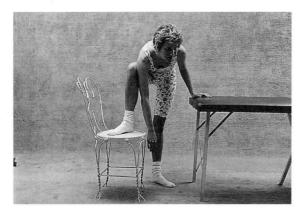

Fig. 42.11   Self-treatment for right anterior ilium. The client places the right foot on a stool with the hip flexed to 90° and abducted to 45°. The client then reaches for the floor with the right hand, which is medial to the right knee. The stretch is performed gently for 2 min. After treatment, retest mobility. *Alternate method*: in sitting, supine or side-lying, bring the knee on the right side to the outside of the right axilla and stretch gently for 2 min. After treatment, retest mobility.

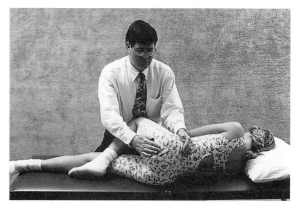

Fig. 42.12   Side-lying treatment for left posterior ilium. *Patient position*: side-lying with the left hip on top flexed 60–90°, assuring that the ilium does not rotate posteriorly. Two or three pillows are placed under the left thigh to keep it both horizontal and comfortable. *Therapist position*: left palmar contact is made on the posterior ilium, 2–4 cm above the level of the PSIS. The patient's left knee rests against the therapist's abdomen. *Treatment*: the therapist takes up the slack by gently pushing the client's femur posteriorly into end-range and pulling the ilium anteriorly into end-range with the left hand. Gently oscillate the ilium anteriorly 10 times with the left hand. After treatment, retest mobility with spring test.

contributes to left lumbar rotation via pull of the right iliolumbar ligament.

   Treatment. See Fig. 42.11.

Left posterior ilium

   Positional dysfunction. ASIS superior, lateral, posterior; anterior iliac shelf superior; posterior iliac shelf inferior; ischial tuberosity inferior; and PSIS posterior.

   Movement dysfunction. Decreased anterior rotation of the left ilium (spring test 4).

   Other findings. Dysfunction of the posterior left ilium does not always follow that of the anterior right ilium, but when present is usually more symptomatic than that of the anterior ilium. Clients usually also have limited and painful lumbar extension, with restricted facet joint movement.

   Treatment. See Figs 42.12 and 42.13.

Type I right inflare/Type I left outflare

   Position dysfunction. Right ASIS medial and anterior; right PSIS lateral and anterior; left ASIS lateral and posterior; left PSIS lateral and posterior.

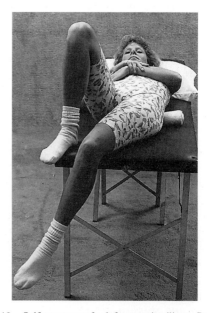

Fig. 42.13   Self-treatment for left posterior ilium. *Patient position*: supine with the left leg off the table. The left hip is maximally adducted. The right hip is flexed and abducted with foot flat on the table. *Treatment*: maintain this position and let it stretch passively for 2 min. The left thigh should literally be suspended above horizontal by the hip capsule and soft tissues, otherwise the degree of adduction is inadequate.

Right inflare — Left outflare

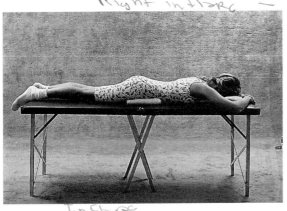

Inflare

Fig. 42.14 *Flare exercise 1.* Lie on your stomach with a 7 cm diameter, 25 cm long rolled towel placed vertically under your right anterior pelvis and thigh for 2 min.

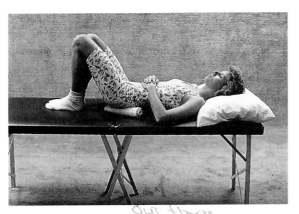

Out flare

Fig. 42.15 *Flare exercise 2.* Lie on your back with the towel roll under the left part of your pelvis at a 30° angle for 2 min. The towel roll should encompass the ilium and the ischium, but not the sacrum. Keep both knees bent and feet flat.

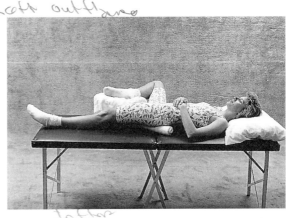

Inflare

Fig. 42.16 *Flare exercise 3.* In the same position as in Fig. 42.15 with the towel roll, bend your right hip to 90° and let it stretch out to the right side for 2 min. Keep your left leg straight. To assist the 90° angle of the hip, you may place a folded pillow under the right foot and lower leg.

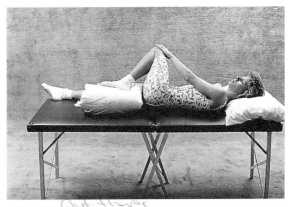

Out flare

Fig. 42.17 *Flare exercise 4.* In the same position as in Fig. 42.15 but without the towel roll, bend your left hip to 90°and with your left hand, push the left thigh to the right. Use a folded pillow under the foot and lower leg if needed to maintain 90° hip flexion, and stretch for 2 min.

Movement dysfunction. Increased anterolateral mobility will be noted when tested at the right posterior ilium in prone (see Fig. 42.6 above). This hypermobility can be subtle. There will be a very apparent decrease of anterolateral mobility as tested in prone at the left posterior ilium.

Other findings. Type I right inflare is a very common pattern. As it is always accompanied by a type I left outflare, treating both sides is mandatory.

Treatment. See Figs 42.14–42.17.

Type II left lumbar flexion movement dysfunction (Greenman 1996)

When the L5–S1 facet has restricted flexion on one side, ipsilateral rotation will be induced when flexion is attempted. If a motion segment cannot flex on the left, it will remain in extension on the left when the rest of the spine flexes. This creates a pathological axis, and the vertebra will extend at the left facet, rotate to the left, and typically side-bend to the left. With flexion movement dysfunction, there may be a slight asymmetry in neutral. With active extension there is no asymmetry; with increasing flexion, there is increasing asymmetry. Palpation through the soft tissues overlying the transverse processes, facets, or laminae will demonstrate increased prominence on the left with flexion. In other words, the side with flexion dysfunction becomes prominent with flexion.

Treating type II left lumbar flexion motion dysfunction

This is by muscle energy treatment (Greenman 1996).

Patient position. Sitting with the lumbar spine in flexion.

Therapist position. Sitting behind the patient. The left thumb palpates the left lumbosacral junction. The right hand is placed in front of the right shoulder.

Treatment. Keep the left ischium in contact with the seating surface. The motion barrier is engaged with flexion from above downwards until the lumbosacral segment attempts to flex. Then side-bending to the right and rotation to the right are added until the L5–S1 segment is again engaged. Resist the patient with contact at the front of the right shoulder as he or she gently attempts to rotate left for 10 s isometrically. Then have the patient relax, and he or she will passively move into the barrier. Repeat three times.

Self-treatment. See Fig. 42.18.

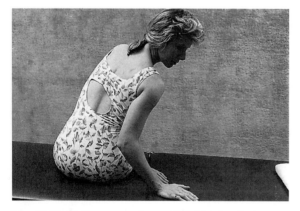

Fig. 42.18 Self-treatment for type II left lumbar flexion motion dysfunction. Keep the left ischium in contact with the seating surface. The patient sits with the lumbar spine in flexion, right side-bending, and right rotation, gently engaging the motion barrier as described above. Gentle active right rotation is repeated 30 times at mid-to-end range.

After treating the lumbar motion dysfunction, it is appropriate to re-evaluate and treat whatever other motion dysfunctions may be present in the lumbar spine, pelvis, and hip, as it is possible that other types of lumbopelvic and hip joint mobility dysfunction may be present (Greenman 1996, Hesch 1996). This is an appropriate time to address muscle function of the spine, pelvis, and hip. Compensation for the lumbopelvic dysfunction can occur in the lower extremity and in the spinal axis as high as the upper cervical spine. Left hip rotator muscle imbalance is almost always present, with shortened left external rotators.

CONCLUSIONS

1. The most common patterns of SIJ dysfunction based on palpation and joint spring tests have been presented. The spring tests may be more appropriate in testing joint play than are gross motion tests that purport to test SIJ motion. Both testing procedures may be more useful in addressing the lumbopelvic structure when used in combination. Additional spring tests are available for more complex presentations, including 12 newly encountered patterns of dysfunction (Hesch 1996).

2. The pelvis is the hub of the body, and movement dysfunction here can contribute to compensatory patterns above and below. Thus, when dysfunction of the lumbopelvic–hip complex is encountered, it is appropriate to evaluate and treat the entire kinetic chain.

3. Continued research on traditional and emerging methods of evaluation and treatment is needed. While research is in progress, we must be aware of what is already known and what new questions need to be answered regarding this complicated and somewhat mysterious articulation. As our understanding of the coupled lumbopelvic–hip complex and its relevance to the rest of the kinetic chain is growing, so must our treatment approaches. We must continue to treat it based on our current understanding, and we must strive diligently for better methods of evaluation and treatment.

REFERENCES

Bernard T 1992 Video presentation on sacroiliac joint injections. First interdisciplinary world congress on low back pain and its relation to the sacroiliac joint. San Diego, CA, 5–6 November

DonTigny R 1993 Mechanics and treatment of the sacroiliac joint. Journal of Manual and Manipulative Therapy 1: 3–12

Ellis T, Moore T, Jackson R, Martin R 1989 Palpation to assess ilial symmetry/asymmetry: isometric mobilization to restore ilial symmetry. In: Proceedings of the Manipulative Therapy Association of Australia 6th biannual conference proceedings. Manipulative Therapist Association of Australia, Adelaide, pp 63–70

Greenman P E 1996 Principles of manual medicine, 2nd edn. Williams & Wilkins, Baltimore

Hesch J 1996 Course workbook – The Hesch method of treating sacroiliac joint dysfunction: an integrated approach. Albuquerque, New Mexico

Hesch J, Aisenbrey J, Guarino J 1992 Manual therapy evaluation of the pelvic joints using palpatory and articular spring tests. In: Vleeming A, Mooney V, Snijders C J, Dorman T (eds) First interdisciplinary world congress on low back pain and its relation to the sacroiliac joint. San Diego, CA, 5–6 November, pp 435–459

Keating J, Matyas T A, Bach T M 1993 The effect of training on physical therapist's ability to apply specific forces of palpation. Physical Therapy 73: 38–46

Lee D 1989 The pelvic girdle. Churchill Livingstone, Edinburgh

Lee D 1992 The relationship between the lumbar spine, pelvic girdle, and hip. In: Vleeming A, Mooney V, Snijders C J, Dorman T (eds) First interdisciplinary world congress on low back pain and its relation to the sacroiliac joint. San Diego, CA, 5–6 November, pp 463–478

Noyes F 1977 Functional properties of knee ligaments and alterations induced by immobilization. Clinical Orthopedics 123: 210

Paris S 1991 Introduction to evaluation and manipulation of the spine. Institute of Graduate Physical Therapy, St Augustine

Porterfield J, DeRosa C 1991 Mechanical low back pain. WB Saunders, Philadelphia

Potter N, Rothstein J 1985 Intertester reliability for selected tests of the sacroiliac joint. Physical Therapy 11: 1671–1677

Vleeming A, Mooney V 1992 Introduction. In: Vleeming A, Mooney V, Snijders C J, Dorman T (eds) Proceedings of the first interdisciplinary world congress on low back pain and its relation to the sacroiliac joint. San Diego, CA, 5–6 November

Vleeming A, Stoeckart R, Snijders C J 1992 General introduction. In: Vleeming A, Mooney V, Snijders C J, Dorman T (eds) Proceedings of the first interdisciplinary world congress on low back pain and its relation to the sacroiliac joint. San Diego, CA, 5–6 November, pp 3–64

Vleeming A, Mooney V, Dorman T, Snijders C J 1995 Second interdisciplinary world congress on low back pain. San Diego, CA, 9–11 November

Walker J M 1992 The sacroiliac joint: a critical review. Physical Therapy 72: 903–916

43. Deep-seated low back pain – a triad of symptoms for pelvic instability

N. A. Broadhurst

INTRODUCTION

Low back pain is ubiquitously experienced by most adults at some time during their life. Such pain is frequently of short duration, probably involves soft tissues, and may not come to attention of the medical profession unless compensation of some kind is involved.

Owing to modern imaging techniques, much attention has recently been paid to compression of the nerve root by a herniated disc and zygapophyseal joint arthropathy as being readily defined sources of low back pain (Jackson et al 1988, Mooney 1987). However, pain arising from these two sources accounts for no more than 30% of cases of low back pain. This means that a significant amount of low back pain has no defined pathological cause. Partly to blame for this dilemma is the inadequate undergraduate teaching given to musculoskeletal dysfunction in our medical schools, where undue emphasis appears to be placed on referred pain being due to nerve root compression (Kirkaldy-Willis & Hill 1979). To improve diagnosis in low back pain, more attention needs to be given to taking a good history and performing a competent clinical examination, which should appropriately reproduce the patient's pain.

It is unfortunate that, throughout the world, there are patients suffering genuine musculoskeletal pain that is unable to be substantiated by recognized pathology, and that in the process of examination, these patients have not had their pain reproduced. After all, it is this pain which has brought the patient to the doctor. It is therefore incumbent on the practitioner to reproduce the pain, preferably by movement and palpation of the structures involved. If in doubt, the area can be blocked by local anesthetic, under image intensification if necessary, thereby at least establishing the existence of the pain and its site.

All musculoskeletal practitioners have been faced with difficult diagnostic challenges concerning patients with chronic musculoskeletal pain who have been told by surgical specialists that their problem is largely functional because radiology has failed to identify the lesion. The patients frequently report that the clinical examination was superficial. These patients become frustrated and disillusioned by the medical profession and begin to shop around for explanations that are likely to add further confusion for the bewildered patient.

The essence of good medical practice in respect to musculoskeletal function must embody the following:

1. On initial consultation, be open minded and give the patient the benefit of any doubt. The malingerer is not hard to identify, but the clinician should be mindful of abnormal illness behavior that is not a conscious effort to defraud.

2. Take a detailed history of how the dysfunction occurred, with particular reference to the presence of initial trauma, effects of cumulative minor trauma, precipitating and relieving factors, and clinical hallmarks of inflammation as opposed to pain of mechanical origin, i.e. morning pain and stiffness versus gradual onset of pain with a particular activity.

3. The musculoskeletal history must be married to careful examination of the structures involved. This can only be achieved when the clinician has a thorough knowledge of the anatomy and biomechanics of these structures.

4. The clinical examination must be under-taken with the patient stripped to underclothes only. The purpose of the clinical examination is to reproduce the patient's pain, preferably by more than one means, i.e. palpation, compression, resisted movement, etc. It is essential to always ask the patient 'Is that your pain?' In other words, is the pain being reproduced in the process of the examination the pain for which the patient has sought medical help?

5. Formulation of a diagnosis is on the basis of the history, a knowledge of anatomy and bio-mechanics and pain reproduction. Blocking the area of pain with small volumes of local anesthetic may help to establish the diagnosis. This may need to be done under image intensification.

6. Formulation of a management plan must follow. Whether the treatment is rest, mobilizing, manipulation, injections, acupuncture, etc., there must be a noticeable response by the patient. Failure to make progress after five or six treat-ment sessions necessitates a review of the whole case. There is no place in good medical practice for 'endless' treatment with no observable improve-ment in function.

Careful adherence to the principles above has revealed a consistent set of symptoms and signs in a small number of patients who had been thought to have low back pain but whose pain arose from damage to specific pelvic structures. These findings have led the author to consider that these patients have an unstable pelvis.

DIAGNOSING PELVIC 'INSTABILITY'

Over a period of 5–6 years, the author accumulated 88 patients whose major complaint was that of deep-seated 'low back pain' that proved to be non-visceral pelvic pain. The major characteristic of these patients was their inability to sit evenly on each buttock, along with significant dimi-nution of their activities of daily living. Table 43.1 shows the patient profile, while the common characteristics of patients suffering pelvic instability as defined in this study are listed below. There is no importance in the order. The eight most common symptoms are:

- history of trauma
- very low back pain

Table 43.1   Study population

	n	Average age	Duration from injury to diagnosis
Female	64	40	2 years 4 months
Male	24	39	2 years 8 months

- favours one buttock
- straight leg raise 70° – no pain
- constant diffuse pelvic discomfort
- cannot fully weight-bear on affected side
- no referred pain beyond the pelvis
- pain down inclines and stairs.

As part of the clinical assessment all patients presenting with lumbar/pelvic musculoskeletal pain are assessed for thoracolumbar functional syndrome as well as the upslips and rotational derangement of the pelvis. None of the 88 patients could be considered to have any of these recognized pathologies.

All these patients had a history of trauma that preceded the onset of their symptoms. Only two patients described the onset following difficult childbirth, all others describing a severe twisting and compression type of accident as one might envisage when a nurse is left to hold a collapsing patient (Table 43.2). The trunk is twisted suddenly in one direction with legs and pelvis pointed in another, causing excessive torque on the pelvis. Motor vehicle accidents are another cause where-by the pelvis can undergo damaging torsion.

From the presenting symptoms common to these patients, as described above, it can be seen that these symptoms could readily fit most causes of lumbar pathology, and it is with this in mind that all these patients had been investigated with either computerized tomography (CT) or magnetic resonance imaging (MRI) of the lumbar spine. The results of these radiological investigations were normal. Not one of these patients had their pain reproduced during the clinical examination, and because no cause to their pain could be found, they were considered to be less than genuine. The fact that all patients except two

Table 43.2   Cause of the impairment

	n
Pregnancy	5
Nursing injury	16
Motor vehicle accident	11
Forceful twist	56

were workers or accident compensation cases added further suffering and indignation when fellow workers learnt that a medical basis for their pain had not been established.

It is unfortunate that much of medical thinking for people with low back pain, whether it is low or very low, invariably concentrates on being related to a dysfunctional disc or zygapophyseal joint. The literature describes many lumbar and pelvic structures as being the source of low back pain even with referred pain patterns (Broudeur et al 1982, Fortin et al 1994, Schwarzer et al 1995). The iliolumbar, sacrospinous, and sacro-tuberous ligaments, hypertonic multifidus and erector spinae muscles, as well as the sacroiliac joints (SIJs) can be responsible for low back and pelvic pain.

By employing the above principles of musculo-skeletal clinical examination, it was found that there was a small group of patients who had deep seated low back pain who had as their major source of pain, sacroiliac (SI) dysfunction coupled with ipsilateral sacrospinous ligament pain. Although these symptoms fit many aspects of low back pain, the cardinal features to alert the clinician as to the possibility of pelvic instability are:

- inability to weight-bear fully or hop with ease on one leg
- habitually favoring one buttock in a sitting position
- exacerbation of pain when going downstairs or inclines.

Stressing the SIJ must be part of the standard assessment of all patients presenting with low back pain. If the provocation tests for the SIJ are positive by reproduction of patient's pain and the patient has had a history of the three symptoms above, he or she becomes a candidate for rectal examination to stress the sacrospinous ligament on the ipsilateral side, comparing it with the one on the contralateral side. All patients with pain reproduction on stressing the SIJ and sacrospinous ligaments in this study displayed an asymptomatic tenderness of the symphysis pubis. Despite this tenderness being unrecognized by the patient, it is important when considering the biomechanics of the problem. These patients were also tender over the sulcus between the posterior superior iliac spine (PSIS) and sacral tuberosities.

A 'GOLD STANDARD' FOR SIJ DYSFUNCTION

To date, there is no gold standard to measure dysfunction of the SIJ. Intertester reliability has been judged as poor when measuring relative movement of the PSISs (Cibulka et al 1988, McCombie et al 1989, Potter & Rothstein 1985). Thus pain provocation was considered the best way to establish the existence of SIJ dysfunction. However, a variety of such tests exists (Laslett & Williams 1994, Walker 1992), so it was decided to assess two tests for the purpose of determining SIJ dysfunction by pain provocation.

A double blind study using a single assessor with 20 patients in the test group and 20 in the placebo group was conducted. In this study, the usual test for lumbar dysfunction (extension, flexion, side-bending, and foraminal compression) did not reproduce pain where the patient normally experienced it. In addition, the functioning of the straight leg raise, femoral nerve stretch testing, hips and knees, were all within normal limits. The two tests chosen for the study were:

1. FABER – **F**lexion, **Ab**duction and **E**xternal **R**otation. This test is also known as Patrick's or the Figure 4 test. The advantage of this test is that it is well known and uses the femur as a lever to move the ilium anteriorly relative to the sacrum while the pelvis is stabilized. However, in this position other structures are also moved or stressed, i.e. iliolumbar ligaments, L5–S1 facet joints, and the soft tissues in the groin. Had these structures been painful, they would have been identified during the clinical examination.

2. FADE or POSH – **F**lexion, **Ad**duction, **E**xtension or **Po**sterior **Sh**ear. This test consists of flexing the hip, adducting the femur to the midline and exerting axial pressure along the femur, thus pushing the ilium posteriorly relative to the sacrum. It must again be noted that other soft tissues are being stressed, especially the sacro-spinous and sacrotuberous ligaments, where pain provocation assists to identify pelvic instability.

Patients whose SI pain was reproduced by these two methods were selected on a randomized basis to receive 4 ml normal saline or 4 ml 1% lidocaine by injection under image intensification. The pain response to the above two tests was measured on a visual analog scale (VAS) of 1 to

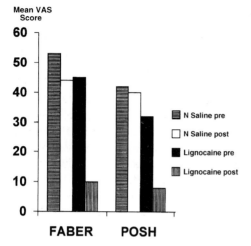

Fig. 43.1 Response of pain provocation for sacroiliac joint dysfunction using the FABER and POSH tests when the joint is injected with either 4ml normal saline or 4ml 1% lignocaine.

100 preinjection and again 15–30 min post injection. Results are shown in Fig. 43.1.

Using the criterion that a successful injection diminished the patient's pain by 75%, the sensitivity was 1.0 and the specificity 0.80 for the FADE test, and 1.0 and 0.77 respectively for the FABER test. The 2 × 2 analysis of variance for each test gave a level of significance of 0.005. It was concluded that these two tests were more than adequate for diagnosing pain arising from the SIJ.

At present, eliciting SI pain by these two tests and blocking such pain with intra-articular injections of 1% local anesthetic is considered a reliable means for establishing SIJ dysfunction. It is now confirmed that there is a small group of deep, very low back pain sufferers who can be said to be suffering from pelvic instability based on this triad of pain provocation in each of the:

• SIJ
• sacrospinous ligament
• symphysis pubis (Broadhurst 1994).

MANAGEMENT

At the time of diagnosis of pelvic instability, all patients were fitted initially with a tightly applied pelvic belt worn just above the greater trochanters. The FABER and FADE tests were repeated and the patients asked whether their pain on provocation had altered or whether they felt a noticeable decrease in their pain. When asked to walk 10 m briskly up and down the passageway with the belt tightly applied, there was a consistent 25–40% reduction in pain measured on VAS change. Many patients remarked that they no longer felt as though their pelvis was falling apart.

A pelvic belt was prescribed for each patient and the belt was to be worn all the time except for toileting and showering. Pelvic floor exercises were also prescribed, whereby the levator ani musculature was contracted for 20 s and released for 20 s. This was repeated for 5 min at least twice a day.

At the 6-week follow-up patients were asked whether the belt had improved their quality of life, made no difference, or had been detrimental. Seventy-six per cent of patients maintained that life had been much more bearable when wearing the belt as directed, whereas 19% said it had not helped. The rest complained that the pain was worse after a day or two of wearing the belt, which was then discarded. It is noted that those patients not happy with the long-term use of the belt had a body mass index (BMI) outside the 20–25 range.

For those patients who were too thin, the belt caused skin and periosteal irritation even though there was padding on the belt, which was then worn over the outside clothing. Unfortunately, the overweight patients had difficulty getting enough lasting pelvic compression because of their adipose tissue, which resulted in the belt slipping upward.

Other treatment options were presented to the patients at the 6-week follow-up, when the triad of tests was again administered and found to be positive. However, in several patients the pain was reduced. Treatment options included dry needling of the trigger points in the buttock muscles, cortisone injection to the SIJ under image intensification, and postisometric exercises for the tender pelvic muscles, i.e. iliopsoas and piriformis. The use of 15% dextrose as a sclerosing agent is not an accepted treatment modality in Australia and was offered to patients after everything else had failed. Only seven patients accepted this option.

Table 43.3 gives a synopsis of the response of the various treatments on the basis of improve, no help or worse. In particular, the responses are as follows:

1. Pelvic belt – still being worn by 63% of patients on a regular basis at the 6-month check,

Table 43.3 Response to treatment after 6 weeks

	Better	No help	Worse
Physiotherapy	18	5	57
Chiropractic	5	0	58
Exercises	33	27	7
Pelvic belt	71	6	11
Injection			
Steroid	32	8	5
5% Dextrose	6	1	0
Hydrotherapy	17	18	0

especially when required to do more than just sitting at home. The rest of the patients had abandoned its use either because it was uncomfortable or because there was lack of progress. Further follow-up was not pursued but at other visits most patients indicated that they resorted to the use of the belt when the pelvis was stressed or their pain for some reason had increased.

2. Pelvic floor exercises – compliance was very poor. After 2–3 weeks, fewer than half of these patients were doing this exercise, and one assumes that they were discontinued by natural attrition. Although the use of these exercises seemed reasonable on the bases of anatomy and biomechanics, the patients obviously do not find them efficacious enough to persevere.

3. Postisometric exercises – these were directed at the two tender muscles often involved in low back pain, i.e. iliopsoas and piriformis (Fishman & Zybert 1992, Lewit 1991). These exercises were done as five repetitions twice a day with the SIJ belt applied. Approximately 37% of patients attributed relief of their pain due to these exercises.

4. Cortisone injections – one vial of a depo-steroid and 2 ml 1% lidocaine – were injected into a painful SIJ under image intensification on 45 occasions, 32 patients saying the injection helped in the overall reduction of their symptoms.

5. Sclerosing using 15% dextrose – this medium has no recognized standing in Australia and has been declared an invalid treatment by compensation and insurance companies. Thus patients were treated using this method only as a 'last ditch stand'. A volume of 10 ml 15% dextrose was applied over the dorsal SI ligaments on four occasions a fortnight apart. Six weeks following the last injection, the patients were assessed for level of pain. Only 7 patients were treated in this way, 1 saying there was no improvement and 6 indicating significant improvement.

RESULTS

It becomes obvious that the entity of pelvic instability involves multiple structures for which neither a single treatment modality nor a combination of treatments are likely to provide effective resolution of the patient's symptoms.

At the end of 3 months, the patients were asked to estimate the success of treatments by indicating the percentage improvement using the VAS. The response of the 88 patients is seen in Fig. 43.2, which indicates that a considerable number of patients continued to experience long-term impairment and worked daily with pain.

The lack of large numbers in this study prevents a reliable statistical analysis being made of the return-to-work status for those who have been diagnosed as having pelvic instability on the basis of the triad of painful symptoms. Unfortunately the work status as the time of the initial consultation was not recorded and was not included in the questionnaire; however, Tables 43.4 and 43.5 are an attempt to categorize the return-to-work status by sex and the level of ongoing discomfort. Nearly 40% of sufferers were unable to work because of the pain suffered in the type of job they occupied. Forty-eight per cent of sufferers had less than a 50% improvement in their pain and this group is noticeable by the fact that 20 females were working, compared with only 4 males. When considering those patients who had 50% or greater improvement, the proportion of males working is increased.

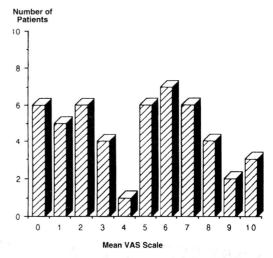

Fig. 43.2 Improvement of the pain score as measured by a VAS 0–10 after 3 months of treatment, which included wearing a SIJ belt and doing pelvic floor exercises.

Table 43.4   Work status after 6 months' treatment

	Female	Male	n
Full time	27	5	32
Part time	17	7	24
Unable	20	12	32

Table 43.5   Distribution of work status improvement by gender

	VAS improvement 0–4		VAS improvement 5–10	
Full time	13		15	
	13F	0M	10F	5M
Part time	11		15	
	7F	4M	12F	3M
Unable	18		16	
	12F	6M	10F	6M

On the basis of the type of industry in which most males were employed, it is obvious that the physical demands of their job meant that they had to have a greater resolution of their injury before they could be gainfully employed. Another explanation could be that females suffer pain and discomfort more stoically than do males.

The questionnaire did not ask whether the patients were self-employed, public servants, in small businesses, or in large corporations. Further investigation needs to be carried out to see whether the figures agree with the study of Greenough and Fraser (1989), whereby injured workers on compensation took longer to return to work than people not on compensation.

CONCLUSIONS

1. People who are subject to considerable pelvic torsion are likely to suffer subsequently from pelvic instability, which can be defined by a triad of painful symptoms emanating from the SIJ, sacrospinous ligament, and symphysis pubis.

2. At present, the major source of relief from suffering is the wearing of a pelvic belt, which in the long term is for most sufferers worn intermittently to minimize the pain when exacerbations are experienced.

3. The continuing absence from the workforce is a constant cause of distress for the worker and family, as well as being a burden on the compensation system. Although the number of sufferers is small, 40% are relatively young and have no likelihood of being gainfully employed.

4. This condition of pelvic instability needs to be recognized as a possible consequence of pelvic trauma. More effort needs to be put into a program to educate physicians of its existence, and better treatment modalities have to be developed in the near future.

ACKNOWLEDGMENTS

The author thanks Professor Jim Taylor of the Australian Neuromuscular Research Institute, Western Australia, and Dr John Durkin, Director of the Alfreda Rehabilitation Service, South Australia, for their willingness to provide helpful and constructive comments.

REFERENCES

Broadhurst N A 1994 Pelvic dysfunction. Journal of Neurology, Orthopaedics Medicine and Surgery 15: 127–129
Broudeur P, Larroque C H, Passeron R et al 1982 Le syndrome ilio-lombaine. Revue du Rhumatisme 49: 693–698
Cibulka M T, Delitto A, Koldehoff R M 1988 Changes in innominate tilt after manipulation of the sacroiliac joint in patients with low back pain. Physical Therapy 68: 1359–1363
Fishman L M, Zybert P L 1992 Electrophyiologic evidence of piriformis syndrome. Archives of Physical Medicine and Rehabilitation 73: 359–364
Fortin J D, Dwyer A D, West S et al 1994 Sacroiliac joint: pain referred maps upon applying a new injection/arthrography technique Parts I and II. Spine 19: 1475–1489
Greenough C G, Fraser R D 1989 The effects of compensation on recovery from low back injury. Spine 14: 947–955
Jackson R P, Jacobs R R, Montesano P X 1988 Facet joint injection in low back pain. Spine 13: 966–971

Kirkaldy-Willis W H, Hill R J 1979 A more precise diagnosis for low back pain. Spine 4: 102–109
Laslett M, Williams M 1994 The reliability of selected pain provocation tests for sacroiliac joint pathology. Spine 19: 1243–1249
Lewit K 1991 Manipulative therapy in rehabilitation of the locomotor system, 2nd end. Butterworth Heinemann, Oxford
McCombie P F, Fairbank J C T, Cockersale B C et al 1989 Reproducibility of physical signs in low back pain. Spine 14: 908–918
Mooney V 1987 Where is the pain coming from. Spine 12: 754–759
Potter N A, Rothstein J M 1985 Intertester reliability for selected clinical tests of the sacroiliac joint. Physical Therapy 65: 1671–1675
Schwarzer A C, Aprill C N, Bogduk N 1995 The sacroiliac joint in chronic low back pain. Spine 20: 31–37
Walker J M 1992 The sacroiliac joint: a critical review. Physical Therapy 72: 903–916

Surgery

44. Surgical fusion of the spine to the sacrum

J. Y. Margulies   V. J. Devlin   J. Gorup
S. A. Caruso

INTRODUCTION

Problems at the lumbopelvic junction date back to the time when humans first stood upright. Even with the advent of modern medicine, the complex anatomy of this region, including the proximity of nerves and other vital structures, has frustrated attempts at satisfactory surgical treatment. While technological advances over the years have improved the success rate of lumbosacral arthrodesis, the search continues for more sophisticated methods that will restore not only general function, but satisfactory motion as well. The enormous forces and long lever arms in this region make arthrodesis difficult to achieve. Solutions to the problems of lumbosacral fusion have emerged only in recent decades as advances in implant design, fusion technique, and anesthesiology have made it possible to achieve consistent success when fusion at the lumbosacral junction is undertaken.

THE ROLE OF FUSION

The decision to perform spine surgery is valid if, and only if, the patient's problem (1) can be defined anatomically and (2) can be solved by neural decompression, tumor excision, correction of deformity, stabilization of unstable segments, or a combination of these procedures. The indications to perform surgery in certain lumbar degenerative disorders is made more difficult owing to the frequent poor correlation between imaging studies and clinical symptomatology, as well as the absence of a universally accepted clinical definition of lumbar spinal instability. In any spine surgery, the last step before closing the incision is to evaluate and treat possible spinal instability, which may be obvious or occult. While certain procedures are performed to correct instability, others, such as extensive decompressive procedures, may create instability. In both cases, the spine must be stabilized prior to closing the incision. Fusion is the most popular means of stabilization. Theoretically, methods other than fusion, for example, muscle strengthening or implanting artificial discs or ligaments, can be used to treat instability. A surgically performed fusion in a patient, however, is evidence that a surgeon encountered a prior instability. Fusion can be employed to treat a single motion segment or the entire spine, depending on the length of the unstable section and considerations of spinal balance. The instability may be of an acute nature, arising from trauma, or it can be caused by surgical decompression. Instability can be chronic, as caused by a degenerative process, or it can be a postural instability, as evident in deformities. In general, fusion is a comprehensive solution to instability as it eliminates pathological motion between neighboring elements. The fusion mass consolidates and includes spinal elements between which a 'fracture situation' has been created, and bone surfaces are permitted to heal into a single unit. It is important to understand that a fusion cannot correct a deformity and that a fusion cannot provide decompression of the spinal canal. A fusion is only a consolidation of the existing situation at the end of a surgical procedure.

THE ROLE OF INSTRUMENTATION

There is a consensus that the main role of instrumentation is to facilitate bone healing by splinting the fusion site. However, there is no consensus regarding the practice of correcting deformities using instrumentation. There is also no consensus regarding non-instrumented in situ fusions that address spinal pathology without attempting anatomic realignment or reduction. The role of instrumentation as a splinting device to provide stable fixation until fusion occurs is well established. Instrumentation permits realignment of the spine during surgery and minimizes spinal motion that may decrease the success of fusion. Fusion of the spine to the sacrum is a considerable mechanical challenge. It requires counteracting the lever arm of the trunk above the pelvis. The bone implant construct achieved in surgery must have sufficient stability to resist collapse under a multitude of loading conditions until fusion occurs. There are currently many techniques and implants available to the spine surgeon that may be utilized to address various types of spinal deformities and spinal instability.

SPINAL STABILITY

The stability of the spine can be predicted if the mechanical behavior is known. The determinants of mechanical behavior vary between individuals. Therefore, the prediction of response to abnormal loading is impossible. A universal definition of instability that includes all variables of mechanical behavior does not exist. The stability of the spine is affected by restraining structures that, if damaged or lax, will lead to altered equilibrium and ultimately instability (Gertzbein et al 1985, Nachemson 1985). A spinal column that is able to maintain alignment when subjected to physiological loads in any plane while protecting the neural elements is considered stable. If displacement of the spinal column is likely to occur, the spinal column is considered unstable (Purcell et al 1981). Most definitions of stability allude to the effect of dynamic loading as well as the presence of deformation over time (Haher et al 1989). Unfortunately, there is no way to restore any kind of dynamic stability at the level of the motion segment. Common practice is to fuse the affected motion segment, sacrificing its mobility altogether, in order to restore the function of the entire spinal column.

PRINCIPLES OF STABILIZATION

Surgical stabilization of the spine may be considered to occur in two stages. In the first stage, a 'fracture situation' is created during surgery in which adjacent bone surfaces are decorticated, bone graft is applied, and spinal instrumentation or external mobilization is utilized to decrease mobility at the surgical site. The second stage begins following surgery and consists of the cascade of events involved in the poorly understood biologic process of fusion consolidation. The surgeon's influence over this process includes the use of meticulous operative technique, selection of the location for fusion (anterior or posterior), as well as the selection of appropriate spinal implants that will adequately support the spine until fusion occurs. The act of stabilization starts, by definition, at an unstable stage that is caused either by the underlying pathology or by the surgeon. The unstable site constitutes a gap in the continuity of a normal functional structure and must be treated in a way that permits growth of a bony bridge across this region. Understanding the mechanics of the spine is crucial in determining exactly where this gap exists. Haher et al (1989) demonstrated that a localized site of mechanical damage to one of the columns of the spine changes the location of the instantaneous axis of rotation (Haher et al 1989). The existence of an axis of rotation in an abnormal location is a sign of instability and may warrant correction. Regardless of how one defines the spinal columns, it is important to augment the unsound column(s) and thus regain the mechanical stability of the spine. Modern surgical technique and technologically advanced implants permit short fusions localized to the unstable columns.

PRINCIPLES OF CORRECTION

Although many revolutionary ideas can be found in Harrington's writings, the posterior system he introduced was designed to treat deformities in the coronal plane. The scoliotic spine was fixed at the end vertebrae with hooks, and distraction was applied through a ratcheted rod that stretched the spine between these hooks. The rod and hooks served as an internal splint until fusion occurred and the construct was generally supplemented by external immobilization with a cast or brace. In an attempt to improve on problems with hook dislodgement and eliminate the need for postoperative external immobilization, Luque developed the sublaminar wiring technique. This technique provided correction in the coronal and sagittal planes via segmental control with wires. It provided for multiple points of fixation, which enhanced deformity correction and decreased the risk of fixation failure. Hybrid methods that combined the techniques of Harrington and Luque evolved and included the Wisconsin construct, with or without Drummond buttons, as well as the use of square-ended rods and special hooks, as introduced by Moe.

Although Wisconsin or 'Harri–Luque' techniques were safe in most hands, the fear of potential neurological injury by wires and the lack of positive reports in the literature led to a search for alternative methods. Since its introduction, Cotrel-Dubousset (CD) instrumentation has become the 'gold standard' for posterior spinal fixation (Cotrel et al 1988). It provides for multiple points of fixation with hooks and avoids the need to place sublaminar wires. CD instrumentation permits correction in the coronal and sagittal planes. It permits kyphosing-distraction and lordotic-compression forces to act along the same rod as a means of simultaneously controlling coronal and sagittal deformities.

The premise that the derotation maneuver proposed by Cotrel and Dubousset realigns the deformed coronal spine into normal sagittal posture was not uniformly accepted. Subsequent studies have shown that the transverse plane 'derotation' achieved with this system is more global than segmental in nature. This led to the development of alternative approaches to achieving curve correction. The principle of maximum control over each affected segment is paramount in the operative correction of spinal deformities. The goal is translation of each vertebra into its desired position by connection to a rod that is prebent to the appropriate sagittal contour. Techniques of segmental fixation have evolved through the use of combinations of hooks, wires, and ultimately pedicle screws. Adequate ancillary instruments may provide efficient lever arms to augment the correction maneuver. This approach is best

represented by the AcroMed Isola (Asher 1993) and Synthes Universal Spine Systems (Aebi 1983).

Another way is to place strong, stiff, but ductile rods on the spine and use the technique of in situ bending to bring the spine to the 'normal' contour. This technique accentuates placing the rods in such a way that, at the end of the correction maneuver, the center of rotation of the whole assembly, which is now in the rods, is as close as possible to the normal center of rotation. The ductility of the rod is crucial to the success of this kind of correction. This approach is promoted by Jackson (Jackson 1994).

Anterior approaches are also utilized for the correction of spinal deformities. In anterior approaches, correction is achieved first through obtaining flexibility as the spine is released via discectomy or osteotomy and subsequently realigned with implants. Global curve derotation as a correction maneuver is possible with the anterior approach. Local curve derotation may be better achieved with the anterior approach than with the posterior approach. Recently, rigid anterior implant systems have been introduced in order to be used as a tool in surgery for derotation, improve fixation strength, and decrease instrumentation failure and pseudarthrosis rates. Control over deformities may be achieved by resection of disc or bone in order to change the relative length of the spinal columns. Shortening the anterior column produces kyphosis; elongating it produces lordosis. Resection or insertion of a wedge can be utilized to align scoliosis or enhance correction of sagittal plane deformities. Structural grafts or implant spacers can be used to restore anterior column height and re-establish the normal relationship between vertebrae. If performed properly, restoration of disc space height provides indirect opening and decompression of neural foramina. Disc height can be restored by posterior lumbar interbody fusion (PLIF), anterior lumbar interbody fusion (ALIF), or a posterior maneuver utilizing a pedicular screw-based construct. The success of posterior pedicle screw-based constructs depends upon the presence of adequate anterior column structural support.

In certain spinal disorders, combined anterior and posterior techniques are required in order to achieve sufficient deformity correction, provide for adequate spinal canal decompression, and increase the likelihood or successful arthrodesis. Harms in Germany advocates the combined approach as the most efficient method of treating a wide variety of spinal problems based on the concepts of the posterior tension band and anterior load-sharing principles (Bohm et al 1990). A relatively thin posterior compression implant, combined with a solid anterior spacer, creates a construct in which 80% of the load is applied to the anterior column and 20% to the posterior column. The logical application of this concept is to the correction of kyphotic deformities and improving lordosis in cases in which it has been lost. A variation of the combined approach consists of an interbody fusion, which may be accomplished as either a PLIF or ALIF and stabilized by posterior instrumentation. In this approach, the purpose of the posterior fixation is to stabilize the interbody graft or cage and a formal posterior fusion is not performed.

In the most extreme and severe deformities, resection and decancellation procedures as advocated by Luque and Bradford may be required. These procedures create circumferential instability and permit subsequent spinal correction through shortening the spinal column. Such techniques permit correction of deformities that are not adequately treated by any other approach. Heinig has applied this concept of creating iatrogenic instability solely through the posterior approach in order to correct severe deformities, and has termed this the eggshell procedure.

ANATOMIC CONSIDERATIONS

The biomechanical situation at the lumbosacral junction does not favor fusion. Since the L5–S1 disc is positioned at 45° to the gravity line and is subject to shear forces, there are no direct natural compressive forces buttressing the fusion site. The lever arm on the fusion zone is enormous. External immobilization is cumbersome and frequently ineffective. With regard to anatomic considerations, two points must be stressed.

First, the lumbopelvic articulation not only includes the L5–S1 junction, but also consists of the distal lumbar vertebrae, the sacrum, and those parts in proximity to the sacroiliac joints (SIJs). It has an osteoarticular axis, is powered by musculofascial elements, and is traversed by neurovascular structures. The articulation has relationships with the neighboring anatomic regions and shares mechanical functions with the rest of the vertebral column (Louis 1985).

Second, the pelvis, as an intercalary bony structure between the spine and lower limbs, should be viewed as the 'pelvic vertebra'. It plays a major role in standing and sitting by adjusting balance in order to maintain the head optimally along the body's line of gravity. Three-dimensional posture is made physiologically possible by a chain of motion segments that permit self-adjusting erect posture in response to the effects of gravity on proprioception.

INDICATIONS FOR FUSION TO THE SACRUM

Trauma

Because of the unique anatomic features and mechanical characteristics of the lumbosacral junction, trauma at this site is infrequent. The lumbar spine requires fusion to the sacrum for trauma only in very specific situations where the integrity of the spinal column is grossly disrupted. Most sacral fractures are secondary to pelvic trauma and do not require fusion.

Tumors and infections

The indications for fusion are a function of the amount of destruction and instability caused by the underlying pathological process as well as the instability created in the procedure of spinal canal decompression. Because the spinal canal in the lumbopelvic region has ample space for neural elements, neurological damage of mechanical origin in the case of tumors and infections is rare. When neurologic symptoms do occur, these are typically manifest late in the course of the condition (Sucher et al 1994).

Degenerative disorders

Degenerative changes involving the lumbosacral spine can lead to pain, instability, and deformity.

A solid and balanced fusion that eliminates painful abnormal motion at the lumbosacral joint while restoring structural integrity may reduce pain, stabilize deformity, and improve overall function. Definitions of instability remain controversial.

Pelvic obliquity

Pelvic obliquity is one of a variety of conditions for which fixation to the sacrum may be recommended or even necessary. Pelvic obliquity occurs when the pelvic vertebra is tilted abnormally in the coronal, sagittal, or horizontal plane. Pelvic obliquity can be caused by suprapelvic, intrapelvic, or infrapelvic pathology, and may be fixed or non-fixed.

Spondylolisthesis

Spondylolisthesis remains among the most controversial indications for surgery. The controversy includes the decision when to perform surgery, the need for decompression, the need for instrumentation, the need for realignment, and the indications for circumferential fusions. Instrumented reduction of severe spondylolisthesis is considered to be among the most challenging types of spinal surgery.

FUSION TECHNIQUES

Non-instrumented fusion

Non-instrumented fusion techniques may be classified as:

- spinous process-related fusions
- interlaminar fusions
- posterolateral fusions
- interbody fusions.

The indications for non-instrumented fusion at the L5–S1 junction are limited, due to limited success (Apel et al 1989, Riley et al 1986). Adherence to the technical aspects of these procedures, specifically meticulous bone graft 'carpentry', is crucial to the success of this type of procedure. In the future, the need for internal fixation may be diminished, especially in cases where anatomic alignment is not the primary concern, if bone morphogenetic protein (BMP) and other agents for bone induction and conduction prove efficacious.

Instrumented fusion

Modern posterior spinal fixation systems consist of three basic elements:

- implants attached to the posterior spinal elements
- implants attached to the sacrum or pelvis
- longitudinal members connecting the posterior implants.

There are three basic options for gaining purchase upon the posterior elements of the spine: (1) hooks, (2) wires or cables, and (3) screws. A single hook permits control in one plane, in either a distraction or compression mode. Once the hook is engaged in a construct and combined with other hooks, various corrective forces can be applied to the spine across the entire instrumented segment. The introduction of hook 'claws' has greatly improved upon the fixation achieved by single hooks. Claw fixation combines upgoing and downgoing hooks across a single or adjacent level to achieve a strong mechanical interlock that greatly exceeds the fixation strength achieved by single hooks. Wires may be placed through the spinous process, underneath the lamina or in the subpars position. The amount of force that can be applied to a wire is less than can be applied to a hook owing to the smaller area of contact of the wire with the bone (Haher et al 1989). The introduction of flexible cables as an alternative to wires offers superior mechanical properties and provides a margin of safety owing to their ease of placement. Pedicle screws permit control of the spine in all planes and permit control of all three spinal columns from a single posterior approach.

Distal fixation options when fusion includes the sacrum are more varied. Hooks and wires are of limited value and are not widely used for sacral fixation. Various types of screw fixation techniques using either single or multiple screws to achieve purchase in the sacrum are the most commonly used techniques to achieve distal fixation. Sacral screws may be placed laterally into the sacral ala or medially into the sacral body toward the promontory to reach the upper endplate of the sacrum.

When maximal distal fixation is necessary, methods to enhance sacral fixation include

Galveston fixation, the Jackson technique, and iliosacral screw fixation. The Galveston method engages the ilium in the construct by utilizing a post that may consist of either a smooth rod or a screw. The post extends within the ilium and is placed in the column of bone located just above the sciatic notch. The Jackson technique enhances S1 screw fixation utilizing the concept of the 'iliac buttress' (Jackson & McManus 1993). The distal end of the rods pass through medially directed sacral screws and pass into the sacrum between its two cortices and under the wings of the ilium. Iliosacral screws are placed from the ilium into the body of the sacrum and engage at least three cortices in their path, thereby constituting a strong foundation for a spinopelvic construct. In most instrumentation constructs, the rods on each side of the spine are linked together with transverse devices in order to convert the unilateral rods to a quadrilateral construct of increased overall strength and rigidity. It is crucial to realize that the goal of the procedure is to achieve a successful fusion and that the spinal instrumentation construct will fail if fusion does not occur.

Anterior spinal fixation options are varied. Selection of the appropriate technique depends upon a variety of factors, which include:

- the type and location of spinal pathology
- the number of levels requiring surgical treatment
- the integrity of the anterior and middle spinal columns
- the goals of the surgical procedure.

The modern anterior spinal fixation options include interbody spacers, intervertebral spacers, screw-plate fixation systems, and screw-rod fixation systems. ALIF has been reported to be mechanically unstable when iliac bone graft alone is utilized without supplemental spinal fixation (Humphries et al 1961).

In an attempt to improve the success rate of interbody fusion and possibly eliminate the need for adjunctive posterior fixation, a variety of interbody spacers have been introduced. These include allograft femoral rings, cylindrical fusion cages such as the BAK device, Moss titanium fusion cages, as well as carbon fiber anterior fusion devices. This is a rapidly emerging field and many of these devices have shown great promise in early studies.

When an entire vertebral body requires replacement, options include autograft, structural allograft, fusion cages, and polymethylmethacrylate (PMMA). Such constructs are generally used with supplemental spinal fixation either anteriorly, posteriorly, or in a combined anterior–posterior fixation construct.

Anterior fixation options include both screw-plate and screw-rod devices. Anterior screw-plate devices (e.g. Synthes locking plate, Z-plate, and the CASP system) permit in situ spinal fixation. Anterior screw-rod devices (e.g. Kostuik-Harrington, anterior TSRH, and Kaneda) are more versatile and permit both distraction and compression as well as deformity correction, and can be more easily adapted to fixation over multiple levels than screw-plate systems. Placement of bulky fixation devices across the L5–S1 junction is generally discouraged owing to the proximity of vascular structures to the implant device.

Implant materials

The chief implant materials used in spinal surgery are stainless steel and titanium alloys. They provide strength, can be contoured to match bony surfaces, and are biocompatible. Stainless steels are alloys composed mainly of iron (> 58%), chromium (17–20%), and nickel (13–16%). As a class of alloys, they are favored owing to the inexpensive nature of their base elements as well as the wide range of structural and mechanical properties that can be achieved by varying the constituent ratios. Pure titanium is a good material for orthopedic use due to its low density, high ductility, and MRI/CT scan compatibility. Its chief drawback, however, is its low modulus of elasticity. As a result, titanium is usually combined with aluminum and vanadium to produce the alloy Ti-6Al-4V, which has a greater tensile and fatigue strength than stainless steel. Although the modulus of elasticity of this alloy is greater than that of pure titanium, it is still less than the modulus of stainless steel. As a consequence, larger hardware must be used to provide comparable rigidity if titanium is used. The structural properties of titanium alloys are approximately half those of stainless steel alloys (Metals Handbook 1975).

PMMA is sometimes used as an adjunct to internal fixation. PMMA is stiffer than cancellous bone, but less stiff than cortical bone. It is used primarily in cases where bone quality compromises fixation. Several authors have demonstrated the efficacy of PMMA in enhancing screw fixation.

SPECIAL PROBLEMS

Spinal decompensation

Normal spinal balance exists when the head is centered over a level pelvis and shoulders in the coronal and sagittal planes. In the sagittal plane, the normal lordosis of the lumbar spine permits the head to be balanced over the pelvis with the hips in full extension (Lenke et al 1994). Spinal decompensation is the result of any condition in the coronal and/or sagittal plane that alters this normal alignment. The effects of spinal decompensation on the patient are significant. Complaints associated with decompensation include apparent leg length discrepancy, gait abnormalities, back pain, spinal fatigue, decreased standing tolerance, pelvic obliquity, difficulty with sitting, cosmetic deformity, and degenerative changes in adjacent motion segments. The flat back syndrome is an example of spinal decompensation in the sagittal plane. This problem arises following a lumbar fusion that results in a loss of lumbar lordosis with subsequent forward inclination of the trunk and an inability to stand erect without hip or knee flexion. It is generally seen in the adult who has undergone surgical fusion extending below L3. In young patients in whom the sacrum is not part of the fusion, decompensation may occur at the last level of the mobile spine, with a corresponding acute hyperextension that can cause nerve root impingement. Further spinal reconstructive surgery to restore lumbar lordosis through osteotomy procedures is frequently required to treat this disabling condition.

Pediatric disorders

The unique aspects of the pediatric spine that must be taken into consideration are the potential for further growth, the difference in elasticity of ligaments compared with adults, the differences in osseous tissue (thicker, biologically more active periosteum), and the relatively smaller size of the spinal elements. Because pediatric bone has not yet achieved its peak bone mineral density and deforms at lower peak forces, it can absorb more energy to ultimate failure. Vertebral body and sacral growth characteristics may have direct consequences for the disease process, as in spondylolisthesis progression, or may affect treatment, as in the crankshaft phenomenon occurring following posterior fusion.

Revision surgery

Spinal revision surgery may be required to treat a variety of problems such as pseudarthrosis, coronal or sagittal decompensation, or deterioration of motion segments adjacent to a prior fusion. Extension of the fusion and pseudarthrosis repair, as well as osteotomies, may be indicated depending on the underlying problem. The reconstructive spinal surgeon must design internal fixation constructs that create a stable environment for fusion to occur in balanced alignment with adjacent spinal motion segments.

Osteoporosis

Metallic constructs implanted in osteoporotic bone cannot be expected to provide solid mechanical support. This situation poses a serious challenge in the treatment of osteoporotic patients. The number of osteopenic (mainly osteoporotic) patients has grown markedly in the USA and Europe, and the treatment of mechanical insufficiency in this population remains a great challenge. The weak purchase of screws in osteopenic bone precludes the application of forceful corrective maneuvers. It has been demonstrated that hook claws on the laminae may provide for a better grip than screws (Coe et al 1990). In other studies, cement or bone graft has been utilized to augment screw purchase in osteopenic vertebrae (Zindrick et al 1986).

SIJ fusion

The nature and significance of movement in the SIJ as well as the relationship of the SIJ to lumbar pain symptomatology remain controversial. Overlapping innervation and referred pain phenomena make the diagnosis of pain emerging from the SIJ difficult. The basic role of the SIJ is to absorb, with minimal movement, the loads of the axial skeleton. All biomechanical loads, whether they are due to sitting, standing, or walking, must pass through the SIJ. Surgical fusions for SI dysfunction are rarely performed except for SI dysfunction following a major traumatic injury. However, recent studies have demonstrated painful incompetence of the SIJ by radiographically controlled injections, and surgical arthrodesis of the SIJ has been reported to provide satisfactory pain relief in select cases. Another related area of ongoing investigation is the consequence of fusion of the spine to the sacrum in relation to SI function and SI pain symptomatology.

CONCLUSIONS

1. Although spinal arthrodesis is widely practiced and is constantly being perfected, it should be appreciated that fusion is a crude solution to the malfunction of sophisticated anatomic mechanisms that occur in nature.

2. While restoration of function of the patient can be accomplished by eliminating motion at the affected level, restoration of normal function of a pathological motion segment is not possible utilizing present technology. Future approaches may abandon fusion altogether and seek other means of treating painful deformity or instability.

3. Restoration of motion is the objective of reconstructive surgery in other areas of orthopedic surgery.

4. Artificial discs and artificial ligaments may become the state of the art in futuristic orthopedics in the lumbosacral junction in the next century.

REFERENCES

Aebi M 1983 Correction of degenerative scoliosis of the lumbar spine. Clinical Orthopaedics and Related Research 232: 80–86

Apel D M, Lorenz M A, Zindrick M R 1989 Symptomatic spondylolisthesis in adults: four decades later. Spine 14: 345–348

Asher M A 1993 Scoliosis Research Society instrumentation manual. Scoliosis Research Society, Rosemont, IL

Bohm H, Harms J, Donk R, Zielke K 1990 Correction and stabilization of angular kyphosis. Clinical Orthopaedics and Related Research 258: 56–61

Coe J D, Warden K E, Herzig M A, McAfee P C 1990 Influence of bone mineral density on the fixation of thoracolumbar implants: a comparative study of transpedicular screws, laminar hooks, and spinous process wires. Spine 15: 902–907

Cotrel Y, Dubousset J, Guillaumat M 1988 New universal instrumentation in spinal surgery. Clinical Orthopaedics and Related Research 227: 10–23

Gertzbein S D, Seligmen M D, Holtby R et al 1985 Centrode pattern and segmental instability in degenerative disc disease. Spine 10: 257–261

Haher T R, Tozzi J M, Lospinuso M F et al 1989a The contribution of the three columns of the spine to spinal stability: Biomechanical model. Paraplegia 27: 432–439

Haher T R, Felmly W T, Welin D et al 1989b The IAR as a function of the three columns of the spine. Proceedings of the Scoliosis Research Society, Amsterdam, Netherlands

Humphries A W, Hawk W A, Cuthbertson A M 1961 Anterior interbody fusion of the lumbar vertebrae: a surgical technique. Surgery Clinics of North America 41: 1685

Jackson R P 1994 Intrasacral fixation with C–D. In: Brown C W (ed.) Spinal instrumentation technique. Scoliosis Research Society, Rosemont, IL

Jackson R P, McManus A C 1993 The iliac buttress. A computed tomographic study of sacral anatomy. Spine 18(10): 1318–1328

Lenke L G, Bridwell K H, O'Brien M F, Baldus C, Blanke K 1994 Recognition and treatment of the proximal thoracic curve in adolescent idiopathic scoliosis treated with Cotrel–Dubousset instrumentation. Spine 19(14): 1589–1597

Louis R 1985 Fusion of the lumbar and sacral spine by internal fixation with screw plates. Clinical Orthopaedics and Related Research 203: 18–33

Metals Handbook 1975 8th edn, vol. 10, pp 10–26. American Society for Metals, USA

Nachemson A 1985 Lumbar spine instability: a critical update and symptoms summary. Spine 10: 290–291

Purcell G A, Markolf K L, Dawson E G 1981 Twelfth thoracic–first lumbar vertebral mechanical stability of fractures after Harrington rod instrumentation. Journal of Bone and Joint Surgery (US) 63: 71–78

Riley P M, Gillespie R, Koneska J 1986 Severe spondylolisthesis and spondyloptosis: results of posterolateral fusion in children and adolescents. Journal of Bone and Joint Surgery (UK) 68: 856

Sucher E, Margulies J Y, Floman Y, Robin G C 1994 Prognostic factors in anterior decompression for metastatic cord compression: an analysis of results. European Spine Journal 3(2): 70–75

Zindrick M R, Wiltse L L, Widell E H et al 1986 A biomechanical study of intrapeduncular screw fixation in the lumbosacral spine. Clinical Orthopaedics and Related Research 203: 99–112

45. Surgical treatment of chronic painful sacroiliac joint dysfunction

M. R. Moore

INTRODUCTION

Chronic sacroiliac joint (SIJ) dysfunction is increasingly recognized as an important consideration in the differential diagnosis of low back pain and sciatica (Bernard & Cassidy 1991, Bernard & Kirkaldy-Willis 1987, Daum 1995, Jamrich et al 1995, Klein et al 1993, Mooney 1993, Moore 1994, 1995, Schwarzer et al 1995). Although frequently discussed as a common cause of low back pain in the early part of the century (Albee 1909, Baer 1917, Garnet 1927, Goldthwait & Osgood 1905, Pitkin & Pheasant 1936), the medical literature and clinical research efforts became sparse after the popularization of the diagnosis of the herniated nucleus pulposus (HNP) and its relation to low back pain and sciatica (Dandy 1929, Mixter & Barr 1934).

Early reports of arthrodesis of the SIJ for patients with chronic painful dysfunction were all favorable. Smith-Petersen and Rodgers (1926) reported on 26 cases of patients treated with sacroiliac (SI) arthrodesis for low back pain and associated sciatica. They reported a clinical success rate of 89%, with 23 out of 26 patients reporting no pain at follow-up. Gaenslen (1927) reported on the results of arthrodesis in 9 patients. Failure of improvement in symptoms was only noted in 1 case. Campbell (1927) reported on an extra-articular technique used in 7 patients. Five were reported as clinically successful, and the remaining 2 patients were considered to be too near to treatment to comment on their success.

These successful reports, however, failed to distract the orthopedic and neurosurgical communities from their new-found enthusiasm for surgical procedures directed at the lumbar discs.

Several generations of orthopedic surgeons went through their clinical training without any serious consideration of the SIJ as a possible pain generator and without any experience with the technique of SI arthrodesis. After these papers, the next report of a surgical series did not occur until the paper by Waisbrod et al (1987), in which a 70% success rate was achieved. With the development of improved imaging techniques and diagnostic tests that allow distinction between pain arising from SI dysfunction and pain arising from other causes, one would expect comparable or improved results today.

The vast majority of patients with SI pain can be successfully treated by the non-surgical methods described elsewhere in this book. When conservative treatment is ineffective, however, arthrodesis remains a viable consideration. Emphasis is directed towards (1) appropriate diagnosis and patient selection, and (2) appropriate technique.

DIAGNOSIS

Patients with SIJ-mediated pain can present with complaints that appear very similar to those reported in other conditions. Careful evaluation, however, will avoid an error in diagnosis. A key feature of SI pain is that patients will clearly identify the pain as being to one side or the other of the lower back rather than at the lumbosacral junction. Figure 45.1 shows typical pain referral patterns. The pattern in Fig. 45.1A looks very similar to that produced by an L5–S1 herniated disc but may include groin pain. Figure 45.1B is frequently interpreted as a 'hysterical' pattern. It is critical that the clinician does not jump to erroneous conclusions based on a cursory review

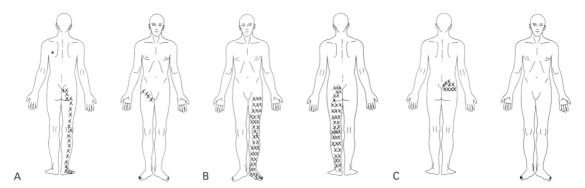

Fig. 45.1 Typical pain drawings of patients with SI dysfunction. (A) Pseudo-S1 radicular pattern. The pattern is similar to that which would be expected for an S1 radiculopathy. The patient may have associated groin pain with this or the other types of pain patterns. (B) Diffuse lower extremity pain often interpreted as 'hysterical'. (C) Pain localized directly over the SIJ and buttock.

of the pain diagrams. Figure 45.1C shows pain localized specifically over the area of the SIJ without radiation to the lower extremity.

The history may be useful in that a majority of patients can identify a specific episode of trauma associated with the onset of their symptoms (Moore 1994). Some patients will report a gradual onset without any precipitating trauma; others report persistent pain after pregnancy. Patients will frequently report difficulty in ascending stairs, and will use a non-reciprocal gait, preferring to advance the leg on the unaffected side.

Multiple physical examination maneuvers are purported to identify a painful SIJ, but several studies have identified the poor reliability of these maneuvers (Bellamy et al 1983, Dreyfuss et al 1995, Potter & Rothstein 1991). Patients with SI dysfunction demonstrate considerable overlap of symptoms with patients suffering from other conditions, such as patients with a symptomatic HNP (Norman & May 1956). Neurocompressive pathology needs to be identified or excluded. Since up to 30% of magnetic resonance imaging (MRI) scans of the lumbar spine will demonstrate some anatomic abnormality (Boden et al 1990), it is crucial to correlate the clinical picture with the results of imaging studies in order to avoid making a serious error. For example, a patient who describes pain in an S1 distribution and whose MRI shows a disc protrusion at L5–S1 should not be considered necessarily to be symptomatic from the disc protrusion. As will be subsequently described, such a patient may very well be symp-

tomatic from SIJ dysfunction, and failure to recognize this in the past has led all too often to a failed discectomy or possibly a lumbar fusion. The author concurs with other investigators that it is necessary to carry out a fluoroscopically or computerized tomography (CT)-guided injection of local anesthetic into the synovial portion of the joint in order to establish the diagnosis (Dreyfuss et al 1995, Haldeman & Soto-Hall 1938, Keating et al 1995, Steindler & Luck 1938).

Injection is accomplished by approaching the inferior portion of the joint by a skin puncture 1 cm below the most inferior portion of the joint as visualized by fluoroscopy with the patient in a prone position. A 3.5 in 25-gauge needle is usually adequate and 1 cm^3 of Isovue 300 is injected to confirm the needle's location within the synovial portion of the joint. The contrast must outline the cartilaginous portion of the joint to be considered an adequate injection. This is followed by injection of 1.5 cm^3 of 0.75% marcaine and 3 mg Celestone. The patient is given a pain diary and asked to record the pain level in the hours subsequent to the injection. Usually more than one injection is recommended, using local anesthetics of differing duration or with saline. If the pain relief is significant and concordant with the local anesthetic used, the diagnosis is considered to be validated. A review of 500 consecutive injections carried out at the Colorado Spine Center showed a positive confirmatory injection in 25% of cases. Thus, when the diagnosis is suspected on the basis of the history and physical examination, it is only confirmed in one case out of four, which further establishes the lack of reliability of the history and physical examination alone.

Radiographic abnormalities are often subtle and seldom diagnostic by themselves. A small association has been found between ventral capsular tears and positive responses to diagnostic injection (Schwarzer et al 1995). Radionuclide imaging has been investigated and found to be inadequate to diagnose SIJ pain, only 19% of patients with SI pain by diagnostic block demonstrating abnormal uptake on technetium-99m phosphate imaging (Slipman et al 1996). The paucity of abnormal findings using radiographic techniques is probably explained by the relative lack of mobility of the joint, even in pathologic hypermobility (Kissling 1995). Diagnostic injection, therefore, remains essential in establishing the diagnosis.

SURGICAL TECHNIQUE

The surgical technique used was a modification of that described by Smith-Petersen (1926). Some modifications were incorporated over the period of the study and are discussed below. The procedure is illustrated in Fig. 45.2.

The patient is positioned prone on chest rolls on an image table. A Foley catheter is placed in the bladder. An image intensifier is used to visualize the joint prior to marking the skin incision. A metal clamp is placed on the posterior superior iliac spine (PSIS). The collector is placed as close as possible to the skin surface in order to obtain the largest field of view. In the anteroposterior (AP) projection in this position, the PSIS will usually overlie the central portion of the joint, although considerable individual variation exists. The central portion of the joint is identified, and a curvilinear incision is planned centered on this point. The length depends upon the size of the patient but is usually 15 cm in length. Figure 45.2A shows a typical incision.

Dissection is carried through subcutaneous tissue with electrocautery until the facial attachments to the posterior iliac crest are identified. The fascia is incised and subperiosteal exposure of the outer table of ilium is carried out (Fig. 45.2B). It is necessary to divide some fibers of the gluteus maximus inferiorly to extend exposure down to the posterior inferior iliac spine. No attempt is made to visualize or divide the posterior SI ligaments. The sciatic notch and inferior extent of the ilium is identified. A Taylor retractor is placed deep in the wound to allow visualization of the surface of the ilium overlying the SIJ.

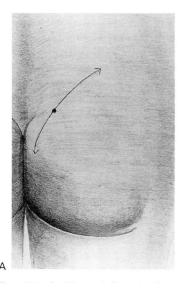 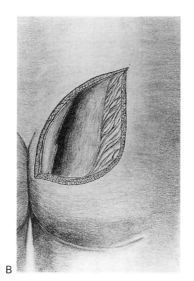 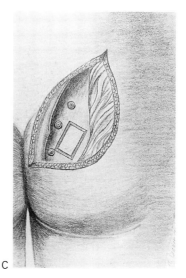

A   B   C

Fig. 45.2 Incision and dissection for posterior SI arthrodesis. (A) Typical incision centered on the PSIS.
(B) The gluteal fascia has been incised and subperiosteal dissection of the outer table of the ilium has been carried out.
(C) Typical location of a transiliac bone window and internal fixation screws.

The superior two-thirds of the joint is ligamentous and is avoided. A Midas Rex AM-8 (Midas Rex Pneumatic Tools Inc., Fort Worth, Texas, USA) dissecting tool is used to score the outer cortex and define a transiliac window overlying the synovial portion of the joint. The dimensions of the window are variable depending upon patient size, but in general the window should be as large as possible while allowing sufficient room for internal fixation screws cephalad and caudad to the window. A 2.5 cm × 3.5 cm rectangular window is usually possible. The window is completed and removed with a combination of straight and curved osteotomes. It is desirable to remove the window with intact subchondral bone and cartilage from the iliac side of the SIJ. It should then be possible to visualize the hyaline cartilage in the depths of the wound on the sacral side of the joint. The subchondral bone and cartilage are removed from the bone window and the resulting block of bone set aside. The subchondral bone and cartilage from the sacral side of the joint are removed with osteotomes and curettes. The anterior, caudad, and posterior cartilage surfaces can be seen with a head light, and these can be removed with a combination of straight and angled curettes or with a power tool. No attempt should be made to extend dissection into the ligamentous portion of the joint as this will lead to further mechanical destabilization of the joint and can theoretically compromise chances of osseous union.

Additional bone graft is harvested from the ipsilateral PSIS with osteotomes and gouges. Cancellous bone is packed through the window into the recesses of the joint. The bone block is then impacted across the joint and cancellous bone packed around it in order to secure an interference fit.

Preparation is then made for internal fixation. Two or three 6.5 mm AO screws with short (16 mm) threads are placed across the joint under image intensifier control. Three cortical surfaces should be felt when drilling the screws. If only three cortical surfaces are drilled, it is impossible to penetrate into the pelvis or into a sacral foramen. It is not recommended to attempt to pass a screw through the graft as the cancellous bone remaining in the sacrum is usually inadequate to allow purchase by the screw. If sufficient bone is packed around the bone plug, its position should be stable without a screw. Figure 45.2C demonstrates the recommended screw placement. A depth gauge is used and cancellous screws of appropriate length are placed with metallic washers. The image intensifier is then used to visualize the screws in PA, inlet, outlet, and oblique planes. No screws should protrude into the pelvis.

The fascia is closed with absorbable suture and a drain placed in the subcutaneous space and brought out through a lateral stab wound. Skin closure is achieved in two layers with an absorbable suture.

POST-OPERATIVE CARE

The patient is mobilized the first postoperative day and is kept non-weight-bearing on the operated side for 8 weeks. The drain is removed at 24–48 h. Patients frequently experience dramatic pain relief in the early (24–48 h) time period and have to be cautioned against early resumption of weight-bearing. Two months after surgery, patients are sent to physical therapy for crutch weaning, gluteal strengthening, and gait normalization.

CRITERIA FOR SURGICAL TREATMENT

After a clear diagnosis is established, an attempt should be made to treat the patient by nonsurgical means. Very specific recommendations for rehabilitation programs are now available (Mooney 1995). Manipulative therapy and prolotherapy have also been reported to have some success, even in chronic cases (Dorman et al 1995, Klein et al 1993). If these measures have been unsuccessful and the patient has severe and disabling symptoms for 6 months or more, arthrodesis may be considered.

EXPERIENCE WITH ARTHRODESIS

Between August 1990 and November 1994, approximately 6500 patients were seen at the Colorado Spine Center. Seventy-seven patients underwent arthrodesis of the SIJ for chronic painful dysfunction and failure of conservative treatment. Data were collected prospectively on all patients, and patients were contacted for a final interview at the time of follow-up. Symptom duration ranged from 6 to 84 months. Minimum follow-up was 1 year and ranged up to 5 years. There were 29 male and 48 female patients. The left side was operated in 47 cases and the right in 27 cases, 3 patients undergoing bilateral procedures.

Patients were considered a clinical success if they were experiencing significant pain relief at follow-up, were satisfied with the operation, and stated that they would recommend the procedure to someone with a similar problem. Sixty-two out of 77 patients were regarded as successes and 15 were considered failures, giving a success rate of 80.5%. There were 28 patients who had isolated SIJ problems, had no prior spine surgery, and had no additional diagnosis related to the lumbar spine, such as discogenic pain. In this group, there were 24 successes, giving a success rate of 86%. Three out of the four failures in this group had a pseudarthrosis.

Forty patients were covered under the worker's compensation scheme. Thirty procedures were clinical successes in this group, giving a success rate of 75%. This was not significantly different from the non-worker's compensation cases (on Chi-square analysis).

Complications

There was one superficial wound infection, which was successfully treated with local care and antibiotics. There were no deep infections. One patient had an intentional penetration of the screw into the pelvis to anchor the bone plug and had radicular irritation as a result. The screw was removed 4 months after surgery, and the patient's radicular pain resolved. Early in the series, there was a fracture into the sciatic notch caused by initiation of the bone window with an osteotome. The fracture was stabilized with a single AO screw and went on to uneventful healing. This problem was eliminated in subsequent cases by scoring the outer cortex with the Midas Rex tool before completing the bone window with an osteotome.

Pseudarthrosis

There were seven pseudarthroses in the entire group. Pseudarthrosis was determined by fine-cut CT scanning. All of these patients were smokers; of the total group, only 40% were smokers. Five patients were reoperated with an attempt to repair the pseudarthrosis. Of the reoperated patients, 2 were successfully repaired and had a good final clinical result. Two patients had a persistent non-union after the second surgery, and remained clinical failures. The remaining patient is too close to the time of the second surgery to assess as a success or failure.

Various options exist for repair of a pesudarthrosis. The joint can be approached anteriorly and a reconstruction plate placed across the joint. The problem with this approach is the danger of damage to the lumbosacral trunk, as well as the difficulty of reaching the synovial portion of the joint and of achieving compression of the joint. The preferred method is to obtain a CT scan of the joint and identify what portions of the joint are available to deposit bone graft. A monopolar EBI stimulator (Electro Biology Inc., Parsippany, NJ, USA) can be used with the wire placed on the sacral side of the joint and the battery placed in a subcutaneous pocket adjacent to the incision. Supplemental bone graft can be harvested from the contralateral PSIS.

Analysis of failures

Of the 15 patients who were failures, 7 had pseudarthroses. Eight of the failures were of unclear cause and were thought to represent either a misdiagnosis or a superimposition of other problems. Six of the early failures were operated before a standardized protocol for diagnostic injection was in place. As was noted above, in patients who had no coexisting spinal problems and no prior surgery, all of the failures were accounted for by pseudarthrosis. Therefore it is clear that it is important to make an accurate diagnosis early and to intervene on the appropriate pathology.

COEXISTENT LUMBAR SPINE PATHOLOGY

It is not uncommon to identify patients with SI

dysfunction who have additional symptomatic lumbar spine pathology. Patients diagnosed with SI dysfunction will not infrequently have additional pathology in the lumbar spine that is identified by a thorough evaluation. When this situation exists, it raises several important issues for the clinician. Which condition is responsible for the patient's complaints? If more than one condition is contributing to the complaint, should these be treated sequentially or simultaneously? Below are given some recommendations for the evaluation of several clinical scenarios.

PAINFUL SI DYSFUNCTION AND COEXISTENT HNP

This is an important case to consider as the presenting symptoms and pain drawing can be very similar. In the author's initial series of 13 patients, 6 had undergone laminectomy that failed to relieve symptoms prior to the diagnosis of SI dysfunction being made. It is widely known that not all HNPs are symptomatic (Boden et al 1990). Fortin (1995) has shown arthrographic evidence of communication between the SIJ capsule and the L5 and S1 root sleeves. Such a communication in some cases could produce a false positive SI injection in the setting of a symptomatic HNP at L4–5 or L5–S1. Such a communication must be sought when determining the actual pain generator in a patient with a coexistent HNP. Conversely, it is important to rule out symptomatic SI dysfunction in a patient with a presumptive diagnosis of a painful HNP. Provocative discography should also be considered as a preoperative study if further clarification is needed.

COEXISTENT SIJ DYSFUNCTION AND DEGENERATIVE DISC DISEASE, WITH OR WITHOUT SPINAL STENOSIS

In the author's experience, this has been the most common multiple pathology situation encountered. Injection of the SIJ alleviates one component of the patient's pain but does not relieve pain experienced in the midline at the lumbosacral junction. Provocative discography reproduces the midline back pain. On occasion, the patient is able to identify one or the other areas of symptomatology as clearly dominant. More commonly, however, the relative contributions to the overall complaint are reported as being nearly equal. Assuming that conservative measures have failed for both problems, a decision must be made about how to proceed. One approach is to treat one problem first, allow the patient to recover from that intervention, and then reassess whether or not the second condition still warrants treatment. Using this approach, we have performed an arthrodesis on the SIJ first, using the rationale that this surgery is easier to perform and has less morbidity than a lumbar spine fusion. Inevitably, when this was done and the SI pain was eliminated, the patient then regarded the midline pain as too troublesome to tolerate, and eventually, a lumbar spine fusion was carried out later. More recently, when coexistent degenerative disc disease and SI dysfunction have been identified, we have offered the patient the option of performing both surgeries at the same setting. In the two patients in whom this has been carried out, early clinical success has been achieved with minimal additional morbidity. The advantage of this approach is that the patient reaches ultimate recovery faster than would be the case if the conditions were treated sequentially (see case example 3 below).

It is also important to avoid jumping to the conclusion that spinal stenosis, as revealed by imaging studies, is responsible for a patient's symptoms. Case example 2 below illustrates a situation in which SI pain was responsible for the patient's complaint, even though significant stenosis was identified in her evaluation. Arthrodesis completely resolved the patient's symptoms, and her stenosis did not require treatment.

CASE EXAMPLES

Case 1

The patient was a 44-year-old female who had slipped on the ice. She had unremitting pain in her low back, buttock, and posterior thigh (Fig. 45.3A). An MRI scan demonstrated degenerative disc disease at L4–5 and L5–S1 (Fig. 45.3B). She underwent a diagnostic injection into the left SIJ and had complete relief of her typical symptoms.

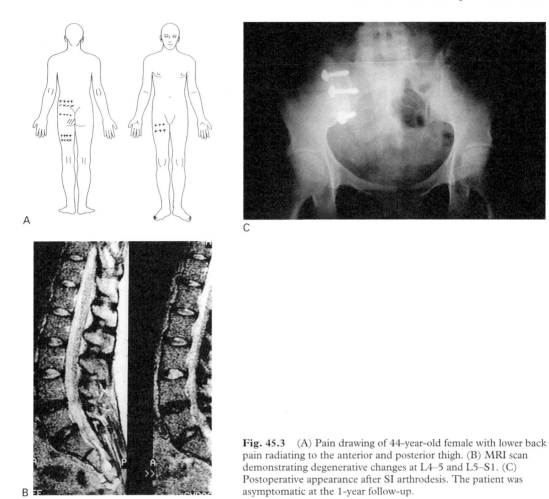

Fig. 45.3   (A) Pain drawing of 44-year-old female with lower back pain radiating to the anterior and posterior thigh. (B) MRI scan demonstrating degenerative changes at L4–5 and L5–S1. (C) Postoperative appearance after SI arthrodesis. The patient was asymptomatic at the 1-year follow-up.

She underwent a left SI arthrodesis (Fig. 45.3C) and at 1 year had no symptoms related to her back or lower extremity.

Case 2

This patient was a 70-year-old female with the complaint of back pain with radiation to the right lower extremity. X-rays demonstrated a grade II degenerative spondylolisthesis of L4 on L5, and an MRI scan demonstrated associated spinal stenosis at that level (Fig. 45.4A–B). However, physical examination suggested SI dysfunction. The patient underwent a series of diagnostic injections into the synovial portion of the SIJ, each of which produced near-complete relief of her typical symptoms. She therefore underwent

an SI arthrodesis (Fig. 45.4). She had immediate relief of her lower extremity pain and 4 months after surgery her ambulation was unlimited. She had minimal or no low back pain, no lower extremity pain, and no claudication.

Case 3

This patient was a 58-year-old female with left-sided lower back pain radiating to the left lower extremity. Her ambulation was limited by leg pain to less than one block. In addition, her physical examination suggested SIJ dysfunction, and maneuvers to stress the left SIJ reproduced her typical left-sided back pain. A CT myelogram demonstrated severe stenosis at the level of L4–5 (Fig. 45.5A–B). An SIJ injection was carried out,

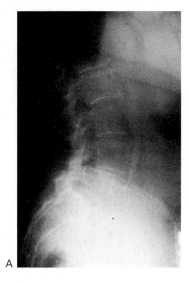

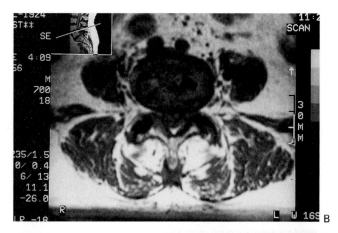

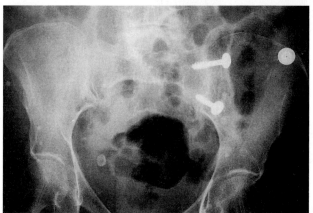

Fig. 45.4   A 70-year-old female with low back pain and sciatica. (A) Grade II degenerative spondylolisthesis. (B) Stenosis at L4–5. (C) Postoperative X-ray after SI fusion.

and while the local anesthetic was acting she was able to ambulate two blocks before she began to experience claudication symptoms.

Because of the apparent coexistent spinal stenosis, symptomatic claudication, lumbar instability, and SIJ dysfunction, it was elected to carry out both a lumbar spine fusion and decompression at the same time as the SIJ arthrodesis (Fig. 45.5C). The patient underwent these procedures and had an excellent outcome with immediate resolution of her SI pain. She was maintained on crutches for 2 months, after which she resumed ambulation and was able to walk 2 miles without any claudication.

CONCLUSIONS

1. SIJ-mediated pain is not uncommon and should be considered in the differential diagnosis of low back pain and sciatica.

2. The majority of patients with painful SIJ dysfunction can be treated by non-surgical means.

3. A small number of patients will not improve with conservative treatment. In the author's experience, this number is approximately 1% of all patients presenting to a spine specialty clinic.

4. Arthrodesis of the SIJ in selected patients produces satisfactory results with minimal complications and morbidity. It should be considered whenever the diagnosis is clear and conservative treatment has failed.

5. If other lumbar spine pathology coexists with SI dysfunction, clinical judgement should be used in planning treatment in a sequential versus a simultaneous manner.

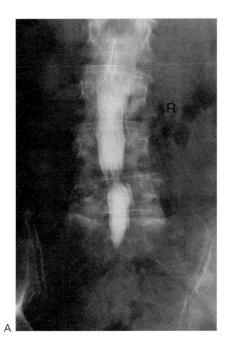

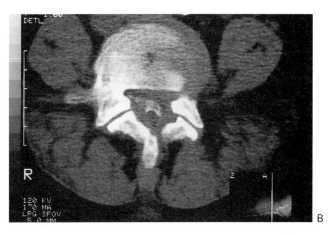

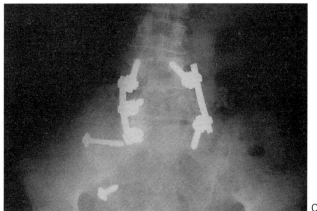

Fig. 45.5 Myelogram (A) and postmyelogram CT (B) demonstrating severe stenosis at the level of L4–5. (C) Postoperative appearance after anterior/posterior spine fusion at L4–S1, decompression, and SI arthrodesis. The patient's pain complaints were resolved and she was able to walk 2 miles without claudication.

REFERENCES

Albee F H 1909 A study of the anatomy and clinical importance of the sacroiliac joint. Journal of the American Medical Association 53: 1273–1276

Baer W S 1917 Sacroiliac strain. Bulletin of the Johns Hopkins Hospital 28: 159–163

Bellamy N, Park W, Rooney P J 1983 What do we know about the sacroiliac joint? Seminars in Arthritis and Rheumatism 12: 282–313

Bernard T N, Cassidy J D 1991 The sacroiliac joint syndrome. In: Frymoyer J W (ed.) The adult spine: principles and practice, Raven Press, New York, pp 2107–2130

Bernard T N, Kirkaldy-Willis W H 1987 Recognizing specific characteristics of nonspecific low back pain. Clinical Orthopaedics and Related Research 217: 266–280

Boden S D, Davis D O, Dina T S, Patronas N J, Wiesel S W 1990 Abnormal magnetic-resonance scans of the lumbar spine in asymptomatic subjects. Journal of Bone and Joint Surgery (US) 72: 403–408

Campbell W C 1927 An operation for extra-articular fusion of the sacro-iliac joint. Surgery, Gynecology and Obstetrics 45: 218–219

Dandy W E 1929 Loose cartilage from intervertebral disk simulating tumor of the spinal cord. Archives of Surgery 19: 660–672

Daum W J 1995 The sacroiliac joint: an underappreciated pain generator. American Journal of Orthopaedics 24: 475–478

Dorman T A, Cohen R E, Dasig D, Jeng S, Fischer N, DeJong A 1995 Energy efficiency during human walking before and after prolotherapy. In: Vleeming A, Mooney V, Dorman T, Snijders C (eds) Second interdisciplinary world congress on low back pain. San Diego, CA, 9–11 November, pp 645–650

Dreyfuss P, Michaelsen M, Pauza K, McLarty J, Bogduk N 1995 The utility of the history and physical examination in diagnosing intraarticular sacroiliac mediated pain as determined by an intraarticular sacroiliac joint anesthetic injection. Addendum to Vleeming A, Mooney V, Dorman T, Snijders C (eds) Second interdisciplinary world congress on low back pain. San Diego, CA, 9–11 November

Fortin J 1995 Sacroiliac joint injection and arthography with imaging correlation. In: Vleeming A, Mooney V, Dorman T, Snijders C (eds) Second interdisciplinary world congress on low back pain. San Diego, CA, 9–11 November, pp 533–544

Gaenslen F J 1927 Sacroiliac arthrodesis. Journal of the American Medical Association 89: 2031–2035

Garnet J H 1927 Chronic strain of the lumbar spine and sacroiliac joints. Annals of Surgery 85: 509–518

Goldthwait J E, Osgood R E 1905 A consideration of the pelvic articulations from an anatomical, pathological and clinical standpoint. Boston Medical and Surgical Journal 152: 593–601

Haldeman K O, Soto-Hall R 1938 The diagnosis and treatment of sacroiliac condition by the injection of procain. Journal of Bone and Joint Surgery (US) 20: 675–685

Jamrich E, Moore M R, Odom J A 1995 Incidence of sacroiliac arthropathy in patients with previous lumbar spine surgery. Paper presented at North American Spine Society Meeting, Washington, DC, October

Keating J G, Sims V, Avillar M 1995 Sacroiliac joint fusion in a chronic low back pain population. In: Vleeming A, Mooney V, Dorman T, Snijders C (eds) Second interdisciplinary world congress on low back pain. San Diego, CA, 9–11 November, pp 359–366

Kissling R O 1995 The mobility of the sacro-iliac joint in healthy subjects. In: Vleeming A, Mooney V, Dorman T, Snijders C (eds) Second interdisciplinary world congress on low back pain. San Diego, CA, 9–11 November, pp 409–422

Klein R G, Eek B C, Delong B, Mooney V 1993 A randomized double blind trial of dextrose–glycerine–phenol injections for chronic low back pain. Journal of Spinal Disorders 6: 23–33

Mixter W J, Barr J S 1934 Rupture of the intervertebral disc, with involvement of the spinal canal. New England Journal of Medicine 211: 210–215

Mooney V 1993 Understanding, examining for, and treating sacroiliac pain. Journal of Musculoskeletal Medicine 10(7): 37–49

Mooney V 1995 Evaluation and treatment of sacroiliac dysfunction. In: Vleeming A, Mooney V, Dorman T, Snijders C (eds) Second interdisciplinary world congress on low back pain. San Diego, CA, 9–11 November, pp 391–407

Moore M 1994 Diagnosis and treatment of chronic sacroiliac arthropathy. Orthopaedic Transactions 18(1): 255

Moore M 1995 Diagnosis and surgical treatment of chronic painful sacroiliac dysfunction. In: Vleeming A, Mooney V, Dorman T, Snijders C (eds) Second interdisciplinary world congress on low back pain. San Diego, CA, 9–11 November, pp 339–354

Norman G F, May A 1956 Sacroiliac conditions simulating intervertebral disc syndrome. Western Journal of Surgery, Obstetrics and Gynecology 64: 461–462

Pitkin H C, Pheasant H C 1936 Sacrarthrogenetic telalgia. Journal of Bone and Joint Surgery (US) 28: 111–133

Potter N A, Rothstein J M 1991 Intertester reliability for selected clinical tests of the sacroiliac joint. Physical Therapy 65: 1671–1675

Schwarzer A C, Aprill C N, Bogduk N 1995 The sacroiliac joint in chronic low back pain. Spine 20: 31–37

Slipman C W, Sterenfeld E B, Chou L H, Herzog R, Vresilovic E J 1996 Sacroiliac joint syndrome: the value of radionuclide imaging in the diagnosis of sacroiliac joint syndrome. Spine 21: 2251–2254

Smith-Peterson M N, Rogers W A 1926 End-result of arthrodesis of the sacro-iliac joint for arthritis – traumatic and non-traumatic. Journal of Bone and Joint Surgery (US) 8: 118–136

Steindler A, Luck J V 1938 Differential diagnosis of pain low in the back. Journal of the American Medical Association 110: 106–113

Waisbrod H, Kainick J U, Gerbershagen H U 1987 Sacroiliac joint arthrodesis for chronic low back pain. Archives of Orthopaedic and Traumatic Surgery 106: 238–240

46. Sacroiliac joint arthrodesis in selected patients with low back pain

J. G. Keating   M. D. Avillar   M. Price

INTRODUCTION

The sacroiliac joint (SIJ) shares with the temporomandibular joint the distinction of having the worst press in the Western medical literature. Both have been widely cited by alternate medical providers as sources of pain and dysfunction and both have stirred controversy in established academia. But the SIJ is the only joint in the body held by many orthopedists to be incapable of producing pain or dysfunction in the absence of horrific trauma or metabolic disorder. Why should this be?

Until the 1930s the SIJ was widely regarded as a source of pain and dysfunction by mainstream orthopedists. Mixter and Barr (1934) with a single operation – discectomy – shifted the focus in the low back toward the nucleus pulposus, where it has remained ever since. There are, of course, many providers who have continued to work with and study the facet joints, the soft tissues surrounding the lumbar spine, and the dynamics of intervertebral motion, but orthopedists have for the most part forgotten about the SIJ. They contend that there is very little motion in the joint; even proponents of the SIJ as a problem admit that this is a relatively immobile joint. They point out that this is a difficult joint to study, and they are right. Plain X-rays, computerized tomography (CT) scans, magnetic resonance imaging (MRI) studies and bone scans have failed to show consistent changes in most patients carrying the diagnosis of SIJ arthrosis. Nevertheless, the relative immobility of the joint and the absence of a single diagnostic test does not explain why this should be the only joint in the body incapable of hurting.

MATERIALS AND METHODS

Between January 1988 and December 1995, approximately 2300 patients were evaluated at The Keating Group for a variety of low back pain complaints. In this patient population, approximately 20% were in the acute stage of the natural healing process (0–6 weeks) for low back pain; these patients were not considered in this evaluation. The diagnosis of chronic SIJ arthrosis (SIJ arthrosis is pain directly coming from the SIJ upon touch or dynamic testing) was evident in 15.5% of these patients. Of these chronic low back pain sufferers diagnosed with SIJ arthrosis, 13.6% (39 patients, 54 SIJs) continued within the SIJ protocol, meeting the necessary criteria for SIJ arthrodesis. This report will cover these patients' pain levels, strength levels, and work status prior to surgery, following surgery, and at 1 year post-SIJ surgery.

The 39 patients who underwent SIJ fusion averaged 28 months of consecutive low back pain prior to the SIJ surgery. Worker's compensation patients made up 85% of the population. There were 28 female and 11 male patients included in this population. The demographic information that was collected for each patient includes: height, weight, age, gender, low back pain history prior to surgery, side(s) of SIJ surgery, and standardized subjective ratings of pain (0–10 scale) (see Fig. 46.3 below). The objective information collected includes a standardized isometric (IM) lumbar strength score (MedX, Ocala, FL, USA), time after SIJ fusion to maximum medical improvement (MMI), and a work status (intensity level of work and the number of hours employed). Table 46.1 gives the basic

Table 46.1   SIJ fusion patient demographics

| | n | Height (cm) | Weight (kg) | Age (years) | LBP (months) | MMI (months) | Workers compensation | Side of surgery | | |
								Right	Left	Bilateral
Male	11	176.9	85.5	40.3	27.7	4.4	9 (82%)	4	5	2
Female	28	168.9	67.3	46.2	29.5	4.0	24 (86%)	6	9	13

LBP = low back pain history; MMI = time after SIJ fusion to maximum medical improvement.

demographic description of the characteristics of the SIJ fusion population for males and females.

DATA COLLECTION

Demographic, pain, and strength information for each patient was collected at three distinct time periods. The data collection times were as follows: prior to entering the SIJ protocol at The Keating Group, at the end of the rehabilitation process following the SIJ fusion surgery (average 4.1 months), and at a 1-year follow-up after the surgery (average 12.7 months).

Prior to entering SIJ protocol

The physician's evaluation at The Keating Group acts as the initial information for patient pain level, work level status, and various other demographic information discussed previously (Table 46.1). The lumbar IM strength data were collected during exercise therapy as part of the initial step of the SIJ protocol (Avillar et al 1995).

Not all the patients in the SIJ fusion set have initial IM strength or final postsurgical IM scores. This incomplete set of strength scores is due to a number of factors: the lumbar IM test was not integrated into the SIJ dysfunction protocol at the time, and a MedX lumbar extension device was not available at the time and/or place of SIJ examination. In the female population, 18 out of 28 patients have initial IM tests. In the male population 10 out of 11 patients have initial IM tests.

End of the rehabilitation process

The end of the postsurgical rehabilitation process is defined as the point at which the patient has reached maximum medical improvement (MMI). At the last physician's visit at which the MMI was assigned, the patient's subjective rating of pain was taken and the work level status assigned. The postsurgical – final rehabilitation (PSF) IM strength test was the last IM test that came closest to this date of MMI.

In the female population, the PSF IM strength scores have been taken in 18 out of 26 possible patients (1 patient is currently in rehabilitation, 1 patient is deceased). In the male population, 8 out of 10 PSF IM strength scores have been taken (1 patient is currently in rehabilitation).

In the strength data in Figs 46.1 and 46.2, the PSI (postsurgical initial) IM test is not to be confused with the PSF IM test. The initial rehabilitation IM score (PSI IM) was performed approximately 1 month after SIJ surgery, and the final rehabilitation score (PSF IM) was performed approximately 4 months after SIJ surgery.

1-year follow-up

At the 1-year follow-up point, 17 out of the 30 eligible patients returned to The Keating Group for a physical examination and strength evaluation (1-year postsurgical IM). Nine patients had questionnaires (Fig. 46.3) and/or phone interviews in questionnaire form conducted, and 4 patients were lost to follow-up.

SACROILIAC PATIENT PAIN SCORING

Patients' subjective reports of pain were recorded at each physicians' visit and at each exercise therapy session. A standardized analog pain scale was utilized to allow patients to describe their pain levels (Fig. 46.3). The patient pain scores were taken at four distinct points in the treatment

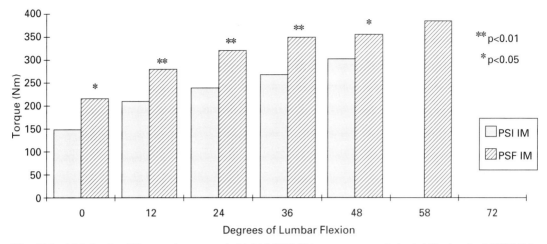

Fig. 46.1   Male lumbar IM strength: postsurgical initial (PSI) IM test to postsurgical rehabilitation final (PSF) IM test.

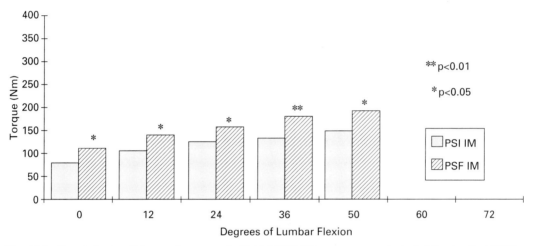

Fig. 46.2   Female lumbar IM strength: postsurgical initial (PSI) IM test to postsurgical rehabilitation final (PSF) IM test.

protocol. The points of data collection were: entrance into the SIJ protocol, prior to SIJ fusion surgery, at the end of rehabilitation from the surgery (MMI), and at the 1-year follow-up point.

Male pain data

Male pain information ANOVA analysis reveals that:

1. There is no significant difference between the entry-to-program pain and the prior-to-surgery pain.

2. There is a significant decrease ($p \leqslant 0.01$) between the prior-to-surgery pain and the end-of-rehabilitation pain.

3. There is no significant difference between the end-of-rehabilitation pain and the 1-year follow-up level of pain.

Female pain data

In the female pain information, ANOVA analysis reveals that:

1. There is a significant decrease ($p \leqslant 0.01$) between the entry-to-program pain and the prior-to-surgery pain.

Please fill this out and return it with the self-addressed envelope! Thank you, your help is greatly appreciated!

Pain level	Description
0	No pain
1–2	Occasional pain
3–4	Mild constant pain
5–6	Moderate constant pain
7–8	Unable to do daily activities
9–10	EMERGENCY: Needs to go to doctor

Name: _____

1. Using the scale above, *what is your everyday level of pain?*_____
2. If you are now employed, *who do you work with?*
3. *How many hours are you working per week?*
4. *How many hours were you working prior to the SIJ surgery?*
5. *Would you have the SI fusion surgery again*, if you could go back in time?
6. *If you are not working at this time, what is the main reason that you are not at work?*
7. Please list any other medicines and doctors (also other procedures that were done) that you have been to after your SI fusion surgery:

Fig. 46.3 Questionnaire sent to all patients at the 1-year follow-up point.

2. There is a significant decrease ($p \leq 0.01$) between the prior-to-surgery pain and the end-of-rehabilitation pain.

3. There is no significant difference between the end-of-rehabilitation pain and the 1-year follow-up level of pain (Table 46.2).

LEG PAIN

A common symptom prior to surgery was numbness in the thighs and numbness radiating below the knee. The upper and lower leg numbness was alleviated in some patients following the surgical procedure (Table 46.3). Upper leg numbness prior to surgery occurred in 35 out of 39 patients, following surgery in 11 out of 36. Lower leg numbness was found prior to surgery in 20 out of 39, and following surgery 11 out of 36 patients. Initial numbness indicator, information obtained from initial pain drawing, is at protocol onset, and the final indicator was at the date of MMI. Upper leg numbness was defined as numbness extending below the gluteal fold; lower leg numbness was defined as numbness radiating below the knee.

WORK DATA

Of the SIJ fusion population described in this text (see Table 46.1 above), 85% are worker's compensation patients, and the others are privately paying patients. The SIJ fusion patients' work status level was assigned at each visit to the physician, which occurred approximately once per month. Work status was assigned at the following levels: 0 = no work, 1 = sedentary duty, 2 = light duty, 3 = medium duty, 4 = regular duty. Work information was collected at three distinct time intervals: work status prior to entering the SIJ protocol (initial work level), at the end of the rehabilitation process (post-protocol – MMI), and at the 1-year follow-up.

In Table 46.4, the SIJ fusion subjects' work levels are illustrated. The most notable change occurs in the number of patients that return to full duty. The proportion of patients who are not at work at the MMI date remains constant to the 1-year follow-up period.

Five out of the ten patients who are not at work displayed Waddell's signs (at MMI) for non-physiologic pain symptoms (Waddell 1980). These signs were absent prior to the SIJ surgery. The other 5 patients not at work not exhibiting Waddell signs described pain relief from the

Table 46.2 Pain averages on a standardized pain scale

	Pain level on entry to program	Pain level prior to surgery	Pain level at end of rehabilitation	Pain level at 1-year follow-up
Male	5.7	4.4	2.2**	2.4
Female	7.1	5.8	2.3**	2.7

**$p < 0.01$, significant difference between prior-to-surgery pain and end-of-rehabilitation pain.

Table 46.3   Upper and lower leg numbness

	Males			Females		
Upper leg numbness						
	Upper leg numbness	No upper leg numbness	Total	Upper leg numbness	No upper leg numbness	Total
Initial	9 (82%)	2	11	26 (93%)	2	28
Final	4 (40%)	6*	10*	7 (27%)	19**	26**
Lower leg numbness						
	Lower leg numbness	No lower leg numbness	Total	Lower leg numbness	No lower leg numbness	Total
Initial	5 (45%)	6	11	15 (54%)	13	28
Final	4 (40%)	6*	10*	7 (27%)	19**	26**

* One male is currently being rehabilitated.
** One female is currently in rehabilitation, one female is deceased.

Table 46.4   Distribution of work status

		At work		No work	
		Male	Female	Male	Female
Initial		7 (70%)	16 (57%)	3 (30%)	12 (43%)
	at full duty	4 of the 7	11 of the 16		
MMI		6 (67%)	19 (73%)	3 (33%)	7 (27%)
	at full duty	5 of the 6	15 of the 19		
At 1 year		5 (71%)	14 (67%)	2 (29%)	7 (33%)
	at full duty	5 of the 5	12 of the 14		

* Female population: at postprotocol (MMI) 1 female is in rehabilitation, 1 female is deceased, 1 female is lost to follow-up at the 1-year mark.
** Male population: at initial work level 1 male was retired prior to program entry; 1 male is currently in rehabilitation; 2 males are lost to follow-up at the 1-year mark.

surgery. All of these patients described relief below the level of 3 (on a 0–10 scale). None of these 5 patients has complaints of leg pain. The 6 privately paying patients have all returned to their prior jobs and lifestyles with pain levels below a level of 4.

IM STRENGTH TESTING

The assessment of patient back strength was determined by the utilization of an isometric strength testing device, the MedX lumbar extension unit (Fig. 46.4). The MedX lumbar unit attempts to isolate the low back muscles through a number of restraints that lock the femur into the hip and theoretically allow only the activation of the lumbar extensors. This design is used to isolate the lumbar extensor muscles. This method of lumbar strength testing has been shown to be of high reliability and validity (Graves et al 1994).

At strength testing, subjects were isometrically tested at their maximal pain-free extension and flexion points. Between these two endpoints, testing was also conducted at a set of standardized points. These standardized points are at 0°, 12°, 24°, 36°, 48°, 60°, and 72° of lumbar flexion.

Strength changes after surgery

The male PSI IM test was performed at an average of 1.2 months after surgery, and the PSF IM test was performed at an average of 4.4 months after surgery. The male strength curve in Fig. 46.1 shows a large torque change from the PSI to PSF tests, the total strength increasing 37%. ANOVA reveals that the angles 0°, 12°, 24°, 36°, and 48° of lumbar flexion underwent a

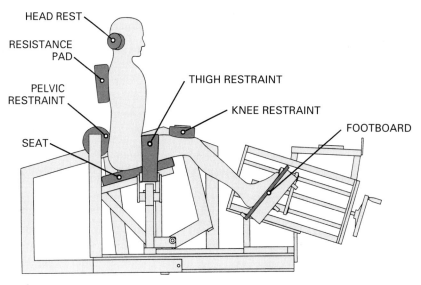

Fig. 46.4   MedX lumbar extension machine restraint system.

significant increase in isometric torque production (see Fig. 46.1 above; Table 46.5). ANOVA shows that the pain-free range of motion (ROM) significantly increased ($p \leqslant 0.05$) from 0–50° at PSI to 0–58° at PSF.

The female PSI IM test was performed at an average of 1.4 months after surgery, and the PSF IM test at an average of 4.0 months after surgery. The female strength curve (see Fig. 46.2 above; Table 46.6) shows a large torque change from the PSI to PSF strength tests, the total strength increasing by 30%. ANOVA reveals that all the standardized female test angles show a significant

strength increase ($p \leqslant 0.05$). No significant difference is seen in female ROM.

Presurgical strength compared with postrehabilitation strength

Comparing the male and female presurgical IM test and the PSF IM test, the lumbar strength scores show little difference. The only significant differences in male ($p \leqslant 0.01$) lumbar strength are seen at 48° and 54° of lumbar flexion (Fig. 46.5). These differences may be due to the fact that earlier in the protocol some patients were

Table 46.5   Male SIJ fusion lumbar IM strength testing: initial IM (at program entry), presurgical initial IM test, postsurgical initial (PSI) IM test, postsurgical rehabilitation final (PSF) IM, and 1-year postsurgery IM test results. Values are means. Pain-free ROM averages are in parentheses

	MedX degrees of lumbar flexion					
Standardized test angle	0°	12°	24°	36°	48°	angle > 48°
Initial IM test torque (Nm) $n = 10$ / ROM (2–53°)	185.1 (2°)	219.8	259.4	271.1	253.6	261.0 (53°)
Presurgical IM test torque (Nm) $n = 11$ / ROM (0—55°)	208.8	255.2	285.8	320.4	286.0	297.2 (55°)
PSI IM test torque (Nm) $n = 10$ / ROM (0–50°)	147.5	207.5	235.5	262.8	296.6	302.8 (50°)
PSF IM test torque (Nm) $n = 8$ / ROM (0–58°)	214.4	275.1	316.4	345.0	349.0	377.1 (58°)
1-year postsurgery torque (Nm) $n = 4$ / ROM (0–60°)	228.9	278.0	327.2	347.8	339.9	378.3 (60°)

Table 46.6 Female SIJ fusion lumbar IM strength testing: initial IM (at program entry), presurgical initial IM test, postsurgical initial (PSI) IM test, postsurgical rehabilitation final (PSF) IM, and 1-year follow-up IM test results. Values are means. Pain-free ROM averages are in parentheses

	MedX degrees of lumbar flexion					
Standardized test angle	0°	12°	24°	36°	48°	angle > 48°
Initial IM test torque (Nm) n = 18 / ROM (2–44°)	73.6 (2°)	97.9	115.3	123.8	135.6 (44°)	
Presurgical IM test torque (Nm) n = 21 / ROM (0–47°)	99.3	128.4	147.1	160.3	177.8 (47°)	
PSI IM test torque (Nm) n = 22 / ROM (0–49°)	76.6	102.8	121.9	131.4	145.6	147.0 (49°)
PSF IM test torque (Nm) n = 18 / ROM (0–51°)	108.2	136.3	153.2	177.6	182.9	187.5 (51°)
1-year postsurgery torque (Nm) n = 13 / ROM (0–59°)	92.5	122.9	141.0	158.2	176.7	195.9 (59°)

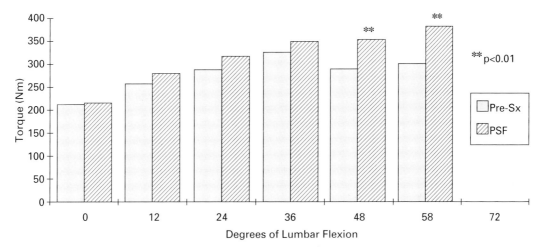

Fig. 46.5 Male lumbar IM strength: presurgery (Pre-Sx) initial IM test to postsurgical rehabilitation final (PSF) IM test.

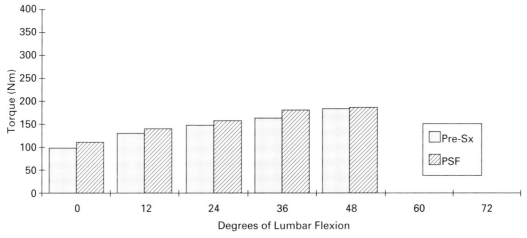

Fig. 46.6 Female lumbar IM strength: presurgery (Pre-Sx) initial IM test to postsurgical rehabilitation final (PSF) IM test.

restricted to only a 0–42° ROM during pre-operative rehabilitation. This restriction could have reduced presurgical IM scores at 48° and beyond. The ROM of the IM tests (presurgical 0–48°, PSF 0–51°) shows no significant difference. The female presurgical test and the female PSF IM test (Fig. 46.6; Table 46.6) show no significant strength differences, as well as no difference in ROM.

In analysing the lumbar isometric strength information, an interesting strength trend emerges. The endpoint of lumbar strength training prior to surgery, and the end point of strength training following surgery yields the same strength results (see Figs 46.5 and 46.6; Tables 46.5 and 46.6). However, prior to surgery and following the SIJ fusion surgery, there is a marked pain and function change even though strength has not been significantly altered. This indicates that lumbar strength in a trained population may not be the mediating factor behind chronic SIJ pain; derangement within the joint itself may be the greatest factor contributing to pain.

DIAGNOSIS

While there may be mechanisms of SIJ injury more common than others, we have found that it is common to find SIJ arthrosis in patients who have not been traumatized. To make the SIJ arthrosis diagnosis, we look to a number of factors, as illustrated in Boxes 46.1–46.3. The

Box 46.1   Common causes of SIJ dysfunction

Repetitive end of range flexion/extension movements
Automobile accident with one leg fully extended
Trauma to buttocks
Postpartum
Repetitive lifting movements
Twisting movements with weight
Overall joint laxity
Shearing type movements
Lift injury in awkward position

Box 46.2   SIJ provocation tests

Distraction	Thigh thrust
Compression	Pelvic torsion right
Iliac shear	Pelvic torsion left
Yeoman's	Figure 4/Patrick's
Posterior	Gaenslen's

Box 46.3   Manual dynamic SIJ dysfunction tests

Sitting flexion test	Standing flexion test
March/stork test	Supine long sit test

factors that need to be observed in order to pinpoint the SIJ arthrosis diagnosis are: common pain and injury patterns for SIJ injuries, specific location of pain (Schwarzer et al 1994), positive static and dynamic tests (Avillar et al 1995), and positive provocation tests (Laslett & Williams 1994, Mooney 1994). After 8 weeks of conservative treatment has failed, a fluoroscopic injection of the SIJ (Fortin et al 1994) will be conducted as a guide to surgical intervention.

TREATMENT

The vast majority of patients diagnosed with chronic (continuous pain for longer than 45 days after initial injury) SIJ arthrosis resolve with non-operative treatment that has been described elsewhere in the SIJ literature (Avillar et al 1995).

In those patients who fail to respond to non-operative treatment, the *sine qua non* for proceeding to the operating room is (1) the absence of Waddell's signs (Waddell 1980), (2) failure of conservative therapy, (3) intractable pain that interferes with the patient's daily activities, and (4) a positive fluoroscopically guided arthrogram and anesthetic injection into the SIJ performed by an interventional radiologist well familiar with the SIJ (Schwarzer et al 1994). An SIJ arthrogram is considered positive if it shows abnormal SI joint morphology, extravasation of dye, and obliteration of the patient's typical pain on provocative tests and in the daily activities for the effective period

Table 46.7 The Keating Group SIJ fusion postoperative protocol

Time	
0–7 days	Crutches/emphasis on increased weight-bearing
1 week	Full weight-bearing
1–2 weeks	Begin walking 3 × 10 min/bike 10 min (3 ×/wk)
2nd–3rd week	Increase all daily activities Piriformis, low back extension, and lower body stretching
3rd–4th week	Full exercise rehabilitation 3 ×/wk
4th week	Begin MedX lumbar extension training Full exercise regime
4–6 weeks	Return to sedentary work level No lifting greater than 10 kg Continue with full exercise regime
8 weeks	Assess for return to regular work status Continual increase of all activities
10–12 weeks	Resume regular work status All sports activities
12 weeks	Anticipate MMI
16 weeks	Discharge at MMI/no sports restrictions

of the local anesthetic agent (Laslett & Williams 1994).

In Table 46.7, the time line for postsurgical rehabilitation of SIJ fusion patients is shown. The most important issue after surgery is the early activation of the patients into activities of daily living, and the start of a walking program, coupled with piriformis stretching. Piriformis stretching continues for 2 months following surgery (Keating et al 1995).

SURGICAL TECHNIQUE

We use a previously undescribed technique for SIJ arthrodesis that employs a combination of surgical debridement and autogenous bone grafting of the inferior–posterior SIJ, with compression screw fixation of the superior joint.

After the anesthesiologist establishes adequate general endotracheal anesthesia, and a Foley catheter has been inserted, the patient is rolled into a prone position on a radiolucent operating table. The surgeon stands on the patient's affected side and, using a C-arm image intensifier coming over from the other side, landmarks are

established: the posterior iliac spine (PSIS), the gluteal notch, and the SIJ. It is extremely important to position the patient on the table so that one can achieve the three views described by Matta (see Chapter 47 in this volume), and a cross-table lateral view.

Marking the skin over the superior inferior aspects of the SIJ, the surgical incision is made over the PSIS and the dissection taken down to the PSIS. Using a combination of bovie dissection and Cobb elevator soft tissue stripping, the PSIS is exposed; this is eventually taken as the autogenous bone graft wedge. Continuing the dissection medially, the posterior medial wall of the ilium is skived down, incising the posterior SI ligament and interosseous ligaments *en route* to the posterior–inferior SIJ.

The SIJ presents with a surprising anatomic variability even in the same patient. The key to establishing one's position in the joint is in identifying the area (Fig. 46.7) directly medial to the posterior inferior iliac spine (PIIS), where the ilium meets the relatively flat surface of the sacrum. The SIJ is by no means always readily visible, so we invariably establish that we are in the joint by placing an 18-gauge spinal needle into the nexus of the ilium and sacrum where we expect the joint to be, and fluoroscope our position (Fig. 46.8).

Once a position in the joint space at the level of the arrow in Fig. 46.7 is established, the PSIS is harvested for eventual use as the autogenous bone graft. That is supplemented with copious cancellous bone harvested from the decorticated iliac crest.

Then, using a combination of rongeur and curette debridement as well as specially built rasps (Fig. 46.9), the cartilage is stripped from the posterior inferior SIJ. We routinely use a headlamp and 3.5 X-loops to ensure that we are stripping the joint itself and not creating a pseudojoint in the posterior surface of the sacrum. This stripping removes 6–8 cm of joint space from superior to inferior and stops approximately 1.0 cm superior to the sciatic notch. The depth of joint debridement is 2.0 cm. Precautions here are taken to avoid the sciatic notch and thereby the superior gluteal artery, and to eschew the temptation to continue joint stripping too

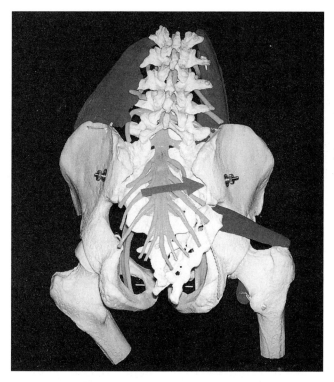

Fig. 46.7 Theoretical alignment of SIJ prior to surgical fusion.

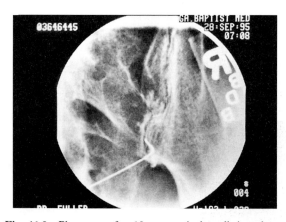

Fig. 46.8 Placement of an 18-gauge spinal needle into the nexus of the ilium and sacrum.

ventrally and thereby go through the anterior SI ligament.

The cancellous bone is then taken from the posterior ilium and packed into the decorticated joint space. Using rongeurs and files, the PSIS is shaped into a wedge, which is placed into the joint and driven home using a tamp.

Satisfied that we have removed the posterior inferior SIJ and packed it tightly with a combination of cancellous bone and cortical wedge, we turn our attention to the superior SIJ where we carry out the percutaneous dual screw fixation.

Using the image intensifier, a guide pin is laid on the buttocks in the orientation necessary to place a guide pin through the lateral iliac wing and across the SIJ into the sacrum, angling distal to proximal. We aim for that portion of the superior sacrum that looks like a pyramid on the image intensifier (Fig. 46.10). This angulation is normally 15° from inferior to superior. Once the proper orientation from inferior to superior has been located, a guide pin is placed three to four finger breadths lateral to the incision (which should be over where the PSIS was) and the skin pierced to push the guide wire through the muscle until it encounters the lateral wall of the iliac wing one finger breadth ventral to the crista glutea (the bony ridge that parallels the PSIS on the lateral ilium; Fig. 46.11). With the guide wire at 90° to the iliac wing and 40° to the floor, a

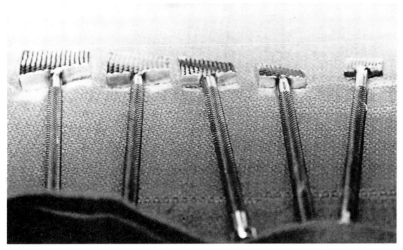

Fig. 46.9   Specially built rasps for SIJ fusion.

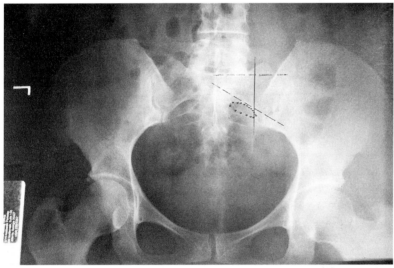

Fig. 46.10   Alignment of superior sacrum into a pyramid configuration upon image intensification.

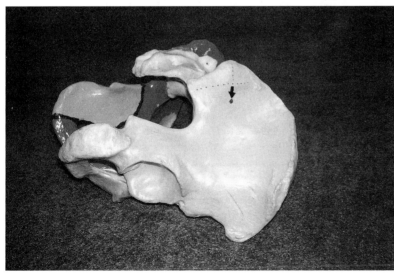

Fig. 46.11   Guide pin lateral to the incision, piercing the skin, pushing the guide wire through muscle until encountering the lateral wall of the iliac wing, ventral to the crista glutea.

drill under fluoroscopic control is used to advance the guide wire through the ilium, across the joint and into the pyramid of the superior sacrum. Progress is checked often using Matta's views plus the cross-table lateral.

It is important to avoid placing the screw medial to an imaginary line drawn along the lateral aspect of the neural foramen (see Fig. 46.10 above). Even using Matta's views with the C-arm, it is easy to place a screw into foramen and crowd a nerve root (Fig. 46.12) unless the imaginary line depicted in Fig. 46.10 above is observed. Once the first guide pin is placed, a second is selected and, paralleling the first 1–2 cm superior and ventral from the first, inserted using the same guidelines. Satisfied that both guide pins are across the joint and contained in the superior sacrum, we slide a spare guide pin down the pins already in place until it hits the iliac

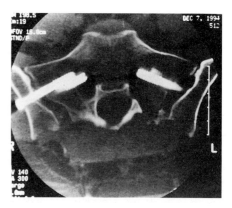

Fig. 46.12   Placement of a screw into the foramen and crowding of a nerve root.

wing; we measure the difference and use that to select the appropriate screw length. Self-tapping cannulated 6.5 mm screws are used, which are

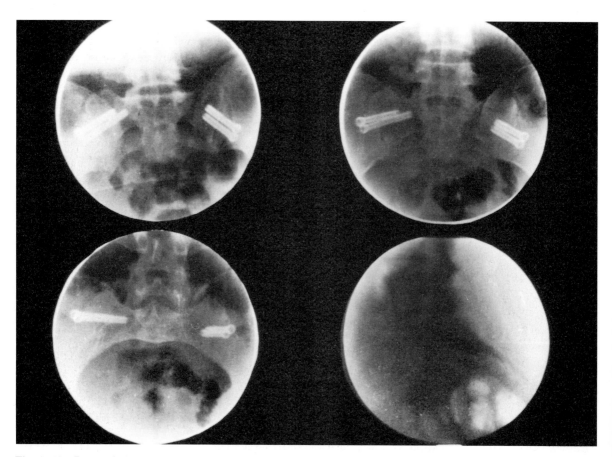

Fig. 46.13   Postsurgical views.

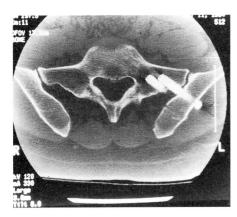

Fig. 46.14 Postoperative CT scan checking screw placement.

advanced using power under fluoroscopic control until we are within a few turns of seating the screw head on the outer table of the ilium, at which point it is screwed home by hand.

A final check of screw placement is made using the four fluoroscopic views and the wound is closed (Fig. 46.13). We rarely drain the incision. Postoperatively, all patients have a CT scan to check screw placement (Fig. 46.14). Most patients go home on the morning of postoperative day 1, and then begin an exercise program at the start of the second postoperative week. This rehabilitation program averages 4 months of exercise therapy until MMI.

Complications

We placed two screws into the S2 neural foramen and a third protruded ventrally adjacent to the S1 nerve root (Fig. 46.15). The intraforaminal screws did not produce any symptoms, but we replaced them. The ventral screw produced an S1 radiculopathy that resolved when we replaced the screw. We have had no misplaced screws since developing the criterion outlined in the surgical technique. One patient had a superficial wound infection; the same patient developed a pulmonary embolus and died.

CONCLUSIONS

1. The SIJ remains a joint of considerable controversy. Laying aside the irrational contention that this is the single major joint in the body that does not commonly cause pain, there are real questions about making such a diagnosis with confidence. The symptoms are highly variable; the signs on physical examination are

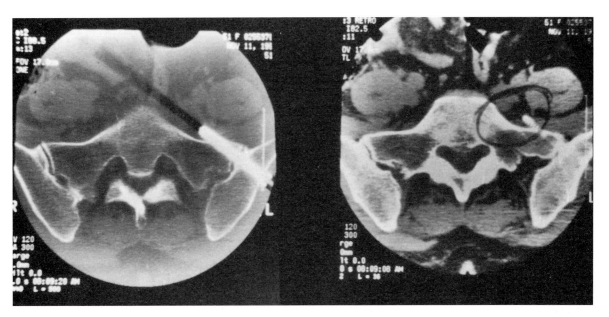

Fig. 46.15 Complications: placement of two screws into the S2 neural foramen and a third protruded ventrally adjacent to the S1 nerve root.

subtle, and moreover there is frequently poor intraexaminer agreement (Laslett & Williams 1994, Potter & Rothstein 1985).

2. Nevertheless, we remain convinced that the SIJ is a common cause for low back, buttock, groin, and lower extremity pain. We have developed an empiric treatment plan that has been effective in the patients we diagnose with chronic SIJ arthrosis who have failed other treatment plans for chronic non-specific low back pain. In that minority of patients we diagnose with chronic SIJ arthrosis who do not resolve with non-operative treatment, we have developed a surgical procedure described here which has proven effective in relieving discomfort and significantly improving function.

REFERENCES

Avillar M D, Sims V, Keating J G, Stinchcomb P, Herrberg J 1995 The effectiveness of a seven week sacroiliac joint mobilization and stabilization program on a low back pain population. In: Vleeming A, Mooney V, Dorman T, Snijders C (eds) Second interdisciplinary world congress on low back pain. San Diego, CA, 9–11 November, pp 305–321

Fortin A, Aprill C, Ponthieux B, Pier J 1994 Sacroiliac joint: pain referral maps upon applying a new injection/arthrography technique. II: Clinical evaluation. Spine 19(13): 1483–1489

Graves J, Webb D, Pollock M et al 1994 Pelvic stabilization during resistance training: its effect on the development of lumbar extension strength. Archives of Physical Medical Rehabilitation 75: 210–215

Keating J G, Sims V, Avillar M D 1995 Sacroiliac joint fusion in a chronic low back pain population. In: Vleeming A, Mooney V, Dorman T, Snijders C (eds) Second interdisciplinary world congress on low back pain. San Diego, CA, 9–11 November, pp 361–365

Laslett M, Williams M 1994 The reliability of selected pain provocation tests for sacroiliac joint pathology. Spine 19(1): 1243–1249

Mixter W J, Barr J S 1934 Rupture of the intervertebral disc with involvement of the spinal canal. New England Journal of Medicine 211: 210–215

Mooney V 1994 Understanding, examining for, and treating sacroiliac pain. Journal of Musculoskeletal Medicine 11(7): 42–44

Potter N, Rothstein J 1985 Intertester reliability for selected clinical tests of the sacroiliac joint. Physical Therapy 65: 1671–1675

Schwarzer A, Aprill C, Bogduk N 1994 The sacroiliac joint in chronic low back pain. Spine 20(1): 31–37

Waddell G 1980 Nonorganic physical signs in low back pain. Spine 5(2): 117–125

FURTHER READING

Moore M 1995 Diagnosis and surgical treatment of chronic painful sacroiliac dysfunction. In: Vleeming A, Mooney V, Dorman T, Snijders C (eds) Second interdisciplinary world congress on low back pain. San Diego, CA, 9–11 November, pp 339–354

Smith-Petersen M, Rogers W 1926 End-result study of arthrodesis of the sacro-iliac joint for arthritis, traumatic and non-traumatic. Journal of Bone and Joint Surgery 8: 118–136

Vernall P J 1926 A bone graft for sacro-iliac fixation. Journal of Bone and Joint Surgery 8: 491–493

47. Percutaneous fixation of the sacroiliac joint

A. B. Lippitt

INTRODUCTION

The diagnosis and management of disorders of the lumbopelvic region is the source of much controversy. Pain is the main reason patients consent to surgery, yet its source is often uncertain. Imaging studies only show anatomy and do not necessarily correlate with the pain source. Injection techniques such as facet blocks, discography, and root sleeve injections may or may not be helpful. Percutaneous stabilization of suspected unstable intervertebral disc segments has been advocated. If the patient achieves pain relief, it is suggested that a spine fusion at the stabilized level will provide permanent pain relief (Jeanneret et al 1994).

The author contends that low back pain that has defied diagnosis by conventional means frequently emanates from the sacroiliac joint (SIJ), and that the pain can be relieved by SIJ stabilization. Stabilization may be achieved by physiotherapy modalities such as muscle strengthening or balancing, by belting, by tightening of the sacroiliac (SI) ligament complex via proliferant injections, or, if these fail, by SIJ fixation or fusion. Fixation can be accomplished by placing screws across the joint.

The initial aim of fixation was to see whether or not pain could be relieved in this manner, and if it could, to convert the fixation to a fusion. Clinical experience with fixation has shown that most patients thus treated had a stable course and did not require further surgery.

APPLIED ANATOMY

The SIJ is a true diarthrodial joint. The concave sacral surface is covered with thick hyaline cartilage, whereas the convex iliac surface is lined with thin fibrocartilage. The articular surfaces are ear-shaped, containing irregular ridges and depressions. This, along with strong posterior ligaments and powerful surrounding muscles, makes the joint very stable.

There is a wide range of segmental innervation, which probably accounts for the variable referred pain patterns in patients with SIJ lesions.

PERTINENT BIOMECHANICS

SIJ movement is not voluntary but is induced by motion occurring at other locations in the body (Dreyfuss et al 1995). This motion consists of rotation and translation. This movement does not occur around a single axis and is very small (<4° rotation and <1.6 mm translation) (Sturesson et al 1989). Nutation refers to the backward rotation of the ilium on the sacrum, whereas counter-nutation is forward movement of the ilium on the sacrum.

The SIJ can withstand 20 times less axial compression and two times less axial torsion than can the lumbar spine, but the SIJs can tolerate 6 times more medially directed force (Bernard & Cassidy 1991).

The SIJ is particularly vulnerable to shear (rotation/translation). Compression of the SIJ with its ridges and depressions allows the joint to resist shear. Those structures that produce joint compression include muscles that cross the joint surface, the interosseous ligaments, and the joint capsule (Snijders et al 1995). Weight-bearing tends to force the sacrum down and rotate it forwards in relation to the ilium (nutation). The sacrotuberous and sacrospinalis ligaments resist

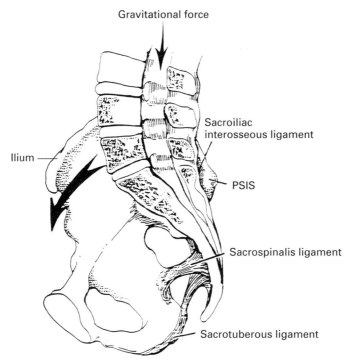

Fig. 47.1   Sagittal section through the pelvis, showing how gravity tends to force the sacrum forward (nutation) and how this is resisted by the sacrotuberous and sacrospinalis ligaments.

this movement (Fig. 47.1). In one-legged standing, the load transfer concentrates on one SIJ.

Any disruption of the ligamentous system leads to SIJ hypermobility, with or without instability.

INCIDENCE OF SIJ DISORDERS

A study by Bernard & Kirkaldy-Willis (1987) suggested that 22.5% of patients with low back pain had SIJ dysfunction in isolation or as part of their pathology. Schwarzer et al (1995) employed diagnostic intra-articular blocks to estimate the prevalence of SIJ pain in a population of patients with chronic low back pain who had defied diagnosis by conventional means. They identified 43 patients who met their criteria, 13 of whom (30%) showed evidence of SIJ pain.

CLASSIFICATION AND ETIOLOGY

SIJ dysfunction should be divided into two categories: intra-articular and extra-articular dysfunctions. True intra-articular pathology includes fracture, infection, tumor, inflammatory spondyloarthropathies, degenerative joint disease, and metabolic conditions. Extra-articular SIJ (EXSIJ) dysfunction is a disorder of abnormal joint movement and alignment owing to disruption of the ligamentous support system. The joint itself may be chronically inflamed but, in and of itself, is structurally normal. Symptoms due to EXSIJ dysfunction are alleviated by restoring stability and alignment.

PATHOPHYSIOLOGY OF EXTRA-ARTICULAR SIJ DYSFUNCTION

The clinical significance of the small motion of the SIJ is till subject to debate. In addition, each SIJ is dependent on the other SIJ and the symphysis pubis. Any change in the characteristics of one joint in the pelvic ring will change the characteristics of the two other joints.

Stability of the SIJ is both static and dynamic. Dynamic stability is muscle dependent. Although no muscle originates from or inserts onto the SIJ, many have fibrous expansions that blend with the SIJ ligament complex. The SIJ ligaments can therefore be affected by muscle activity. Static stability depends upon elevations and depressions on the joint surfaces that interlock and limit mobility, and the thick posterior sacroiliac (SI) ligaments that keep the incongruent sacrum and ilium opposed. In addition, the variation and complexity of the orientation of the SIJ surfaces contributes to static stability (Solonen 1957).

Trauma or hormonal changes, such as those occurring in pregnancy, will allow the SIJ ligaments to become lax and the joint to move beyond its normal range, passing beyond its normal congruity to an area of incongruity. This results in locking between the opposing surfaces of the ilium and sacrum; this locking is unlikely to be restored spontaneously. The joint is particularly vulnerable to locking when the trunk is bent forward and lateral flexion or rotation is superimposed. The joint can remain locked in a neutral or subluxed position. Subluxation can be anterior, posterior, or upwards (Aitken 1986, Fowler 1986, Greenman 1989). Ultimately, the ligamentous stretching produces a hypermobile joint subject to recurrent subluxation into a locked position (Lippitt 1995).

Traumatic causes of SIJ instability include:

- a fall on the buttock
- a dashboard injury that imparts a horizontal force to the SIJ
- a motor vehicle accident in which the affected extremity is extended and the force is transmitted upward to the SIJ, for example the foot on the brake with the knee extended at impact.

Iatrogenic etiologies include:

- instability due to weakening of the joint and ligaments from overzealous bone harvesting for graft (Coventry & Tapper 1972)
- increased force across the joint created secondarily to a spine or hip fusion (Frymoyer et al 1978).

Malposition of the SIJ leads to imbalance in the muscles, ligaments, and fascia. Muscles try to substitute for incompetent ligaments but are usually unsuccessful. The capsule becomes lax,

leading to joint inflammation. The joint itself will not show degenerative changes until late in the process. Due to chronically abnormal spine, pelvis, and lower extremity mechanics, a painful disabling condition ensues. By fixing the joint in its normal position, the normal balance is restored. It should be noted that SIJ subluxation is a clinical observation that has never been proven. It also remains to be proved that altered mobility correlates with symptoms (Bernard & Cassidy 1991).

DIAGNOSIS

The diagnosis of extra-articular SIJ dysfunction is based on a pattern of findings, none of which in and of itself is precise. *One cannot rely on imaging studies.*

Pain is always noted over the posterior superior iliac spine (PSIS), but there is no specific pain referral pattern. Schwarzer et al (1995) compared the pain patterns of patients with SIJ pain confirmed with diagnostic intra-articular blocks with those with non-SIJ pain. They found that the only clinically distinguishing characteristic was the presence of groin pain in those patients with chronic low back pain of SIJ origin. Radiation of pain below the knee was as common in patients with SIJ pain as in those without. Hackett et al (1991) injected hypertonic saline into various ligaments and mapped out the referred pain pattern. SIJ ligament-referred pain follows a distribution similar to that found by Schwarzer. Of special note is the absence of pain referral into the popliteal fossa in patients with attenuated posterior SIJ ligaments.

The physical examination can lead one to suspect SIJ dysfunction, but it does not *per se* allow one to make the diagnosis. Screening tests for SIJ dysfunction are well described elsewhere (Aitken 1986, Fowler 1986, Greenman 1989). These include static palpation of bony landmarks, looking for asymmetry, a one-legged stork (Gillet's) test, a seated flexion (Piedallu) test (Fig. 47.2), and a supine-to-seated test looking for leg length changes ('yo-yo sign') (Fig. 47.3).

It has been shown that these tests are neither reliable nor specific (Dreyfuss et al 1994, Van Deursen et al 1990) and, although positive tests in an individual should raise the index of suspicion

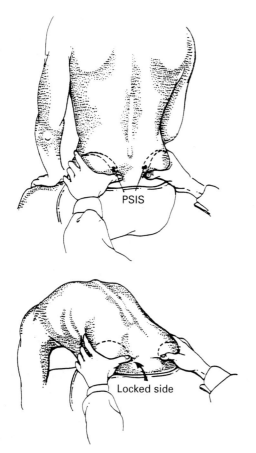

Fig. 47.2 Seated flexion test (Piedallu or lock sign). As one bends forward, the sacrum is locked versus the ilium and is thus brought upward, whereas the free or unlocked side stays down.

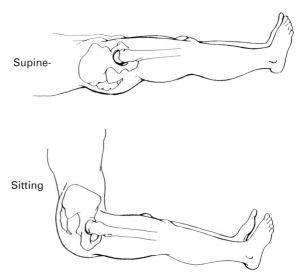

Fig. 47.3 Sit-up test (seated flexion test). As one sits up, leg lengths change ('yo-yo sign').

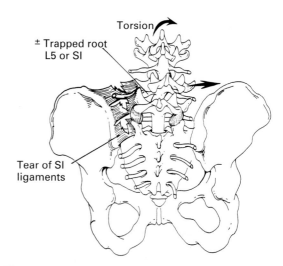

Fig. 47.4 Severe torsion produces ligament and facet capsule disruption, producing torsional instability with resultant nerve root entrapment.

as to the presence of extra-articular SIJ dysfunction, they are not diagnostic.

Symptomatic EXSIJ dysfunction cannot be diagnosed with laboratory or imaging studies. Bone scanning is best to identify occult or stress fractures, infection, or inflammatory disorders (Goldberg et al 1978). The diagnosis of EXSIJ dysfunction must be confirmed by a fluoroscopically controlled SIJ block (Dreyfuss et al 1995, Fortin & Tolchin 1993, Schwarzer et al 1995. However, this technique is probably not effective in anesthetizing a superficial ligament such as the long dorsal SI ligament (see also Chapter 3).

ASSOCIATED CONDITIONS

EXSIJ dysfunction can exist as an isolated disorder or in conjunction with other conditions. The most frequent combined lesion is a torsion injury in which the SI ligaments are torn in conjunction with tearing or stretching of facet capsule, a facet fracture, or tearing of the annulus, with or without disc herniation. Significant ligamentous and facet disruption can lead to a fixed deformity producing nerve root entrapment (Fig. 47.4).

Clinical observation has shown that disruption at L4–5 is more commonly associated with

SIJ dysfunction than are other intervertebral segments.

Piriformis syndrome, greater tronchanteric bursitis, and meralgia paresthetica can be found in conjunction with SIJ dysfunction.

DIFFERENTIAL DIAGNOSIS

Many spine conditions cause pain referral patterns to the SIJ (Table 47.1). These include facet syndrome, herniated disc, lateral spinal stenosis, hip disease, and thoracolumbar facet dysfunction (Maigne syndrome). Imaging studies are helpful in the diagnosis of herniated nucleus pulposus and hip disease, whereas fluoroscopically controlled blocks help to differentiate facet disorders or root entrapment from SIJ dysfunction. It should be noted that these conditions can exist in conjunction with each other.

TREATMENT

The goal of treatment of EXSIJ dysfunction is primarily to restore normal lumbopelvic mechanics. This includes the use of medication or intra-articular steroids for acute or chronic inflammation, manual techniques to reduce SIJ subluxation, muscle strengthening and rebalancing techniques for the muscles involved in SIJ mechanics, and belting or proliferant injections (prolotherapy) to stablilize the joint. Manual methods are well described in the literature (Aitken 1986, Fowler 1986, Greenman 1989). Likewise prolotherapy is covered elsewhere (Hackett et al 1991, Klein et al 1993, Ongley et al 1987, Reeves 1995) (see also Chapter 40). Should these modalities fail, surgical stabilization is indicated.

Criteria for stabilization include the following:

1. Pain must be disabling.
2. Pain must be localized to the SIJ and not relieved by conservative modalities.
3. Pain should be relieved on a transient basis by a fluoroscopically controlled SIJ block.
4. Other causes of lumbopelvic pain such as herniated nucleus pulposus, facet arthropathy, trapped nerve root, spinal stenosis, hip disorders, etc. should be ruled out.
5. Associated conditions must be treated before, in conjunction with, or after treating the SIJ dysfunction.

TECHNIQUE OF SI STABILIZATION

There are several articles describing SIJ fusion (Campbell 1927, Smith-Peterson & Rogers 1926, Waisbrod et al 1987). For EXSIJ dysfunctions, the placement of cannulated screws across a reduced (properly positioned) SIJ is usually adequate. Titanium screws are recommended since they are computerized tomography and magnetic resonance imaging compatible.

SIJ stabilization for traumatic injuries is well described in the orthopedic literature. Matta and Saucedo (1989) suggest that the patient be placed prone on a radiolucent table to allow the use of an image intensifier during surgery. The aim of

Table 47.1   Differential diagnosis

	Imaging study	Pattern	Work-up
Herniated nucleus pulposus	Positive	Better with rest, worse with activity	± Nerve study
Facet arthropathy	Negative	Very stiff in the morning, better as the day goes on	Positive response to facet block
SI dysfunction	Negative	Aggravated by walking, worse with recumbency	Positive response to SI block
Spinal stenosis	±	Aggravated by walking (claudication)	Positive response to epidural block
Trapped nerve root	±	Better with rest, worse with activity; may be helped by a corset	± Positive nerve study, positive root sleeve injection
Spinal instability	±	Worse with ambulation	± Flex/extend lateral X-rays, positive discogram
Hip disorder	Positive	Worse with ambulation	X-ray

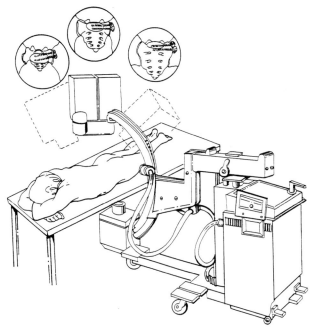

Fig. 47.5 Positioning of the patient and use of the image intensifier for SIJ fixation.

crest. Underlying muscles are stripped from their attachments, exposing the outer iliac table. A point midway between the iliac crest and the sciatic notch, approximately 1.5 mm anterior to the crista glutea, is identified, and a K-wire placed under direct image intensification across the ilium into the sacrum. Anteroposterior (AP) views at 90°, 40° cephalad, and 40° caudad must be obtained to assess proper K-wire placement. If proper placement is achieved, a cannulated screw of appropriate length is then inserted over the K-wire. A second and, if room permits, a third screw are then inserted in a similar manner (Fig. 47.6).

The author has found that the procedure can also be carried out percutaneously. When this is done, it is essential that a lateral view be obtained to ensure that the screws are placed in the sacrum (Fig. 47.7). An external rotation AP view allows one to visualize the joint and outer table to determine that the screws are across the joint and placed all the way to bone.

No postoperative immobilization is required. The patient increases his or her activity to tolerance. Problems with muscle imbalance and spasm are frequent and must be addressed with physical therapy modalities. Associated conditions such as

the operation is to insert cannulated screws from the ilium into the sacrum, monitoring proper placement with an image intensifier (Fig. 47.5). A posterior skin incision is made over the iliac

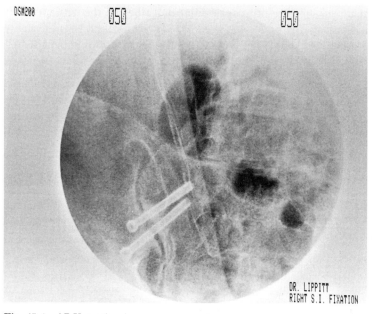

Fig. 47.6 AP X-ray showing proper screw placement.

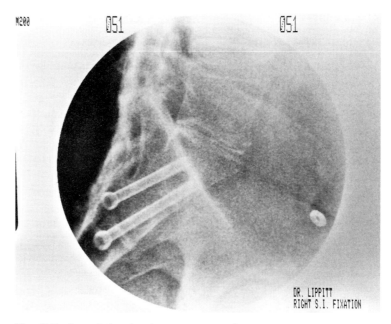

Fig. 47.7 Lateral view showing proper screw placement.

herniated discs, trapped nerve roots, facet arthropathy, segmental instability, piriformis syndrome,
and/or meralgia paresthetica *must also be treated*
for a successful outcome.

To date, no screw has broken or backed
out, and follow-up X-rays have failed to show
evidence of fusion despite continued clinical
improvement.

The procedure has been performed in women
of childbearing potential who are willing to
undergo caesarean section if necessary. To date,
none of those patients has become pregnant.

CONCLUSIONS

1. SIJ fixation is a relatively simple, safe, and
effective treatment in those patients suffering
from EXSIJ dysfunction unresponsive to conservative modalities.

2. It is not necessary to fuse the joint.

REFERENCES

Aitken G S 1986 Syndromes of lumbopelvic dysfunction. In:
   Grieve G (ed.) Modern manual therapy of the vertebral
   column. Churchill Livingstone, Edinburgh, pp 473–478
Bernard T N, Cassidy J O 1991 Sacroiliac joint syndrome:
   pathophysiology diagnosis and management. In: Frymoyer
   J W (ed.) The adult spine: principles and practice. Raven
   Press, New York, pp 2107–2131
Bernard T N, Kirkaldy-Willis W H 1987 Recognizing specific
   characteristics of non specific low back pain. Clinical
   Orthopedics and Related Research 217: 266–280
Campbell W C 1927 An operation for extra articular fusion of
   the sacroiliac joint. Surgery, Gynecology and Obstetrics
   45: 218
Coventry M V, Tapper E H 1972 Pelvic instability: a
   consequence of removing iliac bone for grafting. Journal of
   Bone and Joint Surgery (US) 54: 83–101
Dreyfuss P, Dreyer S, Griffin J, Hoffman J, Walsh N 1994
   Positive sacroiliac screening tests in asymptomatic adults.
   Spine 19: 1138–1143

Dreyfuss P, Cole A J, Pauza K 1995 Sacroiliac joint injection
   techniques. Physical Medicine and Rehabilitation Clinics of
   North America 6: 785–813
Fortin J D, Tolchin R B 1993 Sacroiliac joint provocation
   and arthrography. Archives of Physical Medicine and
   Rehabilitation 74: 1259
Fowler C 1986 Muscle energy techniques for pelvic
   dysfunction. In: Grieve G (ed.) Modern manual therapy of
   the vertebral column. Churchill Livingstone, Edinburgh,
   pp 805–818
Frymoyer J W, Howe J, Kuhlman D 1978 The long term
   effects of spine fusion on the sacroiliac joint. Clinical
   Orthopedics and Related Research 134: 198–201
Goldberg R P, Genant H K, Shimshak R, Shames D 1978
   Applications and limitations of quantitative sacroiliac joint
   scintigraphy. Radiology 128: 683–686
Greenman P 1989 Principles of manual medicine. Williams &
   Wilkins, Baltimore
Hackett G S, Hemwall G A, Montgomery G A 1991
   Ligament and tendon relaxation treated by prolotherapy,
   5th edn. Published by Gustav A. Hemwall MD

Jeanneret B, Jovanovic M, Magerl F 1994 Percutaneous stabilization for low back pain: correlation with results after fusion operation. Clinical Orthopedics and Related Research 304: 130–138

Klein R G, Eek B C, DeLong W B, Mooney V A 1993 Randomized double blind trial of dextrose–glycerine–phenol injections for chronic low back pain. Journal of Spine Disorders 6: 23–33

Lippitt A B 1995 Recurrent subluxation of the sacroiliac joint: diagnosis and treatment. Bulletin of The Hospital for Joint Diseases 54: 94–102

Matta J M, Saucedo T 1989 Internal fixation of pelvic ring fractures. Clinical Orthopedics and Related Research 242: 93

Ongley M J, Klein R G, Dorman T A, Eek B C, Hubert L J 1987 A new approach to the treatment of chronic low back pain. Lancet 2: 143–146

Reeves K D 1995 Prolotherapy present and future applications in soft-tissue pain and disability. Physical Medicine and Rehabilitation Clinics of North America 6: 917–926

Schwarzer A, Aprill C, Bogduk N 1995 The sacroiliac joint in chronic low back pain. Spine 20: 31–37

Solonen V A 1957 The sacroiliac joint in the light of anatomic, roentgenological and clinical studies. Acta Orthopedica Scandinavica 27 (supplement): 1–127

Smith-Peterson M N, Rogers W A 1926 End results of arthrodesis of the scaroiliac joint for arthritis, traumatic and non-traumatic. Journal of Bone and Joint Surgery (US) 8: 118–136

Snijders C J, Vleeming A, Stoeckart R, Kleinrensink G J, Mens J M A 1995 Biomechanics of sacroiliac joint stability: validation experiments on the concept of self-locking. In: Vleeming A, Mooney V, Dorman T, Snijders C J (eds) Second interdisciplinary world congress on low back pain. San Diego, CA, 9–11 November, pp 77–91

Sturesson B, Selvik G, Uden A 1989 Movements of the sacroiliac joint – A roentgen stereophotogrammetric analysis. Spine 14: 162–165

Van Deursen L L, Patijn J M, Ockhutson A L, Vortman B J 1990 The value of some clinical tests of the sacroiliac joint. Journal of Manual Medicine 5: 96–99

Waisbrod J, Krainick J U, Gerbershagen H U 1987 Sacroiliac joint arthrodesis for chronic lower back pain. Archives of Orthopedic and Traumatic Surgery 106: 238–240

Index